MINDMAPS in OPHTHALMOLOGY

MINDMAPS in OPHTHALMOLOGY

Abhishek Sharma

DPhil (Oxon), Fellow of Royal Australian and
New Zealand College of Ophthalmologists
Pediatric Ophthalmology Fellow
Hospital for Sick Children, Toronto
Ontario, Canada

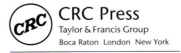

CRC Press
Taylor & Francis Group
Boca Raton London New York

CRC Press is an imprint of the
Taylor & Francis Group, an **informa** business

CRC Press
Taylor & Francis Group
6000 Broken Sound Parkway NW, Suite 300
Boca Raton, FL 33487-2742

© 2015 by Taylor & Francis Group, LLC
CRC Press is an imprint of Taylor & Francis Group, an Informa business

No claim to original U.S. Government works

Printed and bound in India by Replika Press Pvt. Ltd.

Printed on acid-free paper
Version Date: 20141202

International Standard Book Number-13: 978-1-4822-3063-5 (Paperback)

Visit the Taylor & Francis Web site at
http://www.taylorandfrancis.com

and the CRC Press Web site at
http://www.crcpress.com

Contents

Preface

Mind Maps in Ophthalmology provides an overview of clinical ophthalmology using the logical, stepwise format of mind maps. Each page summarizes a topic in the field, with branches that organize the knowledge about the topic.

This book is an excellent rapid-revision tool, suitable for medical students, ophthalmology trainees, orthoptists, optometrists, general practitioners and other health professionals. It should be used in conjunction with a textbook for further elaboration on the topics. Ophthalmologists will find this text a useful teaching tool, simplifying complex topics and providing a structure to teaching.

Acknowledgements

I gratefully acknowledge the creators of the mind map format, including Tony Buzan. These mind maps were created during my final year of training for Fellowship with the Royal Australian & New Zealand College of Ophthalmologists. I am thankful to my fellow trainees in my year group at the Royal Victorian Eye and Ear Hospital, Melbourne, Australia. Thank you to Lance Wobus and the team at Taylor & Francis. I am grateful for the support from my parents and my sister, Anamika.

Thank you to my wife, Nipun, and my beautiful daughters, Anjali and Ameya.

The Author

Abhishek Sharma graduated with a Bachelor of Medicine and Bachelor of Surgery from the University of Tasmania in 2004. He completed a DPhil in Public Health in the field of pediatric ophthalmology in 2009 from the University of Oxford, as a Rhodes Scholar. He completed his ophthalmology training at the Royal Victorian Eye and Ear Hospital in Melbourne, Victoria, Australia in 2013 and successfully completed the Royal Australian & New Zealand College of Ophthalmologists Fellowship examinations in 2013. He is currently completing a fellowship in pediatric ophthalmology at the Hospital for Sick Children, Toronto, Ontario, Canada.

Abbreviations

5FU: 5-fluorouracil
A/W: associated with
AACG: acute angle closure glaucoma
AAION: arteritic anterior ischemic optic neuropathy
AAU: acute anterior uveitis
ABx: antibiotics
AC/A Ratio: (accommodative convergence)/(accommodation)
ACA: anterior cerebral artery
ACC: adenoid cystic carcinoma
ACD: anterior chamber depth
ACE: angiotensin-converting enzyme
ACG: angle closure glaucoma
ACh: acetylcholine
ACIOL: anterior chamber intraocular lens
ACPIOL: anterior chamber phakic intraocular lens
AD: autosomal dominant
AF: atrial fibrillation
AHP: abnormal head posture
AIDS: acquired immunodeficiency syndrome
AION: anterior ischemic optic neuropathy
aka: also known as
AKC: atopic keratoconjuctivitis
ALL: acute lymphoblastic leukemia/lymphoma
AML: acute myelogenous leukemia
ANA: antinuclear antibodies
ANCA: antineutrophil cytoplasmic antibody
Anti-TPO: antithyroid peroxidase
Anti-TSH: antithyroid stimulating hormone
Anti-VEGF: antivascular endothelial growth factor
APMPPE: acute posterior multifocal placoid pigment epitheliopathy
AR: autosomal recessive
ARC: abnormal retinal correspondence
ARMD/AMD: age-related macular degeneration
ARN: acute retinal necrosis
ARPE: acute retinal pigment epithelitis
ASCRS: American Society of Cataract and Refractive Surgery
AVM: arteriovenous malformation
AZOOR: acute zonal occult outer retinopathy
BARN: bilateral acute retinal necrosis
BCC: basal cell carcinoma
BCG vaccine: Bacillus Calmette-Guérin vaccine
BCL: bandage contact lens
BCVA: best corrected visual acuity

BD: twice a day (Latin: *bis die*)
BDUMP: bilateral diffuse uveal melanocytic proliferation
BLRR: bilateral lateral rectus recession
BM: basement membrane
BMI: body mass index
BP: blood pressure
BPES: blepharophimosis epicanthus inversus syndrome
BRAO: branch retinal artery occlusion
BRVO: branch retinal vein occlusion
BSL: blood sugar level
BSS: balanced salt solution
BSV: binocular single vision
BUN: blood urea nitrogen
C3F8 gas: octafluoropropane
Ca: carcinoma
CAR: cancer-associated retinopathy
CCA: common carotid artery
CCF: carotid–cavernous fistula
CCT: central corneal thickness
CDR: cup–disc ratio
cf.: (Latin) compare with
CFEOM: congenital fibrosis of the extraocular muscles
CFF: critical fusion frequency
CHED: congenital hereditary endothelial dystrophy
CHRPE: congenital hypertrophy of the retinal pigment epithelium
CIN: conjunctival/corneal intraepithelial neoplasia
CLE: clear lens exchange
CLL: chronic lymphocytic leukemia
CME: cystoid macular edema
CML: chronic myeloid leukemia
CMN: congenital motor nystagmus
CMV: cytomegalovirus
CN: cranial nerve
CNS: central nervous system
CNV/CNVM: choroidal neovascularization/choroidal neovascular membrane
CPEO: chronic progressive external ophthalmoplegia
CRAO: central retinal artery occlusion
CRP: C-reactive protein
CRVO: central retinal vein occlusion
CSF: cerebrospinal fluid
CSME: clinically significant macular edema
CSNB: congenital stationary night blindness
CSR: central serous retinopathy

CT: connective tissue
CT scan: computed tomography scan
CTA: CT angiogram
CVA: cerebrovascular accident
CVF: confrontational visual field
CWS: cotton wool spot
CXR: chest x-ray
D: diopter
DALK: deep anterior lamellar keratoplasty
DCR: dacryocystorhinostomy
DD: disc diameter
DDx: differential diagnoses
DIDMOAD: diabetes insipidus, diabetes mellitus, optic atrophy, and deafness
DLK: diffuse lamellar keratitis
DM: diabetes mellitus
DNA: deoxyribonucleic acid
DSAEK: Descemet's stripping automated endothelial keratoplasty
dsDNA: double-stranded deoxyribonucleic acid
DVD: dissociated vertical deviation
EBMD: epithelial basement membrane dystrophy
EBV: Epstein–Barr virus
ECA: external carotid artery
ECCE: extracapsular cataract extraction
EDTA: ethylenediaminetetraacetic acid
EKC: epidemic keratoconjunctivitis
ELISA: enzyme-linked immunosorbent assay
EMG: electromyogram/electromyography
ENT: ear, nose & throat
EOG: electro-oculogram
EOM: extraocular muscles
EPG/iEPG: electrophoretogram, hyperviscosity screen
EPO: erythropoietin
ERG: electroretinogram
ERM: epiretinal membrane
ESR: erythrocyte sedimentation rate
ET: esotropia
ETT: endotracheal tube
EUA: examination under anesthesia
EVP: episcleral venous pressure
EW nucleus: Edinger–Westphal nucleus
FAP: familial adenomatous polyposis
FAZ: foveal avascular zone
FB: foreign body
FBC/FBE: full blood count/full blood examination
FDT: frequency doubling technology
FEF: frontal eye fields
FEVR: familial exudative vitreoretinopathy
FFA: fundus fluorescein angiography
FISH: fluorescence in-situ hybridization
FK syndrome: Foster–Kennedy syndrome
FLAIR MRI: fluid attenuated inversion recovery magnetic resonance imaging
FTA-ABS: fluorescent treponemal antibody absorbed
FTMH: full-thickness macular hole

G6PD: glucose-6-phosphate dehydrogenase
GA: general anesthetic
GAGs: glycosaminoglycans
GCA: giant cell arteritis
GDx: glaucoma diagnosis (nerve fiber analyzer from Laser Diagnostic Technologies Inc).
GIT: gastrointestinal tract
GON: glaucomatous optic neuropathy
GP: general physician/general practitioner
GRT: giant retinal tear
GU: genitourinary
GVHD: graft-versus-host disease
HAART: highly active antiretroviral therapy
HIV: human immunodeficiency virus
HSV: herpes simplex virus
HTN: hypertension
HVF: Humphrey visual field
HZO: herpes zoster ophthalmicus
IBD: inflammatory bowel disease
ICA: internal carotid artery
ICE syndrome: iridocorneal endothelial syndrome
ICG: indocyanine green
ICL: implantable collamer lens
ICP: intracranial pressure
ICRB: International Classification of Retinoblastoma
IFN: interferon
IIH: idiopathic intracranial hypertension
IK: interstitial keratitis
ILM: internal limiting membrane
INO: internuclear ophthalmoplegia
IO: inferior oblique
IOFB: intraocular foreign body
IOID: idiopathic orbital inflammatory disease
IOL: intraocular lens
IOOA: inferior oblique over action
IOP: intraocular pressure
IQ: intelligence quotient
IR: inferior rectus
IRMA: intraretinal microvascular abnormalities
IRVAN: idiopathic retinitis, vasculitis, aneurysms, and neuroretinitis
ITC: iridotrabecular contact
IV: intravenous
IVDU: intravenous drug use
IVTA: intravitreal triamcinolone acetonide
JFT: juxtafoveal telangiectasia
JIA: juvenile idiopathic arthritis
JXG: juvenile xanthogranuloma
KPs: keratic precipitates
LA: local anesthetic
LASEK: laser epithelial keratomileusis
LASIK: laser-assisted in situ keratomileusis
LCA: Leber's congenital amaurosis
LFT: liver function test
LG: lacrimal gland
LGV: lymphogranuloma venereum

LL: lower lid
LMN: lower motor neurons
LOC: loss of consciousness
LogMAR: logarithm of the minimum angle of resolution (visual acuity chart)
LP: lumbar puncture
LPS: levator palpebrae superioris
LR: lateral rectus
LRI: limbal relaxing incision
LTS: lateral tarsal strip
M/C/S: microscopy/cultures/sensitivity
MALT: mucosa-associated lymphoid tissue
MAR: melanoma-associated retinopathy
MAs: microaneurysms
MELAS: mitochondrial encephalomyopathy, lactic acidosis, stroke
Mentor B-VAT tester: Mentor Baylor Video Acuity Tester (for stereoacuity)
MEWDS: multiple evanescent white dot syndrome
MFC: multifocal choroiditis
mfERG: multifocal electroretinography
MG: myasthenia gravis
MGJW: Marcus–Gunn jaw-winking
MGUS: monoclonal gammopathy of undetermined significance
MK: microbial keratitis
MLF: medial longitudinal fasiculus
MMC: mitomycin C
MR: medial rectus
MRD: margin reflex distance
MRI: magnetic resonance imaging
MRV: magnetic resonance venogram
MS: multiple sclerosis
mtDNA: mitochondrial DNA
MuSK: muscle-specific kinase (myasthenia due to autoantibodies)
NaCl: sodium chloride
NAD: noradrenaline
NAI: non-accidental injury
NAION: non-arteritic ischemic optic neuropathy
NF: neurofibromatosis
NFL: nerve fiber layer
NL: nasolacrimal
NLDO: nasolacrimal drainage obstruction
NMJ: neuromuscular junction
NMO: neuromyelitis optica
NPDR: nonproliferative diabetic retinopathy
NSAID: non-steroidal anti-inflammatory drug
NTG: normotension glaucoma
NV: neovascularization
NVA: neovascularization angle
NVD: neovascularization disc
NVE: neovascularization elsewhere
NVI: neovascularization iris (rubeosis iridis)
OB/GYN: obstetrics/gynecology
OAG: open angle glaucoma

OCD: obsessive compulsive disorder
OCP: ocular cicatricial pemphigoid
OCT: optical coherence tomography
OHS: ocular histoplasmosis syndrome
OHT: ocular hypertension
OIS: ocular ischemic syndrome
ONH: optic nerve head
OPA1: optic atrophy 1 gene
OSSN: ocular surface squamous neoplasia
PAC: primary angle closure
PACG: primary angle closure glaucoma
PACS: primary angle closure suspect
PAM: primary acquired melanosis
PAN: polyarteritis nodosa
PAS: peripheral anterior synechiae
PC: posterior capsule
PCA: posterior cerebral artery
PCIOL: posterior chamber intraocular lens
PCNSL: primary CNS lymphoma
PCR: polymerase chain reaction
PCRV: polycythemia rubra vera (hyperviscosity cause)
PD: prism diopters
PDG: pigmentary dispersion glaucoma
PDR: proliferative diabetic retinopathy
PDS: pigment dispersion syndrome
PDT: photodynamic therapy
PED: pigment epithelial detachment
PERT: pre-enucleation radiotherapy
PESS: postenucleation socket syndrome
PET: positron emission tomography
PF: palpebral fissure
PHACE syndrome: posterior fossa brain malformations, hemangiomas, cardiovascular anomalies
PHMB: polyhexamethylene biguanide
PHPV: persistent hyperplastic primary vitreous
PI: peripheral iridotomy
PIC: punctate inner choroiditis
PIOL: primary intraocular lymphoma
PION: posterior ischemic optic neuropathy
PK: penetrating keratoplasty
PLGF: placental growth factor
PML: progressive multifocal leukoencephalopathy
POAG: primary open angle glaucoma
POHS: presumed ocular histoplasmosis syndrome
PORN: progressive outer retinal necrosis
PPD: purified protein derivative (tuberculosis test)
PPMD: posterior polymorphous corneal dystrophy
PPRF: paramedian pontine reticular formation
PRK: photorefractive keratectomy
PRP: panretinal photocoagulation
PSCC: posterior subcapsular cataract
PSD: pattern standard deviation
PSP: progressive supranuclear palsy
PTK: phototherapeutic keratectomy
PUD: peptic ulcer disease
PUK: peripheral ulcerative keratitis

PVD: posterior vitreous detachment
PVR: proliferative vitreoretinopathy
PXF: pseudoexfoliation syndrome
QID: four times a day (Latin: *quater in die*)
RA: rheumatoid arthritis
RAPD: relative afferent pupillary defect
RBC: red blood cells
RE: refractive error
REES: recurrent epithelial erosion syndrome
RF: rheumatoid factor
riMLF: rostral interstitial nucleus of medial longitudinal fasciculus
RNA: ribonucleic acid
RNFL: retinal nerve fiber layer
ROP: retinopathy of prematurity
RP: retinitis pigmentosa
RPE: retinal pigment epithelium
RRD: rhegmatogenous retinal detachment
Rx: treatment
SALT: sequential aggressive local therapy
SCC: squamous cell carcinoma
SCI: subcutaneous injection
SF6: sulfur hexafluoride gas
SGC: sebaceous gland carcinoma
SITA: Swedish interactive threshold algorithm
SLE: systemic lupus erythematosus
SLK: superior limbic keratoconjunctivitis
SLT: selective laser trabeculoplasty
SNP: single nucleotide polymorphism
SO: superior oblique
SOAL: secondary ocular adnexal lymphoma
SPK: superficial punctate keratitis
SR: superior rectus
SRF: subretinal fluid
SRK: Sanders, Retzlaff & Kraft IOL formula
SS antibodies: Sjögren syndrome antibodies
SSPE: subacute sclerosing panencephalitis virus
SSRI: selective serotonin reuptake inhibitor
STD: sexually transmitted disease
SWAP: short wavelength automated perimetry
SXR: skull x-ray
TASS: toxic anterior segment syndrome
TB: tuberculosis
TCA: tricyclic antidepressant
TDS: three times daily (Latin: *ter die sumendus*)
TED: thyroid eye disease
TEE: transesophageal echocardiogram
TFBUT: tear film break-up time
TIA: transient ischemic attack
TM: trabecular meshwork
tPA: tissue plasminogen activator
Trab: trabeculectomy
TSH: thyroid stimulating hormone
TVO: transient visual obscuration
UBM: ultrasound biomicroscopy
UEC: urea, electrolytes, creatinine

UGH syndrome: uveitis–glaucoma–hyphema syndrome
UL: upper lid
URTI: upper respiratory tract infection
USS: ultrasound scan
UV: ultraviolet
VA: visual acuity
VDRL/RPR: venereal disease research laboratory / rapid plasma reagin
VEGF: vascular endothelial growth factor
VEP: visual evoked potential
VF: visual field
VHL: von Hippel–Lindau disease
VKC: vernal keratoconjunctivitis
VKH syndrome: Vogt–Koyanagi–Harada syndrome
VOR: vestibulocochlear reflex
VZV: varicella-zoster virus
WAGR syndrome: Wilms tumor, aniridia, genitourinary, retardation
WBC: white blood cells
WCC: white cell count
WEBINO: wide-eyed bilateral internuclear ophthalmoplegia
WHO: World Health Organization
XT: exotropia

Studies

ACCORD: Action to Control Cardiovascular Risk in Diabetes
ADVANCE: Action in Diabetes and Vascular Disease: Preterax and Diamicron MR Controlled Evaluation (evaluation of the effects of a fixed combination of perindopril and indapamide on macrovascular and microvascular outcomes in patients with type 2 diabetes mellitus)
AGIS: Advanced Glaucoma Intervention Study
ANCHOR: Anti-VEGF antibody for the treatment of predominantly classic choroidal neovascularisation in AMD
AREDS: Age-Related Eye Disease Study
BEAT-ROP: Bevacizumab Eliminates the Angiogenic Threat of Retinopathy of Prematurity
BENEFIT: Betaferon®/Betaseron® in Newly Emerging Multiple Sclerosis for Initial Treatment
BOLT: A two-year prospective randomized controlled trial of intravitreal Bevacizumab or Laser Therapy (BOLT) in the management of diabetic macular edema
BRAVO: A Study of the Efficacy and Safety of Ranibizumab Injection in Patients with Macular Edema Secondary to Branch Retinal Vein Occlusion
BVOS: Branch Vein Occlusion Study
CATT: Comparison of Age-Related Macular Degeneration Treatments Trials
CHAMPS: The Controlled High Risk Avonex® Multiple Sclerosis Trial
CIGTS: Collaborative Initial Glaucoma Treatment Study

CNTGS: Collaborative Normal Tension Glaucoma Study

COMS: Collaborative Ocular Melanoma Study

CRASH: Corticosteroid Randomisation after Significant Head Injury

CRUISE: A Study of the Efficacy and Safety of Ranibizumab Injection in Patients with Macular Edema Secondary to Central Retinal Vein Occlusion

CRYO-ROP: Cryotherapy for Retinopathy of Prematurity

CVOS: Central Vein Occlusion Study

DCCT: Diabetes Control and Complications Trial

DIRECT: DIabetic REtinopathy Candesartan Trials

DRCR.net: The Diabetic Retinopathy Clinical Research Network

DRS: Diabetic Retinopathy Study

DRVS: Diabetic Retinopathy Vitrectomy Study

EGPS: European Glaucoma Prevention Study

EMGT: Early Manifest Glaucoma Treatment Study

ESCRS: European Society of Cataract & Refractive Surgeons Study (prophylaxis of postoperative endophthalmitis after cataract surgery)

ETDRS: Early Treatment of Diabetic Retinopathy Study

ETOMS: Early Treatment of Multiple Sclerosis Study

ETROP: Early Treatment for Retinopathy of Prematurity

EUGOGO: European Group on Graves' Orbitopathy

EVEREST: Efficacy and safety of verteporfin photodynamic therapy in combination with ranibizumab or alone versus ranibizumab monotherapy in patients with symptomatic macular polypoidal choroidal vasculopathy

EVS: Endophthalmitis Vitrectomy Study

FFSS: Fluorouracil Filtering Surgery Study

FIELD: Fenofibrate Intervention and Event Lowering in Diabetes

GLT: Glaucoma Laser Trial

IATSG: Infant Aphakia Treatment Study Group

IONTS: International Optic Nerve Trauma Study

MARINA: The Minimally Classic/Occult Trial of Anti-VEGF Antibody Ranibizumab in the Treatment of Neovascular AMD

MOTAS: Monitored Occlusion Treatment of Amblyopia Study

MPS: Macular Photocoagulation Study

NASCET: North American Symptomatic Carotid Endarterectomy Trial

NASCIS: National Acute Spinal Cord Injury Study

OHTS: Ocular Hypertension Treatment Study

ONTT: Optic Neuritis Treatment Trial

PEDIG: Pediatric Eye Disease Investigator Group – Amylopia Studies

PIER: Portland Identification and Early Referral (randomized, double-masked, sham-controlled trial of ranibizumab for neovascular ARM)

PRONTO: Prospective Optical coherence tomography imaging of patients with Neovascular AMD Treated with intra-Ocular ranibizumab

RASS: Renin-Angiotensin System Study

READ: Ranibizumab for Edema of the mAcula in Diabetes study

RESOLVE: Safety & Efficacy of Ranibizumab in Diabetic Macular Edema

RESTORE Study: Ranibizumab monotherapy or combined with laser versus laser monotherapy for diabetic macular edema

RISE and RIDE Studies: Prospective, double-masked, phase 3 trials, compared the use of monthly ranibizumab to sham injections in patients with vision loss and diabetic macular edema

SAILOR: Safety Assessment of Intravitreal Lucentis for AMD

SCORE: Standard Care vs. Corticosteroid for Retinal Vein Occlusion

STOP-ROP: Supplemental Therapeutic Oxygen for Prethreshold Retinopathy of Prematurity

UKPDS: The United Kingdom Prospective Diabetes Study

VIEW: VEGF Trap-Eye: Investigation of Efficacy and Safety in Wet Age-Related Macular Degeneration

WESDR: Wisconsin Epidemiologic Study of Diabetic Retinopathy

References

Banta JT, Farris BK. Pseudotumor cerebri and optic nerve sheath decompression. *Ophthalmology* 2000;107(10):1907–12.

Ciulla TA, Starr MB, Masket S. Bacterial endophthalmitis prophylaxis for cataract surgery: an evidence-based update. *Ophthalmology* 2002;109(1):13–24.

Clark WL, Kaiser PK, Flynn HW, Jr., Belfort A, Miller D, Meisler DM. Treatment strategies and visual acuity outcomes in chronic postoperative Propionibacterium acnes endophthalmitis. *Ophthalmology* 1999;106(9):1665–70.

Dawson EL, Marshman WE, Lee JP. Role of botulinum toxin A in surgically overcorrected exotropia. *JAAPOS* 1999;3(5):269–71.

Ezra DG, Beaconsfield M, Sira M, *et al*. Long-term outcomes of surgical approaches to the treatment of floppy eyelid syndrome. *Ophthalmology* 2010;117(4):839–46.

Fisson S, Ouakrim H, Touitou V, *et al*. Cytokine profile in human eyes: contribution of a new cytokine combination for differential diagnosis between intraocular lymphoma or uveitis. *PloS One* 2013;8(2):e52385.

Gillies MC, Simpson JM, Gaston C, *et al*. Five-year results of a randomized trial with open-label extension of triamcinolone acetonide for refractory diabetic macular edema. *Ophthalmology* 2009;116(11):2182–7.

Grogan PM, Gronseth GS. Practice parameter: Steroids, acyclovir, and surgery for Bell's palsy (an evidence-based review): report of the Quality Standards Subcommittee of the American Academy of Neurology. *Neurology* 2001;56(7):830–6.

NICE: Murray A, Jones L, Milne A, Fraser C, Lourenço T, Burr J. A systematic review of the safety and efficacy of elective photorefractive surgery for the correction of refractive error. Review Body Report submitted to the Interventional Procedures Programme, NICE, 2005.

Settas G, Settas C, Minos E, Yeung I. Photorefractive keratectomy (PRK) versus laser assisted in situ keratomileusis (LASIK) for hyperopia correction. *Cochrane Database Syst Rev* 2012;6:CD007112.

Palay DA, Sternberg P, Jr., Davis J, *et al*. Decrease in the risk of bilateral acute retinal necrosis by acyclovir therapy. Am J Ophthalmol 1991;112(3):250–5.

Watzke RC, Burton TC, Leaverton PE. Ruby laser photocoagulation therapy of central serous retinopathy. I. A controlled clinical study. II. Factors affecting prognosis. *Trans Am Acad Ophthalmol Otolaryngol* 1974;78(2):OP205–11.

Woo KI, Yi K, Kim Y-D. Surgical correction for lower lid epiblepharon in Asians. *BJO* 2000;84(12):1407–10.

Yu-Wai-Man P, Griffiths PG. Steroids for traumatic optic neuropathy. *Cochrane Database Syst Rev* 2007;17(4).

1 Overview

Overview

1.1 Management Principles

1.2 Ophthalmic Emergencies

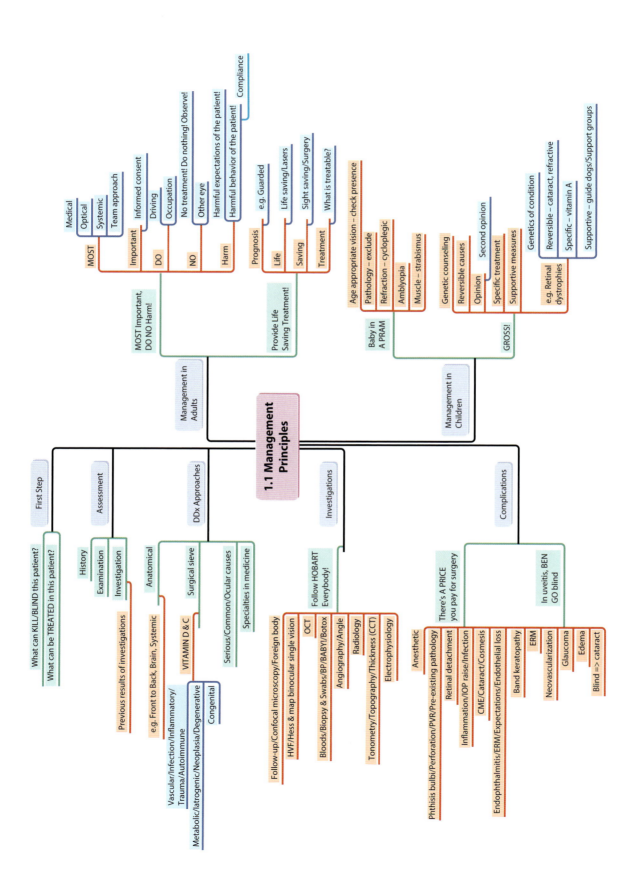

1.1 Management Principles

Management in Adults

MOST Important, DO NO Harm!

- MOST
  - Medical
  - Optical
  - Systemic
  - Team approach
- Important
  - Informed consent
  - Driving
  - Occupation
- DO
  - No treatment! Do nothing! Observe!
- NO
  - Other eye
  - Harmful expectations of the patient!
- Harm
  - Harmful behavior of the patient! — Compliance

Provide Life Saving Treatment!

- Prognosis — e.g. Guarded
- Life — Life saving/Lasers
- Saving — Sight saving/Surgery
- Treatment — What is treatable?

Management in Children

Baby in A PRAM

- Age appropriate vision – check presence
- Pathology – exclude
- Refraction – cycloplegic
- Amblyopia
- Muscle – strabismus

GROSS!

- Genetic counseling
- Reversible causes
- Opinion — Second opinion
- Specific treatment
- Supportive measures
  - Genetics of condition
  - Reversible – cataract, refractive
  - Specific – vitamin A
  - Supportive – guide dogs/Support groups
- e.g. Retinal dystrophies

First Step

- What can KILL/BLIND this patient?
- What can be TREATED in this patient?

Assessment

- History
- Examination
- Investigation
  - Previous results of investigations

DDx Approaches

- Anatomical
  - **VITAMIN D & C**
    - Vascular/Infection/Inflammatory/Trauma/Autoimmune
    - Metabolic/Iatrogenic/Neoplasia/Degenerative
    - Congenital
  - e.g. Front to Back, Brain, Systemic
- Surgical sieve
- Serious/Common/Ocular causes
- Specialties in medicine

Investigations

Follow HOBART Everybody!

- Follow-up/Confocal microscopy/Foreign body
- HVF/Hess & map binocular single vision
- OCT
- Bloods/Biopsy & Swabs/BP/BABY!/Botox
- Angiography/Angle
- Radiology
- Tonometry/Topography/Thickness (CCT)
- Electrophysiology

Complications

There's A PRICE you pay for surgery

- Anesthetic
- Phthisis bulbi/Perforation/PVR/Pre-existing pathology
- Retinal detachment
- Inflammation/IOP raise/Infection
- CME/Cataract/Cosmesis
- Endophthalmitis/ERM/Expectations/Endothelial loss

In uveitis, BEN GO blind

- Band keratopathy
- ERM
- Neovascularization
- Glaucoma
- Edema
- Blind => cataract

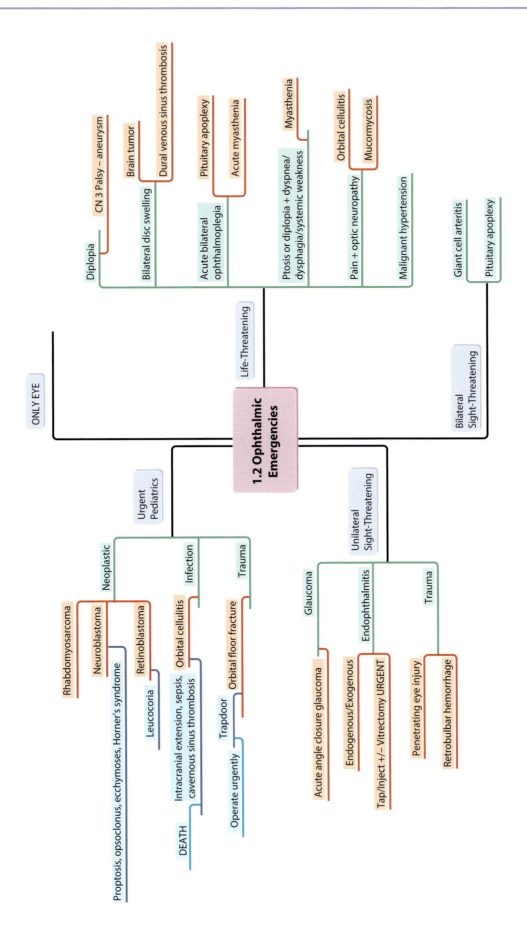

1.2 Ophthalmic Emergencies

ONLY EYE

Life-Threatening

Diplopia
- CN 3 Palsy – aneurysm
- Brain tumor

Bilateral disc swelling
- Dural venous sinus thrombosis

Acute bilateral ophthalmoplegia
- Pituitary apoplexy
- Acute myasthenia

Ptosis or diplopia + dyspnea/dysphagia/systemic weakness
- Myasthenia

Pain + optic neuropathy
- Orbital cellulitis
- Mucormycosis

Malignant hypertension

Bilateral Sight-Threatening
- Giant cell arteritis
- Pituitary apoplexy

Urgent Pediatrics

Neoplastic
- Rhabdomyosarcoma
- Neuroblastoma
  - Proptosis, opsoclonus, ecchymoses, Horner's syndrome
- Retinoblastoma
  - Leucocoria

Infection
- Orbital cellulitis
  - Intracranial extension, sepsis, cavernous sinus thrombosis
  - DEATH

Trauma
- Orbital floor fracture
  - Trapdoor
  - Operate urgently

Unilateral Sight-Threatening

Glaucoma
- Acute angle closure glaucoma

Endophthalmitis
- Endogenous/Exogenous
- Tap/Inject +/– Vitrectomy URGENT

Trauma
- Penetrating eye injury
- Retrobulbar hemorrhage

2 Cataract and Refractive Surgery

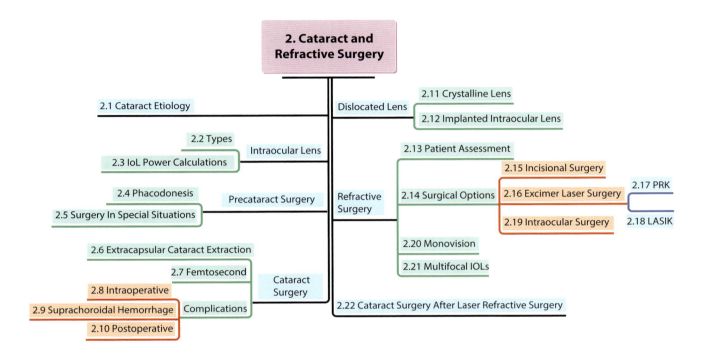

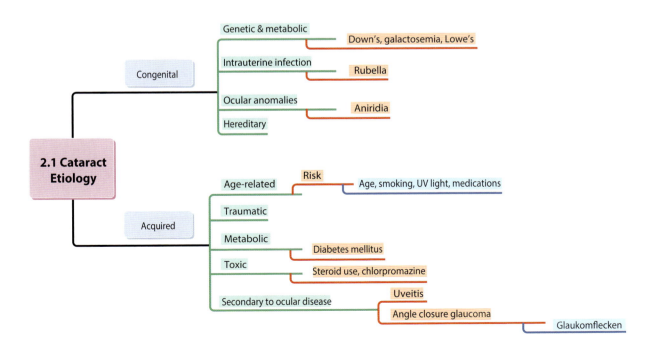

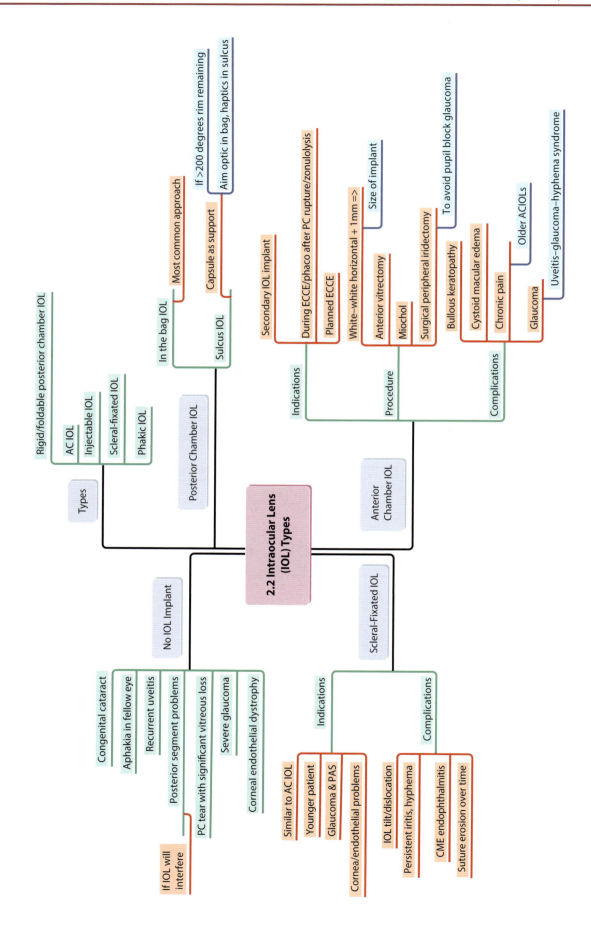

2.2 Intraocular Lens (IOL) Types

Posterior Chamber IOL

Types
- Rigid/foldable posterior chamber IOL
- AC IOL
- Injectable IOL
- Scleral-fixated IOL
- Phakic IOL

In the bag IOL
- Most common approach

Sulcus IOL
- Capsule as support
- If >200 degrees rim remaining
- Aim optic in bag, haptics in sulcus

Anterior Chamber IOL

Indications
- Secondary IOL implant
- During ECCE/phaco after PC rupture/zonulolysis
- Planned ECCE

Procedure
- White–white horizontal + 1mm => Size of implant
- Anterior vitrectomy
- Miochol
- Surgical peripheral iridectomy
- To avoid pupil block glaucoma

Complications
- Bullous keratopathy
- Cystoid macular edema
- Chronic pain
- Glaucoma — Older ACIOLs
- Uveitis–glaucoma–hyphema syndrome

No IOL Implant
- Congenital cataract
- Aphakia in fellow eye
- Recurrent uveitis
- Posterior segment problems
- PC tear with significant vitreous loss
- Severe glaucoma
- Corneal endothelial dystrophy
- If IOL will interfere

Scleral-Fixated IOL

Indications
- Similar to AC IOL
- Younger patient
- Glaucoma & PAS
- Cornea/endothelial problems

Complications
- IOL tilt/dislocation
- Persistent iritis, hyphema
- CME endophthalmitis
- Suture erosion over time

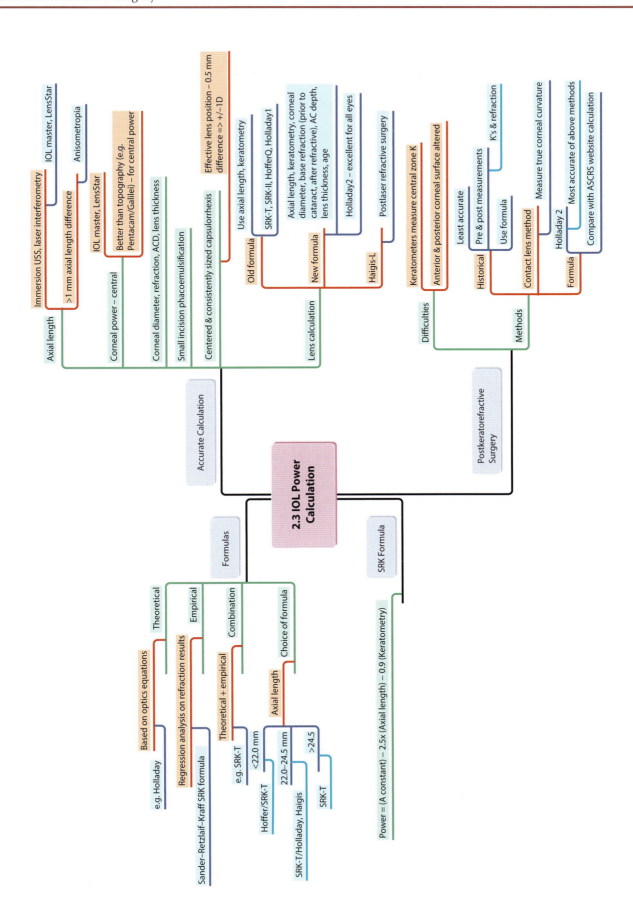

2.3 IOL Power Calculation

Accurate Calculation

Axial length
- Immersion USS, laser interferometry
  - IOL master, LensStar
- >1 mm axial length difference
  - Anisometropia
  - IOL master, LensStar

Corneal power – central
- Better than topography (e.g. Pentacam/Galilei) – for central power

Corneal diameter, refraction, ACD, lens thickness

Small incision phacoemulsification

Centered & consistently sized capsulorrhexis
- Effective lens position – 0.5 mm difference => +/-1D

Lens calculation
- Old formula
  - Use axial length, keratometry
- New formula
  - SRK-T, SRK-II, HofferQ, Holladay1
  - Axial length, keratometry, corneal diameter, base refraction (prior to cataract, after refractive), AC depth, lens thickness, age
  - Holladay2 – excellent for all eyes
- Haigis-L
  - Postlaser refractive surgery

Postkeratorefractive Surgery

Difficulties
- Keratometers measure central zone K
- Anterior & posterior corneal surface altered

Methods
- Historical
  - Least accurate
  - Pre & post measurements
  - Use formula
  - K's & refraction
- Contact lens method
  - Measure true corneal curvature
- Formula
  - Holladay 2
  - Most accurate of above methods
  - Compare with ASCRS website calculation

Formulas

Theoretical
- Based on optics equations
  - e.g. Holladay

Empirical
- Regression analysis on refraction results
  - Sander–Retzlaff–Kraff SRK formula

Combination
- Theoretical + empirical
  - e.g. SRK-T

Choice of formula
- Axial length
  - <22.0 mm
    - Hoffer/SRK-T
  - 22.0–24.5 mm
    - SRK-T/Holladay, Haigis
  - >24.5
    - SRK-T

SRK Formula

Power = (A constant) – 2.5x (Axial length) – 0.9 (Keratometry)

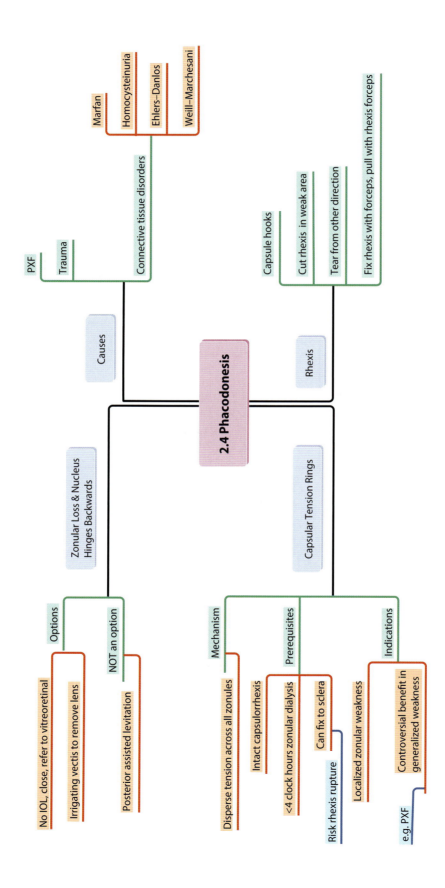

2.4 Phacodonesis

Causes

- PXF
- Trauma
- Connective tissue disorders
  - Marfan
  - Homocysteinuria
  - Ehlers–Danlos
  - Weill–Marchesani

Rhexis

- Capsule hooks
- Cut rhexis in weak area
- Tear from other direction
- Fix rhexis with forceps, pull with rhexis forceps

Zonular Loss & Nucleus Hinges Backwards

- Options
  - No IOL, close, refer to vitreoretinal
  - Irrigating vectis to remove lens
- NOT an option
  - Posterior assisted levitation

Capsular Tension Rings

- Mechanism
  - Disperse tension across all zonules
- Prerequisites
  - Intact capsulorrhexis
  - <4 clock hours zonular dialysis
  - Can fix to sclera
    - Risk rhexis rupture
- Indications
  - Localized zonular weakness
  - Controversial benefit in generalized weakness
    - e.g. PXF

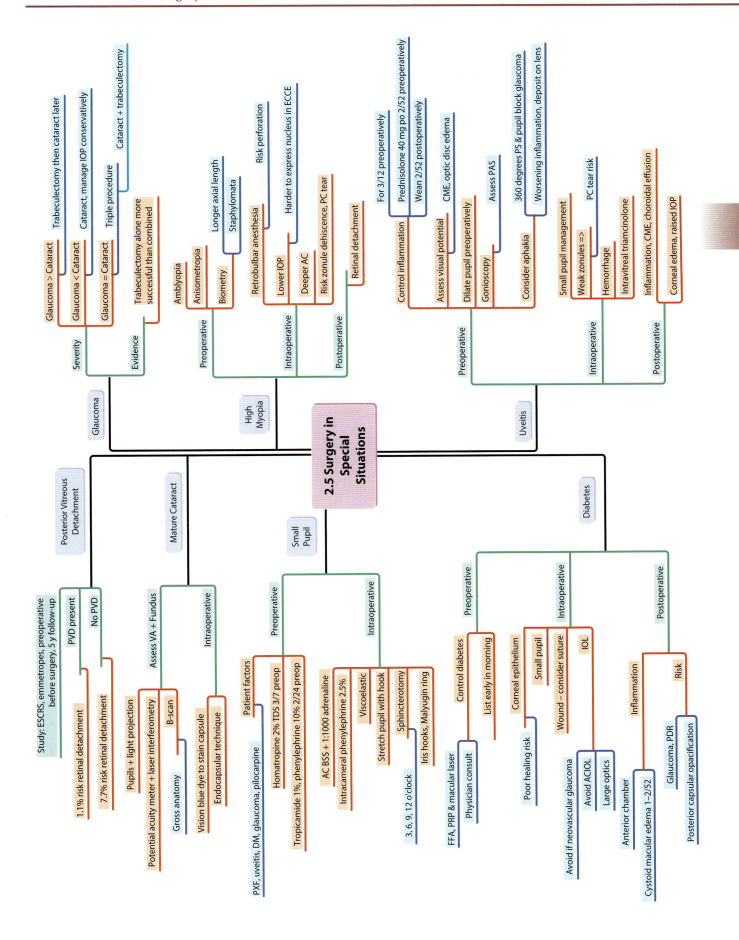

2.5 Surgery in Special Situations

Glaucoma

Severity
- Glaucoma > Cataract — Trabeculectomy then cataract later
- Glaucoma < Cataract — Cataract, manage IOP conservatively
- Glaucoma = Cataract — Triple procedure — Cataract + trabeculectomy

Evidence
- Trabeculectomy alone more successful than combined

High Myopia

Preoperative
- Amblyopia
- Anisometropia
- Biometry — Longer axial length, Staphylomata

Intraoperative
- Retrobulbar anesthesia — Risk perforation
- Lower IOP
- Deeper AC — Harder to express nucleus in ECCE
- Risk zonule dehiscence, PC tear

Postoperative
- Retinal detachment

Uveitis

Preoperative
- Control inflammation — For 3/12 preoperatively, Prednisolone 40 mg po 2/52 preoperatively, Wean 2/52 postoperatively
- Assess visual potential — CME, optic disc edema
- Dilate pupil preoperatively
- Gonioscopy — Assess PAS
- Consider aphakia

Intraoperative
- 360 degrees PS & pupil block glaucoma
- Worsening inflammation, deposit on lens
- Small pupil management
- Weak zonules => — PC tear risk
- Hemorrhage
- Intravitreal triamcinolone

Postoperative
- Inflammation, CME, choroidal effusion
- Corneal edema, raised IOP

Posterior Vitreous Detachment

Study: ESCRS, emmetropes, preoperative before surgery, 5 y follow-up
- PVD present — 1.1% risk retinal detachment
- No PVD — 7.7% risk retinal detachment

Mature Cataract

Assess VA + Fundus
- Pupils + light projection
- Potential acuity meter + laser interferometry
- B-scan — Gross anatomy

Intraoperative
- Vision blue dye to stain capsule
- Endocapsular technique

Small Pupil

Preoperative
- Patient factors — PXF, uveitis, DM, glaucoma, pilocarpine
- Homatropine 2% TDS 3/7 preop
- Tropicamide 1%, phenylephrine 10% 2/24 preop

Intraoperative
- AC BSS + 1:1000 adrenaline
- Intracameral phenylephrine 2.5%
- Viscoelastic
- Stretch pupil with hook
- Sphincterotomy — 3, 6, 9, 12 o'clock
- Iris hooks, Malyugin ring

Diabetes

Preoperative
- Control diabetes — FFA, PRP & macular laser, Physician consult
- List early in morning

Intraoperative
- Corneal epithelium — Poor healing risk
- Small pupil
- Wound – consider suture
- IOL — Avoid if neovascular glaucoma, Avoid ACIOL, Large optics

Postoperative
- Inflammation — Anterior chamber, Cystoid macular edema 1–2/52
- Risk — Glaucoma, PDR, Posterior capsular opacification

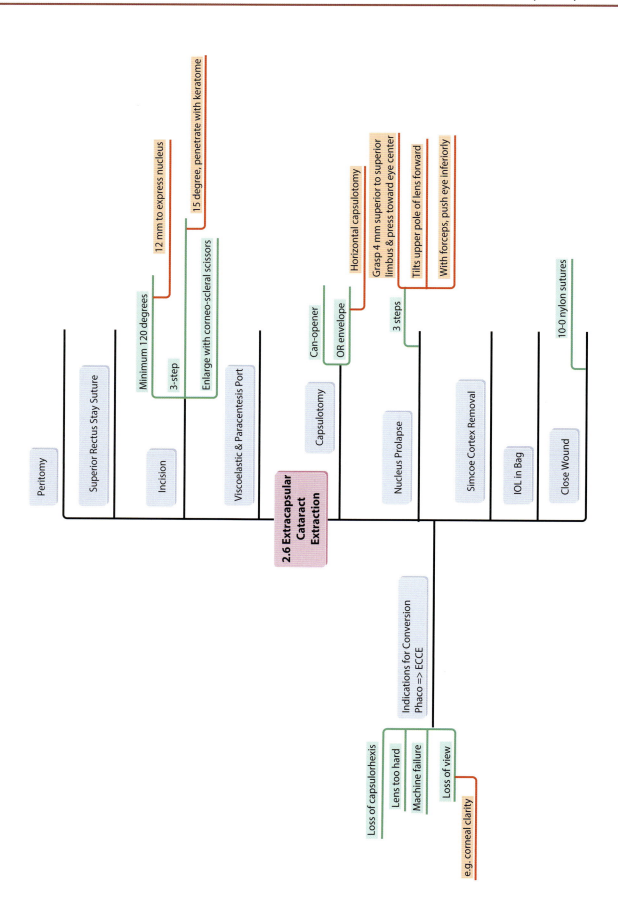

2.6 Extracapsular Cataract Extraction

- Peritomy
- Superior Rectus Stay Suture
- Incision
  - Minimum 120 degrees
    - 12 mm to express nucleus
  - 3-step
    - 15 degree, penetrate with keratome
  - Enlarge with corneo-scleral scissors
- Viscoelastic & Paracentesis Port
- Capsulotomy
  - Can-opener
  - OR envelope
    - Horizontal capsulotomy
    - Grasp 4 mm superior to superior limbus & press toward eye center
    - Tilts upper pole of lens forward
    - With forceps, push eye inferiorly
- Nucleus Prolapse
  - 3 steps
- Simcoe Cortex Removal
- IOL in Bag
- Close Wound
  - 10-0 nylon sutures

Indications for Conversion Phaco => ECCE
- Loss of capsulorhexis
- Lens too hard
- Machine failure
- Loss of view
  - e.g. corneal clarity

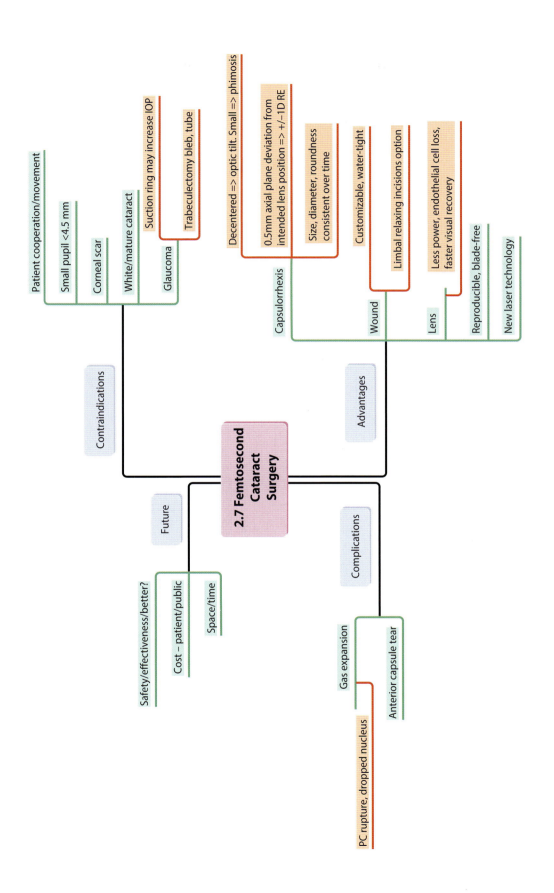

2.7 Femtosecond Cataract Surgery

Contraindications
- Patient cooperation/movement
- Small pupil <4.5 mm
- Corneal scar
- White/mature cataract
- Glaucoma
  - Suction ring may increase IOP
  - Trabeculectomy bleb, tube

Advantages
- Capsulorrhexis
  - Decentered => optic tilt. Small => phimosis
  - 0.5mm axial plane deviation from intended lens position => +/−1D RE
  - Size, diameter, roundness consistent over time
- Wound
  - Customizable, water-tight
  - Limbal relaxing incisions option
- Lens
  - Less power, endothelial cell loss, faster visual recovery
- Reproducible, blade-free
- New laser technology

Future
- Safety/effectiveness/better?
- Cost – patient/public
- Space/time

Complications
- Gas expansion
  - PC rupture, dropped nucleus
- Anterior capsule tear

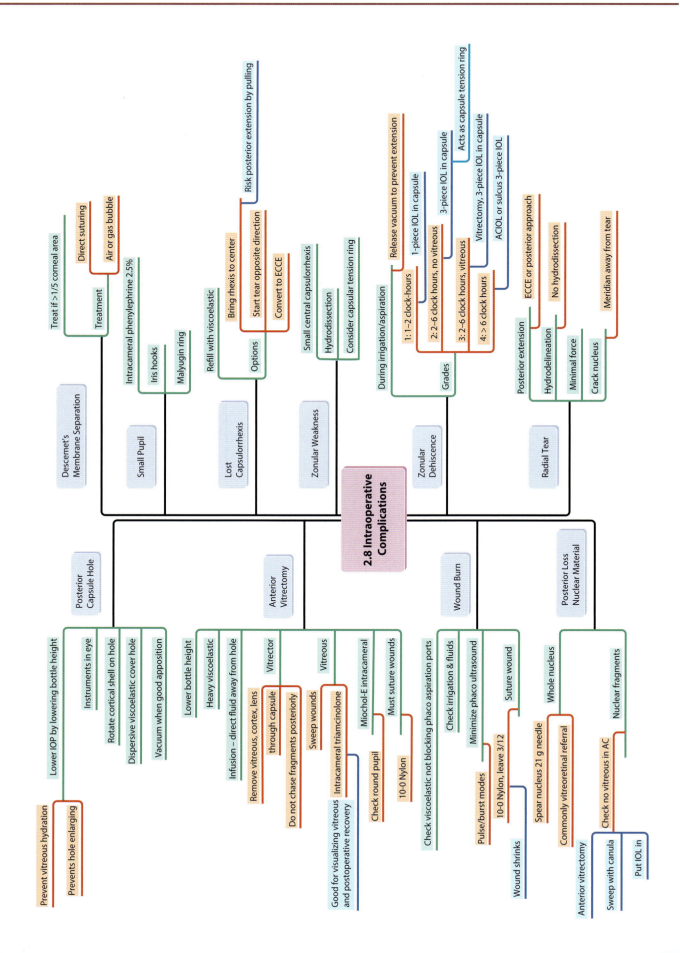

2.8 Intraoperative Complications

Descemet's Membrane Separation
- Treatment
  - Treat if >1/5 corneal area
  - Direct suturing
  - Air or gas bubble

Small Pupil
- Intracameral phenylephrine 2.5%
- Iris hooks
- Malyugin ring

Lost Capsulorrhexis
- Refill with viscoelastic
- Options
  - Bring rhexis to center
  - Start tear opposite direction
    - Risk posterior extension by pulling
  - Convert to ECCE

Zonular Weakness
- Small central capsulorrhexis
- Hydrodissection
- Consider capsular tension ring

Zonular Dehiscence
- During irrigation/aspiration
  - Release vacuum to prevent extension
- Grades
  - 1: 1–2 clock-hours
    - 1-piece IOL in capsule
  - 2: 2–6 clock hours, no vitreous
    - 3-piece IOL in capsule
      - Acts as capsule tension ring
  - 3: 2–6 clock hours, vitreous
    - Vitrectomy, 3-piece IOL in capsule
  - 4: > 6 clock hours
    - ACIOL or sulcus 3-piece IOL

Radial Tear
- Posterior extension
  - ECCE or posterior approach
- Hydrodelineation
  - No hydrodissection
- Minimal force
- Crack nucleus
  - Meridian away from tear

Posterior Capsule Hole
- Lower IOP by lowering bottle height
  - Prevent vitreous hydration
  - Prevents hole enlarging
- Instruments in eye
- Rotate cortical shell on hole
- Dispersive viscoelastic cover hole
- Vacuum when good apposition

Anterior Vitrectomy
- Lower bottle height
- Heavy viscoelastic
- Infusion – direct fluid away from hole
- Vitrector
  - Remove vitreous, cortex, lens through capsule
  - Do not chase fragments posteriorly
- Vitreous
  - Sweep wounds
  - Intracameral triamcinolone
    - Good for visualizing vitreous and postoperative recovery
  - Miochol-E intracameral
    - Check round pupil
  - Must suture wounds
    - 10-0 Nylon

Wound Burn
- Check viscoelastic not blocking phaco aspiration ports
- Check irrigation & fluids
- Minimize phaco ultrasound
  - Pulse/burst modes
- Suture wound
  - 10-0 Nylon, leave 3/12
  - Spear nucleus 21 g needle
  - Wound shrinks

Posterior Loss Nuclear Material
- Whole nucleus
  - Commonly vitreoretinal referral
- Nuclear fragments
  - Anterior vitrectomy
  - Sweep with canula
    - Check no vitreous in AC
    - Put IOL in

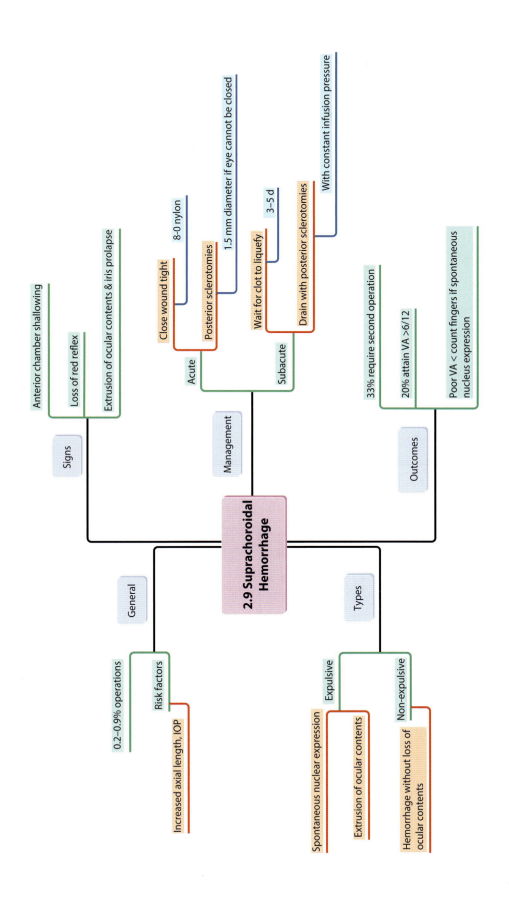

2.9 Suprachoroidal Hemorrhage

Signs
- Anterior chamber shallowing
- Loss of red reflex
- Extrusion of ocular contents & iris prolapse

Management
- Acute
  - Close wound tight
    - 8-0 nylon
  - Posterior sclerotomies
    - 1.5 mm diameter if eye cannot be closed
- Subacute
  - Wait for clot to liquefy
    - 3–5 d
  - Drain with posterior sclerotomies
    - With constant infusion pressure

Outcomes
- 33% require second operation
- 20% attain VA >6/12
- Poor VA < count fingers if spontaneous nucleus expression

General
- Risk factors
  - 0.2–0.9% operations
  - Increased axial length, IOP

Types
- Expulsive
  - Spontaneous nuclear expression
  - Extrusion of ocular contents
- Non-expulsive
  - Hemorrhage without loss of ocular contents

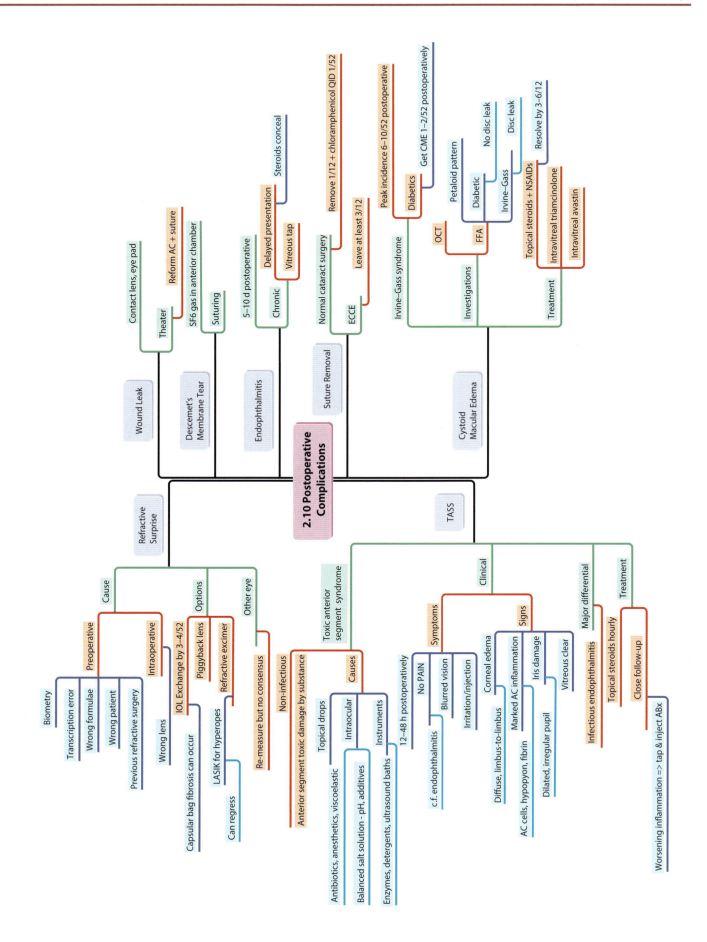

2.10 Postoperative Complications

Wound Leak
- Theater
  - Contact lens, eye pad
  - Reform AC + suture
- SF6 gas in anterior chamber

Descemet's Membrane Tear
- Suturing

Endophthalmitis
- 5–10 d postoperative
- Chronic
  - Delayed presentation
    - Steroids conceal
  - Vitreous tap

Suture Removal
- Normal cataract surgery
  - Remove 1/12 + chloramphenicol QID 1/52
- ECCE
  - Leave at least 3/12

Cystoid Macular Edema
- Irvine–Gass syndrome
  - Peak incidence 6–10/52 postoperative
  - Diabetics
    - Get CME 1–2/52 postoperatively
- Investigations
  - OCT
    - Petaloid pattern
  - FFA
    - No disc leak
      - Diabetic
      - Irvine–Gass
    - Disc leak
      - Resolve by 3–6/12
- Treatment
  - Topical steroids + NSAIDs
  - Intravitreal triamcinolone
  - Intravitreal avastin

Refractive Surprise
- Cause
  - Preoperative
    - Biometry
    - Transcription error
    - Wrong formulae
    - Wrong patient
    - Previous refractive surgery
  - Intraoperative
    - Wrong lens
  - Capsular bag fibrosis can occur
- Options
  - IOL Exchange by 3–4/52
  - Piggyback lens
    - LASIK for hyperopes
  - Refractive excimer
    - Can regress
- Other eye
  - Re-measure but no consensus

TASS
- Toxic anterior segment syndrome
  - Non-infectious
  - Anterior segment toxic damage by substance
  - Causes
    - Topical drops
      - Antibiotics, anesthetics, viscoelastic
    - Intraocular
      - Balanced salt solution - pH, additives
    - Instruments
      - Enzymes, detergents, ultrasound baths
- Clinical
  - Symptoms
    - 12–48 h postoperatively
    - No PAIN
      - c.f. endophthalmitis
    - Blurred vision
    - Irritation/injection
  - Signs
    - Corneal edema
      - Diffuse, limbus-to-limbus
    - Marked AC inflammation
      - AC cells, hypopyon, fibrin
    - Iris damage
      - Dilated, irregular pupil
    - Vitreous clear
- Major differential
  - Infectious endophthalmitis
- Treatment
  - Topical steroids hourly
  - Close follow-up
    - Worsening inflammation => tap & inject ABx

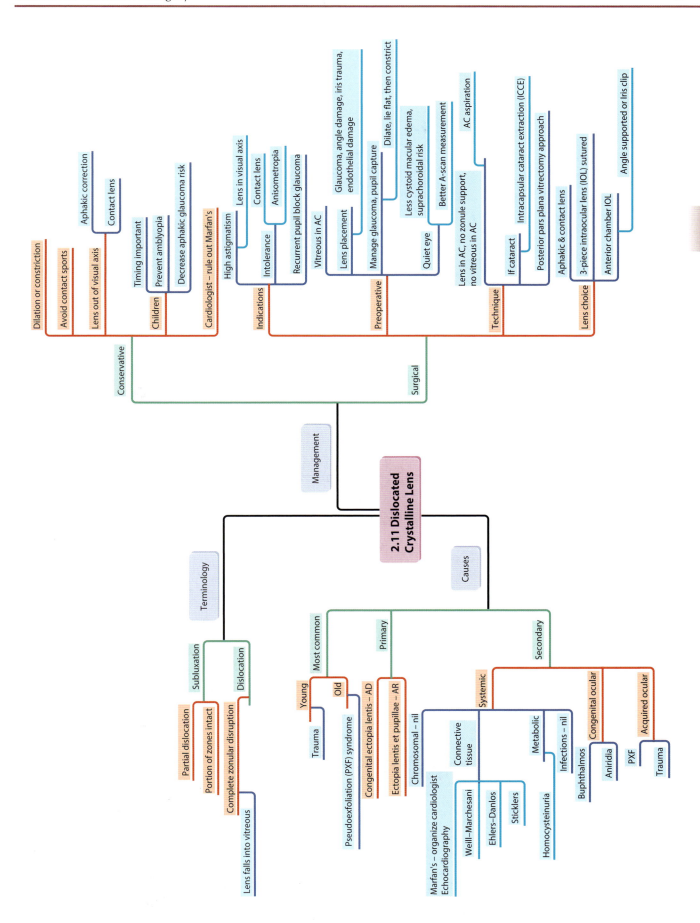

2.11 Dislocated Crystalline Lens

Management

Conservative

- **Dilation or constriction**
- **Avoid contact sports**
- **Lens out of visual axis**
  - Aphakic correction
    - Contact lens
- **Children**
  - Timing important
  - Prevent amblyopia
  - Decrease aphakic glaucoma risk
- **Cardiologist – rule out Marfan's**

Surgical

- **Indications**
  - High astigmatism
  - Lens in visual axis
    - Contact lens
  - Anisometropia
  - Recurrent pupil block glaucoma
  - Intolerance
- **Preoperative**
  - Vitreous in AC
  - Lens placement
    - Glaucoma, angle damage, iris trauma, endothelial damage
  - Manage glaucoma, pupil capture
    - Dilate, lie flat, then constrict
  - Less cystoid macular edema, suprachoroidal risk
  - Quiet eye
    - Better A-scan measurement
  - Lens in AC, no zonule support, no vitreous in AC
    - AC aspiration
- **Technique**
  - If cataract
    - Intracapsular cataract extraction (ICCE)
  - Posterior pars plana vitrectomy approach
- **Lens choice**
  - Aphakic & contact lens
  - 3-piece intraocular lens (IOL) sutured
  - Anterior chamber IOL
    - Angle supported or Iris clip

Terminology

- **Subluxation**
  - Partial dislocation
  - Portion of zones intact
- **Dislocation**
  - Complete zonular disruption
  - Lens falls into vitreous

Causes

- **Primary**
  - **Most common**
    - Young
      - Trauma
    - Old
      - Pseudoexfoliation (PXF) syndrome
  - Congenital ectopia lentis – AD
  - Ectopia lentis et pupillae – AR
- **Secondary**
  - **Systemic**
    - Chromosomal – nil
    - Connective tissue
      - Marfan's – organize cardiologist Echocardiography
      - Weill–Marchesani
      - Ehlers–Danlos
      - Sticklers
    - Metabolic
      - Homocysteinuria
    - Infections – nil
  - **Congenital ocular**
    - Buphthalmos
    - Aniridia
    - PXF
  - **Acquired ocular**
    - Trauma

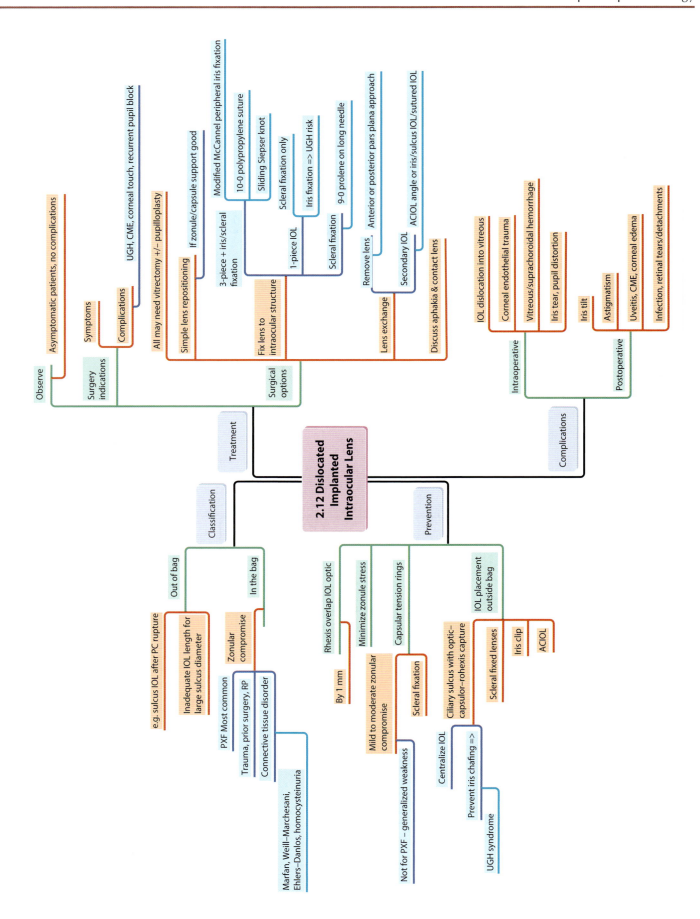

2.12 Dislocated Implanted Intraocular Lens

Treatment

Observe
- Asymptomatic patients, no complications

Surgery indications
- Symptoms
- Complications — UGH, CME, corneal touch, recurrent pupil block

Surgical options
- All may need vitrectomy +/– pupilloplasty
- Simple lens repositioning — If zonule/capsule support good
- Fix lens to intraocular structure
  - 3-piece + iris/scleral fixation
    - Modified McCannel peripheral iris fixation
    - 10-0 polypropylene suture
    - Sliding Siepser knot
  - 1-piece IOL
    - Scleral fixation only
    - Iris fixation => UGH risk
  - Scleral fixation
    - 9-0 prolene on long needle
- Lens exchange
  - Remove lens — Anterior or posterior pars plana approach
  - Secondary IOL
    - ACIOL angle or iris/sulcus IOL/sutured IOL
- Discuss aphakia & contact lens

Complications

Intraoperative
- IOL dislocation into vitreous
- Corneal endothelial trauma
- Vitreous/suprachoroidal hemorrhage
- Iris tear, pupil distortion

Postoperative
- Iris tilt
- Astigmatism
- Uveitis, CME, corneal edema
- Infection, retinal tears/detachments

Classification

Out of bag
- e.g. sulcus IOL after PC rupture
- Inadequate IOL length for large sulcus diameter
- Zonular compromise
  - PXF Most common
  - Trauma, prior surgery, RP
  - Connective tissue disorder
    - Marfan, Weill–Marchesani, Ehlers–Danlos, homocysteinuria

In the bag

Prevention

- Rhexis overlap IOL optic — By 1 mm
- Minimize zonule stress
- Capsular tension rings
  - Mild to moderate zonular compromise
  - Scleral fixation — Not for PXF – generalized weakness
- IOL placement outside bag
  - Ciliary sulcus with optic–capsulor–rohexis capture — Centralize IOL
  - Scleral fixed lenses — Prevent iris chafing =>
  - Iris clip — UGH syndrome
  - ACIOL

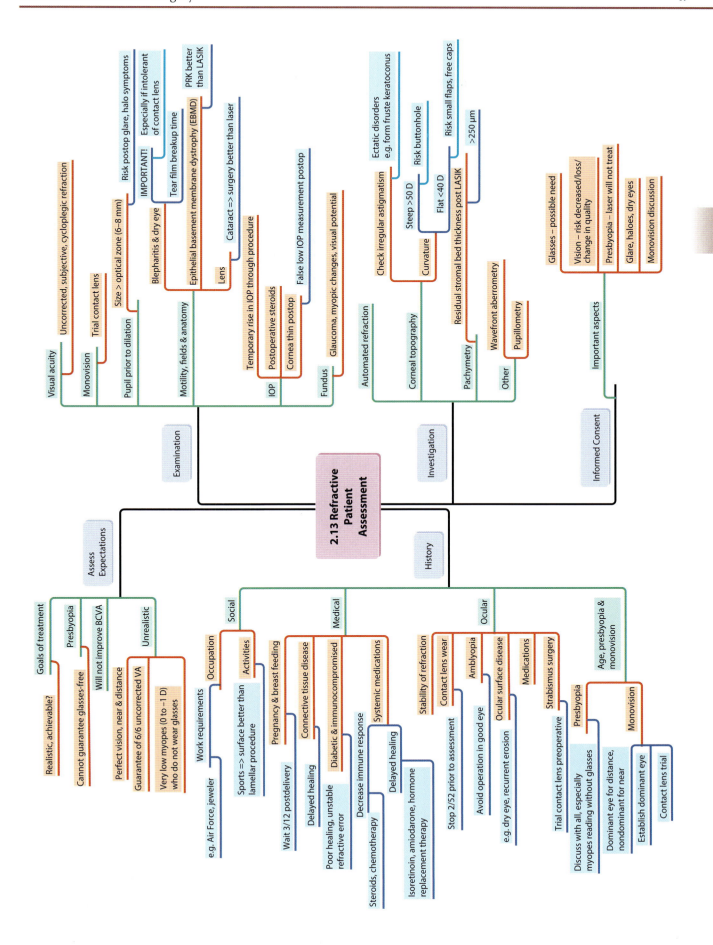

2.13 Refractive Patient Assessment

Examination

Visual acuity
- Uncorrected, subjective, cycloplegic refraction

Monovision
- Trial contact lens

Pupil prior to dilation
- Size > optical zone (6–8 mm)
  - Risk postop glare, halo symptoms
  - IMPORTANT!
    - Especially if intolerant of contact lens
    - PRK better than LASIK
  - Tear film breakup time

Motility, fields & anatomy
- Blepharitis & dry eye
- Epithelial basement membrane dystrophy (EBMD)
- Lens
  - Cataract => surgery better than laser

IOP
- Temporary rise in IOP through procedure
- Postoperative steroids
- Cornea thin postop
  - False low IOP measurement postop

Fundus
- Glaucoma, myopic changes, visual potential

Investigation

Automated refraction
- Check irregular astigmatism
  - Ectatic disorders e.g. form fruste keratoconus

Corneal topography
- Curvature
  - Steep >50 D
    - Risk buttonhole
  - Flat <40 D
    - Risk small flaps, free caps

Pachymetry
- Residual stromal bed thickness post LASIK
  - >250 µm

Other
- Wavefront aberrometry
- Pupillometry

Informed Consent

Important aspects
- Glasses – possible need
- Vision – risk decreased/loss/ change in quality
- Presbyopia – laser will not treat
- Glare, haloes, dry eyes
- Monovision discussion

Assess Expectations

Goals of treatment
- Realistic, achievable?
- Cannot guarantee glasses-free

Presbyopia
- Will not improve BCVA

Will not improve BCVA
- Perfect vision, near & distance
- Guarantee of 6/6 uncorrected VA

Unrealistic
- Very low myopes (0 to –1 D) who do not wear glasses

History

Social
- Occupation
  - Work requirements
    - e.g. Air Force, jeweler
- Activities
  - Sports => surface better than lamellar procedure

Medical
- Pregnancy & breast feeding
  - Wait 3/12 postdelivery
  - Delayed healing
- Connective tissue disease
  - Poor healing, unstable refractive error
- Diabetic & immunocompromised
  - Decrease immune response
  - Delayed healing
- Systemic medications
  - Steroids, chemotherapy
  - Isoretinoin, amiodarone, hormone replacement therapy

Ocular
- Stability of refraction
- Contact lens wear
  - Stop 2/52 prior to assessment
- Amblyopia
  - Avoid operation in good eye
- Ocular surface disease
  - e.g. dry eye, recurrent erosion
- Medications
- Strabismus surgery

Age, presbyopia & monovision
- Presbyopia
  - Trial contact lens preoperative
  - Discuss with all, especially myopes reading without glasses
- Monovision
  - Dominant eye for distance, nondominant for near
  - Establish dominant eye
  - Contact lens trial

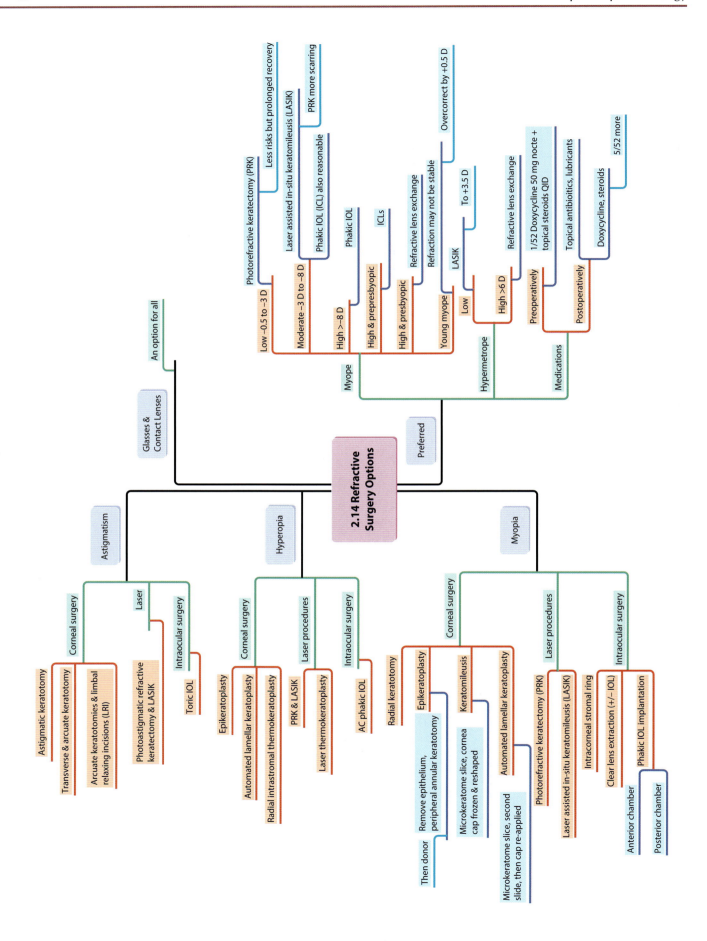

2.14 Refractive Surgery Options

Glasses & Contact Lenses
- An option for all

Preferred
- Myope
  - Low −0.5 to −3 D
    - Photorefractive keratectomy (PRK)
      - Less risks but prolonged recovery
    - Laser assisted in-situ keratomileusis (LASIK)
      - PRK more scarring
  - Moderate −3 D to −8 D
    - Phakic IOL (ICL) also reasonable
  - High >−8 D
    - Phakic IOL
  - High & prepresbyopic
    - ICLs
  - High & presbyopic
    - Refractive lens exchange
  - Young myope
    - Refraction may not be stable
- Hypermetrope
  - Low
    - LASIK
      - Overcorrect by +0.5 D
      - To +3.5 D
  - High >6 D
    - Refractive lens exchange
- Medications
  - Preoperatively
    - 1/52 Doxycycline 50 mg nocte + topical steroids QID
  - Postoperatively
    - Topical antibiotics, lubricants
    - Doxycycline, steroids
      - 5/52 more

Astigmatism
- Corneal surgery
  - Astigmatic keratotomy
    - Transverse & arcuate keratotomy
    - Arcuate keratotomies & limbal relaxing incisions (LRI)
- Laser
  - Photoastigmatic refractive keratectomy & LASIK
- Intraocular surgery
  - Toric IOL

Hyperopia
- Corneal surgery
  - Epikeratoplasty
  - Automated lamellar keratoplasty
  - Radial intrastromal thermokeratoplasty
- Laser procedures
  - PRK & LASIK
  - Laser thermokeratoplasty
- Intraocular surgery
  - AC phakic IOL

Myopia
- Corneal surgery
  - Radial keratotomy
  - Epikeratoplasty
    - Remove epithelium, peripheral annular keratotomy
    - Then donor
  - Keratomileusis
    - Microkeratome slice, cornea cap frozen & reshaped
    - Microkeratome slice, second slide, then cap re-applied
  - Automated lamellar keratoplasty
- Laser procedures
  - Photorefractive keratectomy (PRK)
  - Laser assisted in-situ keratomileusis (LASIK)
  - Intracorneal stromal ring
- Intraocular surgery
  - Clear lens extraction (+/− IOL)
  - Phakic IOL implantation
    - Anterior chamber
    - Posterior chamber

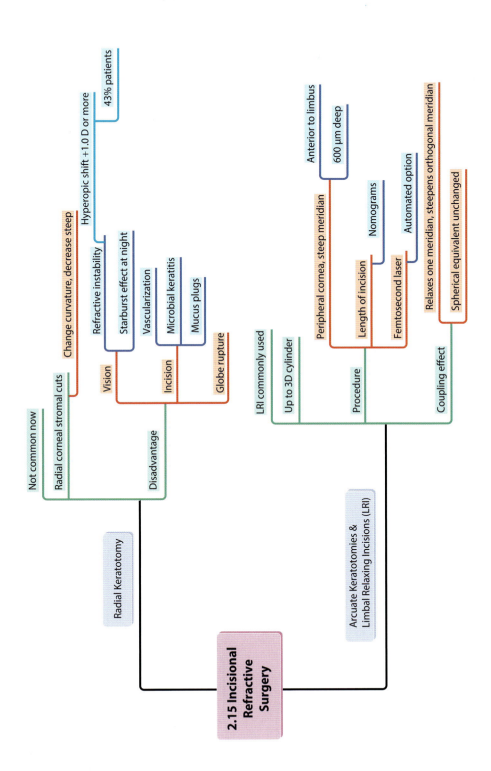

2.15 Incisional Refractive Surgery

Radial Keratotomy
- Not common now
- Radial corneal stromal cuts
  - Vision
    - Change curvature, decrease steep
    - Refractive instability
      - Hyperopic shift +1.0 D or more
        - 43% patients
    - Starburst effect at night
  - Incision
    - Vascularization
    - Microbial keratitis
    - Mucus plugs
  - Disadvantage
    - Globe rupture

Arcuate Keratotomies & Limbal Relaxing Incisions (LRI)
- LRI commonly used
- Up to 3D cylinder
- Procedure
  - Peripheral cornea, steep meridian
    - Anterior to limbus
    - 600 μm deep
  - Length of incision
    - Nomograms
  - Femtosecond laser
    - Automated option
- Coupling effect
  - Relaxes one meridian, steepens orthogonal meridian
  - Spherical equivalent unchanged

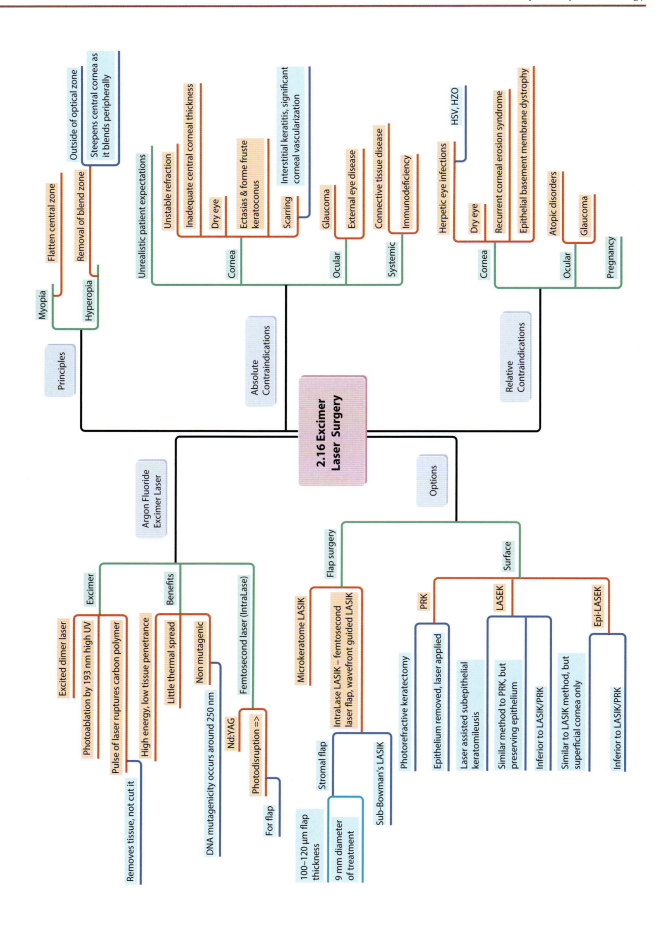

2.16 Excimer Laser Surgery

Principles

Myopia
- Flatten central zone
- Removal of blend zone
  - Outside of optical zone
  - Steepens central cornea as it blends peripherally

Hyperopia

Absolute Contraindications

- Unrealistic patient expectations
- Cornea
  - Unstable refraction
  - Inadequate central corneal thickness
  - Dry eye
  - Ectasias & forme fruste keratoconus
  - Scarring
    - Interstitial keratitis, significant corneal vascularization
- Ocular
  - Glaucoma
  - External eye disease
- Systemic
  - Connective tissue disease
  - Immunodeficiency

Relative Contraindications

- Cornea
  - Herpetic eye infections
    - HSV, HZO
  - Dry eye
  - Recurrent corneal erosion syndrome
  - Epithelial basement membrane dystrophy
- Ocular
  - Atopic disorders
  - Glaucoma
- Pregnancy

Argon Fluoride Excimer Laser

- Excimer
  - Excited dimer laser
  - Photoablation by 193 nm high UV
  - Pulse of laser ruptures carbon polymer
    - Removes tissue, not cut it
- Benefits
  - High energy, low tissue penetrance
  - Little thermal spread
  - Non mutagenic
    - DNA mutagenicity occurs around 250 nm
      - Nd:YAG
- Femtosecond laser (IntraLase)
  - Photodisruption =>
    - For flap

Options

- Flap surgery
  - Microkeratome LASIK
  - IntraLase LASIK – femtosecond laser flap, wavefront guided LASIK
    - Stromal flap
    - Sub-Bowman's LASIK
    - 100–120 μm flap thickness
    - 9 mm diameter of treatment
- Surface
  - PRK
    - Photorefractive keratectomy
    - Epithelium removed, laser applied
  - LASEK
    - Laser assisted subepithelial keratomileusis
    - Similar method to PRK, but preserving epithelium
    - Inferior to LASIK/PRK
  - Epi-LASEK
    - Similar to LASIK method, but superficial cornea only
    - Inferior to LASIK/PRK

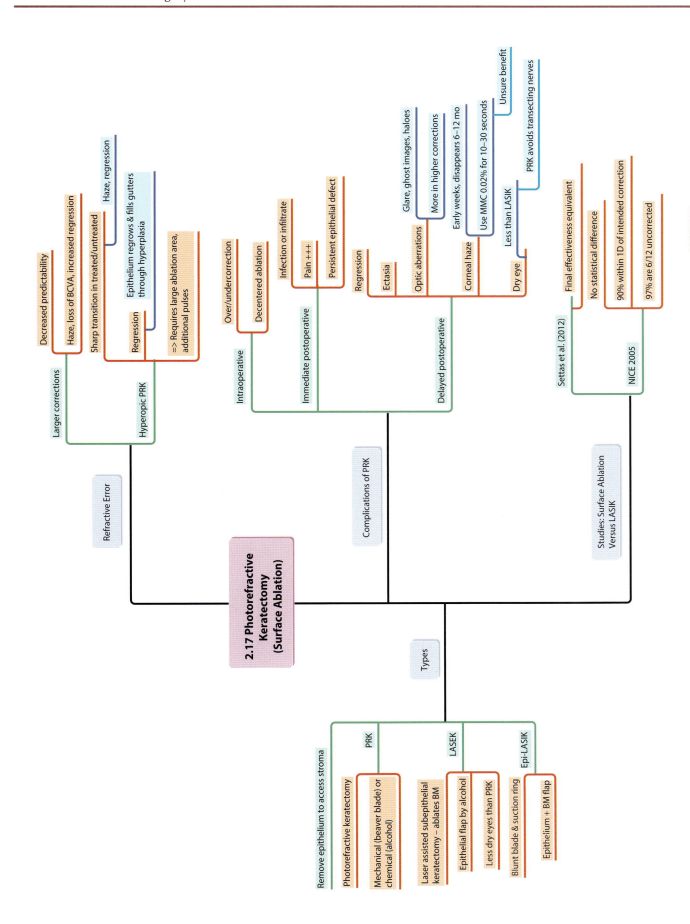

2.17 Photorefractive Keratectomy (Surface Ablation)

Refractive Error

- Larger corrections
  - Decreased predictability
  - Haze, loss of BCVA, increased regression
  - Sharp transition in treated/untreated
    - Haze, regression
- Hyperopic PRK
  - Regression
    - Epithelium regrows & fills gutters through hyperplasia
  - => Requires large ablation area, additional pulses

Complications of PRK

- Intraoperative
  - Over/undercorrection
  - Decentered ablation
- Immediate postoperative
  - Infection or infiltrate
  - Pain +++
  - Persistent epithelial defect
- Delayed postoperative
  - Regression
  - Ectasia
  - Optic aberrations
    - Glare, ghost images, haloes
    - More in higher corrections
  - Corneal haze
    - Early weeks, disappears 6–12 mo
    - Use MMC 0.02% for 10–30 seconds
      - Unsure benefit
  - Dry eye
    - Less than LASIK
      - PRK avoids transecting nerves

Studies: Surface Ablation Versus LASIK

- Settas et al. (2012)
  - Final effectiveness equivalent
  - No statistical difference
- NICE 2005
  - 90% within 1D of intended correction
  - 97% are 6/12 uncorrected

Types

- PRK
  - Remove epithelium to access stroma
  - Photorefractive keratectomy
  - Mechanical (beaver blade) or chemical (alcohol)
- LASEK
  - Laser assisted subepithelial keratectomy – ablates BM
  - Epithelial flap by alcohol
  - Less dry eyes than PRK
- Epi-LASIK
  - Blunt blade & suction ring
  - Epithelium + BM flap

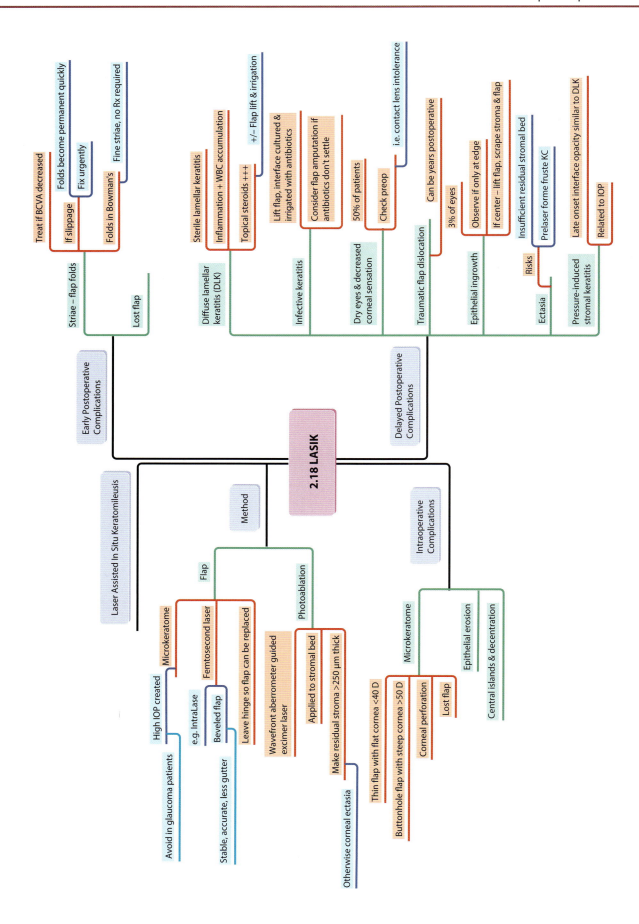

2.18 LASIK

Laser Assisted In Situ Keratomileusis

Method

Flap

- Microkeratome
  - High IOP created
    - Avoid in glaucoma patients
- Femtosecond laser
  - e.g. IntraLase
  - Beveled flap
    - Stable, accurate, less gutter
- Leave hinge so flap can be replaced

Photoablation
- Wavefront aberrometer guided excimer laser
- Applied to stromal bed
- Make residual stroma >250 μm thick
  - Otherwise corneal ectasia

Intraoperative Complications
- Microkeratome
  - Thin flap with flat cornea <40 D
  - Buttonhole flap with steep cornea >50 D
  - Corneal perforation
  - Lost flap
- Epithelial erosion
- Central islands & decentration

Early Postoperative Complications

Striae – flap folds
- Treat if BCVA decreased
  - Folds become permanent quickly
- If slippage
  - Fix urgently
- Folds in Bowman's
  - Fine striae, no Rx required

Lost flap

Delayed Postoperative Complications

Diffuse lamellar keratitis (DLK)
- Sterile lamellar keratitis
- Inflammation + WBC accumulation
- Topical steroids +++
  - +/– Flap lift & irrigation

Infective keratitis
- Lift flap, interface cultured & irrigated with antibiotics
- Consider flap amputation if antibiotics don't settle

Dry eyes & decreased corneal sensation
- 50% of patients
- Check preop

Traumatic flap dislocation
- Can be years postoperative

Epithelial ingrowth
- 3% of eyes
- Observe if only at edge
- If center – lift flap, scrape stroma & flap

Ectasia
- Risks
  - Insufficient residual stromal bed
  - Prelaser forme fruste KC
  - i.e. contact lens intolerance

Pressure-induced stromal keratitis
- Late onset interface opacity similar to DLK
- Related to IOP

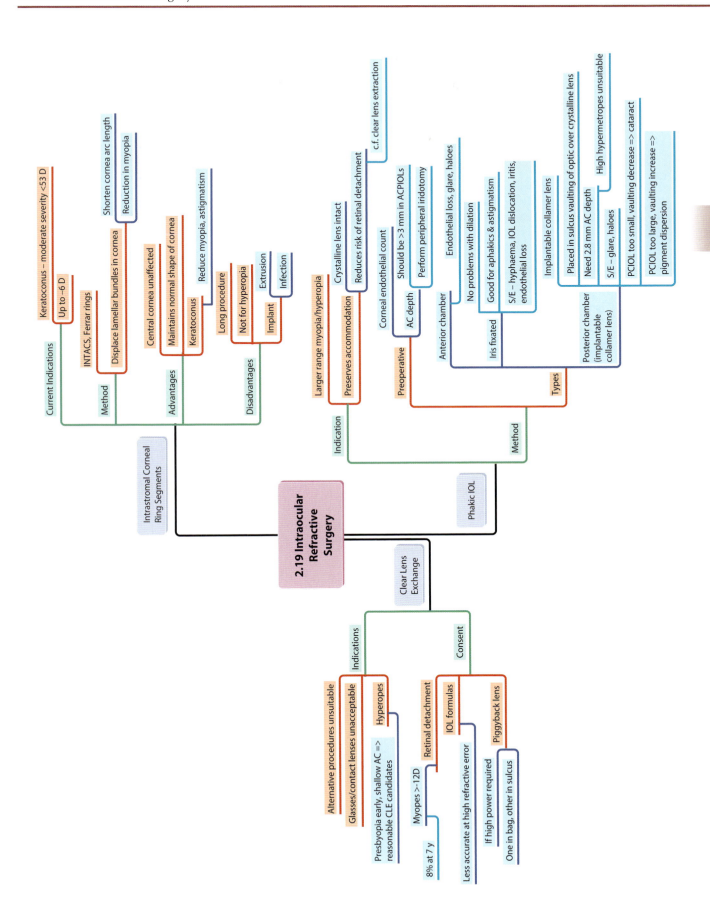

2.19 Intraocular Refractive Surgery

Intrastromal Corneal Ring Segments

Current Indications
- Keratoconus — moderate severity <53 D
- Up to −6 D
- INTACS, Ferrar rings

Method
- Displace lamellar bundles in cornea
  - Shorten cornea arc length
  - Reduction in myopia

Advantages
- Central cornea unaffected
- Maintains normal shape of cornea
- Keratoconus
  - Reduce myopia, astigmatism
- Long procedure
- Not for hyperopia

Disadvantages
- Implant
  - Extrusion
  - Infection

Phakic IOL

Indication
- Larger range myopia/hyperopia
- Preserves accommodation
- Crystalline lens intact
- Reduces risk of retinal detachment
  - c.f. clear lens extraction

Method

Preoperative
- Corneal endothelial count
- AC depth
  - Should be >3 mm in ACPIOLs
  - Perform peripheral iridotomy

Types
- Anterior chamber
  - Endothelial loss, glare, haloes
  - No problems with dilation
  - Good for aphakics & astigmatism
- Iris fixated
  - S/E – hyphaema, IOL dislocation, iritis, endothelial loss
- Posterior chamber (implantable collamer lens)
  - Implantable collamer lens
  - Placed in sulcus vaulting of optic over crystalline lens
    - High hypermetropes unsuitable
  - Need 2.8 mm AC depth
  - S/E – glare, haloes
  - PCIOL too small, vaulting decrease => cataract
  - PCIOL too large, vaulting increase => pigment dispersion

Clear Lens Exchange

Indications
- Alternative procedures unsuitable
- Glasses/contact lenses unacceptable
- Hyperopes
  - Presbyopia early, shallow AC => reasonable CLE candidates
- Myopes >−12D
  - Retinal detachment
    - 8% at 7 y

Consent
- IOL formulas
  - Less accurate at high refractive error
- Piggyback lens
  - If high power required
  - One in bag, other in sulcus

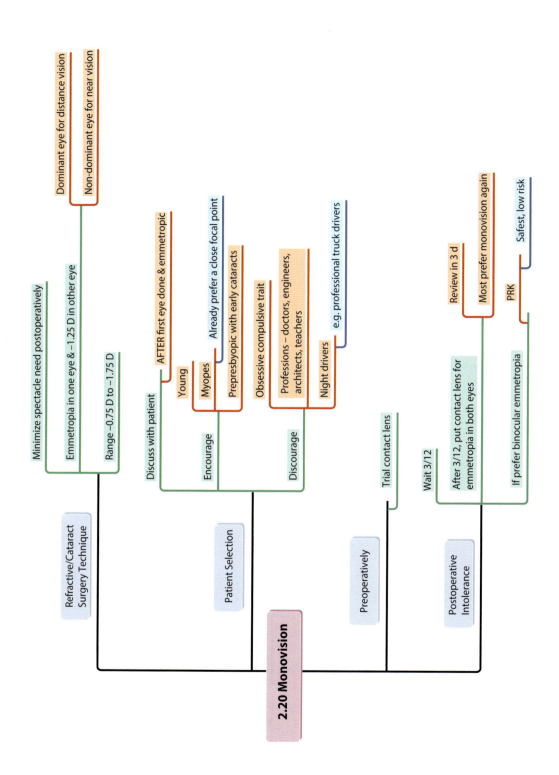

2.20 Monovision

Refractive/Cataract Surgery Technique
- Minimize spectacle need postoperatively
- Emmetropia in one eye & –1.25 D in other eye
  - Range –0.75 D to –1.75 D
- Dominant eye for distance vision
- Non-dominant eye for near vision

Patient Selection
- Discuss with patient
- Encourage
  - AFTER first eye done & emmetropic
  - Young
  - Myopes
    - Already prefer a close focal point
    - Prepresbyopic with early cataracts
- Discourage
  - Obsessive compulsive trait
  - Professions – doctors, engineers, architects, teachers
  - Night drivers
    - e.g. professional truck drivers

Preoperatively
- Trial contact lens

Postoperative Intolerance
- Wait 3/12
- After 3/12, put contact lens for emmetropia in both eyes
- If prefer binocular emmetropia
- Review in 3 d
- Most prefer monovision again
- PRK
  - Safest, low risk

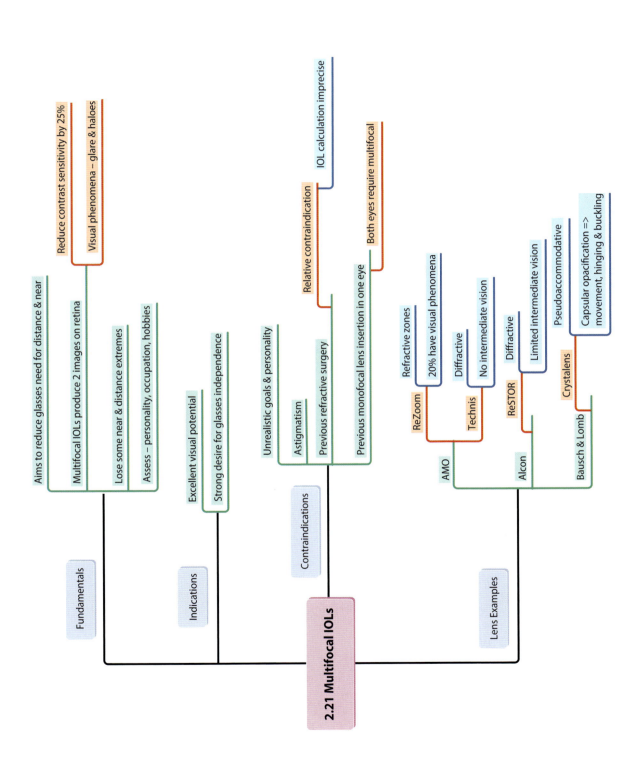

2.21 Multifocal IOLs

Fundamentals
- Aims to reduce glasses need for distance & near
- Multifocal IOLs produce 2 images on retina
  - Reduce contrast sensitivity by 25%
  - Visual phenomena – glare & haloes
- Lose some near & distance extremes
- Assess – personality, occupation, hobbies

Indications
- Excellent visual potential
- Strong desire for glasses independence

Contraindications
- Unrealistic goals & personality
- Astigmatism
- Previous refractive surgery
  - Relative contraindication
    - IOL calculation imprecise
- Previous monofocal lens insertion in one eye
  - Both eyes require multifocal

Lens Examples
- AMO
  - ReZoom
    - Refractive zones
    - 20% have visual phenomena
  - Technis
    - Diffractive
    - No intermediate vision
- Alcon
  - ReSTOR
    - Diffractive
    - Limited intermediate vision
- Bausch & Lomb
  - Crystalens
    - Pseudoaccommodative
    - Capsular opacification => movement, hinging & buckling

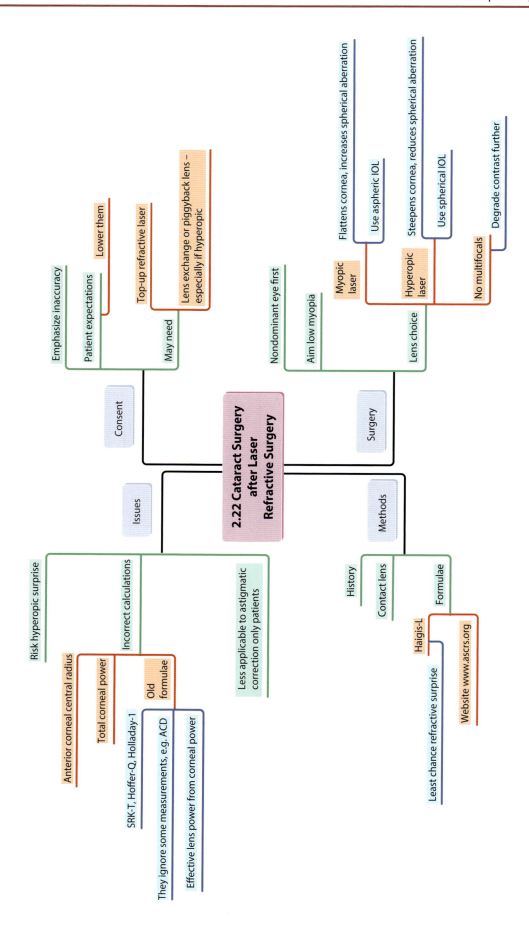

2.22 Cataract Surgery after Laser Refractive Surgery

Consent
- Emphasize inaccuracy
- Patient expectations
  - Lower them
- May need
  - Top-up refractive laser
  - Lens exchange or piggyback lens – especially if hyperopic

Surgery
- Nondominant eye first
- Aim low myopia
- Lens choice
  - Myopic laser
    - Flattens cornea, increases spherical aberration
      - Use aspheric IOL
  - Hyperopic laser
    - Steepens cornea, reduces spherical aberration
      - Use spherical IOL
  - No multifocals
    - Degrade contrast further

Issues
- Risk hyperopic surprise
- Incorrect calculations
  - Anterior corneal central radius
  - Total corneal power
  - Old formulae
    - SRK-T, Hoffer-Q, Holladay-1
    - They ignore some measurements, e.g. ACD
    - Effective lens power from corneal power
- Less applicable to astigmatic correction only patients

Methods
- History
- Contact lens
- Formulae
  - Haigis-L
    - Least chance refractive surprise
  - Website www.ascrs.org

3 Cornea and External Eye

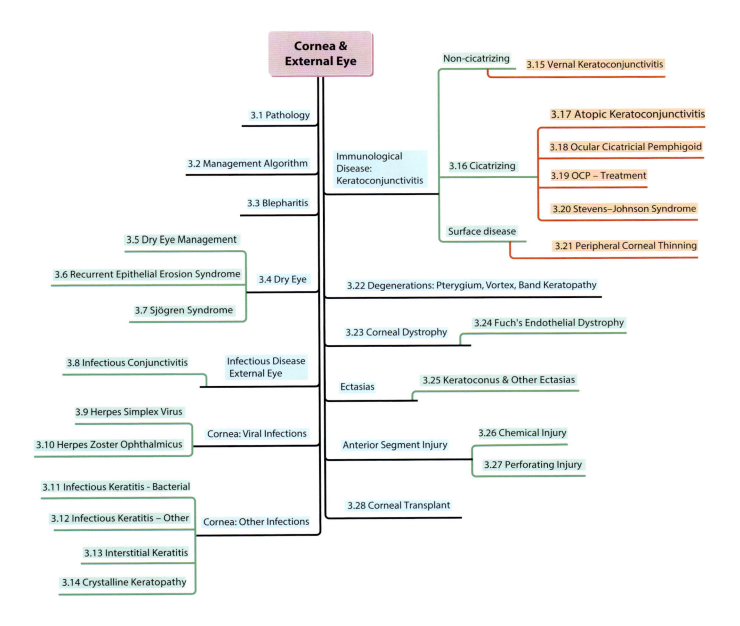

Cornea & External Eye

- 3.1 Pathology
- 3.2 Management Algorithm
- 3.3 Blepharitis
- 3.4 Dry Eye
  - 3.5 Dry Eye Management
  - 3.6 Recurrent Epithelial Erosion Syndrome
  - 3.7 Sjögren Syndrome
- Infectious Disease External Eye
  - 3.8 Infectious Conjunctivitis
- Cornea: Viral Infections
  - 3.9 Herpes Simplex Virus
  - 3.10 Herpes Zoster Ophthalmicus
- Cornea: Other Infections
  - 3.11 Infectious Keratitis - Bacterial
  - 3.12 Infectious Keratitis – Other
  - 3.13 Interstitial Keratitis
  - 3.14 Crystalline Keratopathy

- Immunological Disease: Keratoconjunctivitis
  - Non-cicatrizing
    - 3.15 Vernal Keratoconjunctivitis
  - 3.16 Cicatrizing
    - 3.17 Atopic Keratoconjunctivitis
    - 3.18 Ocular Cicatricial Pemphigoid
    - 3.19 OCP – Treatment
    - 3.20 Stevens–Johnson Syndrome
  - Surface disease
    - 3.21 Peripheral Corneal Thinning
- 3.22 Degenerations: Pterygium, Vortex, Band Keratopathy
- 3.23 Corneal Dystrophy
  - 3.24 Fuch's Endothelial Dystrophy
- Ectasias
  - 3.25 Keratoconus & Other Ectasias
- Anterior Segment Injury
  - 3.26 Chemical Injury
  - 3.27 Perforating Injury
- 3.28 Corneal Transplant

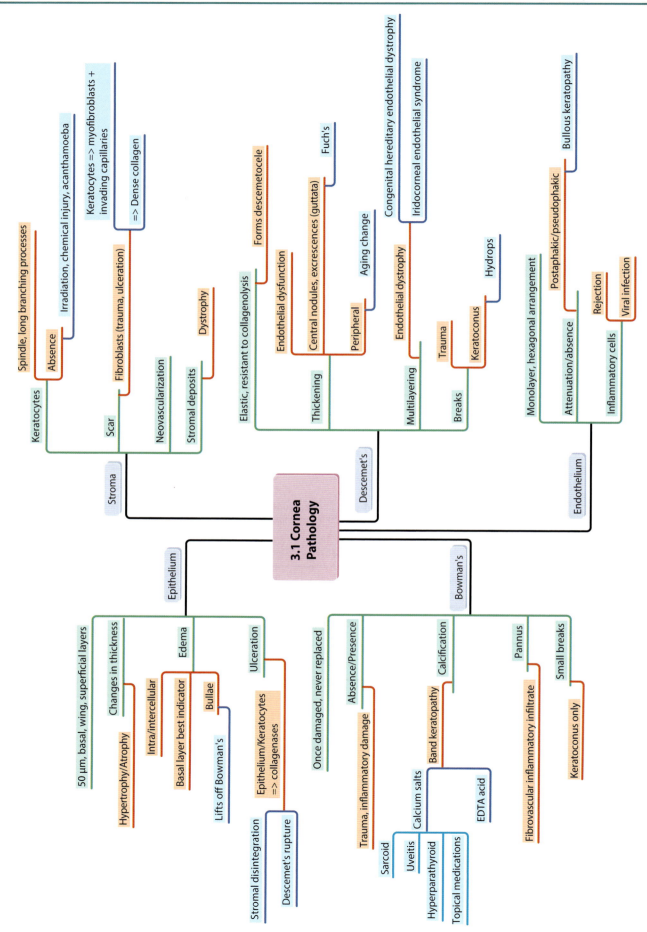

3.1 Cornea Pathology

Stroma
- Keratocytes
  - Spindle, long branching processes
  - Absence
    - Irradiation, chemical injury, acanthamoeba
- Scar
  - Fibroblasts (trauma, ulceration)
    - Keratocytes => myofibroblasts + invading capillaries
    - => Dense collagen
- Neovascularization
- Stromal deposits
  - Dystrophy

Descemet's
- Elastic, resistant to collagenolysis
- Thickening
  - Endothelial dysfunction
    - Forms descemetocele
  - Central nodules, excrescences (guttata)
    - Fuch's
  - Peripheral
    - Aging change
- Multilayering
  - Endothelial dystrophy
    - Congenital hereditary endothelial dystrophy
    - Iridocorneal endothelial syndrome
- Breaks
  - Trauma
  - Keratoconus
    - Hydrops

Endothelium
- Monolayer, hexagonal arrangement
- Attenuation/absence
  - Postaphakic/pseudophakic
    - Bullous keratopathy
- Inflammatory cells
  - Rejection
  - Viral infection

Epithelium
- 50 μm, basal, wing, superficial layers
- Changes in thickness
  - Hypertrophy/Atrophy
- Edema
  - Intra/intercellular
  - Basal layer best indicator
  - Bullae
    - Lifts off Bowman's
- Ulceration
  - Epithelium/Keratocytes => collagenases
    - Stromal disintegration
    - Descemet's rupture

Bowman's
- Absence/Presence
  - Once damaged, never replaced
  - Trauma, inflammatory damage
- Calcification
  - Band keratopathy
    - Calcium salts
      - Sarcoid
      - Uveitis
      - Hyperparathyroid
      - Topical medications
    - EDTA acid
- Pannus
  - Fibrovascular inflammatory infiltrate
- Small breaks
  - Keratoconus only

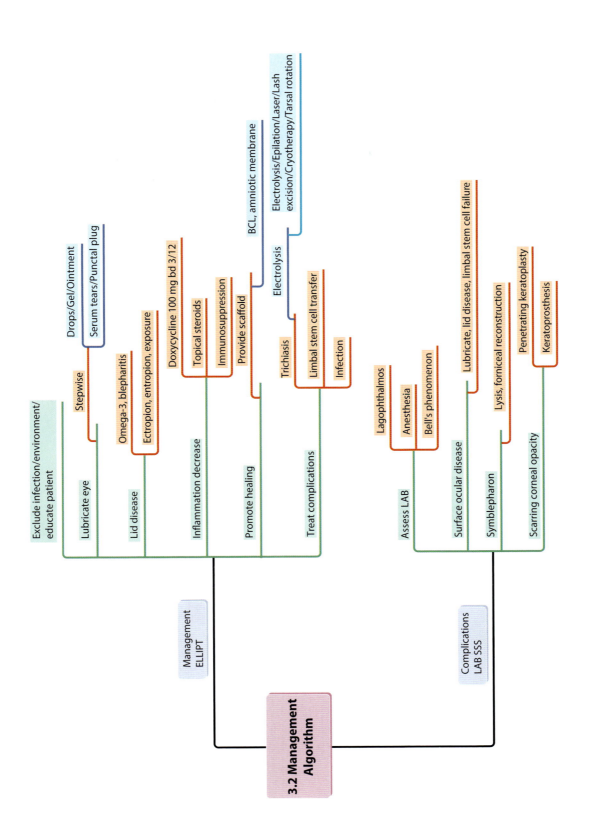

3.2 Management Algorithm

Management ELLIPT

- Exclude infection/environment/educate patient
- Lubricate eye
  - Stepwise
    - Drops/Gel/Ointment
    - Serum tears/Punctal plug
- Lid disease
  - Omega-3, blepharitis
  - Ectropion, entropion, exposure
- Inflammation decrease
  - Doxycycline 100 mg bd 3/12
  - Topical steroids
  - Immunosuppression
- Promote healing
  - Provide scaffold
    - BCL, amniotic membrane
- Treat complications
  - Electrolysis
    - Electrolysis/Epilation/Laser/Lash excision/Cryotherapy/Tarsal rotation
  - Trichiasis
  - Limbal stem cell transfer
  - Infection

Complications LAB SSS

- Assess LAB
  - Lagophthalmos
  - Anesthesia
  - Bell's phenomenon
- Surface ocular disease
  - Lubricate, lid disease, limbal stem cell failure
- Symblepharon
  - Lysis, forniceal reconstruction
- Scarring corneal opacity
  - Penetrating keratoplasty
  - Keratoprosthesis

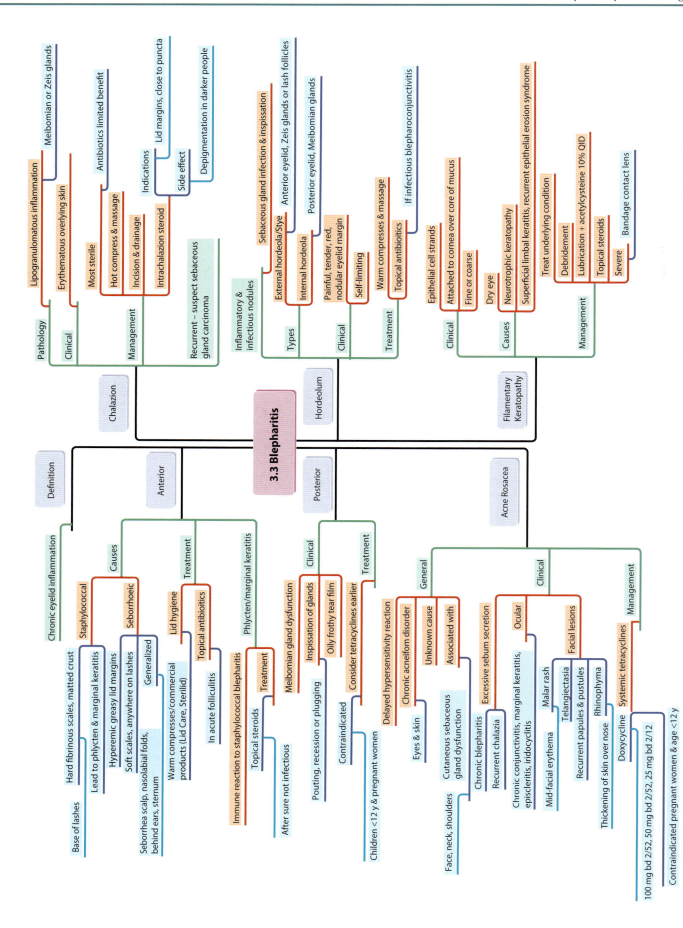

3.3 Blepharitis

Chalazion

Pathology
- Lipogranulomatous inflammation — Meibomian or Zeis glands

Clinical
- Erythematous overlying skin

Management
- Most sterile
- Hot compress & massage
- Incision & drainage
  - Antibiotics limited benefit
- Intrachalazion steroid
  - Indications — Lid margins, close to puncta
  - Side effect — Depigmentation in darker people
- Recurrent – suspect sebaceous gland carcinoma

Hordeolum

Inflammatory & infectious nodules
- Sebaceous gland infection & inspissation

Types
- External hordeola/Stye — Anterior eyelid, Zeis glands or lash follicles
- Internal hordeola — Posterior eyelid, Meibomian glands

Clinical
- Painful, tender, red, nodular eyelid margin
- Self-limiting

Treatment
- Warm compresses & massage
- Topical antibiotics — If infectious blepharoconjunctivitis

Filamentary Keratopathy

Clinical
- Epithelial cell strands
- Attached to cornea over core of mucus
- Fine or coarse

Causes
- Dry eye
- Neurotrophic keratopathy
- Superficial limbal keratitis, recurrent epithelial erosion syndrome

Management
- Treat underlying condition
- Debridement
- Lubrication + acetylcysteine 10% QID
- Topical steroids
- Severe — Bandage contact lens

Definition
- Chronic eyelid inflammation

Anterior

Causes
- Staphylococcal
  - Base of lashes
  - Hard fibrinous scales, matted crust
  - Lead to phlycten & marginal keratitis
  - Hyperemic greasy lid margins
- Seborrhoeic
  - Soft scales, anywhere on lashes
  - Generalized
  - Seborrhea scalp, nasolabial folds, behind ears, sternum

Treatment
- Lid hygiene
  - Warm compresses/commercial products (Lid Care, Sterilid)
- Topical antibiotics
  - In acute folliculitis
- Phlycten/marginal keratitis
  - Immune reaction to staphylococcal blepharitis
  - Treatment
    - Topical steroids
    - After sure not infectious

Posterior

Clinical
- Meibomian gland dysfunction
- Inspissation of glands
  - Pouting, recession or plugging
- Oily frothy tear film

Treatment
- Consider tetracyclines earlier
  - Contraindicated
  - Children <12 y & pregnant women

Acne Rosacea

General
- Delayed hypersensitivity reaction
- Chronic acneiform disorder
- Unknown cause
- Associated with
  - Eyes & skin
  - Cutaneous sebaceous gland dysfunction
  - Excessive sebum secretion

Clinical
- Ocular
  - Chronic blepharitis
  - Recurrent chalazia
  - Chronic conjunctivitis, marginal keratitis, episcleritis, iridocyclitis
- Facial lesions
  - Malar rash
  - Mid-facial erythema
  - Telangiectasia
  - Recurrent papules & pustules
  - Rhinophyma
  - Thickening of skin over nose

Management
- Systemic tetracyclines
  - Doxycycline
  - 100 mg bd 2/52, 50 mg bd 2/52, 25 mg bd 2/12
  - Contraindicated pregnant women & age <12 y
- Face, neck, shoulders

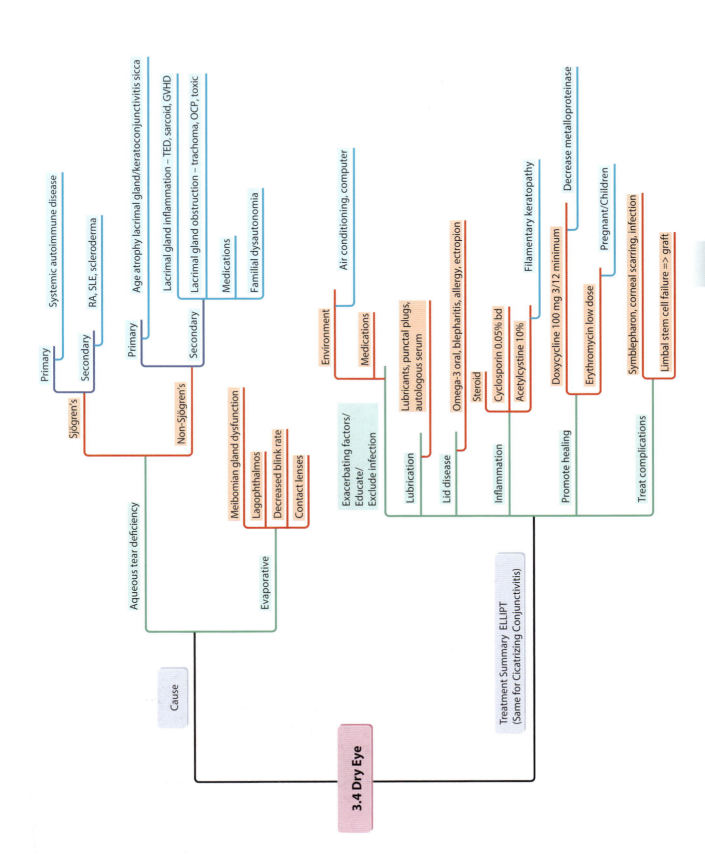

3.4 Dry Eye

Cause

Aqueous tear deficiency
- Sjögren's
  - Primary
  - Secondary
    - Systemic autoimmune disease
    - RA, SLE, scleroderma
- Non-Sjögren's
  - Primary
    - Age atrophy lacrimal gland/keratoconjunctivitis sicca
  - Secondary
    - Lacrimal gland inflammation – TED, sarcoid, GVHD
    - Lacrimal gland obstruction – trachoma, OCP, toxic
    - Medications
    - Familial dysautonomia

Evaporative
- Meibomian gland dysfunction
- Lagophthalmos
- Decreased blink rate
- Contact lenses

Treatment Summary ELLIPT
(Same for Cicatrizing Conjunctivitis)

- Exacerbating factors/Educate/Exclude infection
  - Environment
    - Air conditioning, computer
  - Medications
- Lubrication
  - Lubricants, punctal plugs, autologous serum
- Lid disease
  - Omega-3 oral, blepharitis, allergy, ectropion
- Inflammation
  - Steroid
  - Cyclosporin 0.05% bd
  - Acetylcystine 10%
- Promote healing
  - Doxycycline 100 mg 3/12 minimum
  - Erythromycin low dose
    - Pregnant/Children
  - Decrease metalloproteinase
    - Filamentary keratopathy
- Treat complications
  - Symblepharon, corneal scarring, infection
  - Limbal stem cell failure => graft

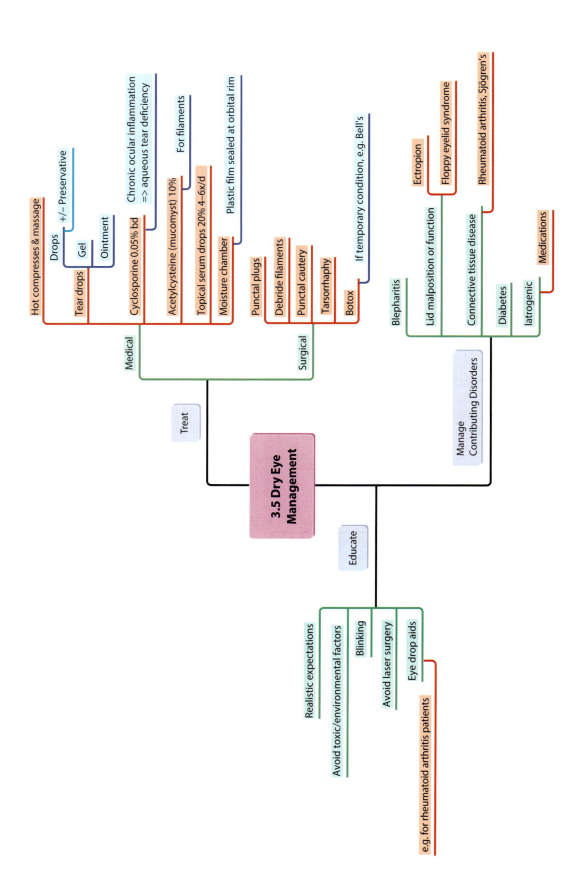

3.5 Dry Eye Management

Treat

Medical
- Hot compresses & massage
- Tear drops
  - Drops — +/– Preservative
  - Gel
  - Ointment
- Cyclosporine 0.05% bd — Chronic ocular inflammation => aqueous tear deficiency
- Acetylcysteine (mucomyst) 10% — For filaments
- Topical serum drops 20% 4–6x/d
- Moisture chamber — Plastic film sealed at orbital rim

Surgical
- Punctal plugs
- Debride filaments
- Punctal cautery
- Tarsorrhaphy
- Botox — If temporary condition, e.g. Bell's

Manage Contributing Disorders
- Blepharitis
- Lid malposition or function
  - Ectropion
  - Floppy eyelid syndrome
- Connective tissue disease — Rheumatoid arthritis, Sjögren's
- Diabetes
- Iatrogenic — Medications

Educate
- Realistic expectations
- Avoid toxic/environmental factors
- Blinking
- Avoid laser surgery
- Eye drop aids — e.g. for rheumatoid arthritis patients

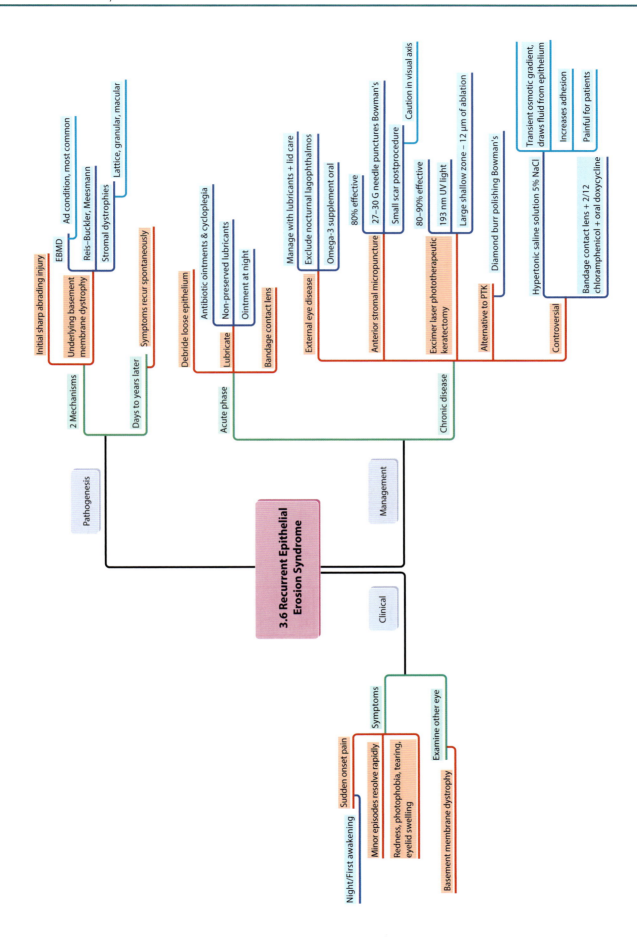

3.6 Recurrent Epithelial Erosion Syndrome

Pathogenesis

2 Mechanisms
- Initial sharp abrading injury
- Underlying basement membrane dystrophy
  - EBMD — Ad condition, most common
  - Reis–Buckler, Meessmann
  - Stromal dystrophies — Lattice, granular, macular

Days to years later
- Symptoms recur spontaneously

Management

Acute phase
- Debride loose epithelium
- Lubricate
  - Antibiotic ointments & cycloplegia
  - Non-preserved lubricants
  - Ointment at night
- Bandage contact lens

Chronic disease
- External eye disease
  - Manage with lubricants + lid care
  - Exclude nocturnal lagophthalmos
  - Omega-3 supplement oral
- Anterior stromal micropuncture
  - 80% effective
  - 27–30 G needle punctures Bowman's
  - Small scar postprocedure
  - Caution in visual axis
- Excimer laser phototherapeutic keratectomy
  - 80–90% effective
  - 193 nm UV light
  - Large shallow zone – 12 μm of ablation
- Alternative to PTK
  - Diamond burr polishing Bowman's
- Controversial
  - Hypertonic saline solution 5% NaCl
    - Transient osmotic gradient, draws fluid from epithelium
    - Increases adhesion
    - Painful for patients
  - Bandage contact lens + 2/12 chloramphenicol + oral doxycycline

Clinical

Symptoms
- Sudden onset pain
- Night/First awakening
- Minor episodes resolve rapidly
- Redness, photophobia, tearing, eyelid swelling
- Examine other eye
- Basement membrane dystrophy

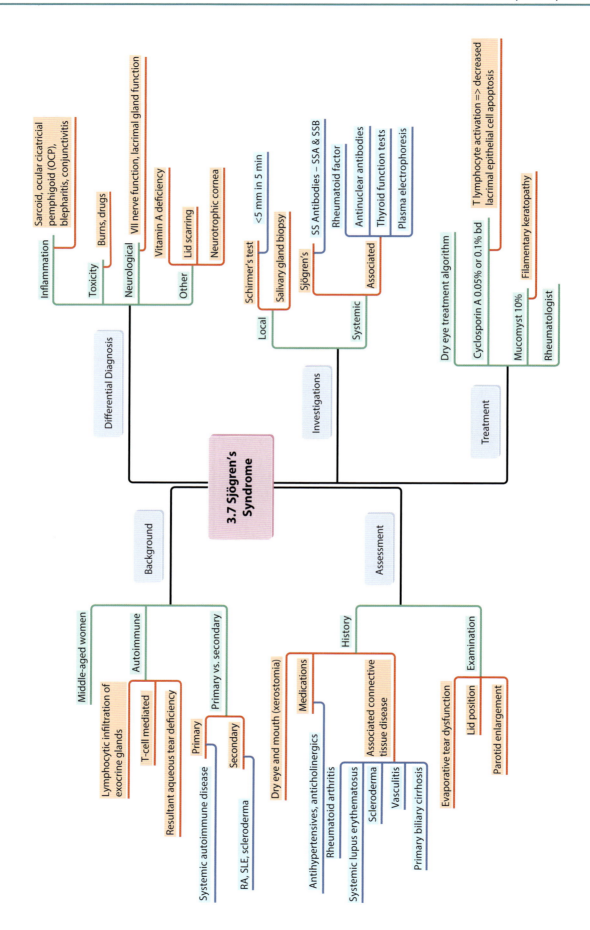

3.7 Sjögren's Syndrome

Differential Diagnosis

- Inflammation
  - Sarcoid, ocular cicatricial pemphigoid (OCP), blepharitis, conjunctivitis
- Toxicity
  - Burns, drugs
- Neurological
  - VII nerve function, lacrimal gland function
- Other
  - Vitamin A deficiency
  - Lid scarring
  - Neurotrophic cornea

Investigations

- Local
  - Schirmer's test
    - <5 mm in 5 min
  - Salivary gland biopsy
- Systemic
  - Sjögren's
    - SS Antibodies – SSA & SSB
  - Associated
    - Rheumatoid factor
    - Antinuclear antibodies
    - Thyroid function tests
    - Plasma electrophoresis

Treatment

- Dry eye treatment algorithm
- Cyclosporin A 0.05% or 0.1% bd
  - T lymphocyte activation => decreased lacrimal epithelial cell apoptosis
- Mucomyst 10%
  - Filamentary keratopathy
- Rheumatologist

Background

- Middle-aged women
- Autoimmune
  - Lymphocytic infiltration of exocrine glands
  - T-cell mediated
  - Resultant aqueous tear deficiency
- Primary vs. secondary
  - Primary
    - Systemic autoimmune disease
  - Secondary
    - RA, SLE, scleroderma

Assessment

- History
  - Dry eye and mouth (xerostomia)
  - Medications
    - Antihypertensives, anticholinergics
  - Associated connective tissue disease
    - Rheumatoid arthritis
    - Systemic lupus erythematosus
    - Scleroderma
    - Vasculitis
    - Primary biliary cirrhosis
- Examination
  - Evaporative tear dysfunction
  - Lid position
  - Parotid enlargement

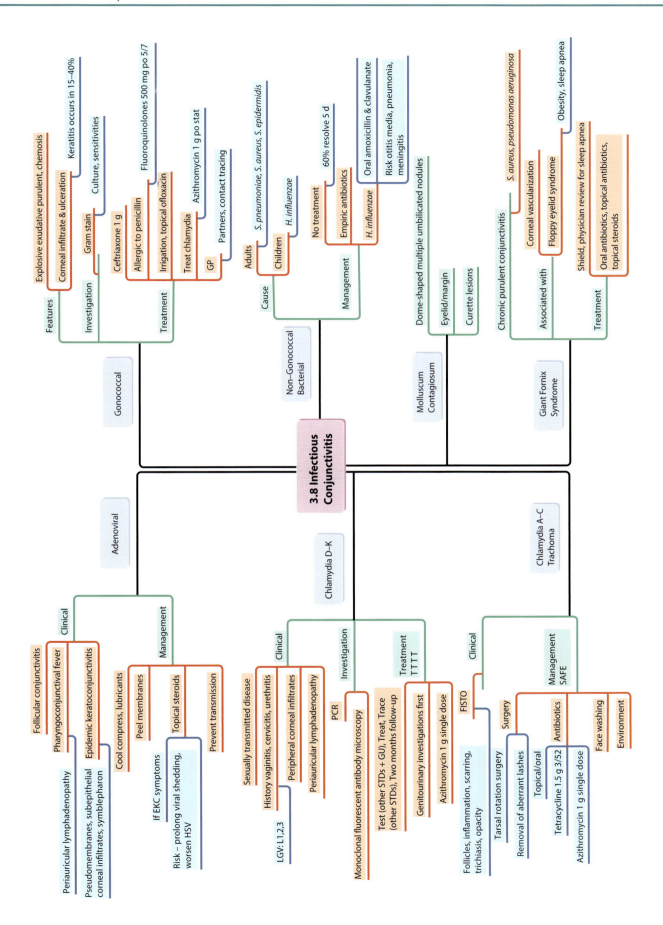

3.8 Infectious Conjunctivitis

Gonococcal

Features
- Explosive exudative purulent, chemosis
- Corneal infiltrate & ulceration
- Keratitis occurs in 15–40%

Investigation
- Gram stain
- Culture, sensitivities

Treatment
- Ceftriaxone 1 g
- Allergic to penicillin
- Irrigation, topical ofloxacin
- Fluoroquinolones 500 mg po 5/7
- Treat chlamydia
- Azithromycin 1 g po stat
- GP
- Partners, contact tracing

Non–Gonococcal Bacterial

Cause
- Adults – S. pneumoniae, S. aureus, S. epidermidis
- Children – H. influenzae

Management
- No treatment – 60% resolve 5 d
- Empiric antibiotics
  - H. influenzae
  - Oral amoxicillin & clavulanate
  - Risk otitis media, pneumonia, meningitis

Molluscum Contagiosum

- Dome-shaped multiple umbilicated nodules
- Eyelid/margin
- Curette lesions

Giant Fornix Syndrome

- Chronic purulent conjunctivitis
- S. aureus, pseudomonas aeruginosa

Associated with
- Corneal vascularization
- Floppy eyelid syndrome
- Obesity, sleep apnea

Treatment
- Shield, physician review for sleep apnea
- Oral antibiotics, topical antibiotics, topical steroids

Adenoviral

Clinical
- Follicular conjunctivitis
- Pharyngoconjunctival fever
  - Periauricular lymphadenopathy
- Epidemic keratoconjunctivitis
  - Pseudomembranes, subepithelial corneal infiltrates, symblepharon

Management
- Cool compress, lubricants
- Peel membranes
- Topical steroids
  - If EKC symptoms
  - Risk – prolong viral shedding, worsen HSV
- Prevent transmission

Chlamydia D–K

Clinical
- Sexually transmitted disease
- History vaginitis, cervicitis, urethritis
- Peripheral corneal infiltrates
- Periauricular lymphadenopathy
  - LGV: L1,2,3

Investigation
- PCR
- Monoclonal fluorescent antibody microscopy

Treatment
TTTT
- Test (other STDs + GU), Treat, Trace (other STDs), Two months follow-up
- Genitourinary investigations first
- Azithromycin 1 g single dose

Chlamydia A–C Trachoma

Clinical
FISTO
- Follicles, inflammation, scarring, trichiasis, opacity

Management
SAFE
- Surgery
  - Tarsal rotation surgery
  - Removal of aberrant lashes
- Antibiotics
  - Topical/oral
  - Tetracycline 1.5 g 3/52
  - Azithromycin 1 g single dose
- Face washing
- Environment

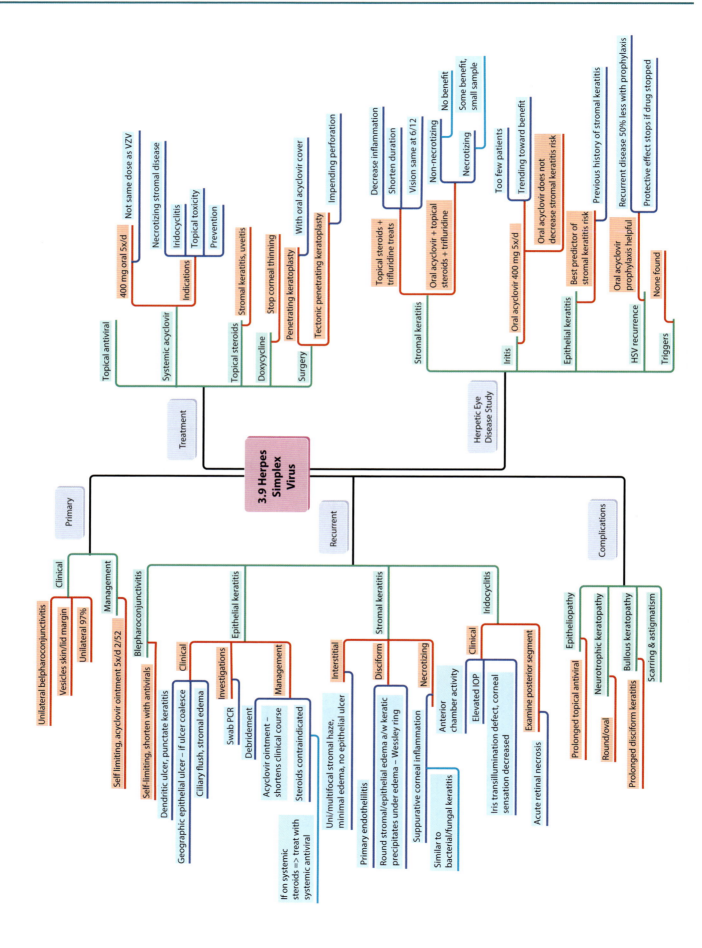

3.9 Herpes Simplex Virus

Treatment

Topical antiviral

Systemic acyclovir
- 400 mg oral 5x/d — Not same dose as VZV
- Indications
  - Necrotizing stromal disease
  - Iridocyclitis
  - Topical toxicity
  - Prevention

Topical steroids — Stromal keratitis, uveitis

Doxycycline — Stop corneal thinning

Penetrating keratoplasty — With oral acyclovir cover

Surgery — Tectonic penetrating keratoplasty — Impending perforation

Herpetic Eye Disease Study

Stromal keratitis
- Topical steroids + trifluridine treats
  - Decrease inflammation
  - Shorten duration
  - Vision same at 6/12
- Oral acyclovir + topical steroids + trifluridine
  - Non-necrotizing — No benefit
  - Necrotizing — Some benefit, small sample

Iritis — Oral acyclovir 400 mg 5x/d
- Too few patients
- Trending toward benefit

Epithelial keratitis — Oral acyclovir does not decrease stromal keratitis risk
- Best predictor of stromal keratitis risk — Previous history of stromal keratitis

HSV recurrence — Oral acyclovir prophylaxis helpful
- Recurrent disease 50% less with prophylaxis
- Protective effect stops if drug stopped

Triggers — None found

Primary

Clinical
- Unilateral belpharoconjunctivitis
- Vesicles skin/lid margin
- Unilateral 97%

Management — Self limiting, acyclovir ointment 5x/d 2/52

Recurrent

Blepharoconjunctivitis — Self-limiting, shorten with antivirals

Epithelial Keratitis
- Clinical
  - Dendritic ulcer, punctate keratitis
  - Geographic epithelial ulcer – if ulcer coalesce
  - Ciliary flush, stromal edema
- Investigations — Swab PCR
- Management
  - Debridement
  - Acyclovir ointment – shortens clinical course
  - Steroids contraindicated
    - If on systemic steroids => treat with systemic antiviral

Stromal keratitis
- Interstitial
  - Uni/multifocal stromal haze, minimal edema, no epithelial ulcer
  - Primary endotheliitis
- Disciform — Round stromal/epithelial edema a/w keratic precipitates under edema – Wessley ring
- Necrotizing
  - Suppurative corneal inflammation
  - Similar to bacterial/fungal keratitis

Iridocyclitis
- Clinical
  - Anterior chamber activity
  - Elevated IOP
  - Iris transillumination defect, corneal sensation decreased
  - Examine posterior segment — Acute retinal necrosis

Complications

- Epitheliopathy — Prolonged topical antiviral
- Neurotrophic keratopathy — Round/oval
- Bullous keratopathy — Prolonged disciform keratitis
- Scarring & astigmatism

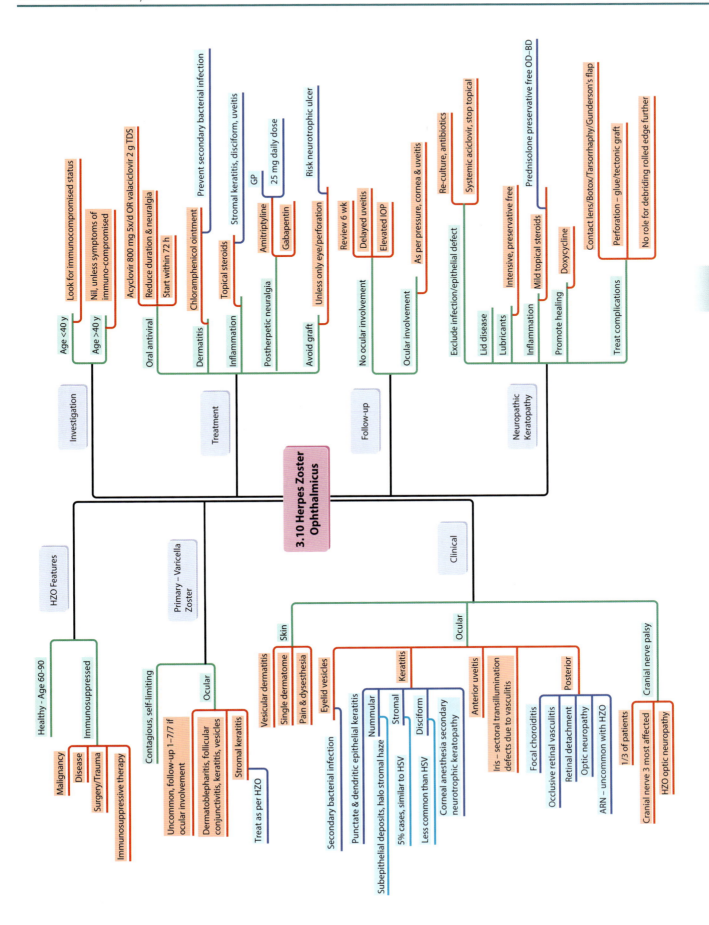

3.10 Herpes Zoster Ophthalmicus

Investigation
- Age <40 y
  - Look for immunocompromised status
- Age >40 y
  - Nil, unless symptoms of immuno-compromised

Treatment
- Oral antiviral
  - Acyclovir 800 mg 5x/d OR valaciclovir 2 g TDS
  - Reduce duration & neuralgia
  - Start within 72 h
- Dermatitis
  - Chloramphenicol ointment
  - Prevent secondary bacterial infection
- Inflammation
  - Topical steroids
  - Stromal keratitis, disciform, uveitis
- Postherpetic neuralgia
  - Amitriptyline
  - Gabapentin
    - GP
    - 25 mg daily dose
- Avoid graft
  - Unless only eye/perforation
  - Risk neurotrophic ulcer

Follow-up
- No ocular involvement
  - Review 6 wk
- Ocular involvement
  - Delayed uveitis
  - Elevated IOP
  - As per pressure, cornea & uveitis

Neuropathic Keratopathy
- Exclude infection/epithelial defect
  - Re-culture, antibiotics
  - Systemic aciclovir, stop topical
- Lid disease
- Lubricants
  - Intensive, preservative free
- Inflammation
  - Mild topical steroids
  - Prednisolone preservative free OD–BD
- Promote healing
  - Doxycycline
- Treat complications
  - Contact lens/Botox/Tarsorrhaphy/Gunderson's flap
  - Perforation – glue/tectonic graft
  - No role for debriding rolled edge further

HZO Features
- Healthy – Age 60–90
- Immunosuppressed
  - Malignancy
  - Disease
  - Surgery/Trauma
  - Immunosuppressive therapy

Primary – Varicella Zoster
- Contagious, self-limiting
- Ocular
  - Uncommon, follow-up 1–7/7 if ocular involvement
  - Dermatoblepharitis, follicular conjunctivitis, keratitis, vesicles
  - Stromal keratitis
    - Treat as per HZO

Clinical
- Skin
  - Vesicular dermatitis
  - Single dermatome
  - Pain & dysesthesia
- Ocular
  - Eyelid vesicles
    - Secondary bacterial infection
  - Keratitis
    - Punctate & dendritic epithelial keratitis
    - Nummular
      - Subepithelial deposits, halo stromal haze
    - Stromal
      - 5% cases, similar to HSV
    - Disciform
      - Less common than HSV
    - Corneal anesthesia secondary neurotrophic keratopathy
  - Anterior uveitis
    - Iris – sectoral transillumination defects due to vasculitis
  - Posterior
    - Focal choroiditis
    - Occlusive retinal vasculitis
    - Retinal detachment
    - Optic neuropathy
    - ARN – uncommon with HZO
  - Cranial nerve palsy
    - 1/3 of patients
    - Cranial nerve 3 most affected
    - HZO optic neuropathy

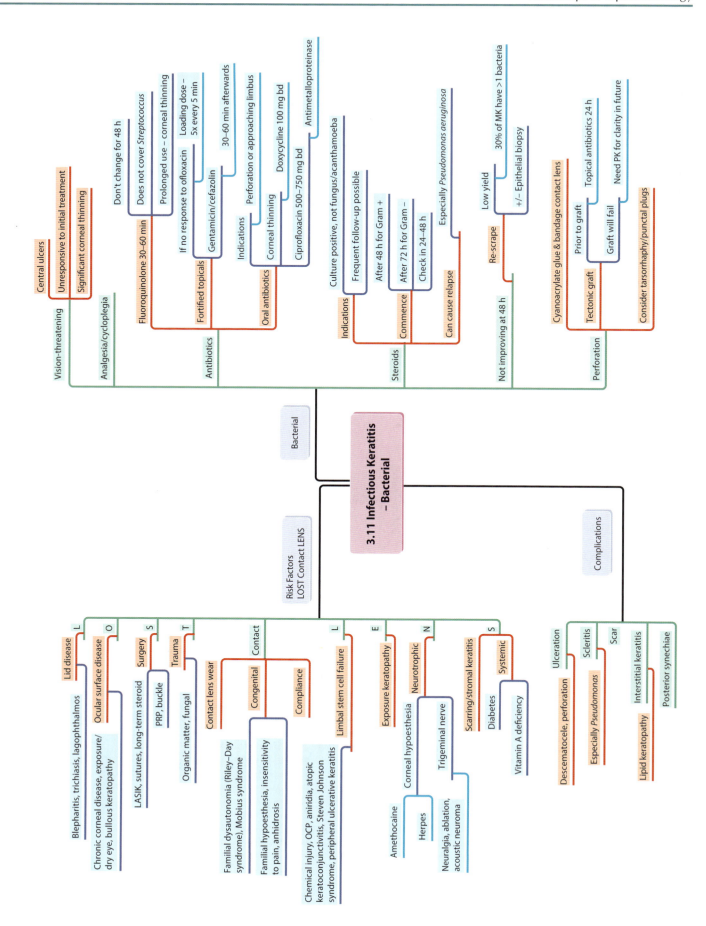

3.11 Infectious Keratitis – Bacterial

Bacterial

Vision-threatening
- Central ulcers
- Unresponsive to initial treatment
- Significant corneal thinning

Analgesia/cycloplegia

Antibiotics
- Fluoroquinolone 30–60 min
  - Don't change for 48 h
  - Does not cover *Streptococcus*
  - Prolonged use – corneal thinning
- Fortified topicals
  - If no response to ofloxacin
    - Loading dose – 5x every 5 min
    - 30–60 min afterwards
  - Gentamicin/cefazolin
- Oral antibiotics
  - Indications
    - Perforation or approaching limbus
  - Corneal thinning
    - Doxycycline 100 mg bd
  - Ciprofloxacin 500–750 mg bd
  - Antimetalloproteinase

Steroids
- Indications
  - Culture positive, not fungus/acanthamoeba
  - Frequent follow-up possible
- Commence
  - After 48 h for Gram +
  - After 72 h for Gram –
  - Check in 24–48 h
- Can cause relapse
  - Especially *Pseudomonas aeruginosa*

Not improving at 48 h
- Re-scrape
  - Low yield
  - 30% of MK have >1 bacteria
  - +/– Epithelial biopsy

Perforation
- Cyanoacrylate glue & bandage contact lens
- Tectonic graft
  - Prior to graft
    - Topical antibiotics 24 h
  - Graft will fail
    - Need PK for clarity in future
- Consider tarsorrhaphy/punctal plugs

Risk Factors
LOST Contact LENS

L – Lid disease
- Blepharitis, trichiasis, lagophthalmos

O – Ocular surface disease
- Chronic corneal disease, exposure/dry eye, bullous keratopathy

S – Surgery
- LASIK, sutures, long-term steroid
- PRP, buckle

T – Trauma
- Organic matter, fungal

Contact – Contact lens wear
- Congenital
  - Familial dysautonomia (Riley–Day syndrome), Mobius syndrome
  - Familial hypoesthesia, insensitivity to pain, anhidrosis
- Compliance

L – Limbal stem cell failure
- Chemical injury, OCP, aniridia, atopic keratoconjunctivitis, Steven Johnson syndrome, peripheral ulcerative keratitis

E – Exposure keratopathy

N – Neurotrophic
- Corneal hypoesthesia
  - Amethocaine
  - Herpes
- Trigeminal nerve
  - Neuralgia, ablation, acoustic neuroma

S – Scarring/stromal keratitis
- Systemic
  - Diabetes
  - Vitamin A deficiency

Complications
- Ulceration
  - Descematocele, perforation
  - Especially *Pseudomonas*
- Scleritis
- Scar
  - Lipid keratopathy
  - Interstitial keratitis
  - Posterior synechiae

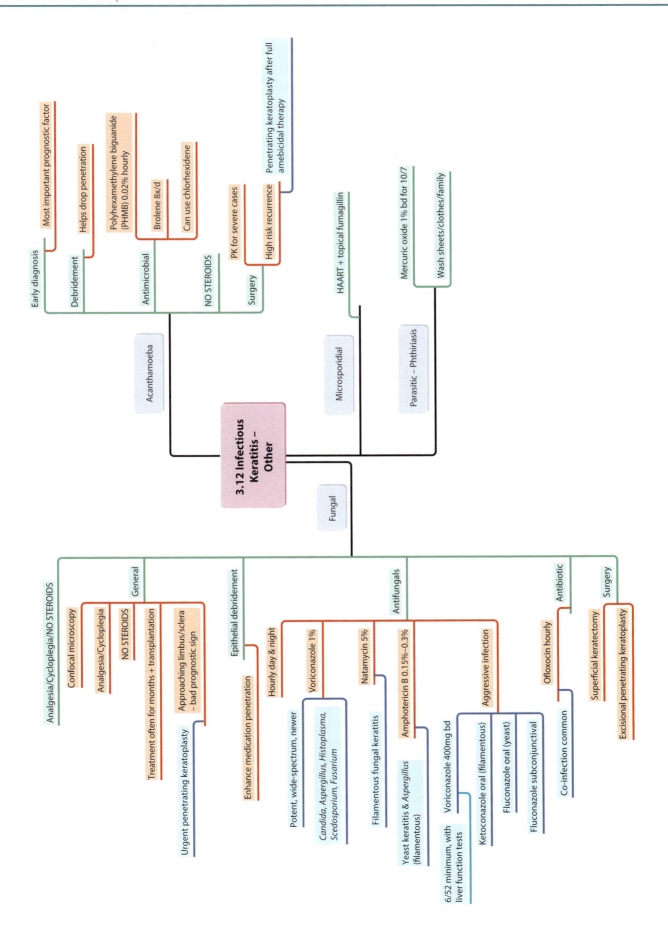

3.12 Infectious Keratitis – Other

Acanthamoeba

- Early diagnosis
  - Most important prognostic factor
- Debridement
  - Helps drop penetration
- Antimicrobial
  - Polyhexamethylene biguanide (PHMB) 0.02% hourly
  - Brolene 8x/d
  - Can use chlorhexidene
- NO STEROIDS
- Surgery
  - PK for severe cases
  - High risk recurrence
    - Penetrating keratoplasty after full amebicidal therapy

Microsporidial

- HAART + topical fumagillin

Parasitic – Phthiriasis

- Mercuric oxide 1% bd for 10/7
- Wash sheets/clothes/family

Fungal

- General
  - Analgesia/Cycloplegia/NO STEROIDS
  - Confocal microscopy
  - Analgesia/Cycloplegia
  - NO STEROIDS
  - Treatment often for months + transplantation
    - Urgent penetrating keratoplasty
  - Approaching limbus/sclera – bad prognostic sign
- Epithelial debridement
  - Enhance medication penetration
- Antifungals
  - Hourly day & night
  - Voriconazole 1%
    - Potent, wide-spectrum, newer
    - Candida, Aspergillus, Histoplasma, Scedosporium, Fusarium
  - Natamycin 5%
    - Filamentous fungal keratitis
  - Amphotericin B 0.15%–0.3%
    - Yeast keratitis & Aspergillus (filamentous)
  - Voriconazole 400mg bd
    - 6/52 minimum, with liver function tests
  - Aggressive infection
    - Ketoconazole oral (filamentous)
    - Fluconazole oral (yeast)
    - Fluconazole subconjunctival
- Antibiotic
  - Ofloxocin hourly
    - Co-infection common
- Surgery
  - Superficial keratectomy
  - Excisional penetrating keratoplasty

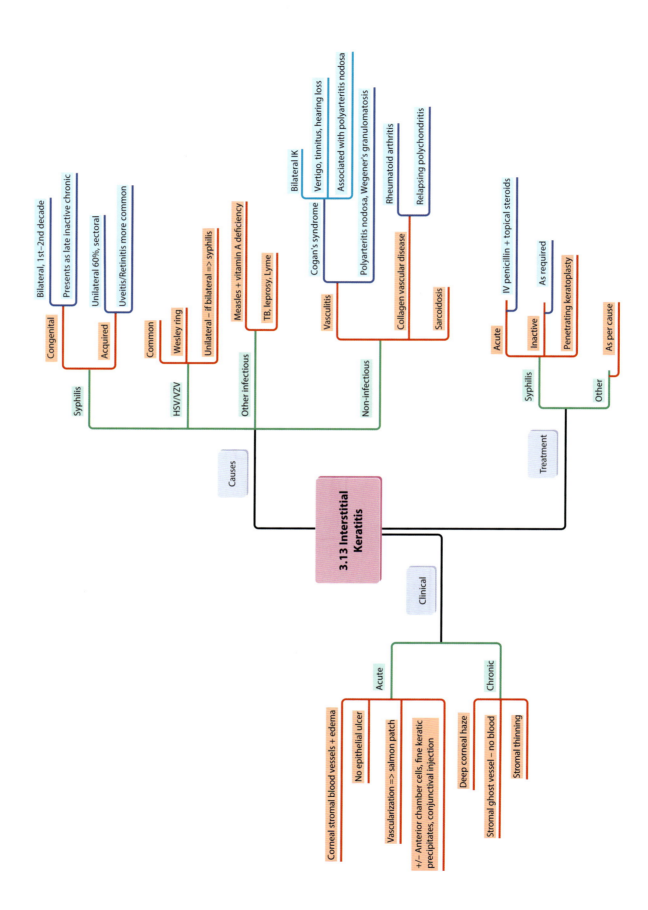

3.13 Interstitial Keratitis

Causes

Syphilis
- Congenital
  - Bilateral, 1st–2nd decade
  - Presents as late inactive chronic
- Acquired
  - Unilateral 60%, sectoral
  - Uveitis/Retinitis more common

HSV/VZV
- Common
- Wesley ring
- Unilateral – if bilateral => syphilis

Other infectious
- Measles + vitamin A deficiency
- TB, leprosy, Lyme

Non-infectious
- Vasculitis
  - Cogan's syndrome
    - Bilateral IK
    - Vertigo, tinnitus, hearing loss
    - Associated with polyarteritis nodosa
  - Polyarteritis nodosa, Wegener's granulomatosis
- Collagen vascular disease
  - Rheumatoid arthritis
  - Relapsing polychondritis
- Sarcoidosis

Treatment

Syphilis
- Acute
  - IV penicillin + topical steroids
- Inactive
  - As required
  - Penetrating keratoplasty

Other
- As per cause

Clinical

Acute
- Corneal stromal blood vessels + edema
- No epithelial ulcer
- Vascularization => salmon patch
- +/– Anterior chamber cells, fine keratic precipitates, conjunctival injection

Chronic
- Deep corneal haze
- Stromal ghost vessel – no blood
- Stromal thinning

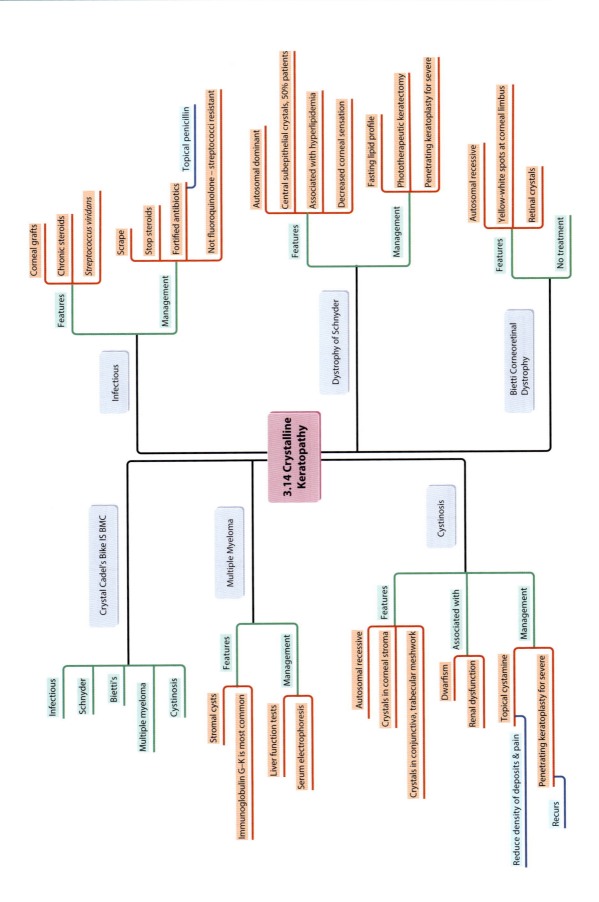

3.14 Crystalline Keratopathy

Crystal Cadel's Bike IS BMC
- Infectious
- Schnyder
- Bietti's
- Multiple myeloma
- Cystinosis

Infectious
- Features
  - Corneal grafts
  - Chronic steroids
  - *Streptococcus viridans*
- Management
  - Scrape
  - Stop steroids
  - Fortified antibiotics
    - Topical penicillin
  - Not fluoroquinolone – streptococci resistant

Dystrophy of Schnyder
- Features
  - Autosomal dominant
  - Central subepithelial crystals, 50% patients
  - Associated with hyperlipidemia
  - Decreased corneal sensation
- Management
  - Fasting lipid profile
  - Phototherapeutic keratectomy
  - Penetrating keratoplasty for severe

Bietti Corneoretinal Dystrophy
- Features
  - Autosomal recessive
  - Yellow-white spots at corneal limbus
  - Retinal crystals
- No treatment

Multiple Myeloma
- Features
  - Stromal cysts
  - Immunoglobulin G–K is most common
- Management
  - Liver function tests
  - Serum electrophoresis

Cystinosis
- Features
  - Autosomal recessive
  - Crystals in corneal stroma
  - Crystals in conjunctiva, trabecular meshwork
- Associated with
  - Dwarfism
  - Renal dysfunction
- Management
  - Topical cystamine
    - Reduce density of deposits & pain
    - Recurs
  - Penetrating keratoplasty for severe

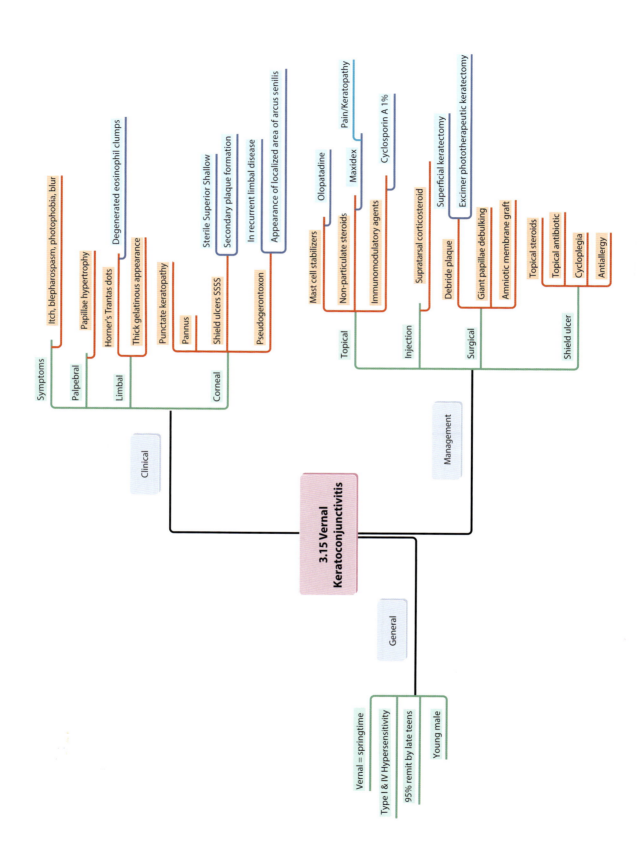

3.15 Vernal Keratoconjunctivitis

Clinical

- **Symptoms**
  - Itch, blepharospasm, photophobia, blur
- **Palpebral**
  - Papillae hypertrophy
  - Horner's Trantas dots
  - Thick gelatinous appearance — Degenerated eosinophil clumps
- **Limbal**
  - Punctate keratopathy
- **Corneal**
  - Pannus
  - Shield ulcers SSSS
    - Sterile Superior Shallow
    - Secondary plaque formation
  - Pseudogerontoxon
    - In recurrent limbal disease
    - Appearance of localized area of arcus senilis

Management

- **Topical**
  - Mast cell stabilizers — Olopatadine
  - Non-particulate steroids — Maxidex — Pain/Keratopathy
  - Immunomodulatory agents — Cyclosporin A 1%
- **Injection**
  - Supratarsal corticosteroid
- **Surgical**
  - Debride plaque
    - Superficial keratectomy
    - Excimer phototherapeutic keratectomy
  - Giant papillae debulking
  - Amniotic membrane graft
- **Shield ulcer**
  - Topical steroids
  - Topical antibiotic
  - Cycloplegia
  - Antiallergy

General

- Vernal = springtime
- Type I & IV Hypersensitivity
- 95% remit by late teens
- Young male

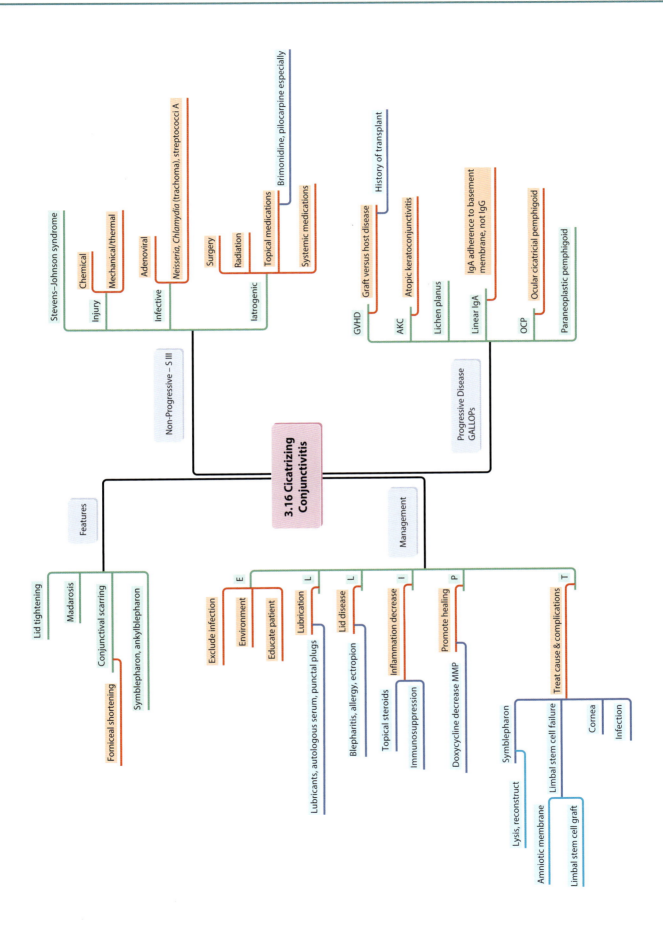

3.16 Cicatrizing Conjunctivitis

Non-Progressive – S III

- Stevens–Johnson syndrome
- Injury
  - Chemical
  - Mechanical/thermal
- Infective
  - Adenoviral
  - Neisseria, Chlamydia (trachoma), streptococci A
- Iatrogenic
  - Surgery
  - Radiation
  - Topical medications
    - Brimonidine, pilocarpine especially
  - Systemic medications

Progressive Disease GALLOPs

- GVHD
  - Graft versus host disease
    - History of transplant
- AKC
  - Atopic keratoconjunctivitis
- Lichen planus
- Linear IgA
  - IgA adherence to basement membrane, not IgG
- OCP
  - Ocular cicatricial pemphigoid
- Paraneoplastic pemphigoid

Features

- Lid tightening
- Madarosis
- Conjunctival scarring
  - Forniceal shortening
  - Symblepharon, ankylblepharon

Management

- E
  - Exclude infection
  - Environment
  - Educate patient
- L
  - Lubrication
    - Lubricants, autologous serum, punctal plugs
- L
  - Lid disease
    - Blepharitis, allergy, ectropion
- I
  - Inflammation decrease
    - Topical steroids
    - Immunosuppression
- P
  - Promote healing
    - Doxycycline decrease MMP
- T
  - Treat cause & complications
    - Symblepharon
      - Lysis, reconstruct
      - Amniotic membrane
    - Limbal stem cell failure
      - Limbal stem cell graft
    - Cornea
    - Infection

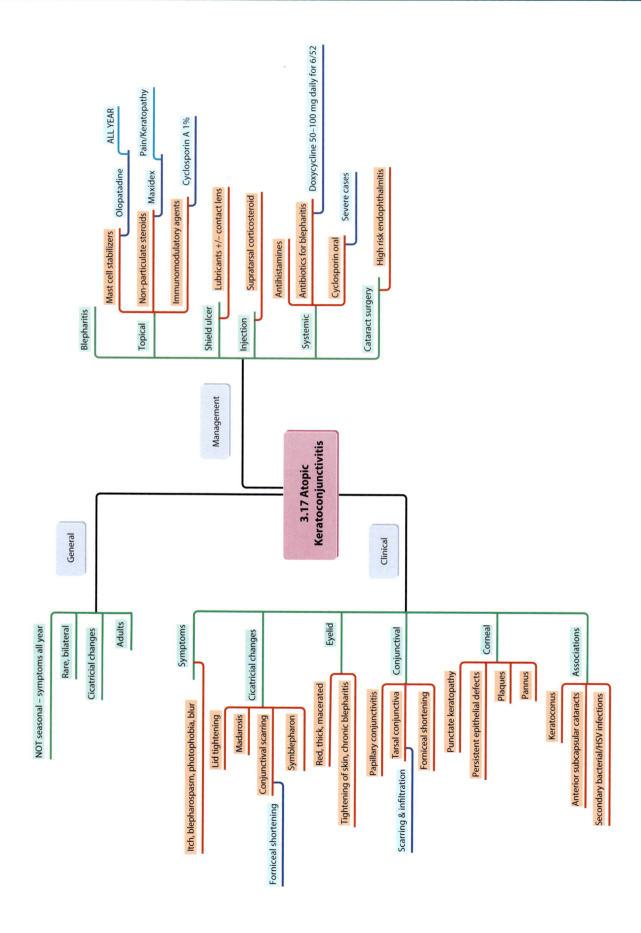

3.17 Atopic Keratoconjunctivitis

Management

Blepharitis

Topical
- Mast cell stabilizers — Olopatadine — ALL YEAR
- Non-particulate steroids — Maxidex — Pain/Keratopathy
- Immunomodulatory agents — Cyclosporin A 1%

Shield ulcer
- Lubricants +/− contact lens

Injection
- Supratarsal corticosteroid

Systemic
- Antihistamines
- Antibiotics for blepharitis — Doxycycline 50–100 mg daily for 6/52
- Cyclosporin oral — Severe cases

Cataract surgery
- High risk endophthalmitis

General
- NOT seasonal – symptoms all year
- Rare, bilateral
- Cicatricial changes
- Adults

Clinical

Symptoms
- Itch, blepharospasm, photophobia, blur

Cicatricial changes
- Lid tightening
- Madarosis
- Conjunctival scarring
- Symblepharon — Forniceal shortening

Eyelid
- Red, thick, macerated
- Tightening of skin, chronic blepharitis

Conjunctival
- Papillary conjunctivitis
- Tarsal conjunctiva — Scarring & infiltration
- Forniceal shortening

Corneal
- Punctate keratopathy
- Persistent epithelial defects
- Plaques
- Pannus

Associations
- Keratoconus
- Anterior subcapsular cataracts
- Secondary bacterial/HSV infections

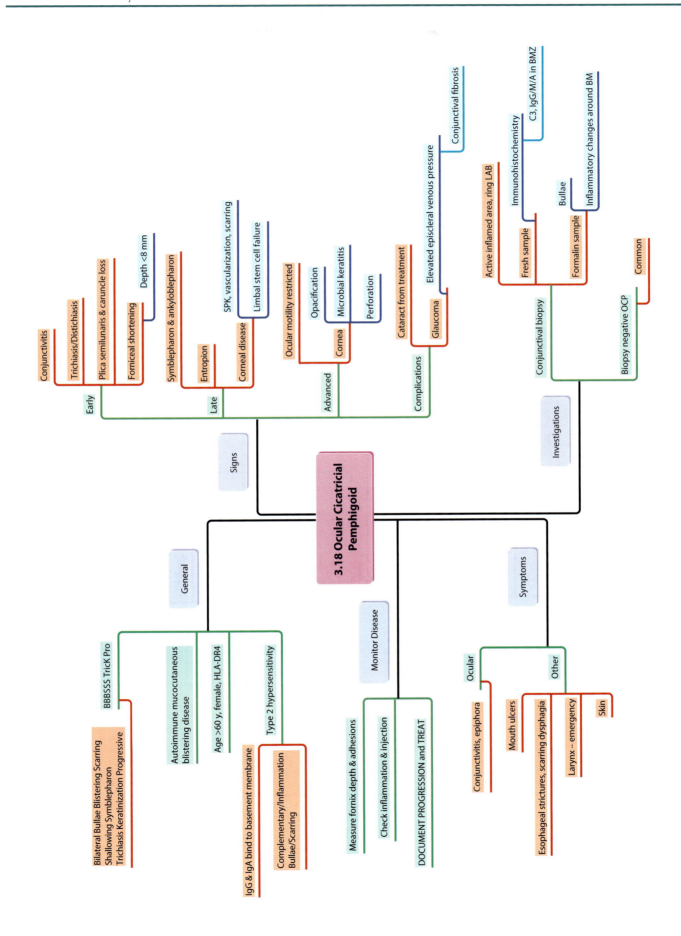

3.18 Ocular Cicatricial Pemphigoid

General

- BBBSSS TricK Pro
  - Bilateral Bullae Blistering Scarring Shallowing Symblepharon Trichiasis Keratinization Progressive
- Autoimmune mucocutaneous blistering disease
- Age >60 y, female, HLA-DR4
- Type 2 hypersensitivity
  - IgG & IgA bind to basement membrane
  - Complementary/Inflammation Bullae/Scarring

Monitor Disease

- Measure fornix depth & adhesions
- Check inflammation & injection
- DOCUMENT PROGRESSION and TREAT

Symptoms

- Ocular
  - Conjunctivitis, epiphora
- Other
  - Mouth ulcers
  - Esophageal strictures, scarring dysphagia
  - Larynx – emergency
  - Skin

Signs

- Early
  - Conjunctivitis
  - Trichiasis/Distichiasis
  - Plica semilunaris & caruncle loss
  - Forniceal shortening
    - Depth <8 mm
- Late
  - Symblepharon & ankyloblepharon
  - Entropion
  - Corneal disease
    - SPK, vascularization, scarring
    - Limbal stem cell failure
- Advanced
  - Ocular motility restricted
  - Cornea
    - Opacification
    - Microbial keratitis
    - Perforation
- Complications
  - Cataract from treatment
  - Glaucoma
    - Elevated episcleral venous pressure
  - Conjunctival fibrosis

Investigations

- Conjunctival biopsy
  - Active inflamed area, ring LAB
  - Fresh sample
    - Immunohistochemistry
      - C3, IgG/M/A in BMZ
  - Formalin sample
    - Bullae
    - Inflammatory changes around BM
- Biopsy negative OCP
  - Common

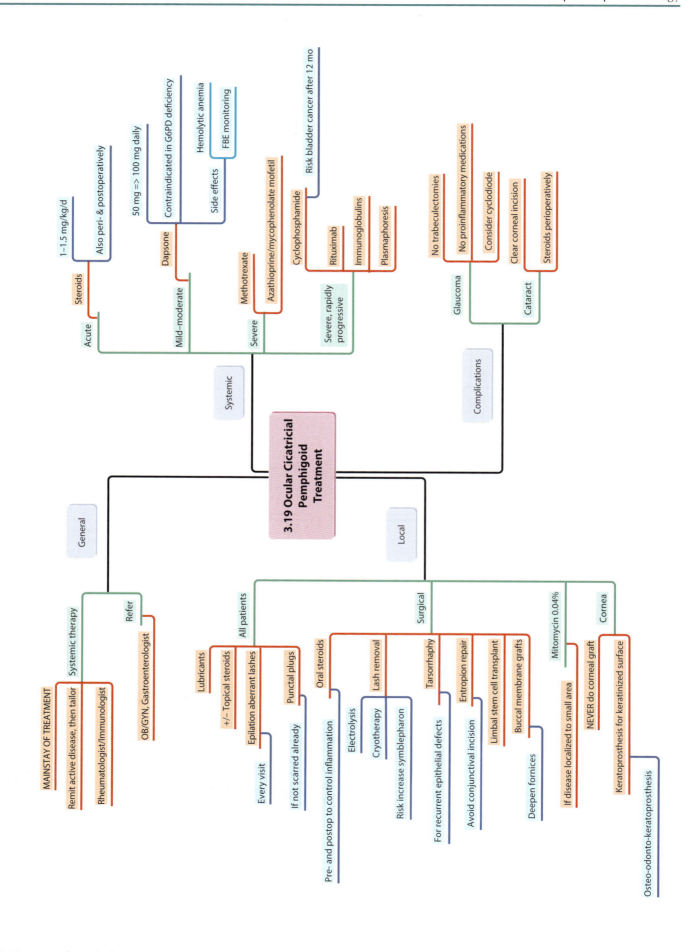

3.19 Ocular Cicatricial Pemphigoid Treatment

Systemic

- Acute
  - Steroids
    - 1–1.5 mg/kg/d
    - Also peri- & postoperatively
- Mild–moderate
  - Dapsone
    - 50 mg => 100 mg daily
    - Contraindicated in G6PD deficiency
    - Side effects
      - Hemolytic anemia
      - FBE monitoring
- Severe
  - Methotrexate
  - Azathioprine/mycophenolate mofetil
- Severe, rapidly progressive
  - Cyclophosphamide
    - Risk bladder cancer after 12 mo
  - Rituximab
  - Immunoglobulins
  - Plasmaphoresis

Complications

- Glaucoma
  - No trabeculectomies
  - No proinflammatory medications
  - Consider cyclodiode
- Cataract
  - Clear corneal incision
  - Steroids perioperatively

General

- Systemic therapy
  - MAINSTAY OF TREATMENT
  - Remit active disease, then tailor
- Refer
  - Rheumatologist/Immunologist
  - OB/GYN, Gastroenterologist

Local

- All patients
  - Lubricants
  - +/− Topical steroids
  - Epilation aberrant lashes
    - Every visit
  - Punctal plugs
    - If not scarred already
  - Oral steroids
    - Pre- and postop to control inflammation
- Surgical
  - Lash removal
    - Electrolysis
    - Cryotherapy
  - Tarsorrhaphy
    - Risk increase symblepharon
  - Entropion repair
    - For recurrent epithelial defects
  - Limbal stem cell transplant
    - Avoid conjunctival incision
  - Buccal membrane grafts
    - Deepen fornices
  - Mitomycin 0.04%
    - If disease localized to small area
- Cornea
  - NEVER do corneal graft
  - Keratoprosthesis for keratinized surface
    - Osteo-odonto-keratoprosthesis

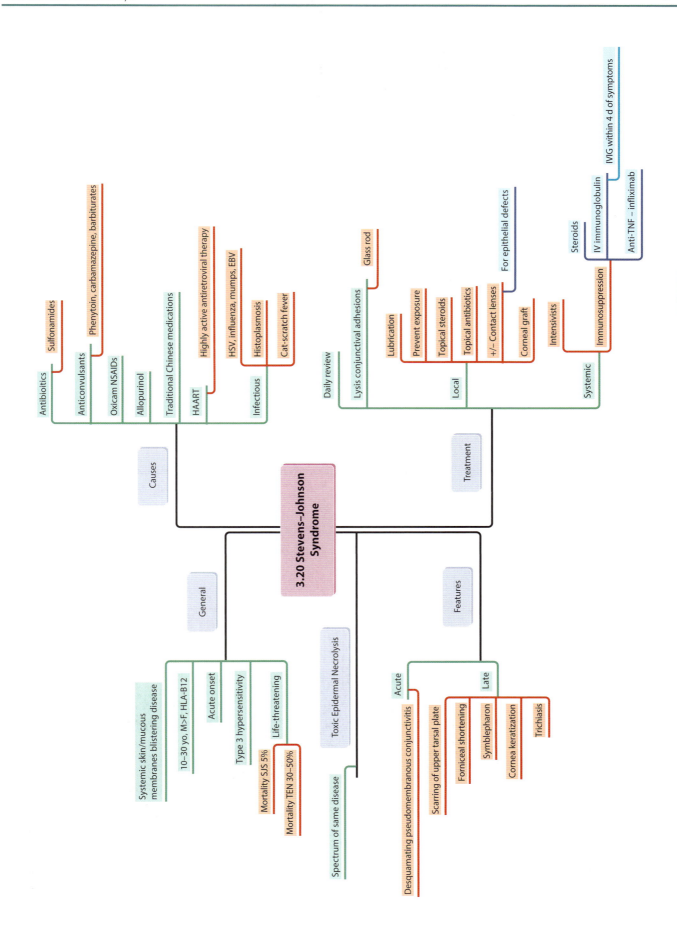

3.20 Stevens–Johnson Syndrome

Causes

Antibiotics
- Sulfonamides

Anticonvulsants
- Phenytoin, carbamazepine, barbiturates

Oxicam NSAIDs

Allopurinol

Traditional Chinese medications

HAART
- Highly active antiretroviral therapy

Infectious
- HSV, influenza, mumps, EBV
- Histoplasmosis
- Cat-scratch fever

Treatment

Daily review

Lysis conjunctival adhesions
- Glass rod

Local
- Lubrication
- Prevent exposure
- Topical steroids
- Topical antibiotics
- +/− Contact lenses
  - For epithelial defects
- Corneal graft

Systemic
- Intensivists
- Immunosuppression
  - Steroids
  - IV immunoglobulin
    - IVIG within 4 d of symptoms
  - Anti-TNF – infliximab

General

Systemic skin/mucous membranes blistering disease

10–30 yo, M>F, HLA-B12

Acute onset

Type 3 hypersensitivity

Life-threatening
- Mortality SJS 5%
- Mortality TEN 30–50%

Toxic Epidermal Necrolysis
- Spectrum of same disease

Features

Acute
- Desquamating pseudomembranous conjunctivitis

Late
- Scarring of upper tarsal plate
- Forniceal shortening
- Symblepharon
- Cornea keratization
- Trichiasis

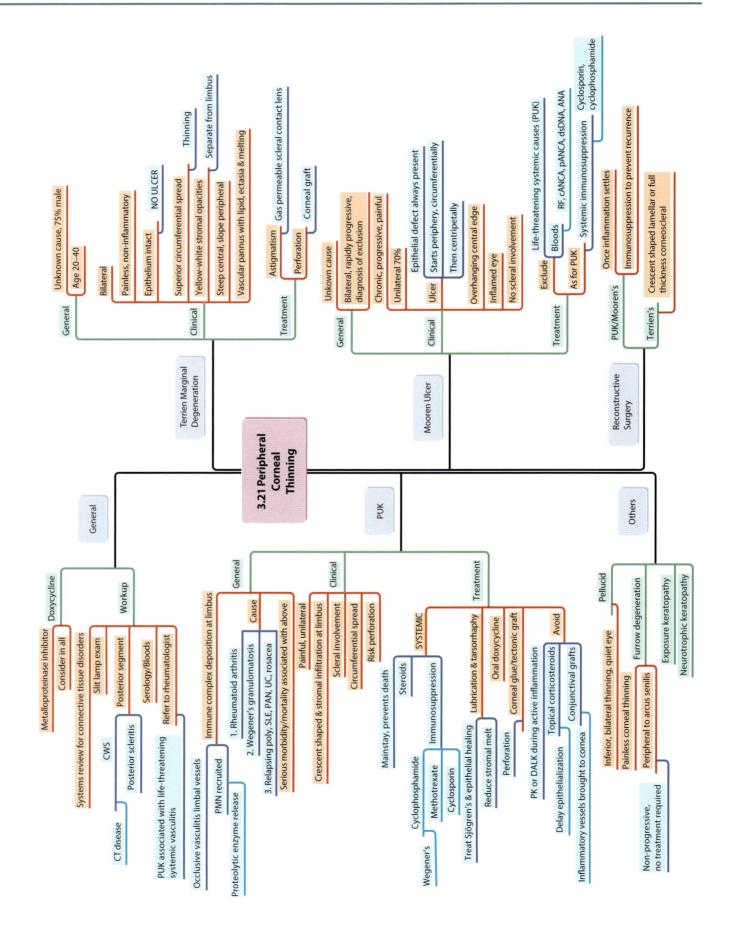

3.21 Peripheral Corneal Thinning

Terrien Marginal Degeneration

General
- Unknown cause, 75% male
- Age 20–40
- Bilateral
- Painless, non-inflammatory

Clinical
- Epithelium intact — NO ULCER
- Superior circumferential spread
  - Thinning
  - Separate from limbus
- Yellow-white stromal opacities
- Steep central, slope peripheral
- Vascular pannus with lipid, ectasia & melting

Treatment
- Astigmatism
  - Gas permeable scleral contact lens
- Perforation
  - Corneal graft

Mooren Ulcer

General
- Unknown cause
- Bilateral, rapidly progressive, diagnosis of exclusion
- Chronic, progressive, painful
- Unilateral 70%

Clinical
- Ulcer
  - Epithelial defect always present
  - Starts periphery, circumferentially
  - Then centripetally
- Overhanging central edge
- Inflamed eye
- No scleral involvement

Treatment
- Exclude
  - Life-threatening systemic causes (PUK)
- Bloods
  - RF, cANCA, pANCA, dsDNA, ANA
- As for PUK
  - Systemic immunosuppression
    - Cyclosporin, cyclophosphamide

Reconstructive Surgery

PUK/Mooren's
- Immunosuppression to prevent recurrence
- Once inflammation settles

Terrien's
- Crescent shaped lamellar or full thickness corneoscleral

General

- Doxycycline
  - Metalloproteinase inhibitor
  - Consider in all
- Systems review for connective tissue disorders
- Slit lamp exam
  - CWS
  - Posterior scleritis
- Posterior segment
- Workup
  - Serology/Bloods
  - Refer to rheumatologist
- PUK associated with life-threatening systemic vasculitis
  - CT disease
  - Occlusive vasculitis limbal vessels
  - PMN recruited
  - Proteolytic enzyme release

PUK

General
- Immune complex deposition at limbus
- Cause
  1. Rheumatoid arthritis
  2. Wegener's granulomatosis
  3. Relapsing poly, SLE, PAN, UC, rosacea
- Serious morbidity/mortality associated with above

Clinical
- Painful, unilateral
- Crescent shaped & stromal infiltration at limbus
- Scleral involvement
- Circumferential spread
- Risk perforation

Treatment
- SYSTEMIC
  - Steroids
    - Mainstay, prevents death
  - Immunosuppression
    - Cyclophosphamide — Wegener's
    - Methotrexate
    - Cyclosporin
- Lubrication & tarsorrhaphy
  - Treat Sjögren's & epithelial healing
- Oral doxycycline
  - Reduce stromal melt
- Corneal glue/tectonic graft
  - Perforation
  - PK or DALK during active inflammation
- Avoid
  - Topical corticosteroids
    - Delay epithelialization
  - Conjunctival grafts
    - Inflammatory vessels brought to cornea

Others

- Pellucid
  - Inferior, bilateral thinning, quiet eye
- Furrow degeneration
  - Painless corneal thinning
  - Peripheral to arcus senilis
  - Non-progressive, no treatment required
- Exposure keratopathy
- Neurotrophic keratopathy

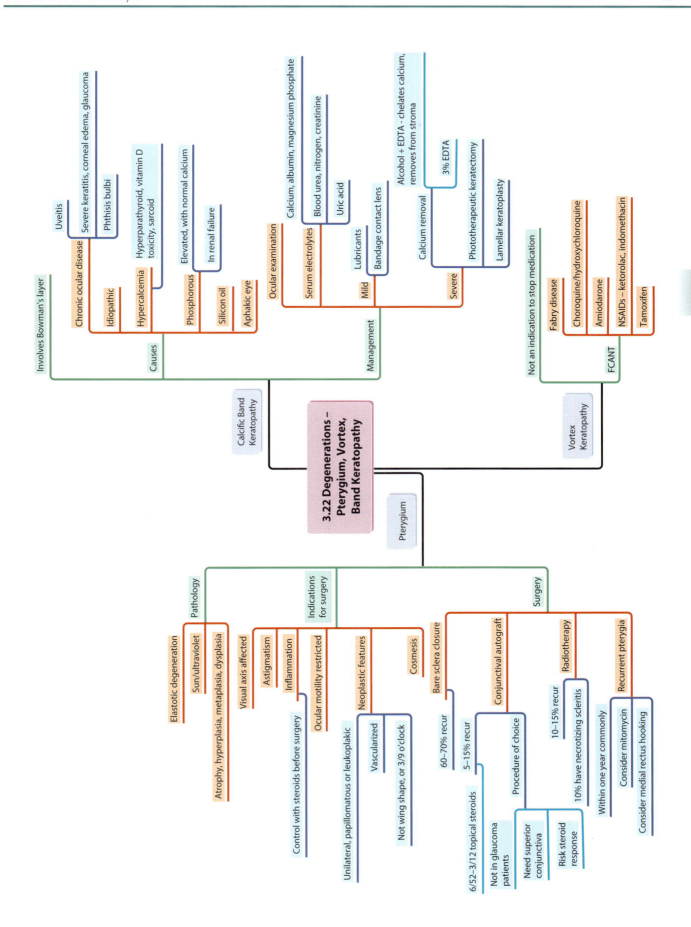

3.22 Degenerations – Pterygium, Vortex, Band Keratopathy

Calcific Band Keratopathy

Involves Bowman's layer

Causes
- Chronic ocular disease
  - Uveitis
  - Severe keratitis, corneal edema, glaucoma
  - Phthisis bulbi
- Idiopathic
- Hypercalcemia
  - Hyperparathyroid, vitamin D toxicity, sarcoid
- Phosphorous
  - Elevated, with normal calcium
  - In renal failure
- Silicon oil
- Aphakic eye

Management
- Ocular examination
  - Calcium, albumin, magnesium phosphate
- Serum electrolytes
  - Blood urea, nitrogen, creatinine
  - Uric acid
- Mild
  - Lubricants
  - Bandage contact lens
- Severe
  - Calcium removal
    - Alcohol + EDTA - chelates calcium, removes from stroma
    - 3% EDTA
  - Phototherapeutic keratectomy
  - Lamellar keratoplasty

Vortex Keratopathy

Not an indication to stop medication

FCANT
- Fabry disease
- Choroquine/hydroxychloroquine
- Amiodarone
- NSAIDs – ketorolac, indomethacin
- Tamoxifen

Pterygium

Pathology
- Elastotic degeneration
- Sun/ultraviolet
- Atrophy, hyperplasia, metaplasia, dysplasia

Indications for surgery
- Visual axis affected
- Astigmatism
- Inflammation
  - Control with steroids before surgery
- Ocular motility restricted
- Neoplastic features
  - Unilateral, papillomatous or leukoplakic
  - Vascularized
  - Not wing shape, or 3/9 o'clock
- Cosmesis

Surgery
- Bare sclera closure
  - 60–70% recur
  - 5–15% recur
    - 6/52–3/12 topical steroids
    - Not in glaucoma patients
- Conjunctival autograft
  - Procedure of choice
    - Need superior conjunctiva
    - Risk steroid response
- Radiotherapy
  - 10–15% recur
  - 10% have necrotizing scleritis
    - Within one year commonly
- Recurrent pterygia
  - Consider mitomycin
  - Consider medial rectus hooking

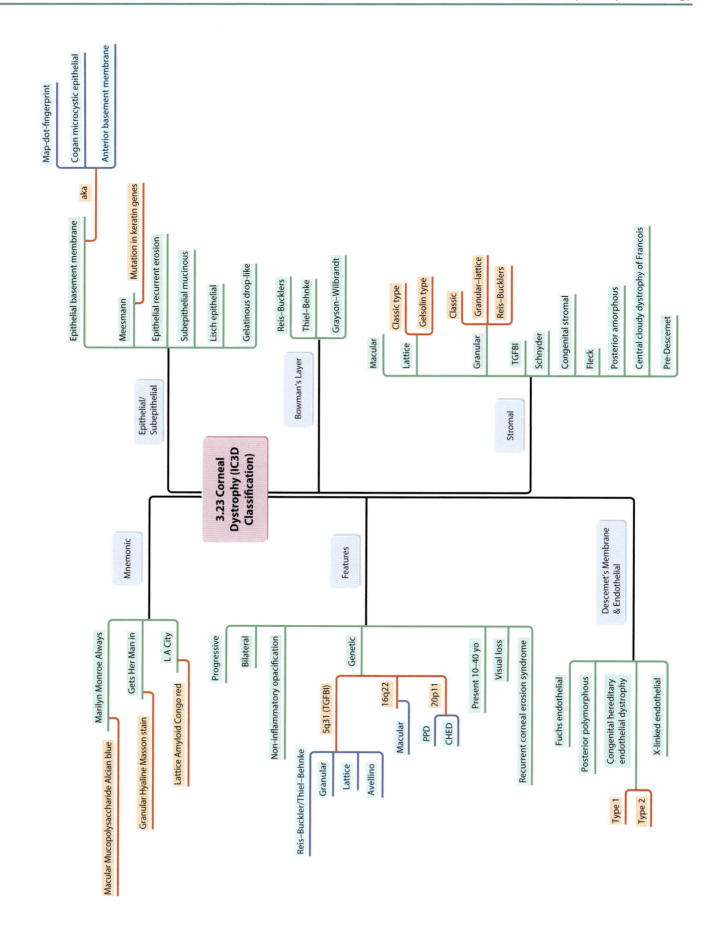

3.23 Corneal Dystrophy (IC3D Classification)

Epithelial/Subepithelial
- Epithelial basement membrane — aka
  - Map-dot-fingerprint
  - Cogan microcystic epithelial
  - Anterior basement membrane
- Meesmann — Mutation in keratin genes
- Epithelial recurrent erosion
- Subepithelial mucinous
- Lisch epithelial
- Gelatinous drop-like

Bowman's Layer
- Reis–Bucklers
- Thiel–Behnke
- Grayson–Wilbrandt

Stromal
- Macular
- Lattice
  - Classic type
  - Gelsolin type
- Granular
  - Classic
  - Granular–lattice
  - Reis–Bucklers
- TGFBI
- Schnyder
- Congenital stromal
- Fleck
- Posterior amorphous
- Central cloudy dystrophy of Francois
- Pre-Descemet

Mnemonic
- Macular Mucopolysaccharide Alcian blue
- Marilyn Monroe Always
- Granular Hyaline Masson stain
- Gets Her Man in
- Lattice Amyloid Congo red
- L A City

Features
- Progressive
- Bilateral
- Non-inflammatory opacification
- Genetic
  - 5q31 (TGFBI)
    - Reis–Buckler/Thiel–Behnke
    - Granular
    - Lattice
    - Avellino
  - 16q22
    - Macular
  - 20p11
    - PPD
    - CHED
- Present 10–40 yo
- Visual loss
- Recurrent corneal erosion syndrome

Descemet's Membrane & Endothelial
- Fuchs endothelial
- Posterior polymorphous
- Congenital hereditary endothelial dystrophy
  - Type 1
  - Type 2
- X-linked endothelial

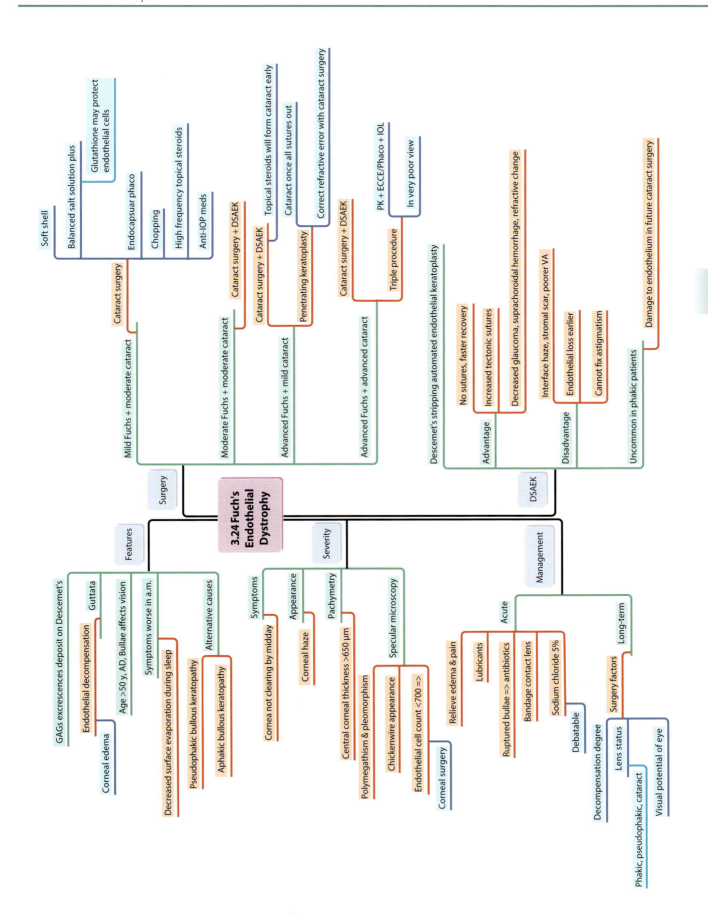

3.24 Fuch's Endothelial Dystrophy

Surgery

Mild Fuchs + moderate cataract
- Cataract surgery
  - Soft shell
  - Balanced salt solution plus
    - Glutathione may protect endothelial cells
  - Endocapsuar phaco
  - Chopping
  - High frequency topical steroids
  - Anti-IOP meds

Moderate Fuchs + moderate cataract
- Cataract surgery + DSAEK

Advanced Fuchs + mild cataract
- Cataract surgery + DSAEK
- Penetrating keratoplasty
  - Topical steroids will form cataract early
  - Cataract once all sutures out
  - Correct refractive error with cataract surgery

Advanced Fuchs + advanced cataract
- Cataract surgery + DSAEK
- Triple procedure
  - PK + ECCE/Phaco + IOL
  - In very poor view

DSAEK
- Descemet's stripping automated endothelial keratoplasty
- Advantage
  - No sutures, faster recovery
  - Increased tectonic sutures
  - Decreased glaucoma, suprachoroidal hemorrhage, refractive change
- Disadvantage
  - Interface haze, stromal scar, poorer VA
  - Endothelial loss earlier
  - Cannot fix astigmatism
- Uncommon in phakic patients
  - Damage to endothelium in future cataract surgery

Features
- GAGs excrescences deposit on Descemet's
- Endothelial decompensation
  - Guttata
  - Corneal edema
- Age >50 y, AD, Bullae affects vision
- Symptoms worse in a.m.
  - Decreased surface evaporation during sleep
- Pseudophakic bullous keratopathy
- Aphakic bullous keratopathy
- Alternative causes

Severity
- Symptoms
  - Cornea not clearing by midday
- Appearance
  - Corneal haze
- Pachymetry
  - Central corneal thickness >650 μm
- Specular microscopy
  - Polymegathism & pleomorphism
  - Chickenwire appearance
  - Endothelial cell count <700 =>
  - Corneal surgery

Management
- Acute
  - Relieve edema & pain
  - Lubricants
  - Ruptured bullae => antibiotics
  - Bandage contact lens
  - Sodium chloride 5%
  - Debatable
- Long-term
  - Surgery factors
    - Decompensation degree
    - Lens status
      - Phakic, pseudophakic, cataract
    - Visual potential of eye

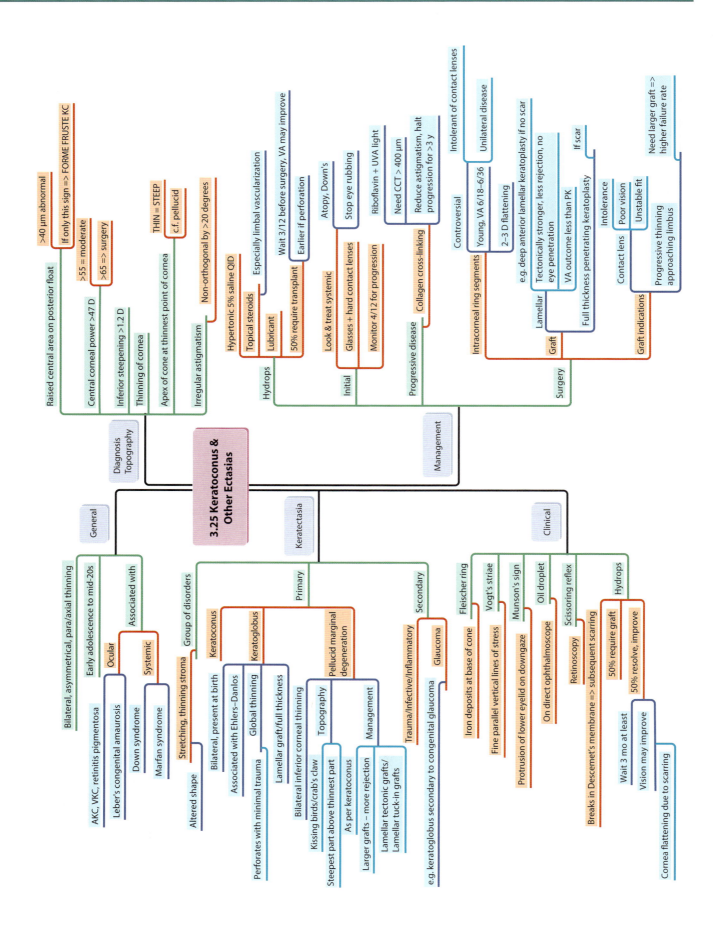

3.25 Keratoconus & Other Ectasias

Diagnosis Topography

- Raised central area on posterior float
  - >40 μm abnormal
  - If only this sign => FORME FRUSTE KC
- Central corneal power >47 D
  - >55 = moderate
  - >65 => surgery
- Inferior steepening >1.2 D
- Thinning of cornea
  - THIN = STEEP
- Apex of cone at thinnest point of cornea
  - c.f. pellucid
- Irregular astigmatism
  - Non-orthogonal by >20 degrees

Management

- Hydrops
  - Hypertonic 5% saline QID
  - Topical steroids
    - Especially limbal vascularization
  - Lubricant
  - 50% require transplant
    - Wait 3/12 before surgery, VA may improve
    - Earlier if perforation
- Initial
  - Look & treat systemic
    - Atopy, Down's
    - Stop eye rubbing
  - Glasses + hard contact lenses
  - Monitor 4/12 for progression
- Progressive disease
  - Collagen cross-linking
    - Riboflavin + UVA light
    - Need CCT > 400 μm
    - Reduce astigmatism, halt progression for >3 y
- Surgery
  - Intracorneal ring segments
    - Controversial
    - Young, VA 6/18–6/36
    - 2–3 D flattening
  - Graft
    - Lamellar
      - e.g. deep anterior lamellar keratoplasty if no scar
      - Tectonically stronger, less rejection, no eye penetration
      - VA outcome less than PK
    - Full thickness penetrating keratoplasty
    - Graft indications
      - Intolerant of contact lenses
      - Unilateral disease
      - If scar
      - Contact lens
        - Intolerance
        - Poor vision
        - Unstable fit
      - Progressive thinning approaching limbus
      - Need larger graft => higher failure rate

General

- Bilateral, asymmetrical, para/axial thinning
- Early adolescence to mid-20s
- Associated with
  - Ocular
    - AKC, VKC, retinitis pigmentosa
    - Leber's congenital amaurosis
  - Systemic
    - Down syndrome
    - Marfan syndrome

Keratectasia

- Group of disorders
  - Stretching, thinning stroma
  - Altered shape
- Primary
  - Keratoconus
    - Bilateral, present at birth
    - Associated with Ehlers–Danlos
  - Keratoglobus
    - Global thinning
    - Lamellar graft/full thickness
    - Bilateral inferior corneal thinning
  - Pellucid marginal degeneration
    - Topography
      - Kissing birds/crab's claw
      - Steepest part above thinnest part
      - As per keratoconus
    - Management
      - Larger grafts – more rejection
      - Lamellar tectonic grafts/ Lamellar tuck-in grafts
- Secondary
  - Trauma/Infective/Inflammatory
    - Perforates with minimal trauma
  - Glaucoma
    - e.g. keratoglobus secondary to congenital glaucoma

Clinical

- Fleischer ring
  - Iron deposits at base of cone
- Vogt's striae
  - Fine parallel vertical lines of stress
- Munson's sign
  - Protrusion of lower eyelid on downgaze
- Oil droplet
  - On direct ophthalmoscope
- Scissoring reflex
  - Retinoscopy
- Hydrops
  - Breaks in Descemet's membrane => subsequent scarring
  - 50% require graft
  - 50% resolve, improve
    - Wait 3 mo at least
    - Vision may improve
    - Cornea flattening due to scarring

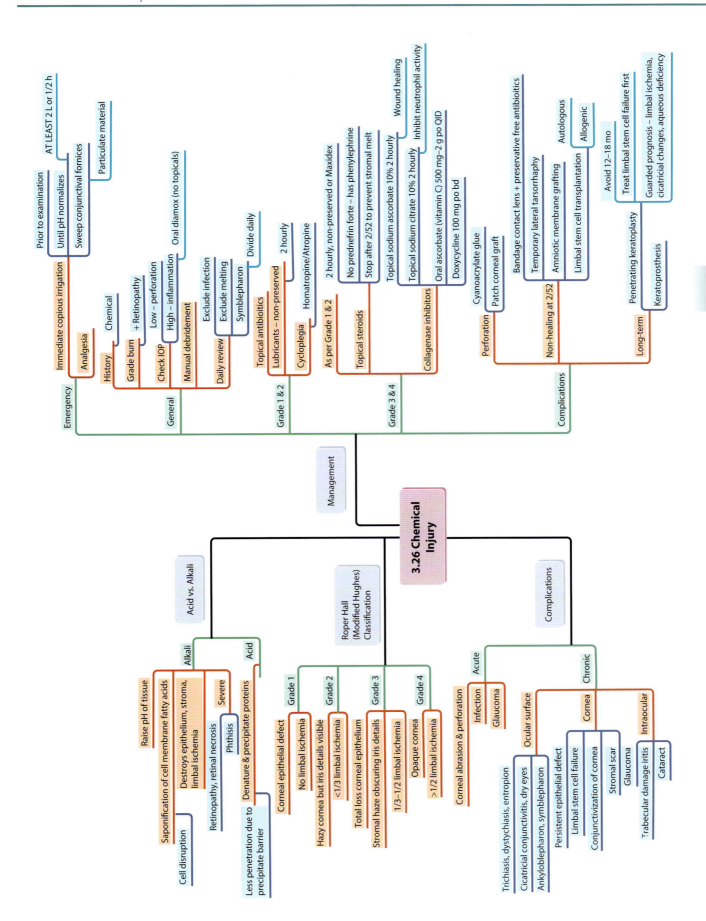

3.26 Chemical Injury

Management

Emergency
- Immediate copious irrigation
  - Prior to examination
  - Until pH normalizes — AT LEAST 2 L or 1/2 h
  - Sweep conjunctival fornices — Particulate material
- Analgesia
- History
  - Chemical
  - Grade burn — + Retinopathy

General
- Check IOP
  - Low – perforation
  - High – inflammation
  - Oral diamox (no topicals)
- Manual debridement
  - Exclude infection
  - Exclude melting
  - Symblepharon
- Daily review — Divide daily

Grade 1 & 2
- Topical antibiotics
- Lubricants – non-preserved — 2 hourly
- Cycloplegia — Homatropine/Atropine

Grade 3 & 4
- As per Grade 1 & 2
- Topical steroids
  - 2 hourly, non-preserved or Maxidex
  - No prednefrin forte – has phenylephrine
  - Stop after 2/52 to prevent stromal melt
- Collagenase inhibitors
  - Topical sodium ascorbate 10% 2 hourly — Wound healing
  - Topical sodium citrate 10% 2 hourly
  - Oral ascorbate (vitamin C) 500 mg–2 g po QID — Inhibit neutrophil activity
  - Doxycycline 100 mg po bd

Complications
- Perforation
  - Cyanoacrylate glue
  - Patch corneal graft
- Non-healing at 2/52
  - Bandage contact lens + preservative free antibiotics
  - Temporary lateral tarsorrhaphy
  - Amniotic membrane grafting
  - Limbal stem cell transplantation
    - Autologous
    - Allogenic
- Long-term
  - Penetrating keratoplasty
    - Avoid 12–18 mo
    - Treat limbal stem cell failure first
    - Guarded prognosis – limbal ischemia, cicatricial changes, aqueous deficiency
  - Keratoprosthesis

Acid vs. Alkali
- Alkali
  - Raise pH of tissue
  - Saponification of cell membrane fatty acids
  - Destroys epithelium, stroma, limbal ischemia
  - Retinopathy, retinal necrosis
  - Severe
    - Phthisis
    - Cell disruption
- Acid
  - Denature & precipitate proteins
  - Less penetration due to precipitate barrier

Roper Hall (Modified Hughes) Classification
- Grade 1
  - Corneal epithelial defect
  - No limbal ischemia
- Grade 2
  - Hazy cornea but iris details visible
  - <1/3 limbal ischemia
- Grade 3
  - Total loss corneal epithelium
  - Stromal haze obscuring iris details
  - 1/3–1/2 limbal ischemia
- Grade 4
  - Opaque cornea
  - >1/2 limbal ischemia

Complications
- Acute
  - Corneal abrasion & perforation
  - Infection
  - Glaucoma
- Chronic
  - Ocular surface
    - Trichiasis, dystychiasis, entropion
    - Cicatricial conjunctivitis, dry eyes
    - Ankyloblepharon, symblepharon
    - Persistent epithelial defect
    - Limbal stem cell failure
  - Cornea
    - Conjunctivization of cornea
    - Stromal scar
    - Glaucoma
  - Intraocular
    - Trabecular damage iritis
    - Cataract

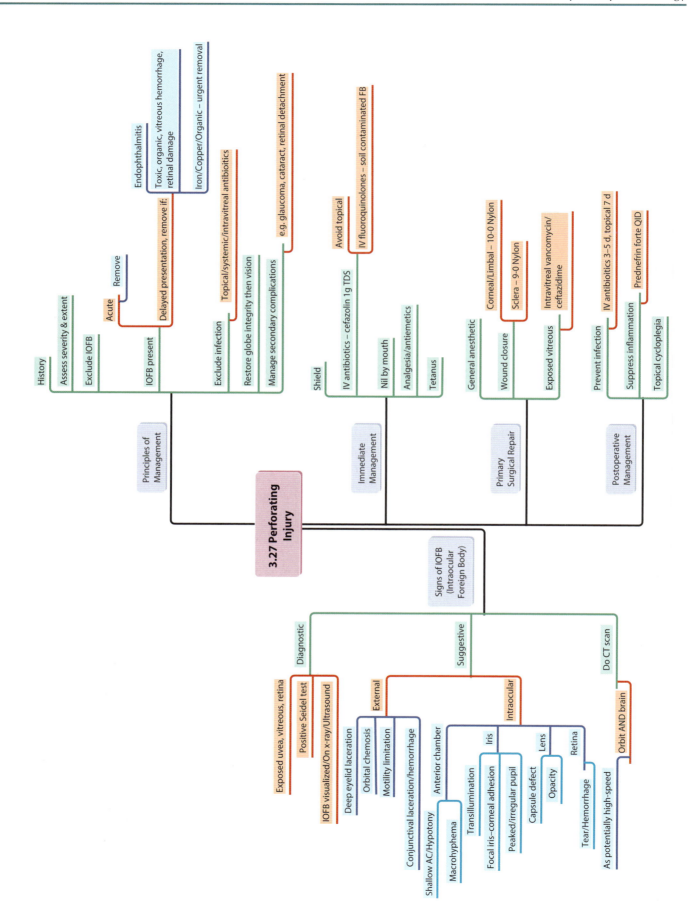

3.27 Perforating Injury

Principles of Management
- History
- Assess severity & extent
- Exclude IOFB
- IOFB present
  - Acute — Remove
  - Delayed presentation, remove if:
    - Endophthalmitis
    - Toxic, organic, vitreous hemorrhage, retinal damage
    - Iron/Copper/Organic – urgent removal
- Exclude infection — Topical/systemic/intravitreal antibiotics
- Restore globe integrity then vision
- Manage secondary complications — e.g. glaucoma, cataract, retinal detachment

Immediate Management
- Shield
- IV antibiotics – cefazolin 1g TDS
  - Avoid topical
  - IV fluoroquinolones – soil contaminated FB
- Nil by mouth
- Analgesia/antiemetics
- Tetanus

Primary Surgical Repair
- General anesthetic
- Wound closure
  - Corneal/Limbal – 10-0 Nylon
  - Sclera – 9-0 Nylon
- Exposed vitreous — Intravitreal vancomycin/ceftazidime

Postoperative Management
- Prevent infection — IV antibiotics 3–5 d, topical 7 d
- Suppress inflammation — Prednefrin forte QID
- Topical cycloplegia

Signs of IOFB (Intraocular Foreign Body)
- Diagnostic
  - Exposed uvea, vitreous, retina
  - Positive Seidel test
  - IOFB visualized/On x-ray/Ultrasound
- Suggestive
  - External
    - Deep eyelid laceration
    - Orbital chemosis
    - Motility limitation
    - Conjunctival laceration/hemorrhage
  - Intraocular
    - Anterior chamber
      - Shallow AC/Hypotony
      - Macrohyphema
      - Transillumination
    - Iris
      - Focal iris–corneal adhesion
      - Peaked/irregular pupil
    - Lens
      - Capsule defect
      - Opacity
    - Retina
      - Tear/Hemorrhage
      - As potentially high-speed
- Do CT scan — Orbit AND brain

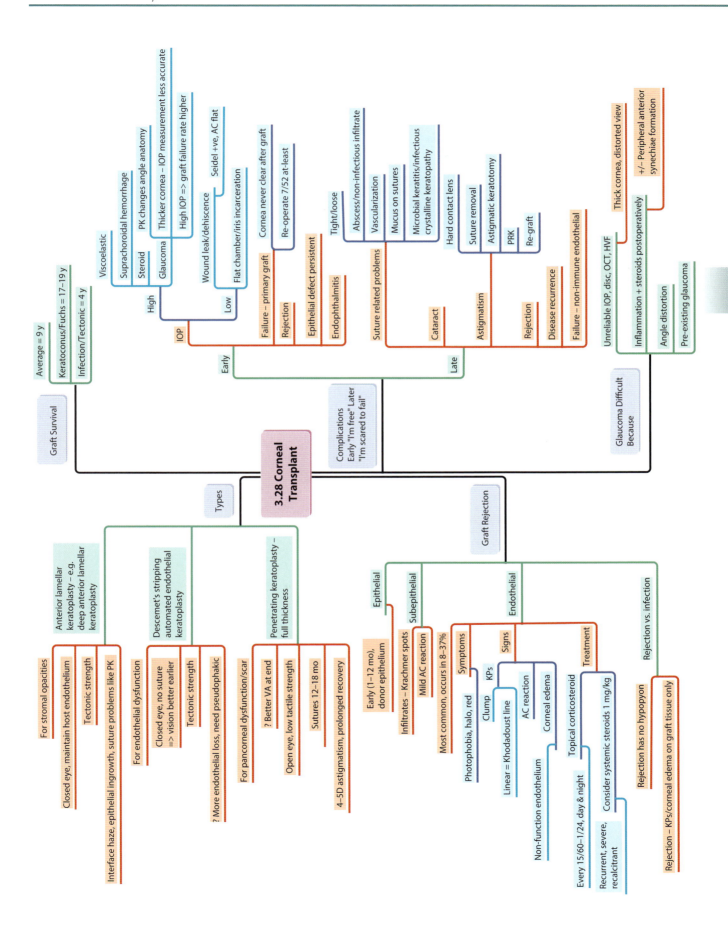

3.28 Corneal Transplant

Graft Survival
- Average = 9 y
- Keratoconus/Fuchs = 17–19 y
- Infection/Tectonic = 4 y

Complications
Early "I'm free" Later "I'm scared to fail"

Early
- IOP
  - High
    - Viscoelastic
    - Suprachoroidal hemorrhage
    - Steroid
    - Glaucoma – PK changes angle anatomy
    - Thicker cornea – IOP measurement less accurate
    - High IOP => graft failure rate higher
  - Low
    - Wound leak/dehiscence – Seidel +ve, AC flat
    - Flat chamber/iris incarceration
- Failure – primary graft
  - Cornea never clear after graft
  - Re-operate 7/52 at-least
- Rejection
- Epithelial defect persistent
- Endophthalmitis

Late
- Suture related problems
  - Tight/loose
  - Abscess/non-infectious infiltrate
  - Vascularization
  - Mucus on sutures
  - Microbial keratitis/infectious crystalline keratopathy
- Cataract
- Astigmatism
  - Hard contact lens
  - Suture removal
  - Astigmatic keratotomy
  - PRK
  - Re-graft
- Rejection
- Disease recurrence
- Failure – non-immune endothelial

Glaucoma Difficult Because
- Unreliable IOP, disc, OCT, HVF
- Inflammation + steroids postoperatively
  - Thick cornea, distorted view
  - +/– Peripheral anterior synechiae formation
- Angle distortion
- Pre-existing glaucoma

Types

Anterior lamellar keratoplasty – e.g. deep anterior lamellar keratoplasty
- For stromal opacities
- Closed eye, maintain host endothelium
- Tectonic strength
- Interface haze, epithelial ingrowth, suture problems like PK

Descemet's stripping automated endothelial keratoplasty
- For endothelial dysfunction
- Closed eye, no suture => vision better earlier
- Tectonic strength
- ? More endothelial loss, need pseudophakic

Penetrating keratoplasty – full thickness
- For pancorneal dysfunction/scar
- ? Better VA at end
- Open eye, low tactile strength
- Sutures 12–18 mo
- 4–5D astigmatism, prolonged recovery

Graft Rejection

- **Epithelial**
  - Early (1–12 mo), donor epithelium
- **Subepithelial**
  - Infiltrates – Krachmer spots
  - Mild AC reaction
- **Endothelial**
  - Most common, occurs in 8–37%
  - Symptoms
    - Photophobia, halo, red
  - Signs
    - KPs
      - Clump
      - Linear = Khodadoust line
    - AC reaction
    - Corneal edema
      - Non-function endothelium
  - Treatment
    - Topical corticosteroid
      - Every 15/60–1/24, day & night
    - Consider systemic steroids 1 mg/kg
      - Recurrent, severe, recalcitrant
  - Rejection vs. infection
    - Rejection has no hypopyon
    - Rejection – KPs/corneal edema on graft tissue only

4 Glaucoma

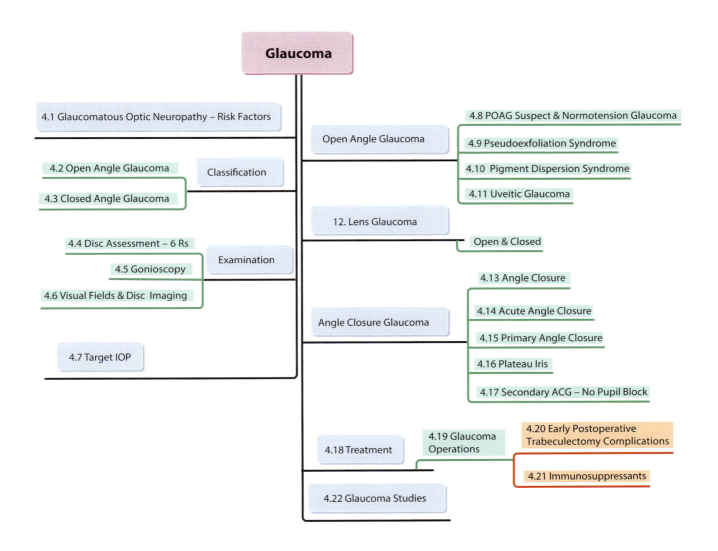

Glaucoma

4.1 Glaucomatous Optic Neuropathy – Risk Factors

4.2 Open Angle Glaucoma

4.3 Closed Angle Glaucoma

Classification

4.4 Disc Assessment – 6 Rs

4.5 Gonioscopy

4.6 Visual Fields & Disc Imaging

Examination

4.7 Target IOP

Open Angle Glaucoma

4.8 POAG Suspect & Normotension Glaucoma

4.9 Pseudoexfoliation Syndrome

4.10 Pigment Dispersion Syndrome

4.11 Uveitic Glaucoma

12. Lens Glaucoma

Open & Closed

Angle Closure Glaucoma

4.13 Angle Closure

4.14 Acute Angle Closure

4.15 Primary Angle Closure

4.16 Plateau Iris

4.17 Secondary ACG – No Pupil Block

4.18 Treatment

4.19 Glaucoma Operations

4.20 Early Postoperative Trabeculectomy Complications

4.21 Immunosuppressants

4.22 Glaucoma Studies

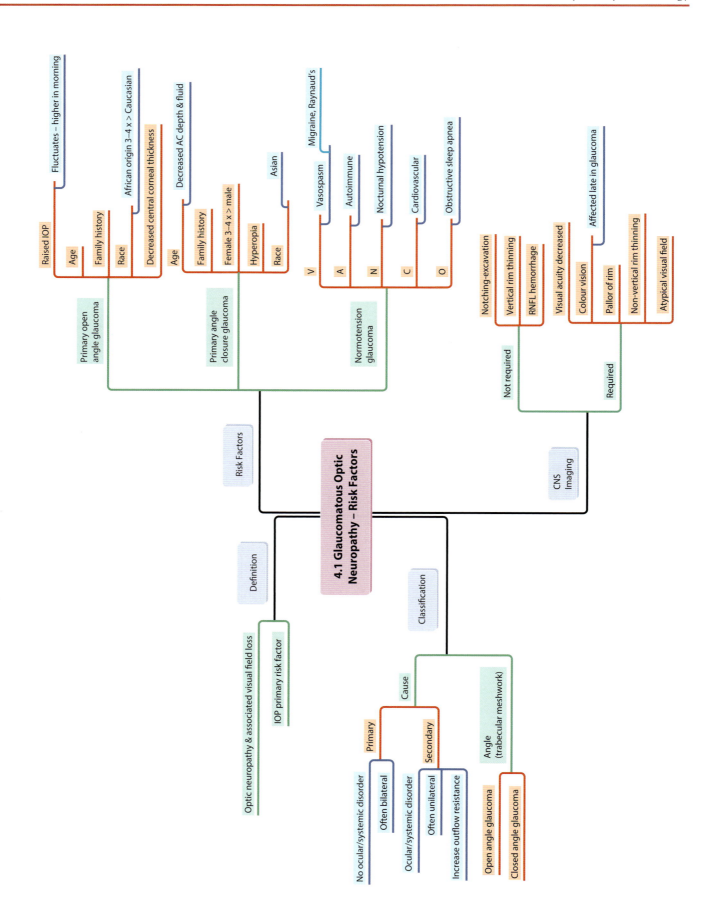

4.1 Glaucomatous Optic Neuropathy – Risk Factors

Definition
- Optic neuropathy & associated visual field loss
- IOP primary risk factor

Risk Factors

Primary open angle glaucoma
- Raised IOP
  - Fluctuates – higher in morning
- Age
- Family history
- Race
  - African origin 3–4 x > Caucasian
- Decreased central corneal thickness

Primary angle closure glaucoma
- Age
  - Decreased AC depth & fluid
- Family history
- Female 3–4 x > male
- Hyperopia
- Race
  - Asian

Normotension glaucoma
- V — Vasospasm
  - Migraine, Raynaud's
- A — Autoimmune
- N — Nocturnal hypotension
- C — Cardiovascular
- O — Obstructive sleep apnea

CNS Imaging

Not required
- Notching-excavation
- Vertical rim thinning
- RNFL hemorrhage

Required
- Visual acuity decreased
- Colour vision
  - Affected late in glaucoma
- Pallor of rim
- Non-vertical rim thinning
- Atypical visual field

Classification

Cause
- Primary
  - No ocular/systemic disorder
  - Often bilateral
- Secondary
  - Ocular/systemic disorder
  - Often unilateral
  - Increase outflow resistance

Angle (trabecular meshwork)
- Open angle glaucoma
- Closed angle glaucoma

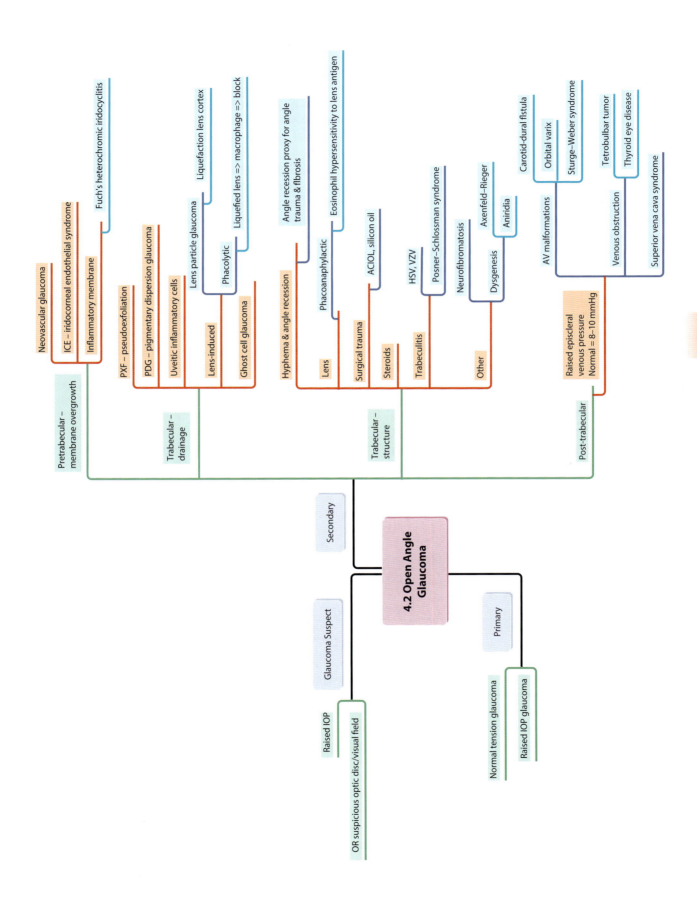

4.2 Open Angle Glaucoma

Glaucoma Suspect
- Raised IOP
- OR suspicious optic disc/visual field

Primary
- Normal tension glaucoma
- Raised IOP glaucoma

Secondary

Pretrabecular – membrane overgrowth
- Neovascular glaucoma
- ICE – iridocorneal endothelial syndrome
- Inflammatory membrane
  - Fuch's heterochromic iridocyclitis

Trabecular – drainage
- PXF – pseudoexfoliation
- PDG – pigmentary dispersion glaucoma
- Uveitic inflammatory cells
- Lens-induced
  - Lens particle glaucoma
  - Phacolytic
    - Liquefaction lens cortex
    - Liquefied lens => macrophage => block
- Ghost cell glaucoma

Trabecular – structure
- Hyphema & angle recession
  - Angle recession proxy for angle trauma & fibrosis
- Lens
  - Phacoanaphylactic
    - Eosinophil hypersensitivity to lens antigen
- Surgical trauma
  - ACIOL, silicon oil
- Steroids
- Trabeculitis
  - HSV, VZV
  - Posner–Schlossman syndrome
- Other
  - Neurofibromatosis
  - Dysgenesis
    - Axenfeld–Rieger
    - Aniridia

Post-trabecular
- Raised episcleral venous pressure Normal = 8–10 mmHg
  - AV malformations
    - Carotid-dural fistula
    - Orbital varix
    - Sturge–Weber syndrome
  - Venous obstruction
    - Tetrobulbar tumor
    - Thyroid eye disease
    - Superior vena cava syndrome

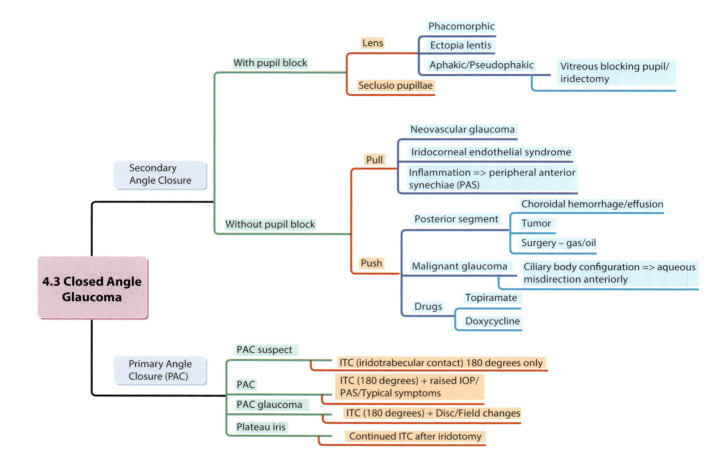

4.3 Closed Angle Glaucoma

Secondary Angle Closure
- With pupil block
  - Lens
    - Phacomorphic
    - Ectopia lentis
    - Aphakic/Pseudophakic
  - Seclusio pupillae
    - Vitreous blocking pupil/iridectomy
- Without pupil block
  - Pull
    - Neovascular glaucoma
    - Iridocorneal endothelial syndrome
    - Inflammation => peripheral anterior synechiae (PAS)
  - Push
    - Posterior segment
      - Choroidal hemorrhage/effusion
      - Tumor
      - Surgery – gas/oil
    - Malignant glaucoma
      - Ciliary body configuration => aqueous misdirection anteriorly
    - Drugs
      - Topiramate
      - Doxycycline

Primary Angle Closure (PAC)
- PAC suspect
  - ITC (iridotrabecular contact) 180 degrees only
- PAC
  - ITC (180 degrees) + raised IOP/PAS/Typical symptoms
- PAC glaucoma
  - ITC (180 degrees) + Disc/Field changes
- Plateau iris
  - Continued ITC after iridotomy

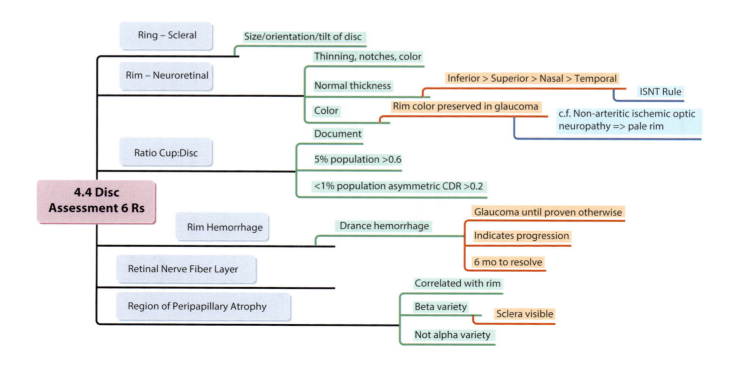

4.4 Disc Assessment 6 Rs

- Ring – Scleral
  - Size/orientation/tilt of disc
- Rim – Neuroretinal
  - Thinning, notches, color
  - Normal thickness
    - Inferior > Superior > Nasal > Temporal
      - ISNT Rule
  - Color
    - Rim color preserved in glaucoma
      - c.f. Non-arteritic ischemic optic neuropathy => pale rim
- Ratio Cup:Disc
  - Document
  - 5% population >0.6
  - <1% population asymmetric CDR >0.2
- Rim Hemorrhage
  - Drance hemorrhage
    - Glaucoma until proven otherwise
    - Indicates progression
    - 6 mo to resolve
- Retinal Nerve Fiber Layer
- Region of Peripapillary Atrophy
  - Correlated with rim
  - Beta variety
    - Sclera visible
  - Not alpha variety

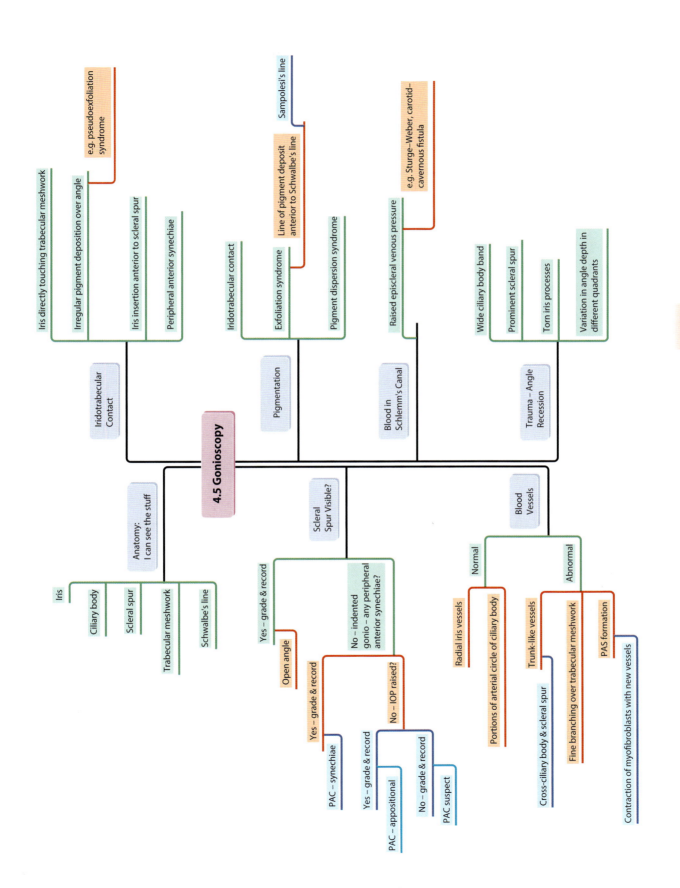

4.5 Gonioscopy

Anatomy: I can see the stuff
- Iris
- Ciliary body
- Scleral spur
- Trabecular meshwork
- Schwalbe's line

Iridotrabecular Contact
- Iris directly touching trabecular meshwork
- Irregular pigment deposition over angle
  - e.g. pseudoexfoliation syndrome
- Iris insertion anterior to scleral spur
- Peripheral anterior synechiae

Pigmentation
- Iridotrabecular contact
- Exfoliation syndrome
  - Line of pigment deposit anterior to Schwalbe's line
  - Sampolesi's line
- Pigment dispersion syndrome

Blood in Schlemm's Canal
- Raised episcleral venous pressure
  - e.g. Sturge–Weber, carotid–cavernous fistula

Trauma – Angle Recession
- Wide ciliary body band
- Prominent scleral spur
- Torn iris processes
- Variation in angle depth in different quadrants

Scleral Spur Visible?
- Yes – grade & record
  - Open angle
  - No – indented gonio – any peripheral anterior synechiae?
    - Yes – grade & record
      - PAC – synechiae
    - No – IOP raised?
      - Yes – grade & record
        - PAC – appositional
      - No – grade & record
        - PAC suspect

Blood Vessels
- Normal
  - Radial iris vessels
  - Portions of arterial circle of ciliary body
- Abnormal
  - Trunk-like vessels
    - Cross-ciliary body & scleral spur
  - Fine branching over trabecular meshwork
  - PAS formation
    - Contraction of myofibroblasts with new vessels

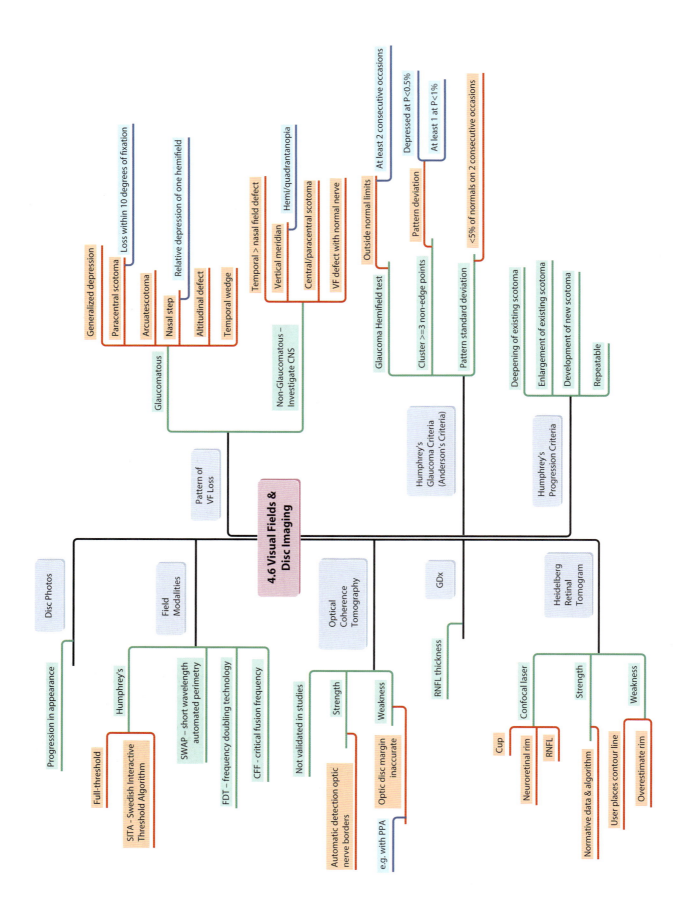

4.6 Visual Fields & Disc Imaging

Pattern of VF Loss

- Glaucomatous
  - Generalized depression
  - Paracentral scotoma
    - Loss within 10 degrees of fixation
  - Arcuatescotoma
  - Nasal step
    - Relative depression of one hemifield
  - Altitudinal defect
  - Temporal wedge
- Non-Glaucomatous – Investigate CNS
  - Temporal > nasal field defect
  - Vertical meridian
    - Hemi/quadrantanopia
  - Central/paracentral scotoma
  - VF defect with normal nerve

Humphrey's Glaucoma Criteria (Anderson's Criteria)
- Outside normal limits
  - At least 2 consecutive occasions
- Glaucoma Hemifield test
- Pattern deviation
  - Depressed at P<0.5%
  - At least 1 at P<1%
- Cluster >=3 non-edge points
- Pattern standard deviation
  - <5% of normals on 2 consecutive occasions

Humphrey's Progression Criteria
- Deepening of existing scotoma
- Enlargement of existing scotoma
- Development of new scotoma
- Repeatable

Disc Photos
- Progression in appearance

Field Modalities
- Humphrey's
  - Full-threshold
  - SITA - Swedish Interactive Threshold Algorithm
- SWAP – short wavelength automated perimetry
- FDT – frequency doubling technology
- CFF – critical fusion frequency

Optical Coherence Tomography
- Strength
  - Automatic detection optic nerve borders
- Weakness
  - Not validated in studies
  - Optic disc margin inaccurate
    - e.g. with PPA

GDx
- RNFL thickness

Heidelberg Retinal Tomogram
- Confocal laser
  - Cup
  - Neuroretinal rim
  - RNFL
- Strength
  - Normative data & algorithm
- Weakness
  - User places contour line
  - Overestimate rim

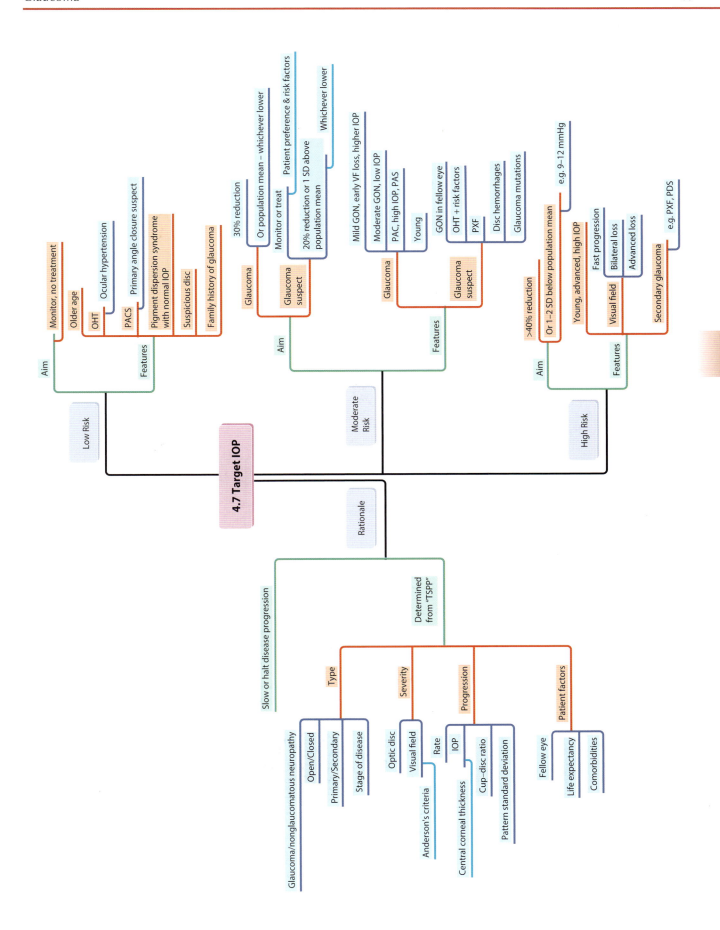

4.7 Target IOP

Low Risk

Aim
- Monitor, no treatment

Features
- Older age
- OHT
  - Ocular hypertension
- PACS
  - Primary angle closure suspect
- Pigment dispersion syndrome with normal IOP
- Suspicious disc
- Family history of glaucoma

Moderate Risk

Aim
- Glaucoma
  - 30% reduction
  - Or population mean – whichever lower
- Glaucoma suspect
  - Monitor or treat
  - 20% reduction or 1 SD above population mean
    - Patient preference & risk factors
  - Whichever lower

Features
- Glaucoma
  - Mild GON, early VF loss, higher IOP
  - Moderate GON, low IOP
  - PAC, high IOP, PAS
  - Young
- Glaucoma suspect
  - GON in fellow eye
  - OHT + risk factors
  - PXF
  - Disc hemorrhages
  - Glaucoma mutations

High Risk

Aim
- >40% reduction
- Or 1–2 SD below population mean
  - e.g. 9–12 mmHg

Features
- Young, advanced, high IOP
- Visual field
  - Fast progression
  - Bilateral loss
  - Advanced loss
- Secondary glaucoma
  - e.g. PXF, PDS

Rationale

- Slow or halt disease progression
- Determined from "TSPP"
  - Type
    - Glaucoma/nonglaucomatous neuropathy
    - Open/Closed
    - Primary/Secondary
    - Stage of disease
  - Severity
    - Optic disc
    - Visual field
      - Anderson's criteria
    - Central corneal thickness
    - Cup–disc ratio
    - Pattern standard deviation
  - Progression
    - Rate
    - IOP
  - Patient factors
    - Fellow eye
    - Life expectancy
    - Comorbidities

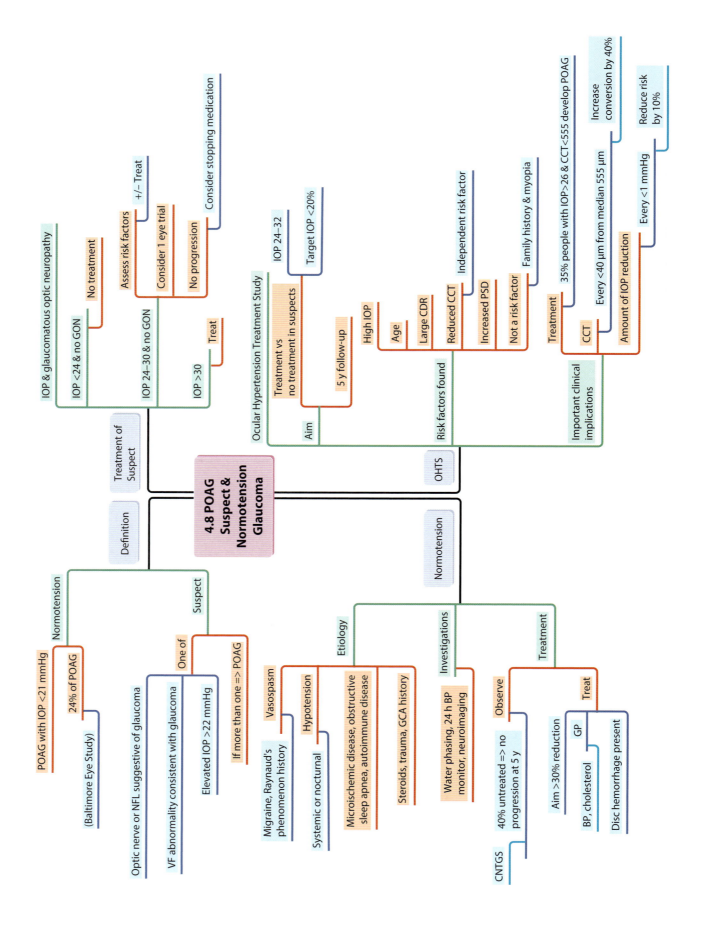

4.8 POAG Suspect & Normotension Glaucoma

Definition
- Normotension
  - POAG with IOP <21 mmHg
  - 24% of POAG
    - (Baltimore Eye Study)
- Suspect
  - One of
    - Optic nerve or NFL suggestive of glaucoma
    - VF abnormality consistent with glaucoma
    - Elevated IOP >22 mmHg
  - If more than one => POAG

Treatment of Suspect
- IOP & glaucomatous optic neuropathy
  - IOP <24 & no GON
    - No treatment
  - IOP 24–30 & no GON
    - Assess risk factors
      - +/– Treat
    - Consider 1 eye trial
    - No progression
      - Consider stopping medication
  - IOP >30
    - Treat

OHTS
- Ocular Hypertension Treatment Study
  - Aim
    - Treatment vs no treatment in suspects
      - IOP 24–32
        - Target IOP <20%
    - 5 y follow-up
  - Risk factors found
    - High IOP
    - Age
    - Large CDR
    - Reduced CCT
      - Independent risk factor
    - Increased PSD
    - Not a risk factor
      - Family history & myopia
  - Important clinical implications
    - Treatment
      - 35% people with IOP>26 & CCT<555 develop POAG
    - CCT
      - Every <40 μm from median 555 μm
        - Increase conversion by 40%
    - Amount of IOP reduction
      - Every <1 mmHg
        - Reduce risk by 10%

Normotension
- Etiology
  - Vasospasm
    - Migraine, Raynaud's phenomenon history
  - Hypotension
    - Systemic or nocturnal
  - Microischemic disease, obstructive sleep apnea, autoimmune disease
  - Steroids, trauma, GCA history
- Investigations
  - Water phasing, 24 h BP monitor, neuroimaging
- Treatment
  - Observe
    - 40% untreated => no progression at 5 y
      - CNTGS
  - Treat
    - Aim >30% reduction
    - GP
      - BP, cholesterol
    - Disc hemorrhage present

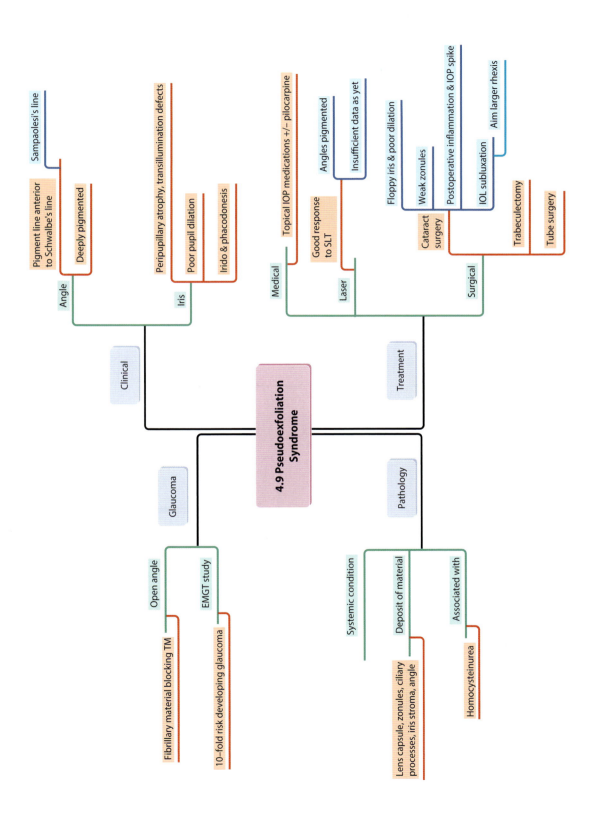

4.9 Pseudoexfoliation Syndrome

Clinical

Angle
- Pigment line anterior to Schwalbe's line
  - Sampaolesi's line
- Deeply pigmented

Iris
- Peripupillary atrophy, transillumination defects
- Poor pupil dilation
- Irido & phacodonesis

Glaucoma
- Open angle
  - Fibrillary material blocking TM
- EMGT study
  - 10-fold risk developing glaucoma

Treatment

Medical
- Topical IOP medications +/- pilocarpine

Laser
- Good response to SLT
  - Angles pigmented
  - Insufficient data as yet

Surgical
- Cataract surgery
  - Floppy iris & poor dilation
  - Weak zonules
  - Postoperative inflammation & IOP spike
  - IOL subluxation
  - Aim larger rhexis
- Trabeculectomy
- Tube surgery

Pathology

Systemic condition

Deposit of material
- Lens capsule, zonules, ciliary processes, iris stroma, angle

Associated with
- Homocysteinurea

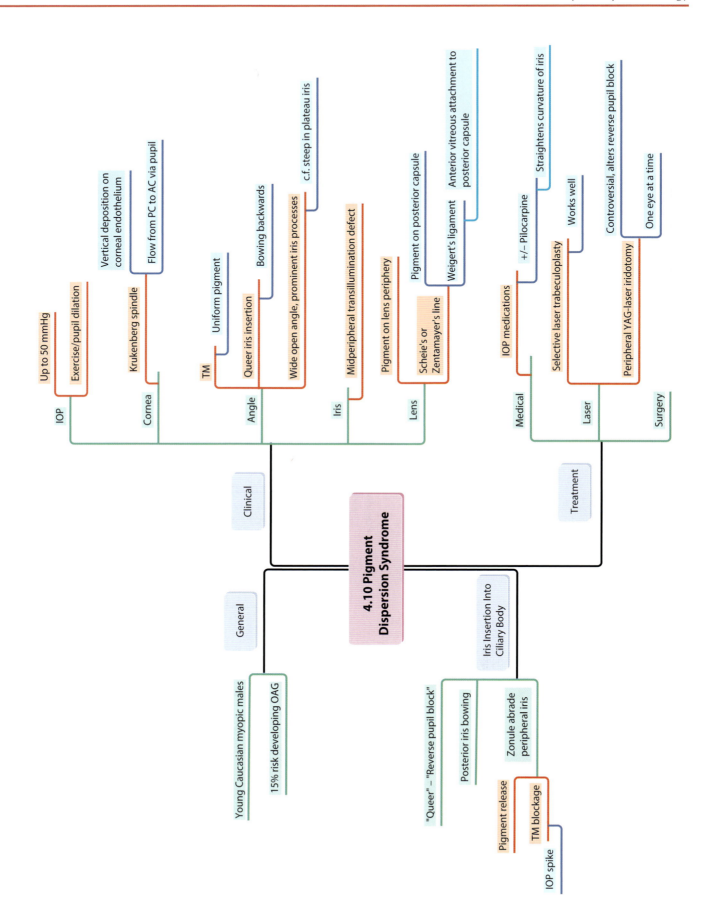

4.10 Pigment Dispersion Syndrome

Clinical

IOP
- Up to 50 mmHg
- Exercise/pupil dilation

Cornea
- Krukenberg spindle
  - Vertical deposition on corneal endothelium
  - Flow from PC to AC via pupil

Angle
- TM
  - Uniform pigment
- Queer iris insertion
  - Bowing backwards
- Wide open angle, prominent iris processes
  - c.f. steep in plateau iris

Iris
- Midperipheral transillumination defect

Lens
- Pigment on lens periphery
- Scheie's or Zentamayer's line
  - Pigment on posterior capsule
  - Weigert's ligament
    - Anterior vitreous attachment to posterior capsule

General

- Young Caucasian myopic males
- 15% risk developing OAG

Iris Insertion Into Ciliary Body
- "Queer" – "Reverse pupil block"
  - Posterior iris bowing
- Zonule abrade peripheral iris
  - Pigment release
    - TM blockage
      - IOP spike

Treatment

Medical
- IOP medications
  - +/– Pilocarpine
    - Straightens curvature of iris
    - Works well

Laser
- Selective laser trabeculoplasty
- Peripheral YAG-laser iridotomy
  - Controversial, alters reverse pupil block
  - One eye at a time

Surgery

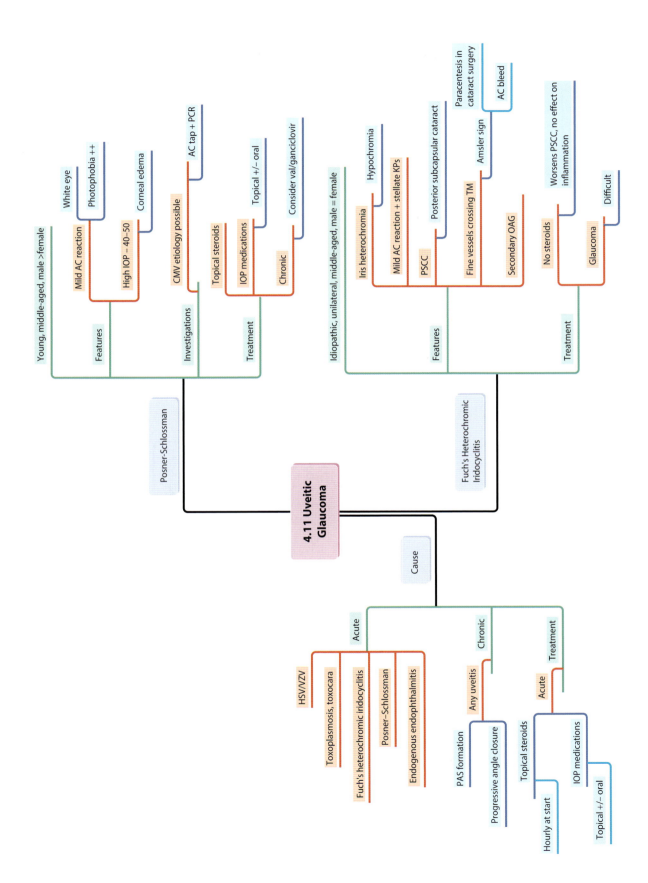

4.11 Uveitic Glaucoma

Posner-Schlossman

Features
- Young, middle-aged, male >female
- White eye
- Mild AC reaction — Photophobia ++
- High IOP – 40–50 — Corneal edema

Investigations
- CMV etiology possible — AC tap + PCR

Treatment
- Topical steroids
- IOP medications — Topical +/- oral
- Chronic — Consider val/ganciclovir

Fuch's Heterochromic Iridocyclitis

Features
- Idiopathic, unilateral, middle-aged, male = female
- Iris heterochromia — Hypochromia
- Mild AC reaction + stellate KPs
- PSCC — Posterior subcapsular cataract
- Fine vessels crossing TM — Amsler sign — Paracentesis in cataract surgery — AC bleed
- Secondary OAG

Treatment
- No steroids — Worsens PSCC, no effect on inflammation
- Glaucoma — Difficult

Cause

Acute
- HSV/VZV
- Toxoplasmosis, toxocara
- Fuch's heterochromic iridocyclitis
- Posner–Schlossman
- Endogenous endophthalmitis

Chronic
- Any uveitis — PAS formation
- Progressive angle closure

Treatment
- Acute — Topical steroids — Hourly at start
- IOP medications — Topical +/- oral

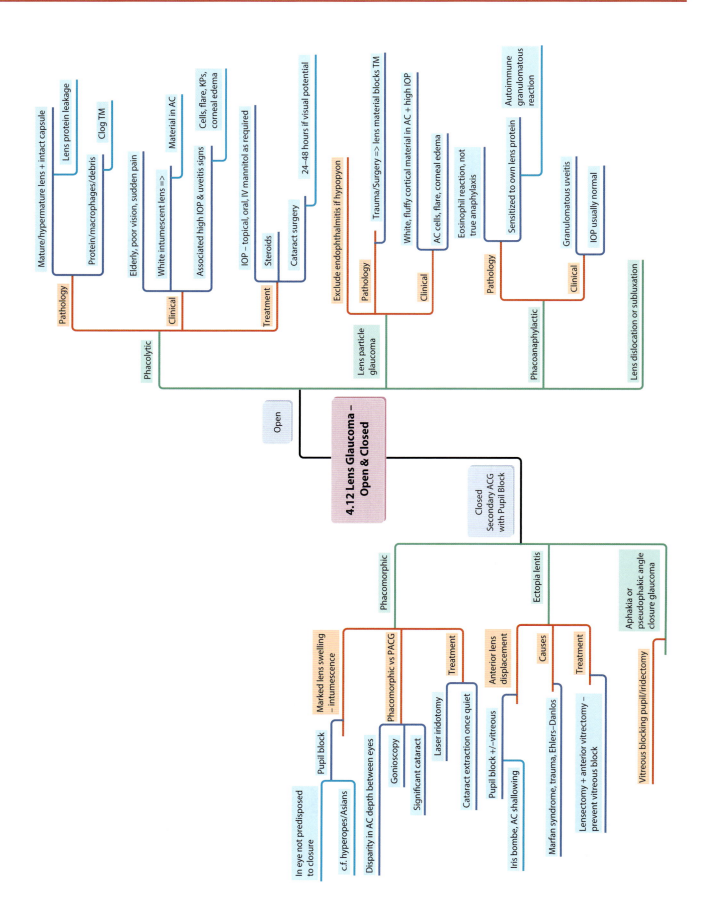

4.12 Lens Glaucoma – Open & Closed

Open

Phacolytic
- Pathology
  - Mature/hypermature lens + intact capsule
    - Lens protein leakage
    - Clog TM
  - Protein/macrophages/debris
- Clinical
  - Elderly, poor vision, sudden pain
  - White intumescent lens =>
    - Material in AC
  - Associated high IOP & uveitis signs
    - Cells, flare, KPs, corneal edema
- Treatment
  - IOP – topical, oral, IV mannitol as required
  - Steroids
  - Cataract surgery
    - 24–48 hours if visual potential

Lens particle glaucoma
- Exclude endophthalmitis if hypopyon
- Pathology
  - Trauma/Surgery => lens material blocks TM
- Clinical
  - White, fluffy cortical material in AC + high IOP
  - AC cells, flare, corneal edema

Phacoanaphylactic
- Pathology
  - Eosinophil reaction, not true anaphylaxis
  - Sensitized to own lens protein
  - Autoimmune granulomatous reaction
- Clinical
  - Granulomatous uveitis
  - IOP usually normal

Lens dislocation or subluxation

Closed
Secondary ACG with Pupil Block

Phacomorphic
- Marked lens swelling – intumescence
  - Pupil block
    - In eye not predisposed to closure
    - c.f. hyperopes/Asians
    - Disparity in AC depth between eyes
- Phacomorphic vs PACG
  - Gonioscopy
  - Significant cataract
- Treatment
  - Laser iridotomy
  - Cataract extraction once quiet

Ectopia lentis
- Anterior lens displacement
  - Pupil block +/–vitreous
  - Iris bombe, AC shallowing
- Causes
  - Marfan syndrome, trauma, Ehlers–Danlos
- Treatment
  - Lensectomy + anterior vitrectomy – prevent vitreous block

Aphakia or pseudophakic angle closure glaucoma
- Vitreous blocking pupil/iridectomy

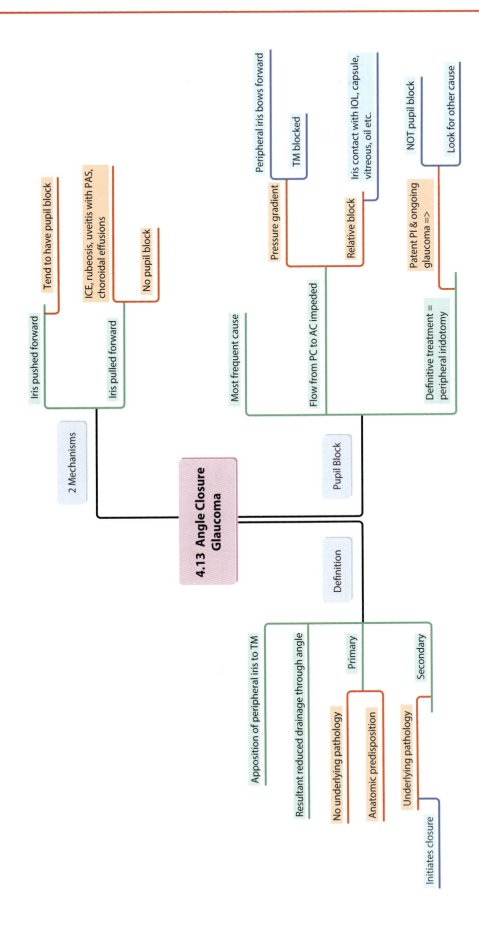

4.13 Angle Closure Glaucoma

2 Mechanisms

- Iris pushed forward
  - Tend to have pupil block
  - ICE, rubeosis, uveitis with PAS, choroidal effusions
- Iris pulled forward
  - No pupil block

Pupil Block

- Most frequent cause
- Flow from PC to AC impeded
  - Pressure gradient
    - Peripheral iris bows forward
    - TM blocked
  - Relative block
    - Iris contact with IOL, capsule, vitreous, oil etc.
- Definitive treatment = peripheral iridotomy
  - Patent PI & ongoing glaucoma =>
    - NOT pupil block
    - Look for other cause

Definition

- Apposition of peripheral iris to TM
- Resultant reduced drainage through angle
- Primary
  - No underlying pathology
  - Anatomic predisposition
- Secondary
  - Underlying pathology
    - Initiates closure

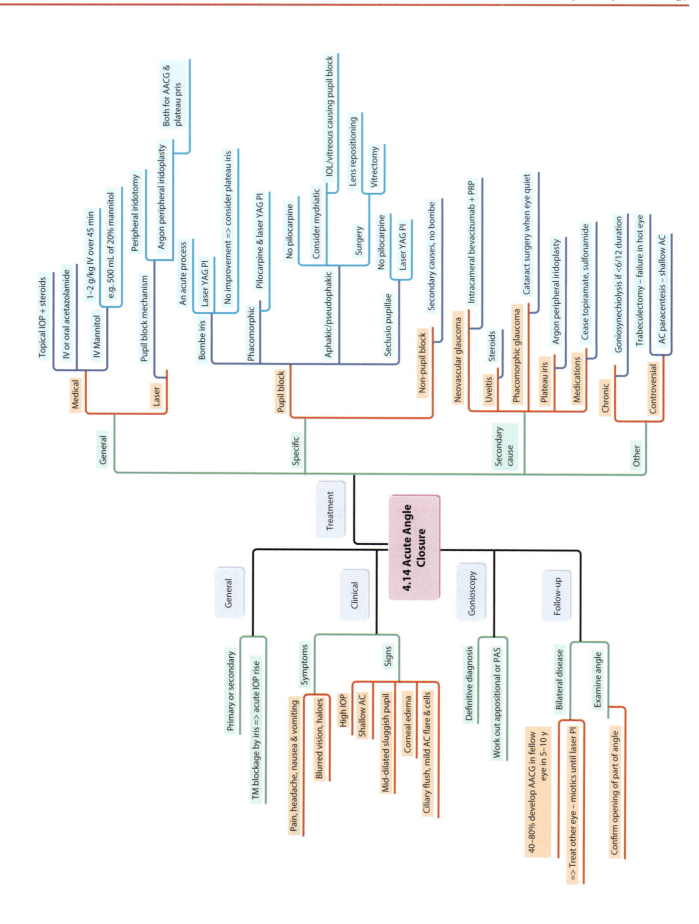

4.14 Acute Angle Closure

Treatment

General
- Medical
  - Topical IOP + steroids
  - IV or oral acetazolamide
  - IV Mannitol
    - 1–2 g/kg IV over 45 min
    - e.g. 500 mL of 20% mannitol
- Laser
  - Peripheral iridotomy
  - Argon peripheral iridoplasty
    - Both for AACG & plateau iris

Specific
- Pupil block
  - An acute process
  - Bombe iris
    - Laser YAG PI
    - No improvement => consider plateau iris
  - Phacomorphic
    - Pilocarpine & laser YAG PI
  - Aphakic/pseudophakic
    - No pilocarpine
    - Consider mydriatic
    - IOL/vitreous causing pupil block
    - Lens repositioning
    - Surgery
    - Vitrectomy
  - Seclusio pupillae
    - No pilocarpine
    - Laser YAG PI
- Non-pupil block
  - Secondary causes, no bombe

Secondary cause
- Neovascular glaucoma
  - Intracameral bevacizumab + PRP
  - Uveitis
    - Steroids
  - Phacomorphic glaucoma
    - Cataract surgery when eye quiet
- Plateau iris
  - Argon peripheral iridoplasty
- Medications
  - Cease topiramate, sulfonamide

Other
- Chronic
  - Goniosynechiolysis if <6/12 duration
  - Trabeculectomy – failure in hot eye
- Controversial
  - AC paracentesis – shallow AC

Clinical

General
- Primary or secondary
- TM blockage by iris => acute IOP rise

Symptoms
- Pain, headache, nausea & vomiting
- Blurred vision, haloes

Signs
- High IOP
- Shallow AC
- Mid-dilated sluggish pupil
- Corneal edema
- Ciliary flush, mild AC flare & cells

Gonioscopy
- Definitive diagnosis
- Work out appositional or PAS

Follow-up
- Bilateral disease
  - 40–80% develop AACG in fellow eye in 5–10 y
  - => Treat other eye – miotics until laser PI
- Examine angle
  - Confirm opening of part of angle

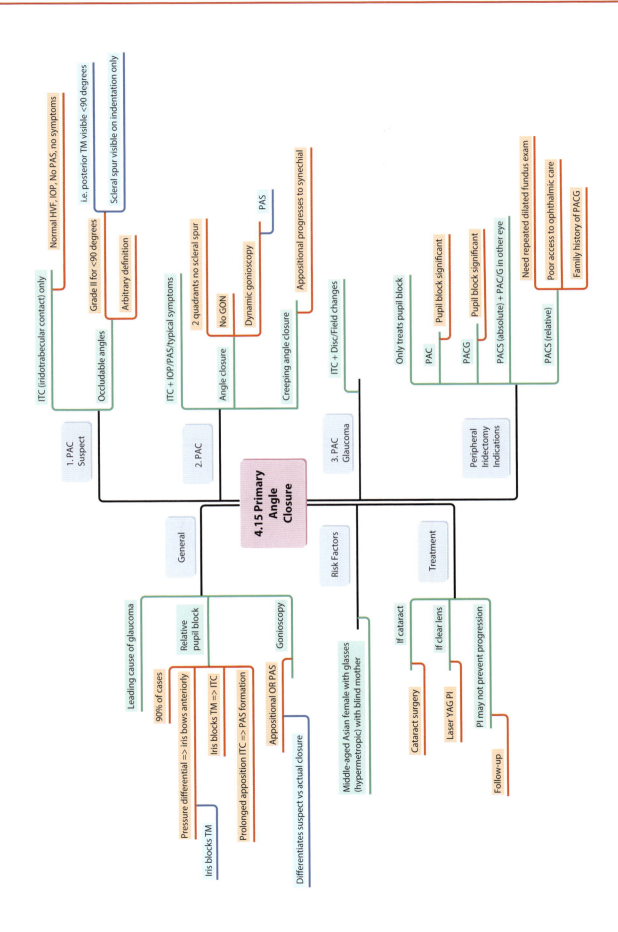

4.15 Primary Angle Closure

General
- Leading cause of glaucoma
  - 90% of cases
- Relative pupil block
  - Iris blocks TM
  - Pressure differential => iris bows anteriorly
  - Iris blocks TM => ITC
  - Prolonged apposition ITC => PAS formation
- Gonioscopy
  - Appositional OR PAS
  - Differentiates suspect vs actual closure

1. PAC Suspect
- ITC (iridotrabecular contact) only
  - Normal HVF, IOP, No PAS, no symptoms
- Occludable angles
  - Grade II for <90 degrees
    - i.e. posterior TM visible <90 degrees
  - Arbitrary definition
    - Scleral spur visible on indentation only

2. PAC
- ITC + IOP/PAS/typical symptoms
- Angle closure
  - 2 quadrants no scleral spur
  - No GON
  - Dynamic gonioscopy
    - PAS
- Creeping angle closure
  - Appositional progresses to synechial

3. PAC Glaucoma
- ITC + Disc/Field changes

Peripheral Iridectomy Indications
- Only treats pupil block
- PAC
  - Pupil block significant
- PACG
  - Pupil block significant
- PACS (absolute) + PAC/G in other eye
- PACS (relative)
  - Need repeated dilated fundus exam
  - Poor access to ophthalmic care
  - Family history of PACG

Risk Factors
- Middle-aged Asian female with glasses (hypermetropic) with blind mother

Treatment
- If cataract
  - Cataract surgery
- If clear lens
  - Laser YAG PI
- PI may not prevent progression
  - Follow-up

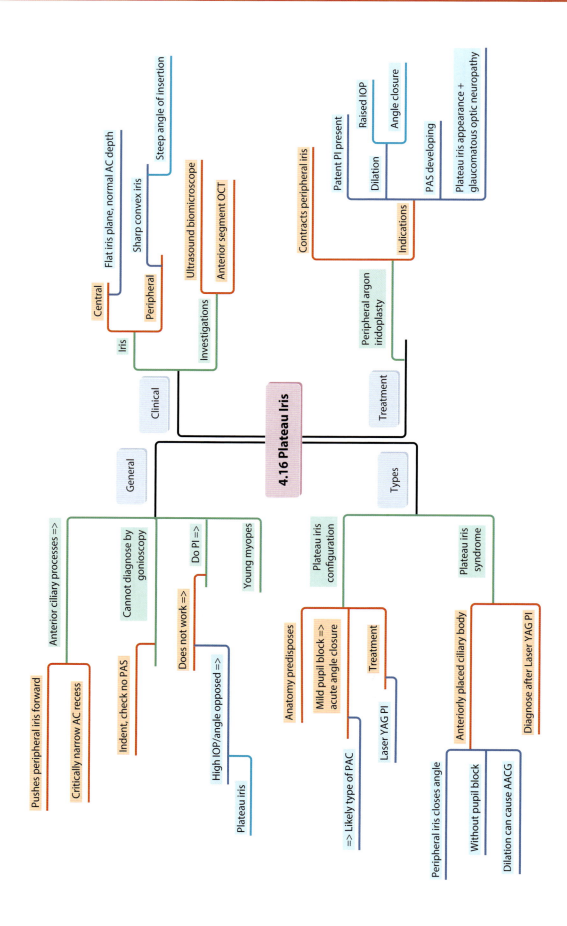

4.16 Plateau Iris

Clinical

Iris
- Central
  - Flat iris plane, normal AC depth
  - Sharp convex iris
  - Steep angle of insertion
- Peripheral

Investigations
- Ultrasound biomicroscope
- Anterior segment OCT

Treatment
- Peripheral argon iridoplasty
  - Contracts peripheral iris
  - Indications
    - Patent PI present
      - Dilation
        - Raised IOP
        - Angle closure
    - PAS developing
    - Plateau iris appearance + glaucomatous optic neuropathy

General

- Anterior ciliary processes =>
  - Pushes peripheral iris forward
  - Critically narrow AC recess
- Cannot diagnose by gonioscopy
  - Indent, check no PAS
- Do PI =>
  - Does not work =>
  - High IOP/angle opposed =>
    - Plateau iris
- Young myopes

Types

Plateau iris configuration
- Anatomy predisposes
- Mild pupil block => acute angle closure
  - => Likely type of PAC
- Treatment
  - Laser YAG PI

Plateau iris syndrome
- Anteriorly placed ciliary body
  - Peripheral iris closes angle
  - Without pupil block
  - Dilation can cause AACG
- Diagnose after Laser YAG PI

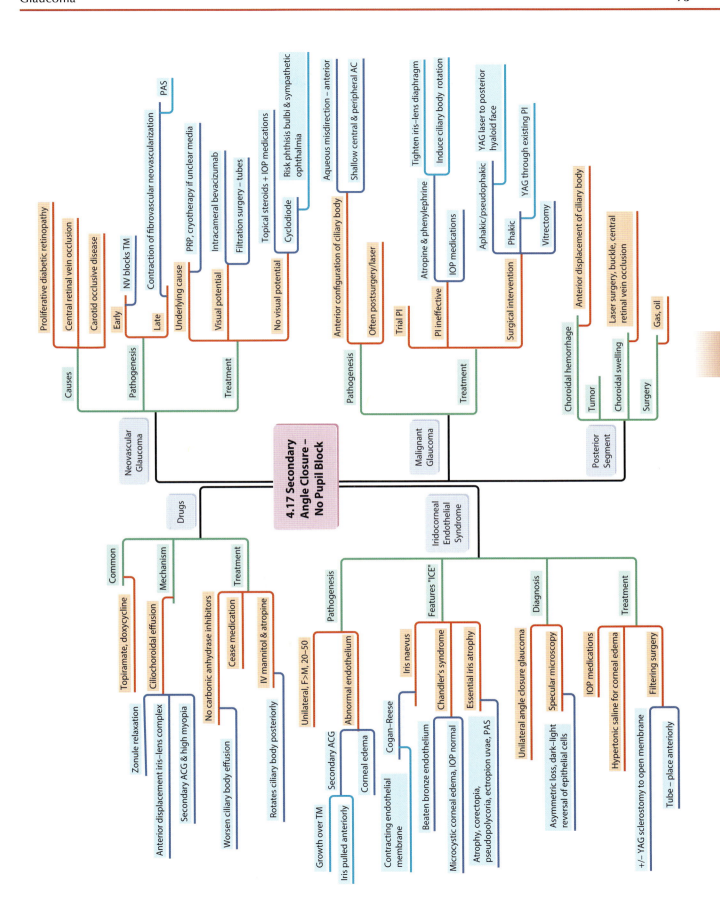

4.17 Secondary Angle Closure – No Pupil Block

Neovascular Glaucoma

Causes
- Proliferative diabetic retinopathy
- Central retinal vein occlusion
- Carotid occlusive disease

Pathogenesis
- Early
  - NV blocks TM
- Late
  - Contraction of fibrovascular neovascularization
    - PAS

Treatment
- Underlying cause
  - PRP, cryotherapy if unclear media
  - Intracameral bevacizumab
- Visual potential
  - Filtration surgery – tubes
  - Topical steroids + IOP medications
- No visual potential
  - Cyclodiode
  - Risk phthisis bulbi & sympathetic ophthalmia

Malignant Glaucoma

Pathogenesis
- Anterior configuration of ciliary body
  - Aqueous misdirection – anterior
  - Shallow central & peripheral AC
- Often postsurgery/laser

Treatment
- Trial PI
- PI ineffective
  - Atropine & phenylephrine
  - IOP medications
- Surgical intervention
  - Aphakic/pseudophakic
    - YAG laser to posterior hyaloid face
    - YAG through existing PI
  - Phakic
    - Tighten iris–lens diaphragm
    - Induce ciliary body rotation
  - Vitrectomy

Posterior Segment

- Choroidal hemorrhage
  - Anterior displacement of ciliary body
- Tumor
- Choroidal swelling
  - Laser surgery, buckle, central retinal vein occlusion
- Surgery
  - Gas, oil

Drugs

Common
- Topiramate, doxycycline
- Ciliochoroidal effusion

Mechanism
- Zonule relaxation
- Anterior displacement iris–lens complex
- Secondary ACG & high myopia
- No carbonic anhydrase inhibitors
- Worsen ciliary body effusion
- Rotates ciliary body posteriorly

Treatment
- Cease medication
- IV mannitol & atropine

Iridocorneal Endothelial Syndrome

Pathogenesis
- Unilateral, F>M, 20–50
- Abnormal endothelium
  - Growth over TM
  - Iris pulled anteriorly
  - Secondary ACG
  - Corneal edema
  - Contracting endothelial membrane

Features "ICE"
- Iris naevus
  - Cogan–Reese
  - Beaten bronze endothelium
- Chandler's syndrome
  - Microcystic corneal edema, IOP normal
- Essential iris atrophy
  - Atrophy, corectopia, pseudopolycoria, ectropion uvae, PAS

Diagnosis
- Unilateral angle closure glaucoma
- Specular microscopy
  - Asymmetric loss, dark–light reversal of epithelial cells

Treatment
- IOP medications
- Hypertonic saline for corneal edema
- Filtering surgery
  - +/– YAG sclerostomy to open membrane
  - Tube – place anteriorly

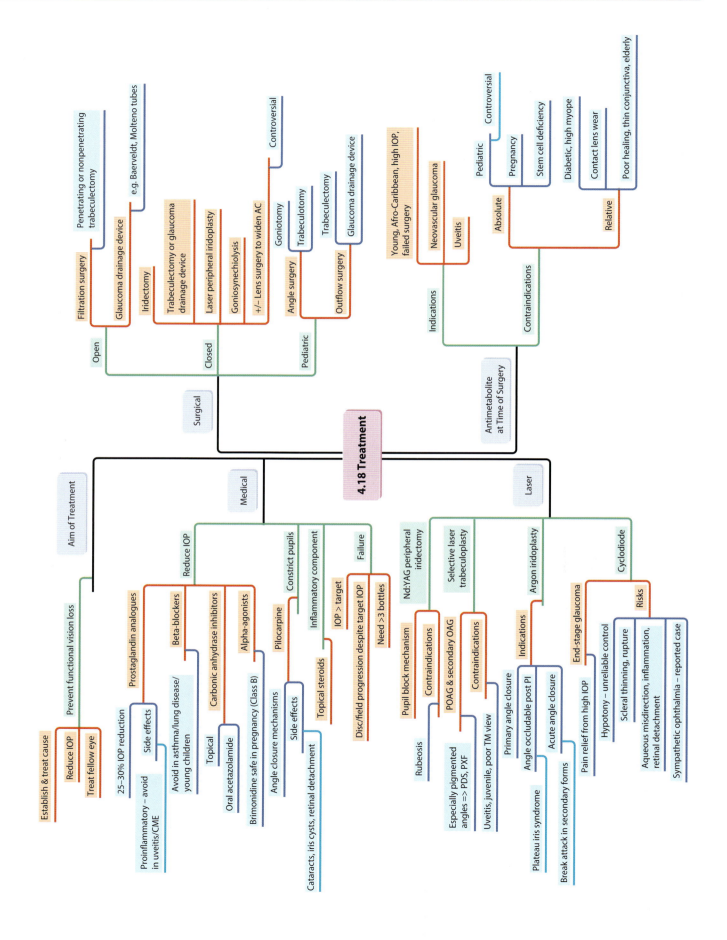

4.18 Treatment

Surgical

Open
- Filtration surgery
  - Penetrating or nonpenetrating trabeculectomy
- Glaucoma drainage device
  - e.g. Baerveldt, Molteno tubes

Closed
- Iridectomy
- Trabeculectomy or glaucoma drainage device
- Laser peripheral iridoplasty
- Goniosynechiolysis
- +/- Lens surgery to widen AC — Controversial

Pediatric
- Angle surgery
  - Goniotomy
  - Trabeculotomy
  - Trabeculectomy
- Outflow surgery
  - Glaucoma drainage device

Antimetabolite at Time of Surgery
- Indications
  - Young, Afro-Caribbean, high IOP, failed surgery
  - Neovascular glaucoma
  - Uveitis
- Contraindications
  - Absolute
    - Pediatric — Controversial
    - Pregnancy
    - Stem cell deficiency
  - Relative
    - Diabetic, high myope
    - Contact lens wear
    - Poor healing, thin conjunctiva, elderly

Aim of Treatment
- Prevent functional vision loss
- Establish & treat cause
- Reduce IOP
- Treat fellow eye

Medical

Reduce IOP
- Prostaglandin analogues
  - 25–30% IOP reduction
  - Side effects
    - Proinflammatory – avoid in uveitis/CME
- Beta-blockers
  - Avoid in asthma/lung disease/ young children
- Carbonic anhydrase inhibitors
  - Topical
  - Oral acetazolamide
- Alpha-agonists
  - Brimonidine safe in pregnancy (Class B)
- Pilocarpine
  - Angle closure mechanisms
  - Side effects
    - Cataracts, iris cysts, retinal detachment

Constrict pupils

Inflammatory component
- Topical steroids

Failure
- IOP > target
- Disc/field progression despite target IOP
- Need >3 bottles

Laser
- Nd:YAG peripheral iridectomy
  - Pupil block mechanism
  - Contraindications
    - Rubeosis
- Selective laser trabeculoplasty
  - POAG & secondary OAG
    - Especially pigmented angles => PDS, PXF
  - Contraindications
    - Uveitis, juvenile, poor TM view
- Argon iridoplasty
  - Indications
    - Primary angle closure
      - Angle occludable post PI
    - Acute angle closure
      - Plateau iris syndrome
      - Break attack in secondary forms
- Cyclodiode
  - End-stage glaucoma
    - Pain relief from high IOP
  - Risks
    - Hypotony – unreliable control
    - Scleral thinning, rupture
    - Aqueous misdirection, inflammation, retinal detachment
    - Sympathetic ophthalmia – reported case

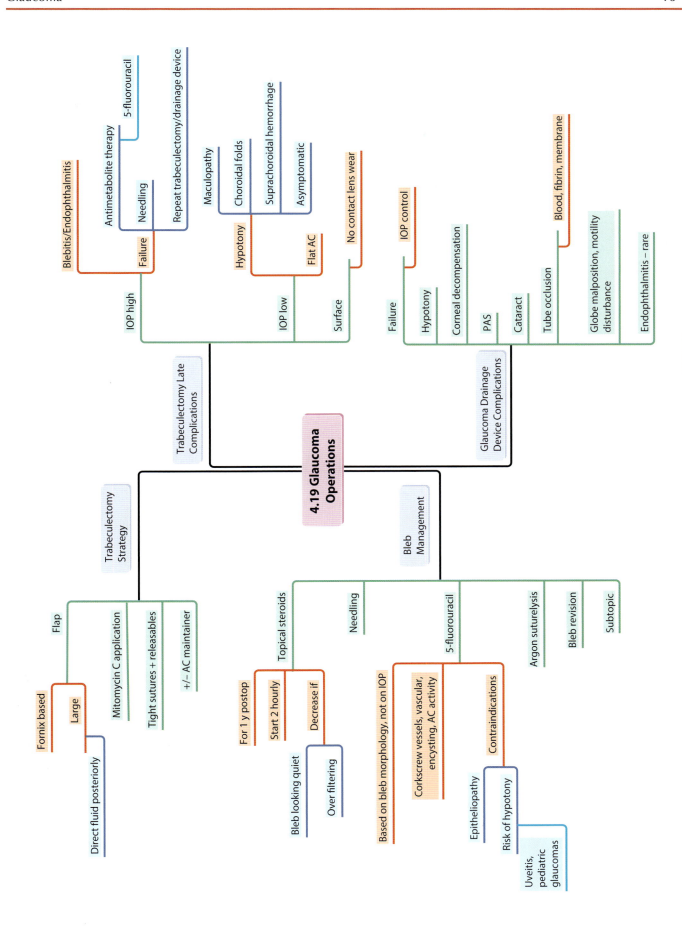

4.19 Glaucoma Operations

Trabeculectomy Late Complications

IOP high
- Blebitis/Endophthalmitis
- Failure
  - Antimetabolite therapy
    - 5-fluorouracil
  - Needling
  - Repeat trabeculectomy/drainage device

IOP low
- Maculopathy
- Hypotony
  - Choroidal folds
  - Suprachoroidal hemorrhage
  - Asymptomatic
- Flat AC

Surface
- No contact lens wear

Glaucoma Drainage Device Complications
- Failure
  - IOP control
- Hypotony
- Corneal decompensation
- PAS
- Cataract
- Tube occlusion
  - Blood, fibrin, membrane
- Globe malposition, motility disturbance
- Endophthalmitis – rare

Trabeculectomy Strategy

Flap
- Fornix based
- Large
  - Direct fluid posteriorly
- Mitomycin C application
- Tight sutures + releasables
- +/– AC maintainer

Bleb Management

Topical steroids
- For 1 y postop
- Start 2 hourly
- Decrease if
  - Bleb looking quiet
  - Over filtering

Needling

5-fluorouracil
- Based on bleb morphology, not on IOP
- Corkscrew vessels, vascular, encysting, AC activity
- Contraindications
  - Epitheliopathy
  - Risk of hypotony
    - Uveitis, pediatric glaucomas

Argon suturelysis

Bleb revision

Subtopic

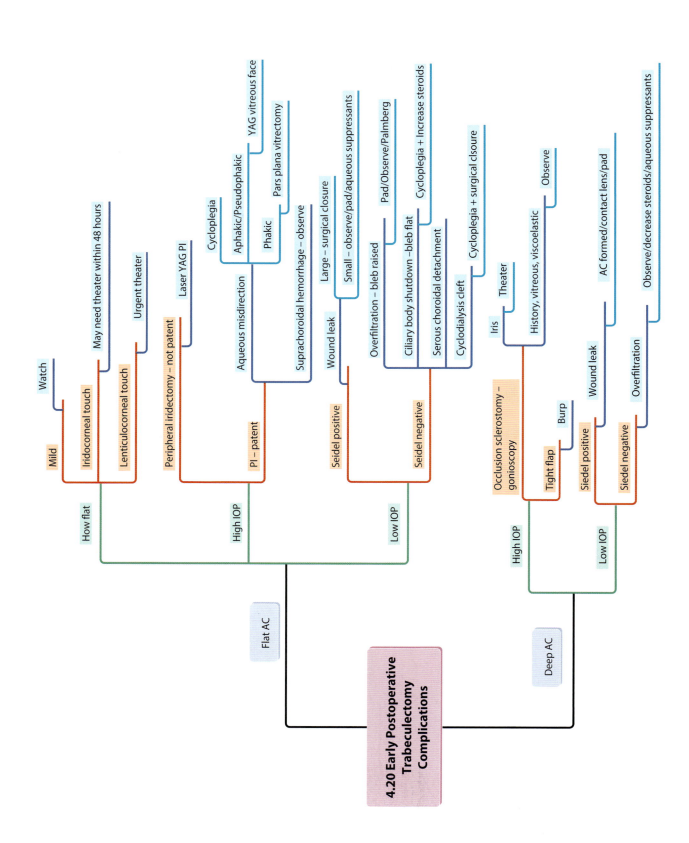

4.20 Early Postoperative Trabeculectomy Complications

Flat AC

How flat
- Mild
  - Watch
- Iridocorneal touch
  - May need theater within 48 hours
- Lenticulocorneal touch
  - Urgent theater

High IOP
- Peripheral iridectomy – not patent
  - Laser YAG PI
- PI – patent
  - Aqueous misdirection
    - Cycloplegia
    - Aphakic/Pseudophakic
      - YAG vitreous face
    - Phakic
      - Pars plana vitrectomy
  - Suprachoroidal hemorrhage – observe

Low IOP
- Seidel positive
  - Wound leak
    - Large – surgical closure
    - Small – observe/pad/aqueous suppressants
- Seidel negative
  - Overfiltration – bleb raised
    - Pad/Observe/Palmberg
  - Ciliary body shutdown – bleb flat
    - Cycloplegia + Increase steroids
  - Serous choroidal detachment
    - Cycloplegia + surgical clsoure
  - Cyclodialysis cleft
    - Cycloplegia + surgical clsoure

Deep AC

High IOP
- Occlusion sclerostomy – gonioscopy
  - Iris
    - Theater
  - History, vitreous, viscoelastic
    - Observe
- Tight flap
  - Burp

Low IOP
- Siedel positive
  - Wound leak
    - AC formed/contact lens/pad
- Siedel negative
  - Overfiltration
    - Observe/decrease steroids/aqueous suppressants

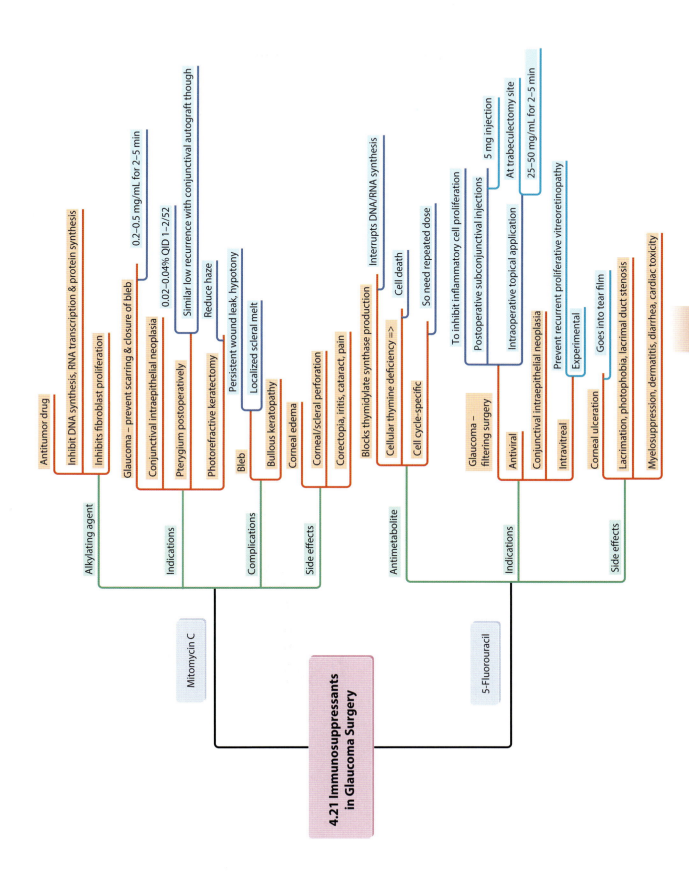

4.21 Immunosuppressants in Glaucoma Surgery

Mitomycin C

- Alkylating agent
  - Antitumor drug
  - Inhibit DNA synthesis, RNA transcription & protein synthesis
  - Inhibits fibroblast proliferation
- Indications
  - Glaucoma – prevent scarring & closure of bleb — 0.2–0.5 mg/mL for 2–5 min
  - Conjunctival intraepithelial neoplasia
  - Pterygium postoperatively — 0.02–0.04% QID 1–2/52
  - Photorefractive keratectomy
    - Similar low recurrence with conjunctival autograft though
    - Reduce haze
- Complications
  - Bleb
    - Persistent wound leak, hypotony
    - Localized scleral melt
  - Bullous keratopathy
  - Corneal edema
  - Corneal/scleral perforation
  - Corectopia, iritis, cataract, pain
- Side effects

5-Fluorouracil

- Antimetabolite
  - Blocks thymidylate synthase production
  - Interrupts DNA/RNA synthesis
  - Cellular thymine deficiency =>
    - Cell death
  - Cell cycle-specific
    - So need repeated dose
- Indications
  - Glaucoma – filtering surgery
    - To inhibit inflammatory cell proliferation
    - Postoperative subconjunctival injections — 5 mg injection
    - Intraoperative topical application — At trabeculectomy site — 25–50 mg/mL for 2–5 min
  - Antiviral
  - Conjunctival intraepithelial neoplasia
  - Intravitreal
    - Prevent recurrent proliferative vitreoretinopathy
    - Experimental
- Side effects
  - Corneal ulceration
    - Goes into tear film
  - Lacrimation, photophobia, lacrimal duct stenosis
  - Myelosuppression, dermatitis, diarrhea, cardiac toxicity

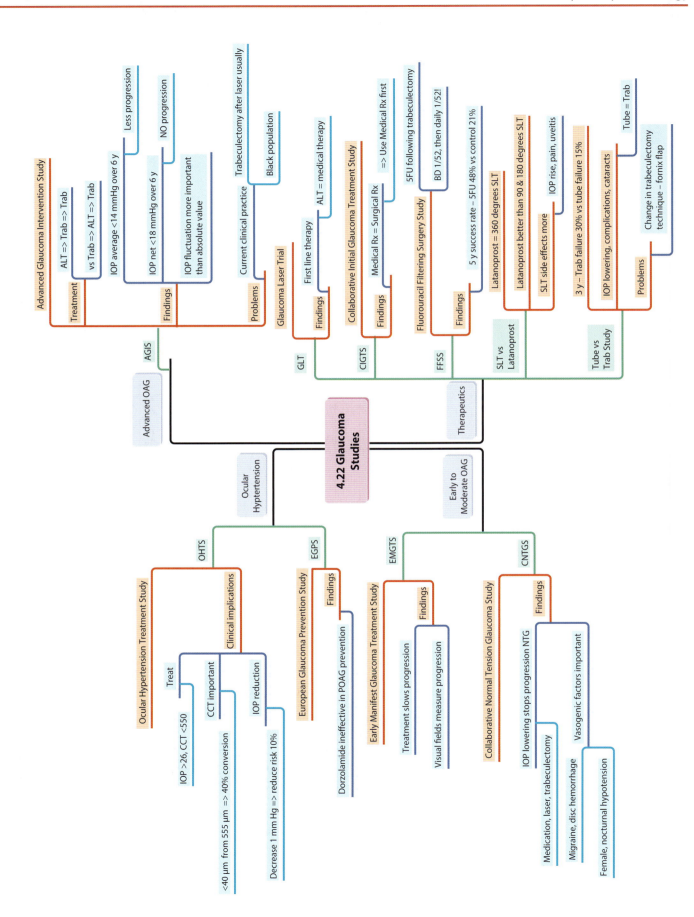

4.22 Glaucoma Studies

Advanced OAG

AGIS — Advanced Glaucoma Intervention Study
- Treatment
  - ALT => Trab => Trab
  - vs Trab => ALT => Trab
- Findings
  - IOP average <14 mmHg over 6 y
    - Less progression
    - NO progression
  - IOP net <18 mmHg over 6 y
  - IOP fluctuation more important than absolute value
- Problems
  - Current clinical practice
  - Trabeculectomy after laser usually
  - Black population

Therapeutics

GLT — Glaucoma Laser Trial
- Findings
  - First line therapy
  - ALT = medical therapy

CIGTS — Collaborative Initial Glaucoma Treatment Study
- Findings
  - Medical Rx = Surgical Rx
  - => Use Medical Rx first

FFSS — Fluorouracil Filtering Surgery Study
- Findings
  - 5FU following trabeculectomy
  - BD 1/52, then daily 1/52!
  - 5 y success rate – 5FU 48% vs control 21%

SLT vs Latanoprost
- Latanoprost = 360 degrees SLT
- Latanoprost better than 90 & 180 degrees SLT
- SLT side effects more
  - IOP rise, pain, uveitis

Tube vs Trab Study
- 3 y – Trab failure 30% vs tube failure 15%
- IOP lowering, complications, cataracts
- Problems
  - Tube = Trab
  - Change in trabeculectomy technique – fornix flap

Ocular Hypertension

OHTS — Ocular Hypertension Treatment Study
- Treat
  - IOP >26, CCT <550
- Clinical implications
  - CCT important
    - <40 μm from 555 μm => 40% conversion
  - IOP reduction
    - Decrease 1 mm Hg => reduce risk 10%

EGPS — European Glaucoma Prevention Study
- Findings
  - Dorzolamide ineffective in POAG prevention

Early to Moderate OAG

EMGTS — Early Manifest Glaucoma Treatment Study
- Findings
  - Treatment slows progression
  - Visual fields measure progression

CNTGS — Collaborative Normal Tension Glaucoma Study
- Findings
  - IOP lowering stops progression NTG
    - Medication, laser, trabeculectomy
  - Vasogenic factors important
    - Migraine, disc hemorrhage
    - Female, nocturnal hypotension

5 Neuro-Ophthalmology

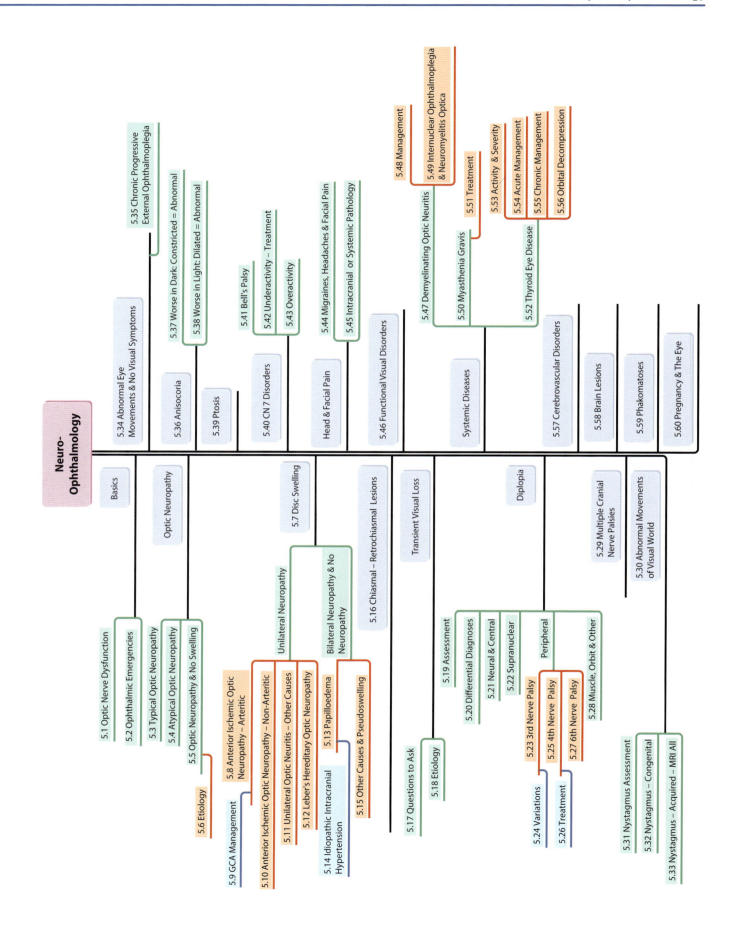

Neuro-Ophthalmology

Basics
- 5.1 Optic Nerve Dysfunction
- 5.2 Ophthalmic Emergencies

Optic Neuropathy
- 5.3 Typical Optic Neuropathy
- 5.4 Atypical Optic Neuropathy
- 5.5 Optic Neuropathy & No Swelling
  - 5.6 Etiology

Unilateral Neuropathy
- 5.8 Anterior Ischemic Optic Neuropathy – Arteritic
  - 5.9 GCA Management
- 5.10 Anterior Ischemic Optic Neuropathy – Non-Arteritic
- 5.11 Unilateral Optic Neuritis – Other Causes
- 5.12 Leber's Hereditary Optic Neuropathy

Bilateral Neuropathy & No Neuropathy
- 5.13 Papilloedema
- 5.14 Idiopathic Intracranial Hypertension
- 5.15 Other Causes & Pseudoswelling

5.7 Disc Swelling

5.16 Chiasmal – Retrochiasmal Lesions

Transient Visual Loss
- 5.17 Questions to Ask
- 5.18 Etiology

Diplopia
- 5.19 Assessment
- 5.20 Differential Diagnoses
- 5.21 Neural & Central
- 5.22 Supranuclear

Peripheral
- 5.23 3rd Nerve Palsy
  - 5.24 Variations
- 5.25 4th Nerve Palsy
  - 5.26 Treatment
- 5.27 6th Nerve Palsy
- 5.28 Muscle, Orbit & Other

5.29 Multiple Cranial Nerve Palsies

5.30 Abnormal Movements of Visual World
- 5.31 Nystagmus Assessment
- 5.32 Nystagmus – Congenital
- 5.33 Nystagmus – Acquired – MRI All

Abnormal Eye Movements & No Visual Symptoms
- 5.34 Abnormal Eye Movements & No Visual Symptoms
- 5.35 Chronic Progressive External Ophthalmoplegia

Anisocoria
- 5.36 Anisocoria
- 5.37 Worse in Dark: Constricted = Abnormal
- 5.38 Worse in Light: Dilated = Abnormal

Ptosis
- 5.39 Ptosis

CN 7 Disorders
- 5.40 CN 7 Disorders
- 5.41 Bell's Palsy
- 5.42 Underactivity – Treatment
- 5.43 Overactivity

Head & Facial Pain
- 5.44 Migraines, Headaches & Facial Pain
- 5.45 Intracranial or Systemic Pathology

Functional Visual Disorders
- 5.46 Functional Visual Disorders

5.47 Demyelinating Optic Neuritis
- 5.48 Management
- 5.49 Internuclear Ophthalmoplegia & Neuromyelitis Optica

Systemic Diseases
- 5.50 Myasthenia Gravis
  - 5.51 Treatment
- 5.52 Thyroid Eye Disease
  - 5.53 Activity & Severity
  - 5.54 Acute Management
  - 5.55 Chronic Management
  - 5.56 Orbital Decompression

Cerebrovascular Disorders
- 5.57 Cerebrovascular Disorders

5.58 Brain Lesions

5.59 Phakomatoses

5.60 Pregnancy & The Eye

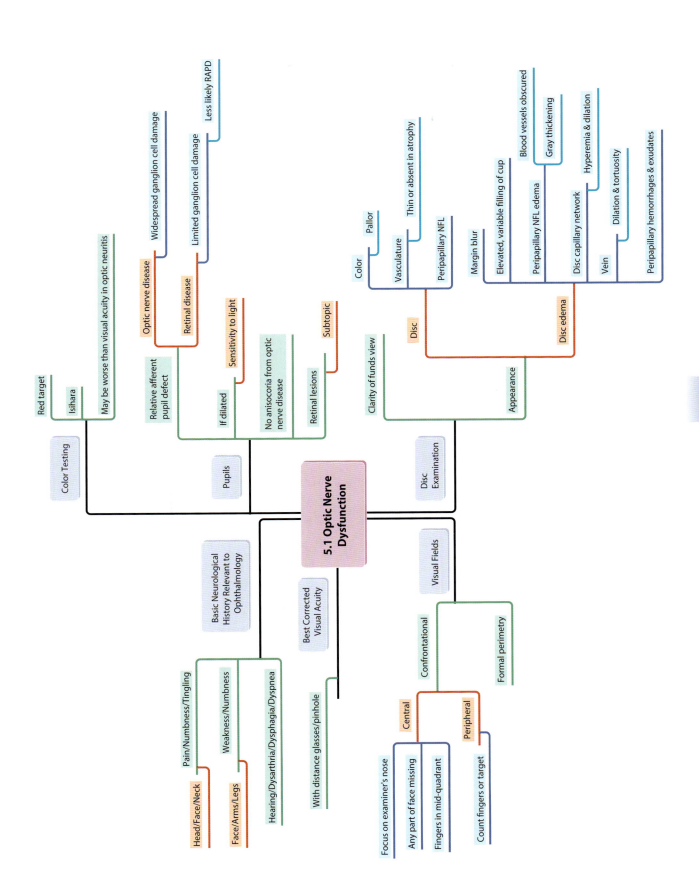

5.1 Optic Nerve Dysfunction

Color Testing
- Red target
- Isihara
- May be worse than visual acuity in optic neuritis

Pupils
- Relative afferent pupil defect
  - Optic nerve disease
    - Widespread ganglion cell damage
    - Limited ganglion cell damage
      - Less likely RAPD
  - Retinal disease
- Sensitivity to light
  - If dilated
- No anisocoria from optic nerve disease
- Retinal lesions
  - Subtopic

Disc Examination
- Clarity of funds view
- Appearance
  - Disc
    - Color
      - Pallor
    - Vasculature
      - Thin or absent in atrophy
    - Peripapillary NFL
  - Disc edema
    - Margin blur
    - Elevated, variable filling of cup
    - Peripapillary NFL edema
      - Blood vessels obscured
      - Gray thickening
    - Disc capillary network
      - Hyperemia & dilation
    - Vein
      - Dilation & tortuosity
    - Peripapillary hemorrhages & exudates

Basic Neurological History Relevant to Ophthalmology
- Pain/Numbness/Tingling
  - Head/Face/Neck
- Weakness/Numbness
  - Face/Arms/Legs
- Hearing/Dysarthria/Dysphagia/Dyspnea

Best Corrected Visual Acuity
- With distance glasses/pinhole

Visual Fields
- Confrontational
  - Central
    - Focus on examiner's nose
    - Any part of face missing
    - Fingers in mid-quadrant
  - Peripheral
    - Count fingers or target
- Formal perimetry

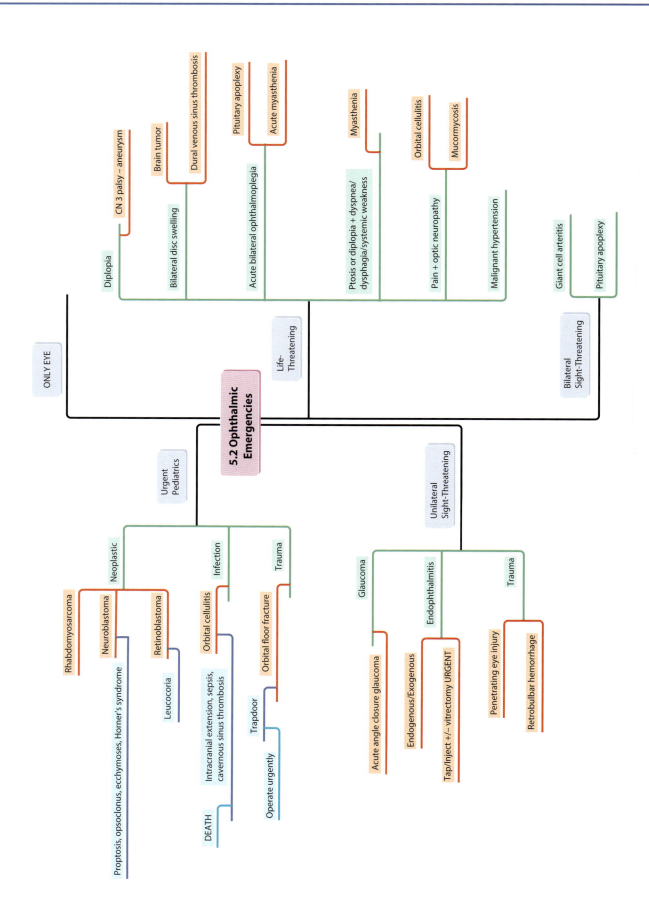

5.2 Ophthalmic Emergencies

ONLY EYE

Diplopia
- CN 3 palsy – aneurysm
- Brain tumor

Bilateral disc swelling
- Dural venous sinus thrombosis

Acute bilateral ophthalmoplegia
- Pituitary apoplexy
- Acute myasthenia

Life-Threatening

Ptosis or diplopia + dyspnea/dysphagia/systemic weakness
- Myasthenia

Pain + optic neuropathy
- Orbital cellulitis
- Mucormycosis

Malignant hypertension

Bilateral Sight-Threatening

Giant cell arteritis

Pituitary apoplexy

Urgent Pediatrics

Neoplastic
- Rhabdomyosarcoma
- Neuroblastoma — Proptosis, opsoclonus, ecchymoses, Horner's syndrome
- Retinoblastoma — Leucocoria

Infection
- Orbital cellulitis — Intracranial extension, sepsis, cavernous sinus thrombosis — DEATH

Trauma
- Orbital floor fracture — Trapdoor — Operate urgently

Unilateral Sight-Threatening

Glaucoma
- Acute angle closure glaucoma

Endophthalmitis
- Endogenous/Exogenous
- Tap/Inject +/− vitrectomy URGENT

Trauma
- Penetrating eye injury
- Retrobulbar hemorrhage

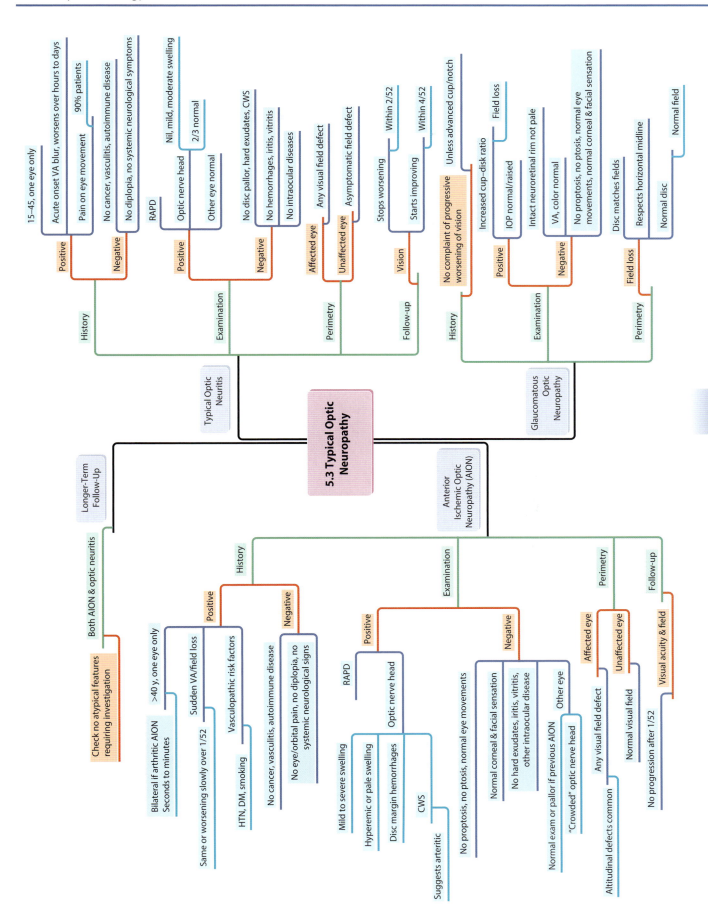

5.3 Typical Optic Neuropathy

Typical Optic Neuritis

History
- Positive
  - 15–45, one eye only
  - Acute onset VA blur, worsens over hours to days
  - Pain on eye movement — 90% patients
- Negative
  - No cancer, vasculitis, autoimmune disease
  - No diplopia, no systemic neurological symptoms

Examination
- Positive
  - RAPD
  - Optic nerve head — Nil, mild, moderate swelling — 2/3 normal
  - Other eye normal
- Negative
  - No disc pallor, hard exudates, CWS
  - No hemorrhages, iritis, vitritis
  - No intraocular diseases

Perimetry
- Affected eye — Any visual field defect
- Unaffected eye — Asymptomatic field defect

Follow-up
- Vision
  - Stops worsening — Within 2/52
  - Starts improving — Within 4/52

Glaucomatous Optic Neuropathy

History
- No complaint of progressive worsening of vision — Unless advanced cup/notch

Examination
- Positive
  - Increased cup–disk ratio — Field loss
  - IOP normal/raised
- Negative
  - Intact neuroretinal rim not pale
  - VA, color normal
  - No proptosis, no ptosis, normal eye movements, normal corneal & facial sensation

Perimetry
- Field loss
  - Disc matches fields
  - Respects horizontal midline
- Normal disc — Normal field

Anterior Ischemic Optic Neuropathy (AION)

History
- Positive
  - >40 y, one eye only
  - Bilateral if arthritic AION
  - Seconds to minutes
  - Same or worsening slowly over 1/52
  - Sudden VA/field loss
  - Vasculopathic risk factors — HTN, DM, smoking
- Negative
  - No cancer, vasculitis, autoimmune disease
  - No eye/orbital pain, no diplopia, no systemic neurological signs

Examination
- Positive
  - RAPD
  - Optic nerve head
    - Mild to severe swelling
    - Hyperemic or pale swelling
    - Disc margin hemorrhages
    - CWS — Suggests arteritic
- Negative
  - No proptosis, no ptosis, normal eye movements
  - Normal corneal & facial sensation
  - No hard exudates, iritis, vitritis, other intraocular disease
  - Other eye
    - Normal exam or pallor if previous AION
    - "Crowded" optic nerve head

Perimetry
- Affected eye — Any visual field defect — Altitudinal defects common
- Unaffected eye — Normal visual field

Follow-up
- Visual acuity & field — No progression after 1/52

Longer-Term Follow-Up
- Both AION & optic neuritis — Check no atypical features requiring investigation

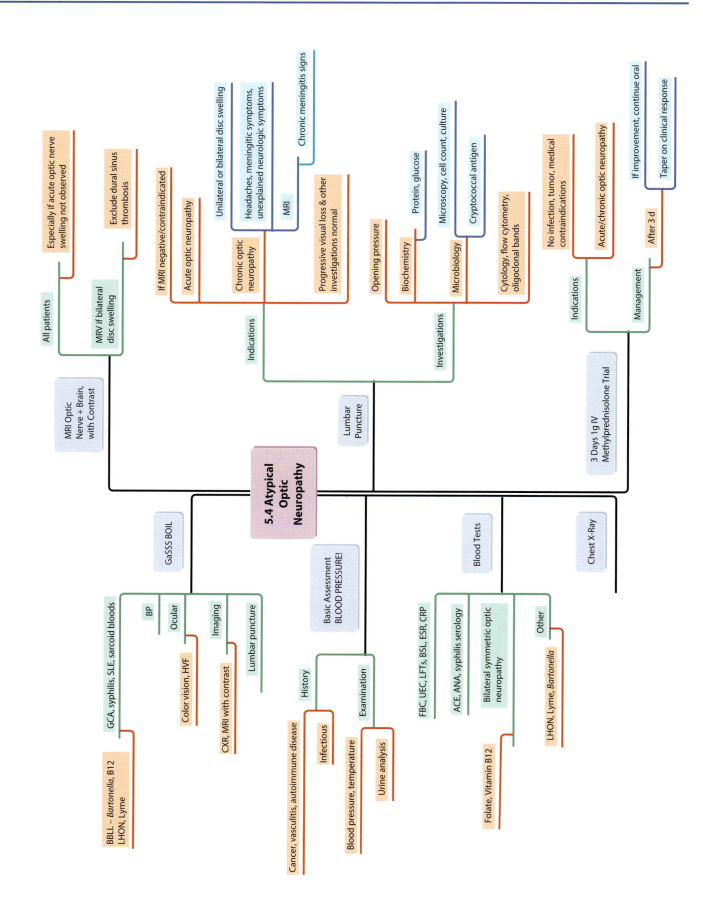

5.4 Atypical Optic Neuropathy

MRI Optic Nerve + Brain, with Contrast
- All patients
  - Especially if acute optic nerve swelling not observed
- MRV if bilateral disc swelling
  - Exclude dural sinus thrombosis

Lumbar Puncture
- Indications
  - Acute optic neuropathy
    - If MRI negative/contraindicated
  - Chronic optic neuropathy
    - Unilateral or bilateral disc swelling
    - Headaches, meningitic symptoms, unexplained neurologic symptoms
    - MRI
    - Chronic meningitis signs
  - Progressive visual loss & other investigations normal
- Investigations
  - Opening pressure
  - Biochemistry
    - Protein, glucose
  - Microbiology
    - Microscopy, cell count, culture
    - Cryptococcal antigen
  - Cytology, flow cytometry, oligoclonal bands

3 Days 1g IV Methylprednisolone Trial
- Indications
  - No infection, tumor, medical contraindications
  - Acute/chronic optic neuropathy
- Management
  - After 3 d
    - If improvement, continue oral
    - Taper on clinical response

GaSSS BOIL
- GCA, syphilis, SLE, sarcoid bloods
  - BBLL – *Bartonella*, B12 LHON, Lyme
- BP
- Ocular
  - Color vision, HVF
- Imaging
  - CXR, MRI with contrast
- Lumbar puncture

Basic Assessment BLOOD PRESSURE!
- History
  - Infectious
  - Cancer, vasculitis, autoimmune disease
- Examination
  - Blood pressure, temperature
  - Urine analysis

Blood Tests
- FBC, UEC, LFTs, BSL, ESR, CRP
- ACE, ANA, syphilis serology
- Bilateral symmetric optic neuropathy
  - Folate, Vitamin B12
- Other
  - LHON, Lyme, *Bartonella*

Chest X-Ray

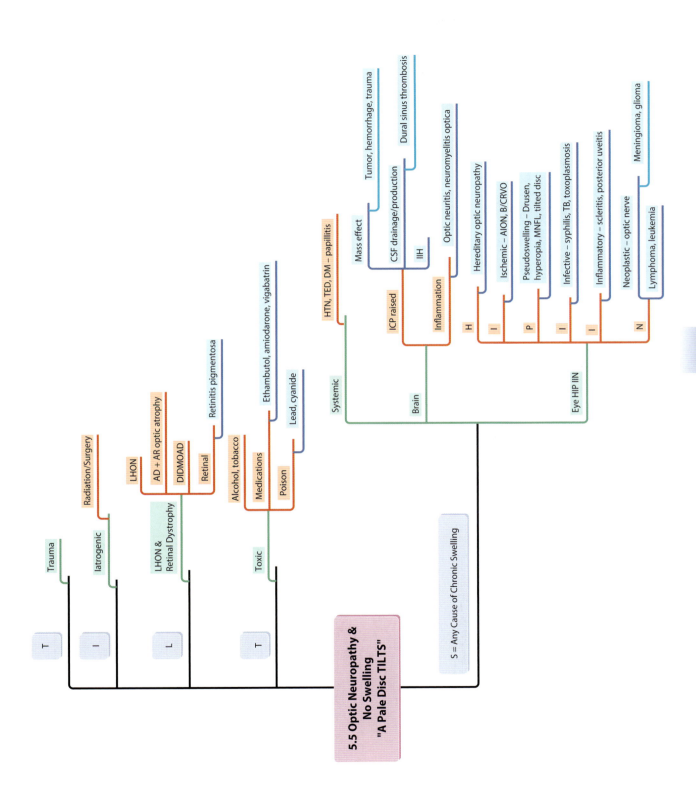

5.5 Optic Neuropathy & No Swelling "A Pale Disc TILTS"

T

- Trauma
- Iatrogenic
  - Radiation/Surgery

I

L — LHON & Retinal Dystrophy
- LHON
- AD + AR optic atrophy
- DIDMOAD
- Retinal
  - Retinitis pigmentosa

T — Toxic
- Alcohol, tobacco
- Medications
  - Ethambutol, amiodarone, vigabatrin
- Poison
  - Lead, cyanide

S = Any Cause of Chronic Swelling

Systemic
- HTN, TED, DM – papillitis

Brain
- ICP raised
  - Mass effect
    - Tumor, hemorrhage, trauma
  - CSF drainage/production
    - Dural sinus thrombosis
  - IIH
- Inflammation
  - Optic neuritis, neuromyelitis optica

Eye HIP IIN
- H — Hereditary optic neuropathy
- I — Ischemic – AION, B/CRVO
- P — Pseudoswelling – Drusen, hyperopia, MNFL, tilted disc
- I — Infective – syphilis, TB, toxoplasmosis
- I — Inflammatory – scleritis, posterior uveitis
- N — Neoplastic – optic nerve
  - Meningioma, glioma
  - Lymphoma, leukemia

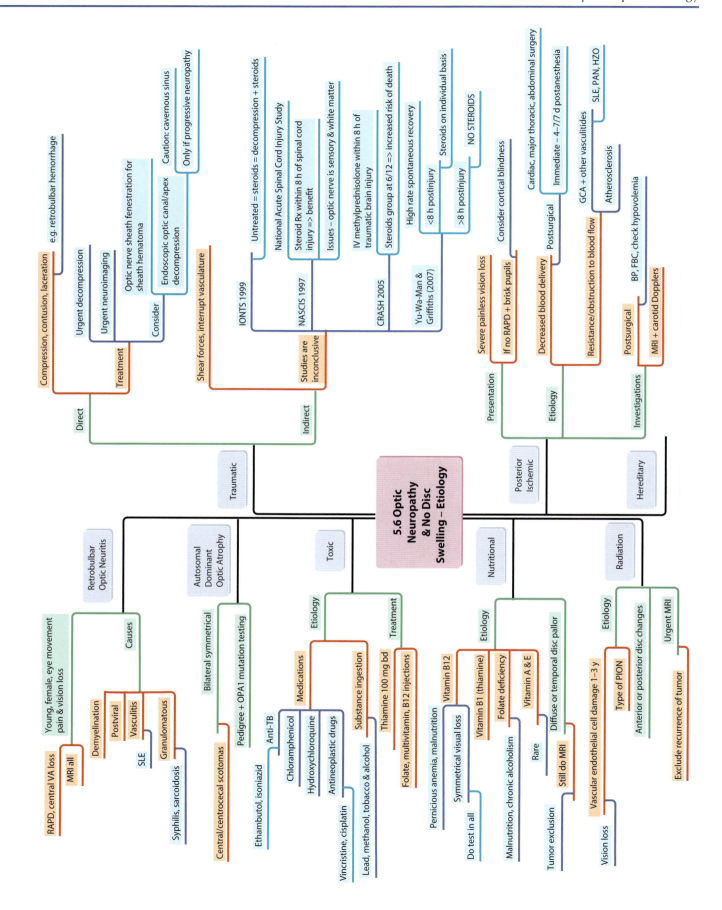

5.6 Optic Neuropathy & No Disc Swelling – Etiology

Traumatic

Direct
- Compression, contusion, laceration — e.g. retrobulbar hemorrhage
- Treatment
  - Urgent decompression
  - Urgent neuroimaging
  - Consider
    - Optic nerve sheath fenestration for sheath hematoma
    - Endoscopic optic canal/apex decompression — Caution: cavernous sinus
      - Only if progressive neuropathy

Indirect
- Shear forces, interrupt vasculature
- Studies are inconclusive
  - IONTS 1999
    - Untreated = steroids = decompression + steroids
  - NASCIS 1997 — National Acute Spinal Cord Injury Study
    - Steroid Rx within 8 h of spinal cord injury => benefit
    - Issues – optic nerve is sensory & white matter
  - CRASH 2005
    - IV methylprednisolone within 8 h of traumatic brain injury
    - Steroids group at 6/12 => increased risk of death
    - High rate spontaneous recovery
  - Yu-Wa-Man & Griffiths (2007)
    - <8 h postinjury — Steroids on individual basis
    - >8 h postinjury — NO STEROIDS

Posterior Ischemic
- Presentation
  - Severe painless vision loss
  - If no RAPD + brisk pupils — Consider cortical blindness
- Etiology
  - Decreased blood delivery
    - Postsurgical — Cardiac, major thoracic, abdominal surgery
    - Immediate – 4–7/7 d postanesthesia
  - Resistance/obstruction to blood flow
    - GCA + other vasculitides — SLE, PAN, HZO
    - Atherosclerosis
- Investigations
  - Postsurgical — BP, FBC, check hypovolemia
  - MRI + carotid Dopplers

Retrobulbar Optic Neuritis
- Young, female, eye movement pain & vision loss
  - RAPD, central VA loss
  - MRI all
- Causes
  - Demyelination
  - Postviral
  - Vasculitis — SLE
  - Granulomatous — Syphilis, sarcoidosis

Autosomal Dominant Optic Atrophy
- Bilateral symmetrical
  - Central/centrocecal scotomas
  - Pedigree + OPA1 mutation testing

Toxic
- Etiology
  - Medications
    - Anti-TB — Ethambutol, isoniazid
    - Chloramphenicol
    - Hydroxychloroquine
    - Antineoplastic drugs — Vincristine, cisplatin
  - Substance ingestion — Lead, methanol, tobacco & alcohol
- Treatment
  - Thiamine 100 mg bd
  - Folate, multivitamin, B12 injections

Nutritional
- Etiology
  - Vitamin B12 — Pernicious anemia, malnutrition
  - Vitamin B1 (thiamine) — Symmetrical visual loss
    - Malnutrition, chronic alcoholism
    - Do test in all
  - Folate deficiency
  - Vitamin A & E — Rare
  - Diffuse or temporal disc pallor
    - Tumor exclusion
    - Still do MRI

Radiation
- Etiology
  - Vascular endothelial cell damage 1–3 y
    - Vision loss
  - Type of PION
  - Anterior or posterior disc changes
- Urgent MRI — Exclude recurrence of tumor

Hereditary

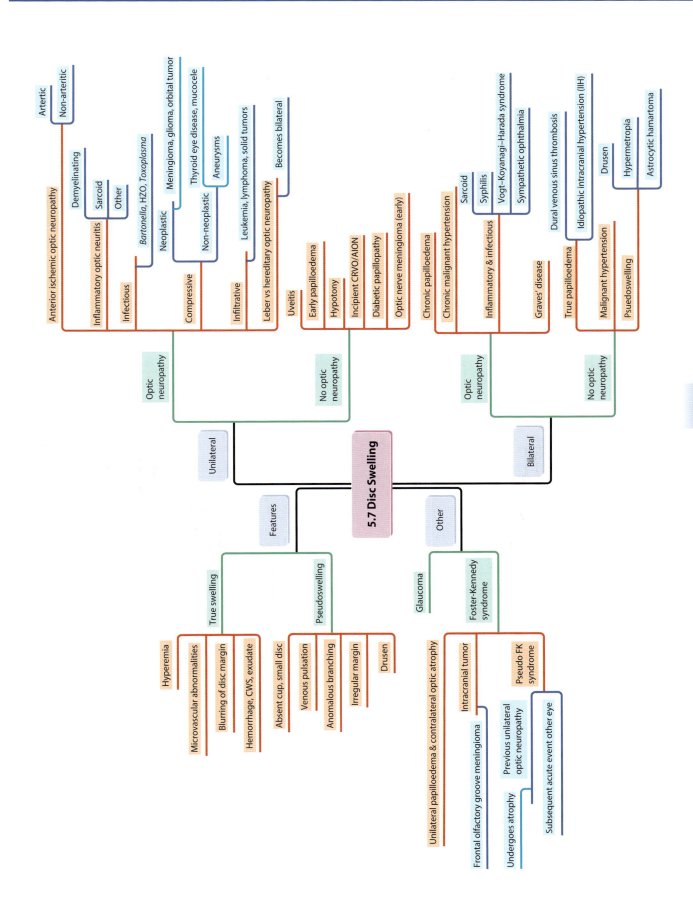

5.7 Disc Swelling

Unilateral

Optic neuropathy
- Anterior ischemic optic neuropathy
  - Arteritic
  - Non-arteritic
- Inflammatory optic neuritis
  - Demyelinating
  - Sarcoid
  - Other
- Infectious
  - Bartonella, HZO, Toxoplasma
- Compressive
  - Neoplastic
    - Meningioma, glioma, orbital tumor
    - Thyroid eye disease, mucocele
  - Non-neoplastic
    - Aneurysms
- Infiltrative
  - Leukemia, lymphoma, solid tumors
- Leber vs hereditary optic neuropathy
  - Becomes bilateral

No optic neuropathy
- Uveitis
- Early papilloedema
- Hypotony
- Incipient CRVO/AION
- Diabetic papillopathy
- Optic nerve meningioma (early)

Bilateral

Optic neuropathy
- Chronic papilloedema
- Chronic malignant hypertension
- Inflammatory & infectious
  - Sarcoid
  - Syphilis
  - Vogt–Koyanagi–Harada syndrome
  - Sympathetic ophthalmia
- Graves' disease

No optic neuropathy
- True papilloedema
  - Dural venous sinus thrombosis
  - Idiopathic intracranial hypertension (IIH)
- Malignant hypertension
- Psuedoswelling
  - Drusen
  - Hypermetropia
  - Astrocytic hamartoma

Features

True swelling
- Hyperemia
- Microvascular abnormalities
- Blurring of disc margin
- Hemorrhage, CWS, exudate

Pseudoswelling
- Absent cup, small disc
- Venous pulsation
- Anomalous branching
- Irregular margin
- Drusen

Other

Glaucoma

Foster-Kennedy syndrome
- Unilateral papilloedema & contralateral optic atrophy
- Intracranial tumor
  - Frontal olfactory groove meningioma
- Pseudo FK syndrome
  - Previous unilateral optic neuropathy
    - Undergoes atrophy
  - Subsequent acute event other eye

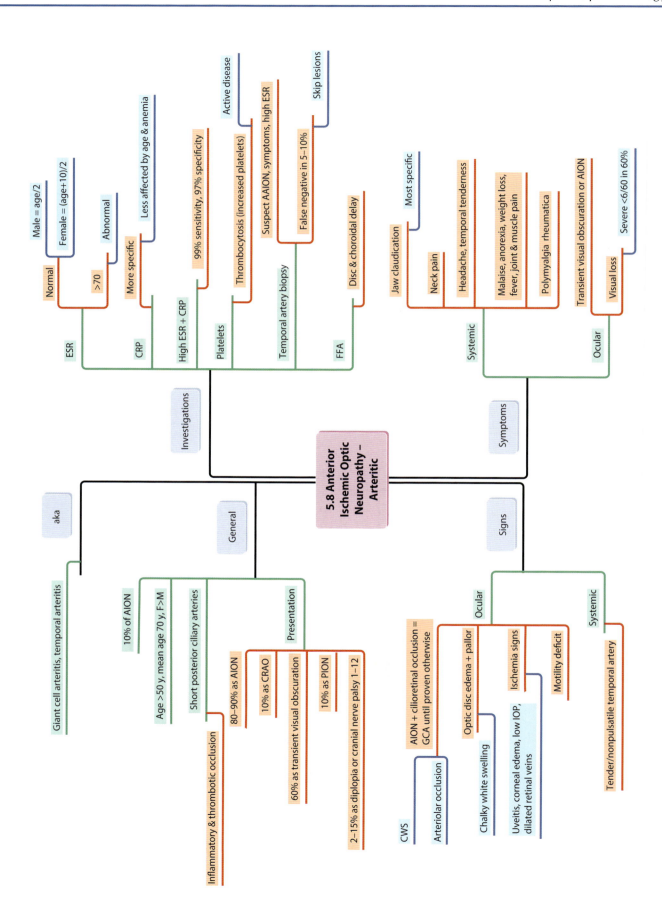

5.8 Anterior Ischemic Optic Neuropathy – Arteritic

Investigations

ESR
- Normal
  - Male = age/2
  - Female = (age+10)/2
- Abnormal
  - >70
- More specific
  - Less affected by age & anemia

CRP
- 99% sensitivity, 97% specificity

High ESR + CRP

Platelets
- Thrombocytosis (increased platelets)

Temporal artery biopsy
- Active disease
- Suspect AAION, symptoms, high ESR
- False negative in 5–10%
- Skip lesions

FFA
- Disc & choroidal delay

Symptoms

Systemic
- Jaw claudication
  - Most specific
- Neck pain
- Headache, temporal tenderness
- Malaise, anorexia, weight loss, fever, joint & muscle pain
- Polymyalgia rheumatica

Ocular
- Transient visual obscuration or AION
- Visual loss
  - Severe <6/60 in 60%

aka
- Giant cell arteritis, temporal arteritis

General
- 10% of AION
- Age >50 y, mean age 70 y, F>M
- Short posterior ciliary arteries
- Inflammatory & thrombotic occlusion
- Presentation
  - 80–90% as AION
  - 10% as CRAO
  - 60% as transient visual obscuration
  - 10% as PION
  - 2–15% as diplopia or cranial nerve palsy 1–12

Signs

Ocular
- AION + cilioretinal occlusion = GCA until proven otherwise
- Optic disc edema + pallor
  - CWS
  - Arteriolar occlusion
  - Chalky white swelling
- Ischemia signs
  - Uveitis, corneal edema, low IOP, dilated retinal veins
- Motility deficit

Systemic
- Tender/nonpulsatile temporal artery

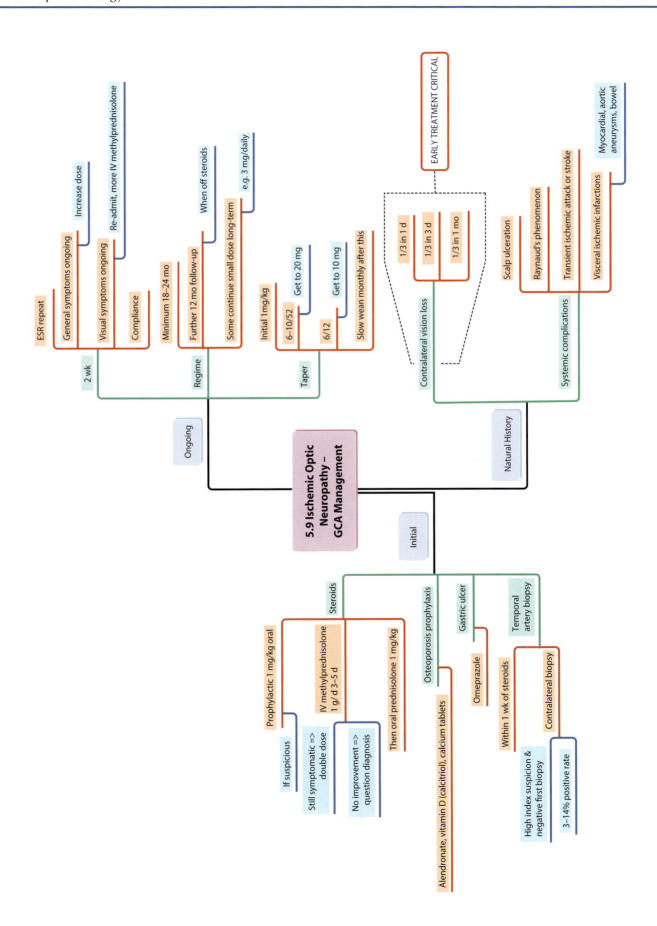

5.9 Ischemic Optic Neuropathy – GCA Management

Ongoing

2 wk
- ESR repeat
- General symptoms ongoing → Increase dose
- Visual symptoms ongoing → Re-admit, more IV methylprednisolone
- Compliance

Regime
- Minimum 18–24 mo
- Further 12 mo follow-up — When off steroids
- Some continue small dose long-term — e.g. 3 mg/daily

Taper
- Initial 1 mg/kg
- 6–10/52 — Get to 20 mg
- 6/12 — Get to 10 mg
- Slow wean monthly after this

Natural History

Contralateral vision loss
- 1/3 in 1 d
- 1/3 in 3 d
- 1/3 in 1 mo
→ EARLY TREATMENT CRITICAL

Systemic complications
- Scalp ulceration
- Raynaud's phenomenon
- Transient ischemic attack or stroke
- Visceral ischemic infarctions → Myocardial, aortic aneurysms, bowel

Initial

Steroids
- Prophylactic 1 mg/kg oral — If suspicious
- IV methylprednisolone 1 g/d 3–5 d
  - Still symptomatic => double dose
  - No improvement => question diagnosis
- Then oral prednisolone 1 mg/kg

Osteoporosis prophylaxis
- Alendronate, vitamin D (calcitriol), calcium tablets

Gastric ulcer
- Omeprazole

Temporal artery biopsy
- Within 1 wk of steroids
- Contralateral biopsy
  - High index suspicion & negative first biopsy
  - 3–14% positive rate

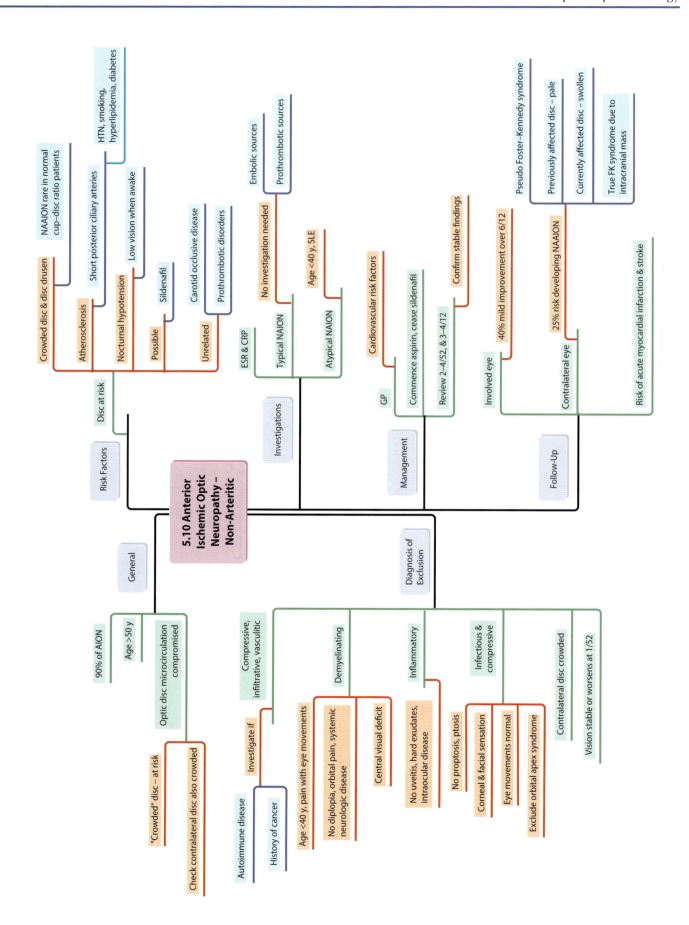

5.10 Anterior Ischemic Optic Neuropathy – Non-Arteritic

Risk Factors

Disc at risk
- Crowded disc & disc drusen
  - NAAION rare in normal cup–disc ratio patients
- Atherosclerosis
  - Short posterior ciliary arteries
  - HTN, smoking, hyperlipidemia, diabetes
- Nocturnal hypotension
  - Low vision when awake
- Possible
  - Sildenafil
- Unrelated
  - Carotid occlusive disease
  - Prothrombotic disorders

Investigations

- ESR & CRP
- Typical NAION
  - Embolic sources
  - Prothrombotic sources
  - No investigation needed
- Atypical NAION
  - Age <40 y, SLE

Management

- GP
  - Cardiovascular risk factors
- Commence aspirin, cease sildenafil
- Review 2–4/52, & 3–4/12
  - Confirm stable findings

Follow-Up

- Involved eye
  - 40% mild improvement over 6/12
- Contralateral eye
  - 25% risk developing NAAION
- Risk of acute myocardial infarction & stroke

- Pseudo Foster–Kennedy syndrome
  - Previously affected disc – pale
  - Currently affected disc – swollen
  - True FK syndrome due to intracranial mass

General

- 90% of AION
- Age >50 y
- Optic disc microcirculation compromised
  - "Crowded" disc – at risk
  - Check contralateral disc also crowded

Diagnosis of Exclusion

- Compressive, infiltrative, vasculitic
  - Investigate if
    - Autoimmune disease
    - History of cancer
- Demyelinating
  - Age <40 y, pain with eye movements
  - No diplopia, orbital pain, systemic neurologic disease
  - Central visual deficit
- Inflammatory
  - No uveitis, hard exudates, intraocular disease
- Infectious & compressive
  - No proptosis, ptosis
  - Corneal & facial sensation
  - Eye movements normal
  - Exclude orbital apex syndrome
  - Contralateral disc crowded
  - Vision stable or worsens at 1/52

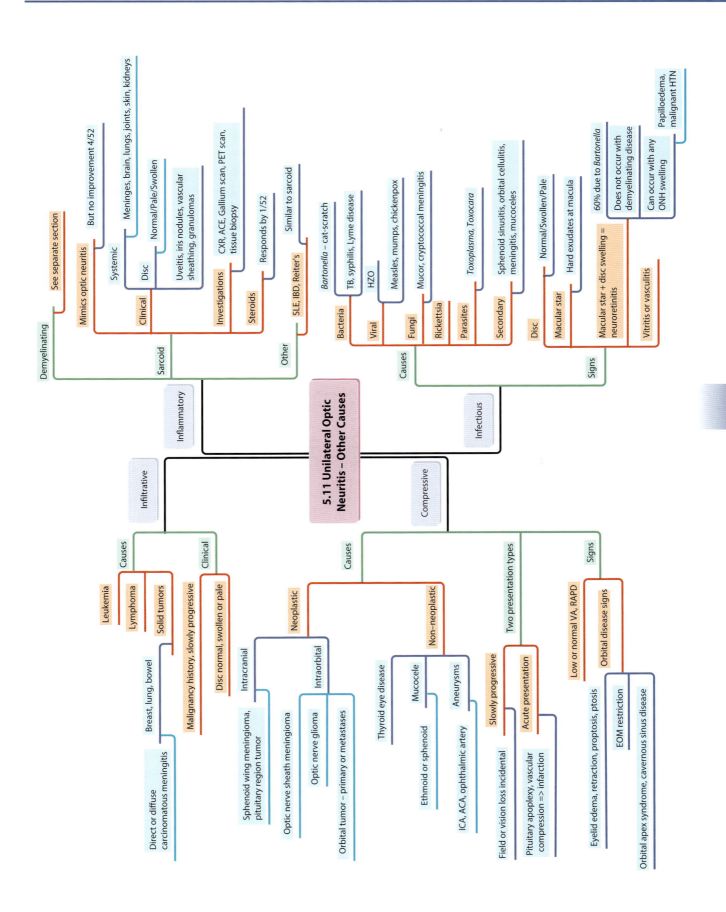

5.11 Unilateral Optic Neuritis – Other Causes

Inflammatory
- Demyelinating
  - See separate section
- Sarcoid
  - Mimics optic neuritis
    - But no improvement 4/52
  - Clinical
    - Systemic
      - Meninges, brain, lungs, joints, skin, kidneys
    - Disc
      - Normal/Pale/Swollen
    - Uveitis, iris nodules, vascular sheathing, granulomas
  - Investigations
    - CXR, ACE, Gallium scan, PET scan, tissue biopsy
  - Steroids
    - Responds by 1/52
- Other
  - SLE, IBD, Reiter's
    - Similar to sarcoid

Infectious
- Causes
  - Bacteria
    - *Bartonella* – cat-scratch
    - TB, syphilis, Lyme disease
  - Viral
    - HZO
    - Measles, mumps, chickenpox
  - Fungi
    - Mucor, cryptococcal meningitis
  - Rickettsia
  - Parasites
    - *Toxoplasma, Toxocara*
  - Secondary
    - Sphenoid sinusitis, orbital cellulitis, meningitis, mucoceles
- Signs
  - Disc
    - Normal/Swollen/Pale
  - Macular star
    - Hard exudates at macula
  - Macular star + disc swelling = neuroretinitis
    - 60% due to *Bartonella*
    - Does not occur with demyelinating disease
    - Can occur with any ONH swelling
      - Papilloedema, malignant HTN
  - Vitritis or vasculitis

Infiltrative
- Causes
  - Leukemia
  - Lymphoma
  - Solid tumors
    - Breast, lung, bowel
    - Direct or diffuse carcinomatous meningitis
- Clinical
  - Malignancy history, slowly progressive
  - Disc normal, swollen or pale

Compressive
- Causes
  - Neoplastic
    - Intracranial
      - Sphenoid wing meningioma, pituitary region tumor
      - Optic nerve sheath meningioma
    - Intraorbital
      - Optic nerve glioma
      - Orbital tumor – primary or metastases
  - Non-neoplastic
    - Thyroid eye disease
    - Mucocele
      - Ethmoid or sphenoid
    - Aneurysms
      - ICA, ACA, ophthalmic artery
- Two presentation types
  - Slowly progressive
    - Field or vision loss incidental
  - Acute presentation
    - Pituitary apoplexy, vascular compression => infarction
- Signs
  - Low or normal VA, RAPD
  - Orbital disease signs
    - Eyelid edema, retraction, proptosis, ptosis
    - EOM restriction
    - Orbital apex syndrome, cavernous sinus disease

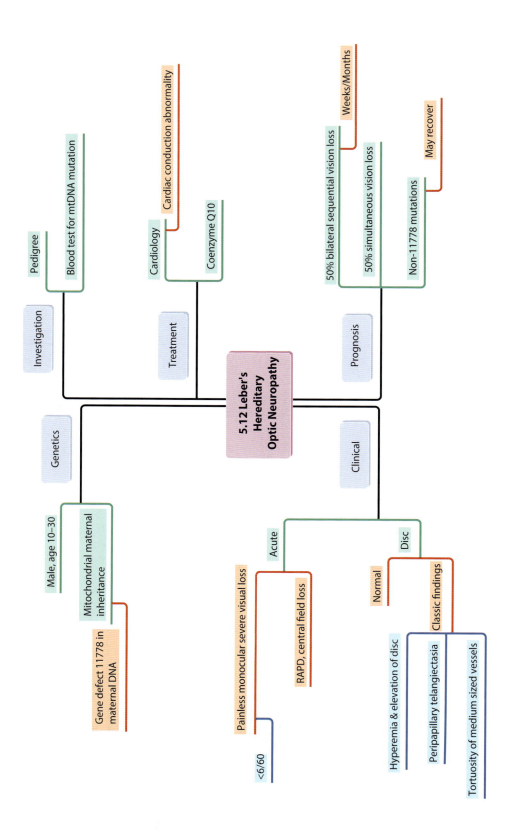

5.12 Leber's Hereditary Optic Neuropathy

Investigation
- Pedigree
- Blood test for mtDNA mutation

Treatment
- Cardiology
  - Cardiac conduction abnormality
- Coenzyme Q10

Prognosis
- 50% bilateral sequential vision loss
  - Weeks/Months
- 50% simultaneous vision loss
- Non-11778 mutations
  - May recover

Genetics
- Male, age 10–30
- Mitochondrial maternal inheritance
  - Gene defect 11778 in maternal DNA

Clinical
- Acute
  - Painless monocular severe visual loss
    - <6/60
  - RAPD, central field loss
- Disc
  - Normal
  - Classic findings
    - Hyperemia & elevation of disc
    - Peripapillary telangiectasia
    - Tortuosity of medium sized vessels

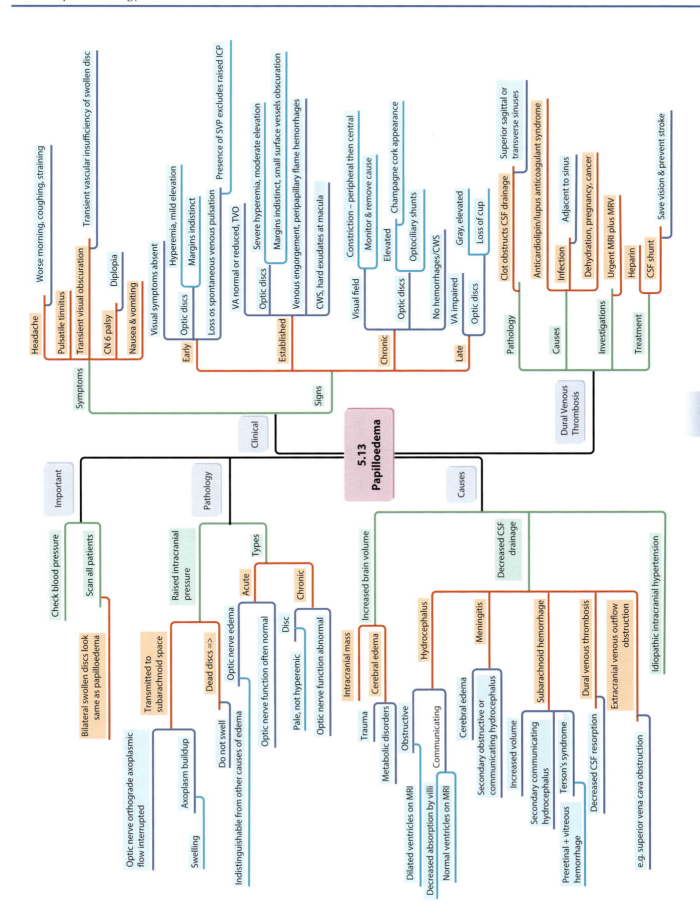

5.13 Papilloedema

Clinical

Symptoms

Headache
- Worse morning, coughing, straining

Pulsatile tinnitus
Transient visual obscuration
- Transient vascular insufficiency of swollen disc

CN 6 palsy
- Diplopia

Nausea & vomiting

Signs

Early
- Visual symptoms absent
- Optic discs
  - Hyperemia, mild elevation
  - Margins indistinct
- Loss os spontaneous venous pulsation
  - Presence of SVP excludes raised ICP

Established
- VA normal or reduced, TVO
- Optic discs
  - Severe hyperemia, moderate elevation
  - Margins indistinct, small surface vessels obscuration
- Venous engorgement, peripapillary flame hemorrhages
- CWS, hard exudates at macula

Chronic
- Visual field
  - Constriction – peripheral then central
  - Monitor & remove cause
- Elevated
- Optic discs
  - Champagne cork appearance
  - Optociliary shunts
- No hemorrhages/CWS

Late
- VA impaired
- Optic discs
  - Gray, elevated
  - Loss of cup

Dural Venous Thrombosis

Pathology
- Clot obstructs CSF drainage
- Superior sagittal or transverse sinuses

Causes
- Anticardiolipin/lupus anticoagulant syndrome
- Infection
  - Adjacent to sinus
- Dehydration, pregnancy, cancer

Investigations
- Urgent MRI plus MRV

Treatment
- Heparin
- CSF shunt
- Save vision & prevent stroke

Important
- Check blood pressure
- Scan all patients
- Bilateral swollen discs look same as papilloedema

Pathology

Raised intracranial pressure
- Transmitted to subarachnoid space
- Dead discs =>
  - Do not swell
  - Indistinguishable from other causes of edema

Optic nerve orthograde axoplasmic flow interrupted
- Axoplasm buildup
- Swelling

Types

Acute
- Optic nerve edema
- Optic nerve function often normal
- Disc
  - Pale, not hyperemic

Chronic
- Optic nerve function abnormal

Causes

Increased brain volume
- Intracranial mass
  - Trauma
  - Metabolic disorders
- Cerebral edema

Hydrocephalus
- Obstructive
  - Secondary obstructive or communicating hydrocephalus
- Communicating
  - Cerebral edema
  - Dilated ventricles on MRI
  - Increased volume
- Meningitis
  - Secondary communicating hydrocephalus
  - Decreased absorption by villi
  - Normal ventricles on MRI

Subarachnoid hemorrhage
- Terson's syndrome
  - Preretinal + vitreous hemorrhage
- Decreased CSF resorption

Decreased CSF drainage
- Dural venous thrombosis
- Extracranial venous outflow obstruction
  - e.g. superior vena cava obstruction
- Idiopathic intracranial hypertension

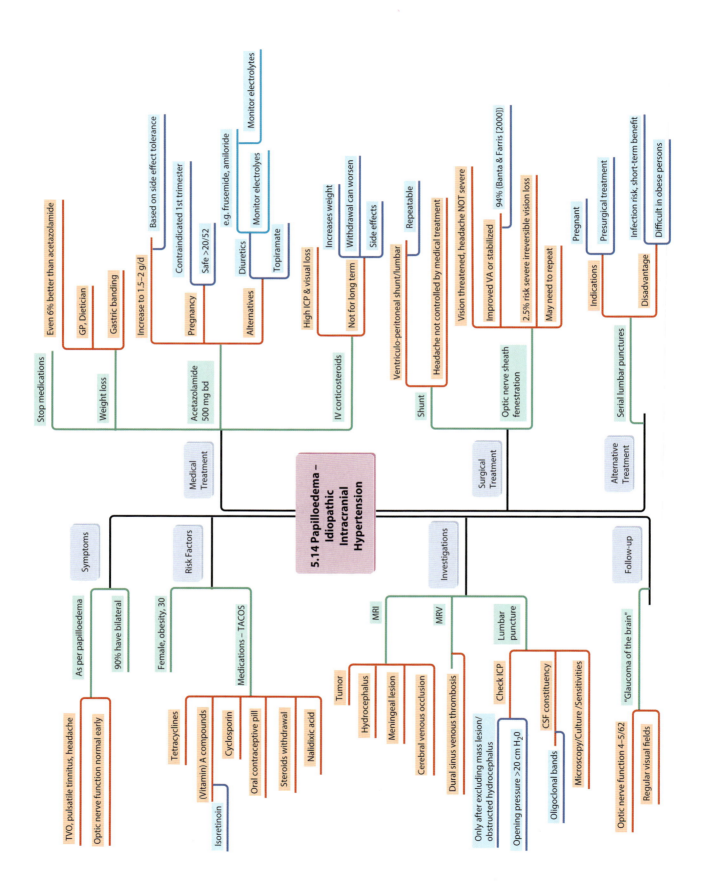

5.14 Papilloedema – Idiopathic Intracranial Hypertension

Medical Treatment

- Stop medications
- Weight loss
  - Even 6% better than acetazolamide
  - GP, Dietician
  - Gastric banding
- Acetazolamide 500 mg bd
  - Increase to 1.5–2 g/d
    - Based on side effect tolerance
  - Pregnancy
    - Contraindicated 1st trimester
    - Safe >20/52
  - Alternatives
    - Diuretics
      - e.g. frusemide, amiloride
      - Monitor electrolyes
    - Topiramate
      - Monitor electrolytes
- IV corticosteroids
  - High ICP & visual loss
  - Not for long term
    - Increases weight
    - Withdrawal can worsen
    - Side effects

Surgical Treatment

- Shunt
  - Ventriculo-peritoneal shunt/lumbar
    - Repeatable
  - Headache not controlled by medical treatment
- Optic nerve sheath fenestration
  - Vision threatened, headache NOT severe
  - Improved VA or stabilized
    - 94% (Banta & Farris [2000])
  - 2.5% risk severe irreversible vision loss
  - May need to repeat

Alternative Treatment

- Serial lumbar punctures
  - Indications
    - Pregnant
    - Presurgical treatment
  - Disadvantage
    - Infection risk, short-term benefit
    - Difficult in obese persons

Symptoms

- As per papilloedema
- 90% have bilateral
- TVO, pulsatile tinnitus, headache
- Optic nerve function normal early

Risk Factors

- Female, obesity, 30
- Medications – TACOS
  - Tetracyclines
  - (Vitamin) A compounds
    - Isoretinoin
  - Cyclosporin
  - Oral contraceptive pill
  - Steroids withdrawal
  - Nalidixic acid

Investigations

- MRI
  - Tumor
  - Hydrocephalus
  - Meningeal lesion
- MRV
  - Cerebral venous occlusion
  - Dural sinus venous thrombosis
- Lumbar puncture
  - Only after excluding mass lesion/ obstructed hydrocephalus
  - Check ICP
    - Opening pressure >20 cm H$_2$O
  - CSF constituency
    - Oligoclonal bands
    - Microscopy/Culture /Sensitivities

Follow-up

- "Glaucoma of the brain"
- Optic nerve function 4–5/62
- Regular visual fields

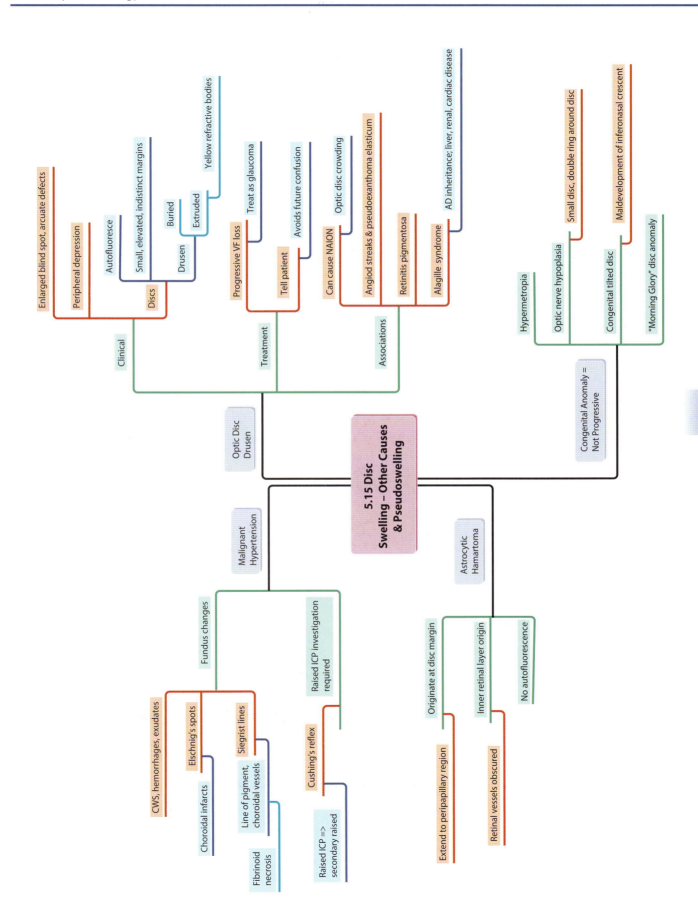

5.15 Disc Swelling – Other Causes & Pseudoswelling

Optic Disc Drusen

- Clinical
  - Enlarged blind spot, arcuate defects
  - Peripheral depression
  - Autofluoresce
  - Discs
    - Small, elevated, indistinct margins
    - Drusen
      - Buried
      - Extruded
        - Yellow refractive bodies
- Treatment
  - Progressive VF loss
    - Treat as glaucoma
  - Tell patient
    - Avoids future confusion
- Associations
  - Optic disc crowding
  - Can cause NAION
  - Angioid streaks & pseudoxanthoma elasticum
  - Retinitis pigmentosa
  - Alagille syndrome
    - AD inheritance; liver, renal, cardiac disease

Congenital Anomaly = Not Progressive
- Hypermetropia
- Optic nerve hypoplasia
  - Small disc, double ring around disc
- Congenital tilted disc
  - Maldevelopment of inferonasal crescent
- "Morning Glory" disc anomaly

Malignant Hypertension
- Fundus changes
  - CWS, hemorrhages, exudates
  - Elschnig's spots
    - Choroidal infarcts
  - Siegrist lines
    - Line of pigment, choroidal vessels
    - Fibrinoid necrosis
- Raised ICP investigation required
  - Cushing's reflex
    - Raised ICP => secondary raised

Astrocytic Hamartoma
- Originate at disc margin
  - Extend to peripapillary region
- Inner retinal layer origin
  - Retinal vessels obscured
- No autofluorescence

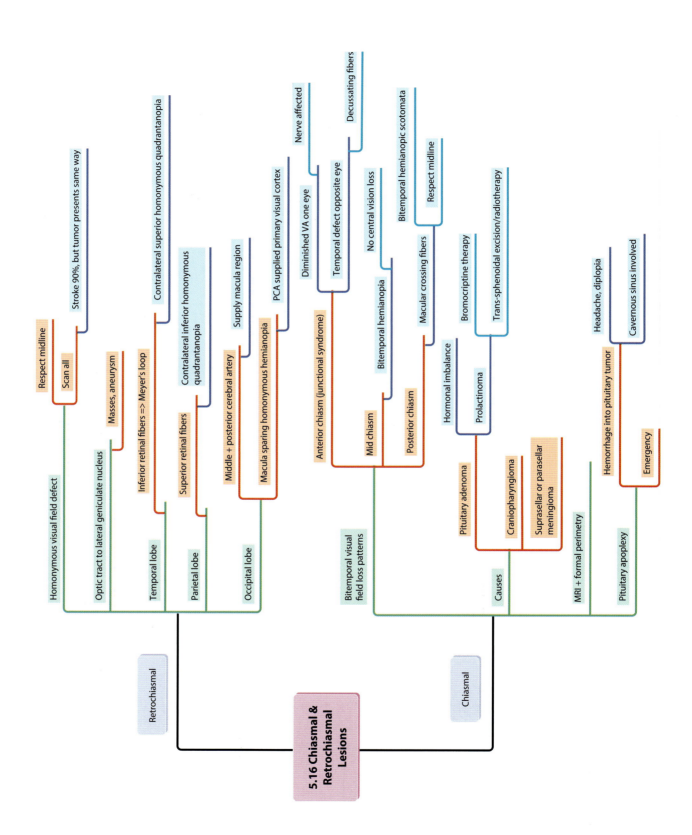

5.16 Chiasmal & Retrochiasmal Lesions

Retrochiasmal

- Homonymous visual field defect
  - Respect midline
  - Scan all
    - Stroke 90%, but tumor presents same way
- Optic tract to lateral geniculate nucleus
  - Masses, aneurysm
- Temporal lobe
  - Inferior retinal fibers => Meyer's loop
    - Contralateral superior homonymous quadrantanopia
- Parietal lobe
  - Superior retinal fibers
    - Contralateral inferior homonymous quadrantanopia
- Occipital lobe
  - Middle + posterior cerebral artery
    - Supply macula region
  - Macula sparing homonymous hemianopia
    - PCA supplied primary visual cortex

Chiasmal

- Bitemporal visual field loss patterns
  - Anterior chiasm (junctional syndrome)
    - Diminished VA one eye
    - Temporal defect opposite eye
      - Nerve affected
  - Mid chiasm
    - Bitemporal hemianopia
      - No central vision loss
      - Bitemporal hemianopic scotomata
      - Respect midline
        - Decussating fibers
  - Posterior chiasm
    - Macular crossing fibers
- Causes
  - Pituitary adenoma
    - Prolactinoma
      - Hormonal imbalance
      - Bromocriptine therapy
      - Trans-sphenoidal excision/radiotherapy
  - Craniopharyngioma
  - Suprasellar or parasellar meningioma
- MRI + formal perimetry
- Pituitary apoplexy
  - Hemorrhage into pituitary tumor
    - Headache, diplopia
    - Cavernous sinus involved
  - Emergency

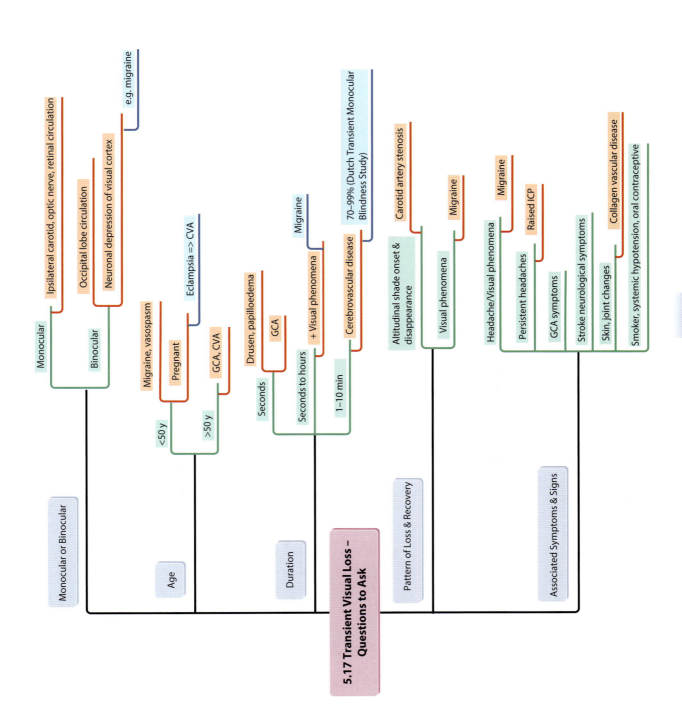

5.17 Transient Visual Loss – Questions to Ask

Monocular or Binocular
- Monocular
  - Ipsilateral carotid, optic nerve, retinal circulation
- Binocular
  - Occipital lobe circulation
  - Neuronal depression of visual cortex
    - e.g. migraine

Age
- <50 y
  - Migraine, vasospasm
  - Pregnant
    - Eclampsia => CVA
- >50 y
  - GCA, CVA

Duration
- Seconds
  - Drusen, papilloedema
  - GCA
- Seconds to hours
  - + Visual phenomena
    - Migraine
- 1–10 min
  - Cerebrovascular disease
    - 70–99% (Dutch Transient Monocular Blindness Study)

Pattern of Loss & Recovery
- Altitudinal shade onset & disappearance
  - Carotid artery stenosis
- Visual phenomena
  - Migraine

Associated Symptoms & Signs
- Headache/Visual phenomena
  - Migraine
- Persistent headaches
  - Raised ICP
- GCA symptoms
- Stroke neurological symptoms
- Skin, joint changes
  - Collagen vascular disease
- Smoker, systemic hypotension, oral contraceptive

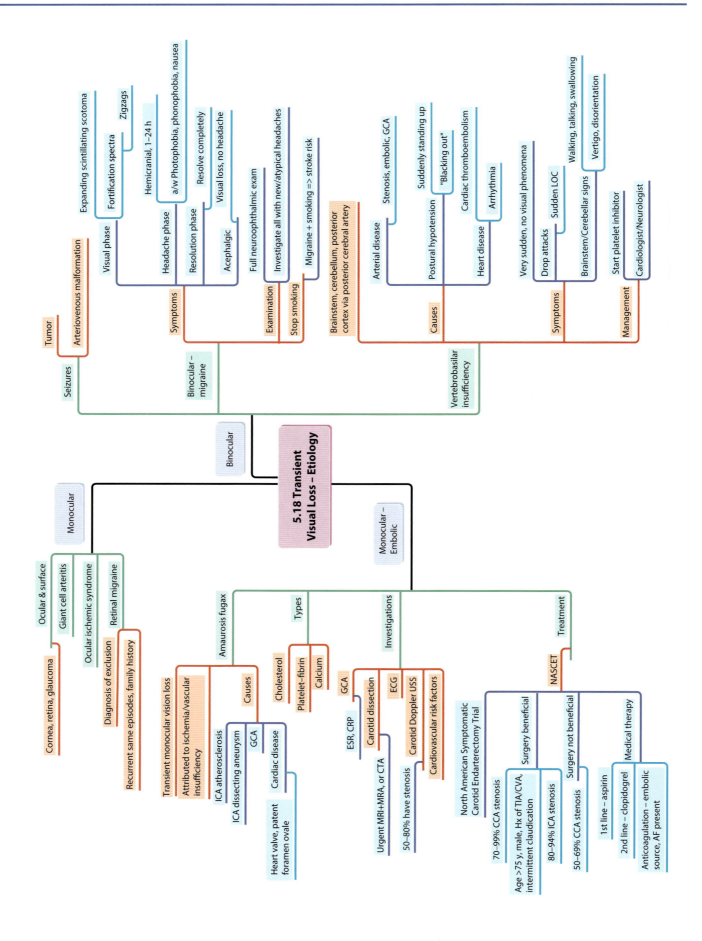

5.18 Transient Visual Loss – Etiology

Binocular

Binocular – migraine
- Tumor
- Seizures
- Arteriovenous malformation
- Symptoms
  - Visual phase
    - Expanding scintillating scotoma
    - Fortification spectra
    - Zigzags
  - Headache phase
    - Hemicranial, 1–24 h
    - a/w Photophobia, phonophobia, nausea
    - Resolve completely
  - Resolution phase
  - Acephalgic
    - Visual loss, no headache
- Examination
  - Full neuroophthalmic exam
  - Investigate all with new/atypical headaches
- Stop smoking
  - Migraine + smoking => stroke risk

Vertebrobasilar insufficiency
- Brainstem, cerebellum, posterior cortex via posterior cerebral artery
- Causes
  - Arterial disease
    - Stenosis, embolic, GCA
  - Postural hypotension
    - Suddenly standing up
    - "Blacking out"
  - Heart disease
    - Cardiac thromboembolism
    - Arrhythmia
- Symptoms
  - Very sudden, no visual phenomena
  - Drop attacks
    - Sudden LOC
  - Brainstem/Cerebellar signs
    - Walking, talking, swallowing
    - Vertigo, disorientation
- Management
  - Start platelet inhibitor
  - Cardiologist/Neurologist

Monocular

- Ocular & surface
  - Cornea, retina, glaucoma
- Giant cell arteritis
- Ocular ischemic syndrome
- Retinal migraine
  - Diagnosis of exclusion
  - Recurrent same episodes, family history

Monocular – Embolic

- Amaurosis fugax
  - Transient monocular vision loss
  - Attributed to ischemia/vascular insufficiency
- Causes
  - ICA atherosclerosis
  - ICA dissecting aneurysm
  - GCA
  - Cardiac disease
    - Heart valve, patent foramen ovale
- Types
  - Cholesterol
  - Platelet–fibrin
  - Calcium
- Investigations
  - GCA
    - ESR, CRP
  - Carotid dissection
    - Urgent MRI+MRA, or CTA
  - Carotid Doppler USS
    - 50–80% have stenosis
  - ECG
  - Cardiovascular risk factors
- Treatment
  - NASCET
    - North American Symptomatic Carotid Endarterectomy Trial
    - Surgery beneficial
      - 70–99% CCA stenosis
      - Age >75 y, male, Hx of TIA/CVA, intermittent claudication
      - 80–94% ICA stenosis
    - Surgery not beneficial
      - 50–69% CCA stenosis
  - Medical therapy
    - 1st line – aspirin
    - 2nd line – clopidogrel
    - Anticoagulation – embolic source, AF present

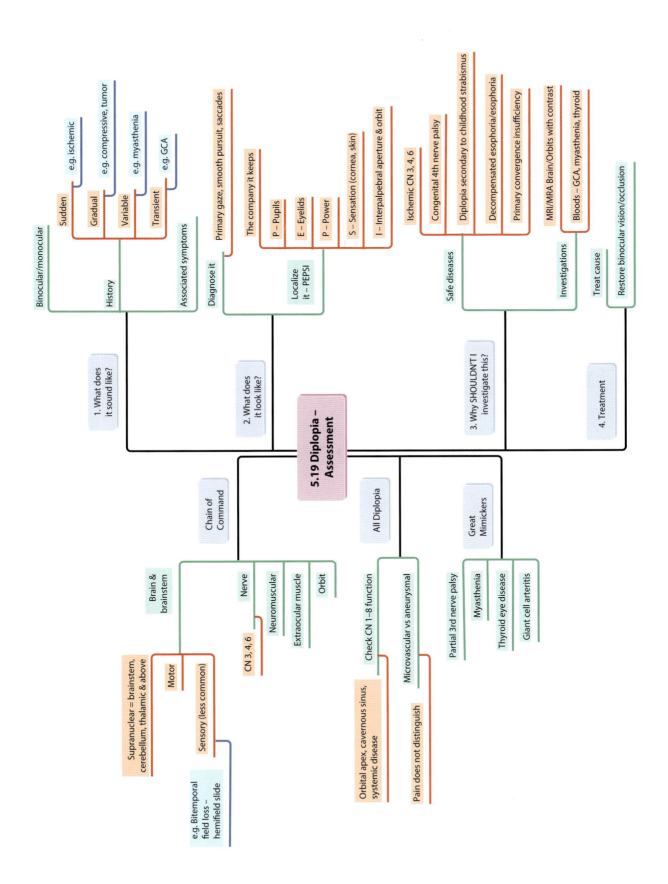

5.19 Diplopia – Assessment

1. What does it sound like?

History
- Binocular/monocular
- History
  - Sudden — e.g. ischemic
  - Gradual — e.g. compressive, tumor
  - Variable — e.g. myasthenia
  - Transient — e.g. GCA
- Associated symptoms

2. What does it look like?

- Diagnose it
  - Primary gaze, smooth pursuit, saccades
  - The company it keeps
- Localize it – PEPSI
  - P – Pupils
  - E – Eyelids
  - P – Power
  - S – Sensation (cornea, skin)
  - I – Interpalpebral aperture & orbit

3. Why SHOULDN'T I investigate this?

- Safe diseases
  - Ischemic CN 3, 4, 6
  - Congenital 4th nerve palsy
  - Diplopia secondary to childhood strabismus
  - Decompensated esophoria/esophoria
  - Primary convergence insufficiency
- Investigations
  - MRI/MRA Brain/Orbits with contrast
  - Bloods – GCA, myasthenia, thyroid

4. Treatment

- Treat cause
- Restore binocular vision/occlusion

Chain of Command

- Brain & brainstem
  - Motor
    - Supranuclear = brainstem, cerebellum, thalamic & above
  - Sensory (less common)
    - e.g. Bitemporal field loss – hemifield slide
- Nerve
  - CN 3, 4, 6
- Neuromuscular
- Extraocular muscle
- Orbit

All Diplopia

- Check CN 1–8 function
  - Orbital apex, cavernous sinus, systemic disease
- Microvascular vs aneurysmal
  - Pain does not distinguish

Great Mimickers

- Partial 3rd nerve palsy
- Myasthenia
- Thyroid eye disease
- Giant cell arteritis

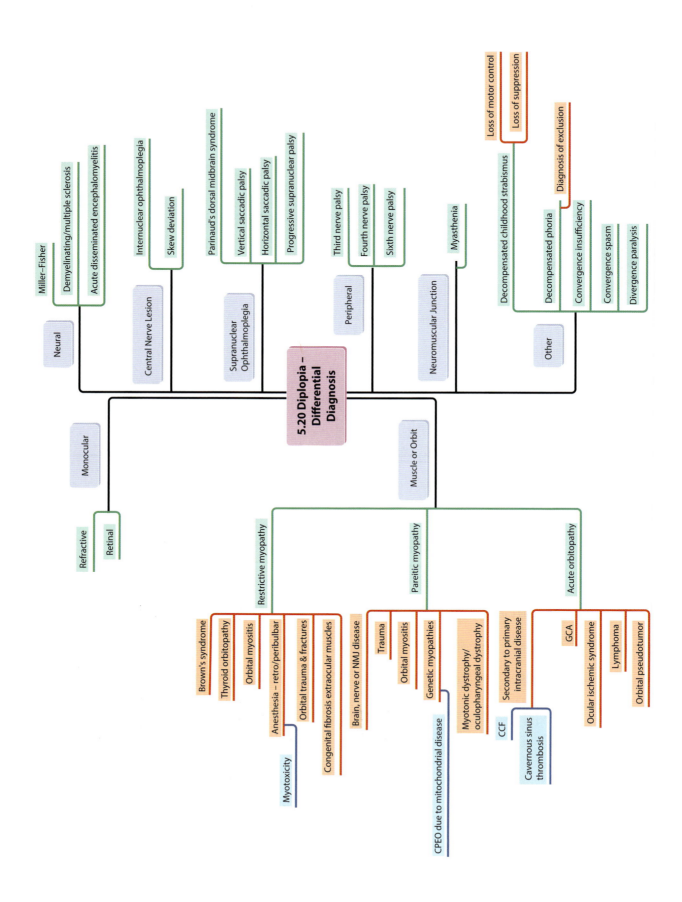

5.20 Diplopia – Differential Diagnosis

Neural
- Miller–Fisher
- Demyelinating/multiple sclerosis
- Acute disseminated encephalomyelitis

Central Nerve Lesion
- Internuclear ophthalmoplegia
- Skew deviation

Supranuclear Ophthalmoplegia
- Parinaud's dorsal midbrain syndrome
- Vertical saccadic palsy
- Horizontal saccadic palsy
- Progressive supranuclear palsy

Peripheral
- Third nerve palsy
- Fourth nerve palsy
- Sixth nerve palsy

Neuromuscular Junction
- Myasthenia

Other
- Decompensated childhood strabismus
  - Loss of motor control
  - Loss of suppression
- Decompensated phoria
- Convergence insufficiency
  - Diagnosis of exclusion
- Convergence spasm
- Divergence paralysis

Monocular
- Refractive
- Retinal

Muscle or Orbit

Restrictive myopathy
- Brown's syndrome
- Thyroid orbitopathy
- Orbital myositis
- Anesthesia – retro/peribulbar
  - Myotoxicity
- Orbital trauma & fractures
- Congenital fibrosis extraocular muscles

Pareitic myopathy
- Brain, nerve or NMJ disease
- Trauma
- Orbital myositis
- Genetic myopathies
  - CPEO due to mitochondrial disease
- Myotonic dystrophy/oculopharyngeal dystrophy

Acute orbitopathy
- Secondary to primary intracranial disease
  - CCF
  - Cavernous sinus thrombosis
- GCA
- Ocular ischemic syndrome
- Lymphoma
- Orbital pseudotumor

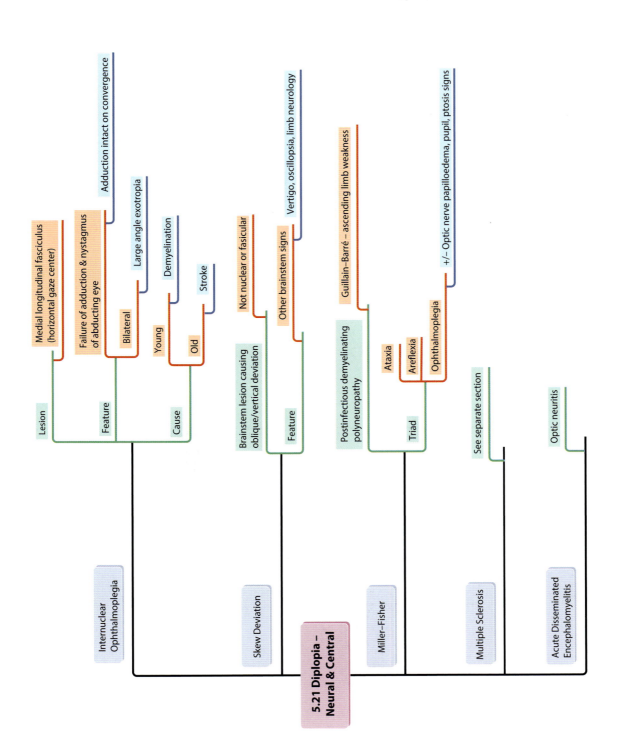

5.21 Diplopia – Neural & Central

Internuclear Ophthalmoplegia
- Lesion: Medial longitudinal fasciculus (horizontal gaze center)
- Feature: Failure of adduction & nystagmus of abducting eye
  - Adduction intact on convergence
  - Bilateral — Large angle exotropia
- Cause:
  - Young — Demyelination
  - Old — Stroke

Skew Deviation
- Brainstem lesion causing oblique/vertical deviation
- Feature:
  - Not nuclear or fasicular
  - Other brainstem signs — Vertigo, oscillopsia, limb neurology

Miller–Fisher
- Postinfectious demyelinating polyneuropathy
  - Guillain–Barré – ascending limb weakness
- Triad:
  - Ataxia
  - Areflexia
  - Ophthalmoplegia — +/- Optic nerve papilloedema, pupil, ptosis signs

Multiple Sclerosis
- See separate section

Acute Disseminated Encephalomyelitis
- Optic neuritis

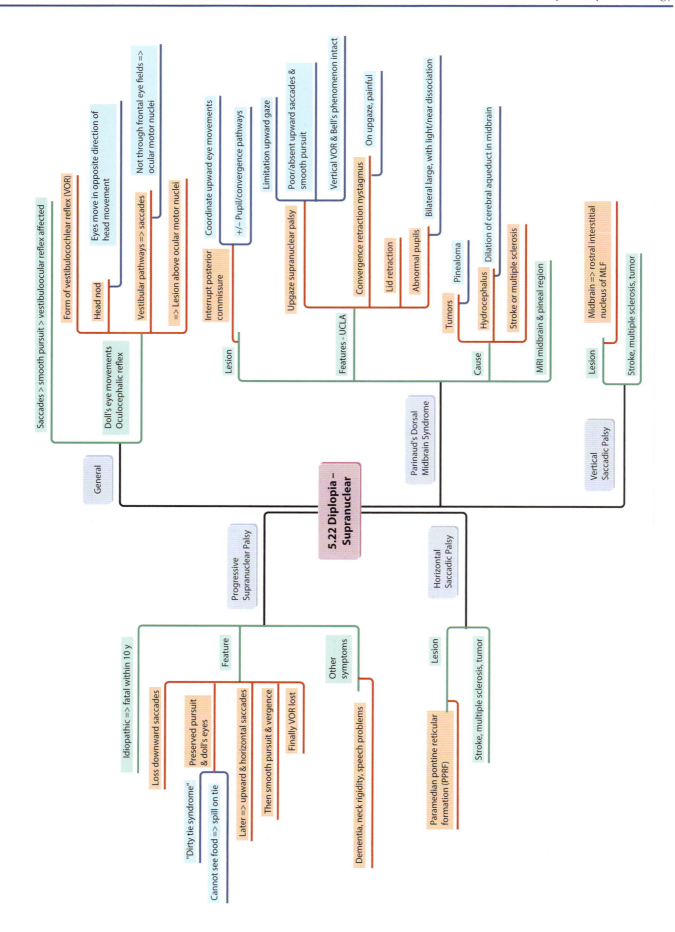

5.22 Diplopia – Supranuclear

General
- Saccades > smooth pursuit > vestibuloocular reflex affected
- Form of vestibulocochlear reflex (VOR)
  - Eyes move in opposite direction of head movement
  - Head nod
  - Vestibular pathways => saccades
    - Not through frontal eye fields => ocular motor nuclei
  - => Lesion above ocular motor nuclei
- Doll's eye movements Oculocephalic reflex

Parinaud's Dorsal Midbrain Syndrome
- Lesion
  - Interrupt posterior commissure
  - Coordinate upward eye movements
  - +/– Pupil/convergence pathways
- Features – UCLA
  - Upgaze supranuclear palsy
    - Limitation upward gaze
    - Poor/absent upward saccades & smooth pursuit
    - Vertical VOR & Bell's phenomenon intact
  - Convergence retraction nystagmus
    - On upgaze, painful
  - Lid retraction
  - Abnormal pupils
    - Bilateral large, with light/near dissociation
- Cause
  - Tumors
    - Pinealoma
  - Hydrocephalus
    - Dilation of cerebral aqueduct in midbrain
  - Stroke or multiple sclerosis
- MRI midbrain & pineal region

Vertical Saccadic Palsy
- Lesion
  - Midbrain => rostral interstitial nucleus of MLF
  - Stroke, multiple sclerosis, tumor

Progressive Supranuclear Palsy
- Idiopathic => fatal within 10 y
- Feature
  - Loss downward saccades
    - "Dirty tie syndrome"
      - Cannot see food => spill on tie
  - Preserved pursuit & doll's eyes
  - Later => upward & horizontal saccades
  - Then smooth pursuit & vergence
  - Finally VOR lost
- Other symptoms
  - Dementia, neck rigidity, speech problems

Horizontal Saccadic Palsy
- Lesion
  - Paramedian pontine reticular formation (PPRF)
  - Stroke, multiple sclerosis, tumor

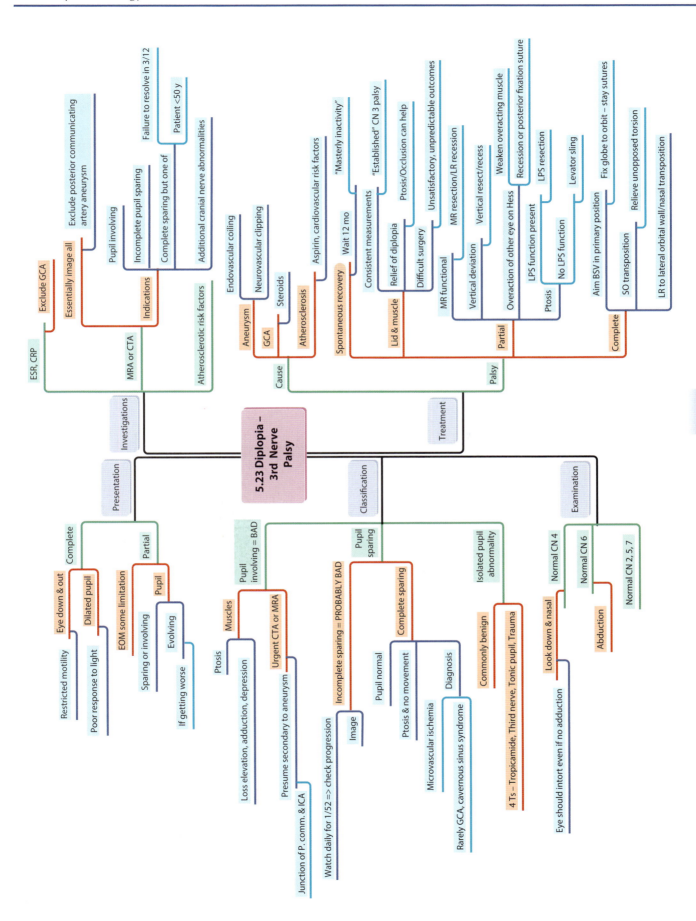

5.23 Diplopia – 3rd Nerve Palsy

Investigations

- ESR, CRP
  - Exclude GCA
  - Essentially image all
    - Exclude posterior communicating artery aneurysm
    - Pupil involving
    - Incomplete pupil sparing
    - Complete sparing but of one
      - Failure to resolve in 3/12
      - Patient <50 y
    - Additional cranial nerve abnormalities
  - Indications
- MRA or CTA
  - Endovascular coiling
  - Neurovascular clipping
  - Aneurysm
  - GCA
    - Steroids
  - Atherosclerosis
    - Aspirin, cardiovascular risk factors
  - Cause
- Atherosclerotic risk factors

Presentation

- Complete
  - Eye down & out
  - Dilated pupil
    - Restricted motility
    - Poor response to light
- Partial
  - EOM some limitation
  - Pupil
    - Sparing or involving
    - Evolving
      - If getting worse

Classification

- Pupil involving = BAD
  - Muscles
    - Ptosis
    - Loss elevation, adduction, depression
  - Urgent CTA or MRA
    - Presume secondary to aneurysm
    - Watch daily for 1/52 => check progression
    - Junction of P. comm. & ICA
- Pupil sparing
  - Incomplete sparing = PROBABLY BAD
    - Image
  - Complete sparing
    - Pupil normal
    - Ptosis & no movement
    - Diagnosis
      - Microvascular ischemia
      - Rarely GCA, cavernous sinus syndrome
- Isolated pupil abnormality
  - Commonly benign
  - 4 Ts – Tropicamide, Third nerve, Tonic pupil, Trauma

Examination

- Normal CN 4
  - Look down & nasal
  - Eye should intort even if no adduction
- Normal CN 6
  - Abduction
- Normal CN 2, 5, 7

Treatment

- Spontaneous recovery
  - Wait 12 mo
  - Consistent measurements
  - "Masterly inactivity"
- Lid & muscle
  - Relief of diplopia
  - Difficult surgery
  - Ptosis/Occlusion can help
  - "Established" CN 3 palsy
  - Unsatisfactory, unpredictable outcomes
- Palsy
  - Partial
    - MR functional
    - Vertical deviation
      - MR resection/LR recession
      - Vertical resect/recess
    - Overaction of other eye on Hess
      - Weaken overacting muscle
      - Recession or posterior fixation suture
    - LPS function present
      - LPS resection
    - Ptosis
    - No LPS function
      - Levator sling
  - Complete
    - Aim BSV in primary position
      - Fix globe to orbit – stay sutures
    - SO transposition
      - Relieve unopposed torsion
    - LR to lateral orbital wall/nasal transposition

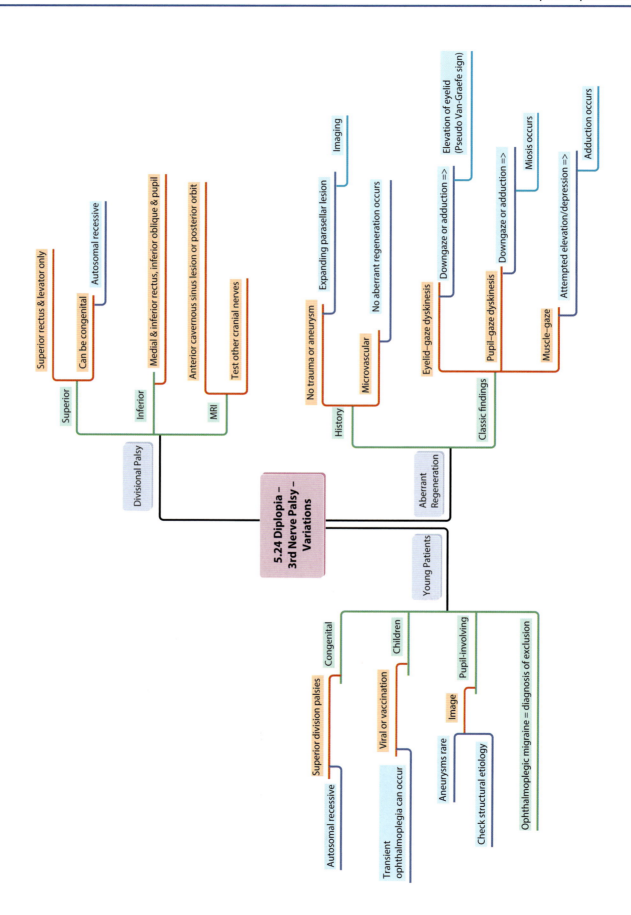

5.24 Diplopia – 3rd Nerve Palsy – Variations

Divisional Palsy

- Superior
  - Superior rectus & levator only
  - Can be congenital
    - Autosomal recessive
- Inferior
  - Medial & inferior rectus, inferior oblique & pupil
- MRI
  - Anterior cavernous sinus lesion or posterior orbit
  - Test other cranial nerves

Aberrant Regeneration

- History
  - No trauma or aneurysm
    - Expanding parasellar lesion
      - Imaging
  - Microvascular
    - No aberrant regeneration occurs
- Classic findings
  - Eyelid–gaze dyskinesis
    - Downgaze or adduction =>
      - Elevation of eyelid (Pseudo Van-Graefe sign)
  - Pupil–gaze dyskinesis
    - Downgaze or adduction =>
      - Miosis occurs
  - Muscle–gaze
    - Attempted elevation/depression =>
      - Adduction occurs

Young Patients

- Congenital
  - Superior division palsies
    - Autosomal recessive
  - Viral or vaccination
    - Transient ophthalmoplegia can occur
- Children
  - Pupil-involving
    - Aneurysms rare
      - Image
        - Check structural etiology
    - Ophthalmoplegic migraine = diagnosis of exclusion

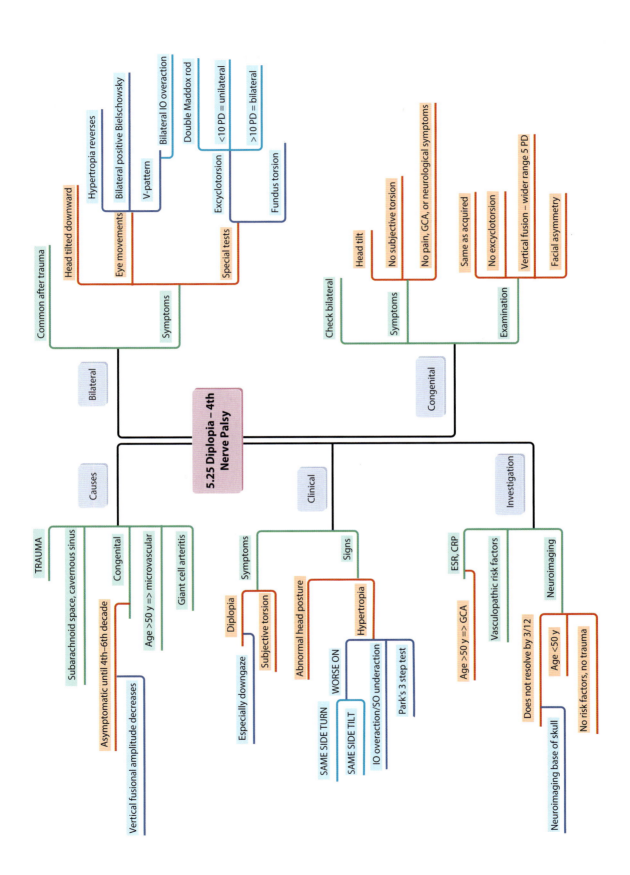

5.25 Diplopia – 4th Nerve Palsy

Bilateral

Symptoms
- Common after trauma
- Head tilted downward
- Eye movements
  - Hypertropia reverses
  - Bilateral positive Bielschowsky
  - V-pattern
  - Bilateral IO overaction
- Special tests
  - Double Maddox rod
    - <10 PD = unilateral
    - >10 PD = bilateral
  - Excyclotorsion
  - Fundus torsion

Congenital

Check bilateral

Symptoms
- Head tilt
- No subjective torsion
- No pain, GCA, or neurological symptoms

Examination
- Same as acquired
- No excyclotorsion
- Vertical fusion – wider range 5 PD
- Facial asymmetry

Causes
- TRAUMA
- Subarachnoid space, cavernous sinus
- Congenital
  - Asymptomatic until 4th–6th decade
  - Vertical fusional amplitude decreases
- Age >50 y => microvascular
- Giant cell arteritis

Clinical

Symptoms
- Diplopia
  - Especially downgaze
- Subjective torsion

Signs
- Abnormal head posture
  - SAME SIDE TURN
  - SAME SIDE TILT
- Hypertropia
  - WORSE ON
  - IO overaction/SO underaction
  - Park's 3 step test

Investigation
- ESR, CRP
  - Age >50 y => GCA
- Vasculopathic risk factors
- Neuroimaging
  - Does not resolve by 3/12
  - Age <50 y
    - Neuroimaging base of skull
    - No risk factors, no trauma

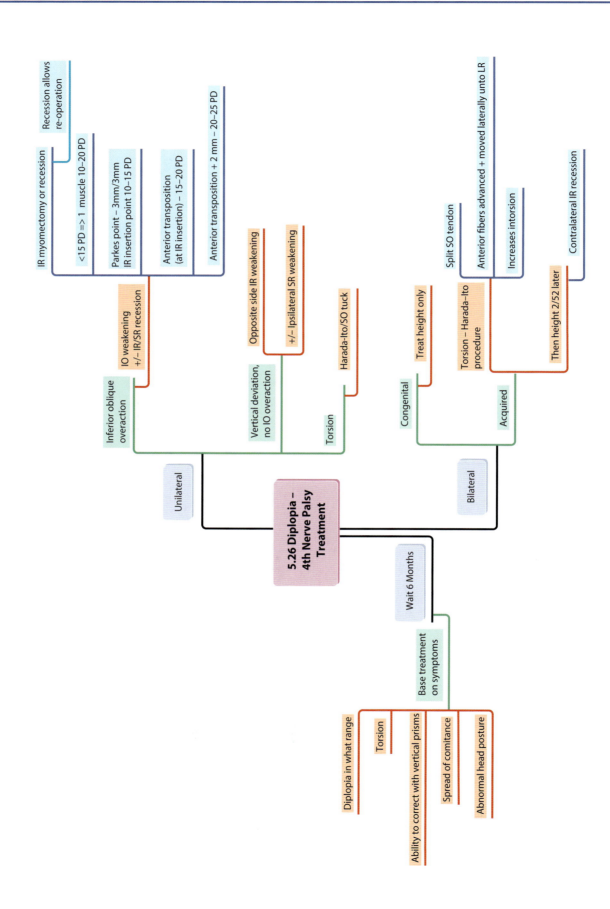

5.26 Diplopia – 4th Nerve Palsy Treatment

Unilateral

Inferior oblique overaction
- IO weakening +/− IR/SR recession
  - IR myomectomy or recession
    - Recession allows re-operation
  - <15 PD => 1 muscle 10–20 PD
  - Parkes point – 3mm/3mm IR insertion point 10–15 PD
  - Anterior transposition (at IR insertion) – 15–20 PD
  - Anterior transposition + 2 mm – 20–25 PD

Vertical deviation, no IO overaction
- Opposite side IR weakening
- +/− Ipsilateral SR weakening

Torsion
- Harada-Ito/SO tuck

Bilateral

Congenital
- Treat height only

Acquired
- Torsion – Harada-Ito procedure
  - Split SO tendon
  - Anterior fibers advanced + moved laterally unto LR
  - Increases intorsion
- Then height 2/52 later
  - Contralateral IR recession

Wait 6 Months

Base treatment on symptoms
- Diplopia in what range
- Torsion
- Ability to correct with vertical prisms
- Spread of comitance
- Abnormal head posture

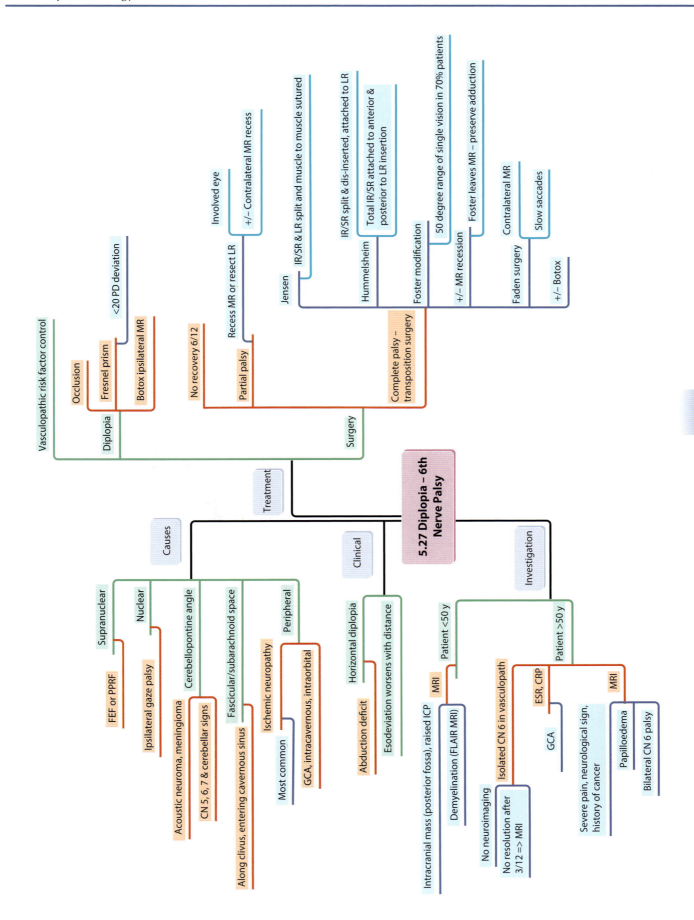

5.27 Diplopia – 6th Nerve Palsy

Treatment

- Diplopia
  - Vasculopathic risk factor control
  - Occlusion
  - Fresnel prism
    - <20 PD deviation
  - Botox ipsilateral MR

- Surgery
  - No recovery 6/12
  - Partial palsy
    - Recess MR or resect LR
      - Involved eye
      - +/– Contralateral MR recess
  - Complete palsy – transposition surgery
    - Jensen
      - IR/SR & LR split and muscle to muscle sutured
    - Hummelsheim
      - IR/SR split & dis-inserted, attached to LR
      - Total IR/SR attached to anterior & posterior to LR insertion
    - Foster modification
      - 50 degree range of single vision in 70% patients
    - +/– MR recession
      - Foster leaves MR – preserve adduction
    - Faden surgery
      - Contralateral MR
      - Slow saccades
    - +/– Botox

Causes

- Supranuclear
  - FEF or PPRF
- Nuclear
  - Ipsilateral gaze palsy
- Cerebellopontine angle
  - Acoustic neuroma, meningioma
  - CN 5, 6, 7 & cerebellar signs
- Fascicular/subarachnoid space
  - Along clivus, entering cavernous sinus
- Peripheral
  - Ischemic neuropathy
    - Most common
  - GCA, intracavernous, intraorbital

Clinical

- Horizontal diplopia
- Abduction deficit
- Esodeviation worsens with distance

Investigation

- Patient <50 y
  - Intracranial mass (posterior fossa), raised ICP
    - MRI
  - Demyelination (FLAIR MRI)
  - No neuroimaging
    - Isolated CN 6 in vasculopath
    - No resolution after 3/12 => MRI
- Patient >50 y
  - ESR, CRP
    - GCA
  - Severe pain, neurological sign, history of cancer
    - MRI
  - Papilloedema
  - Bilateral CN 6 palsy

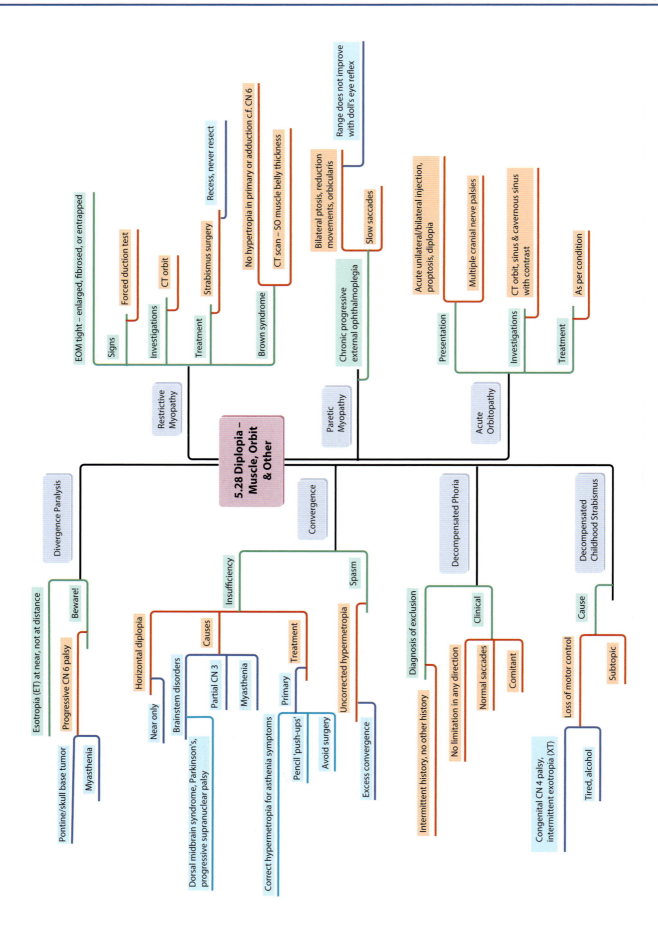

5.28 Diplopia – Muscle, Orbit & Other

Restrictive Myopathy
- Signs
  - EOM tight – enlarged, fibrosed, or entrapped
- Investigations
  - Forced duction test
  - CT orbit
- Treatment
  - Strabismus surgery
    - Recess, never resect
- Brown syndrome
  - No hypertropia in primary or adduction c.f. CN 6
  - CT scan – SO muscle belly thickness

Paretic Myopathy
- Chronic progressive external ophthalmoplegia
  - Bilateral ptosis, reduction movements, orbicularis
  - Slow saccades
    - Range does not improve with doll's eye reflex

Acute Orbitopathy
- Presentation
  - Acute unilateral/bilateral injection, proptosis, diplopia
  - Multiple cranial nerve palsies
- Investigations
  - CT orbit, sinus & cavernous sinus with contrast
- Treatment
  - As per condition

Divergence Paralysis
- Esotropia (ET) at near, not at distance
- Progressive CN 6 palsy
- Beware!
  - Pontine/skull base tumor
  - Myasthenia

Convergence
- Insufficiency
  - Horizontal diplopia
    - Near only
  - Causes
    - Brainstem disorders
      - Dorsal midbrain syndrome, Parkinson's, progressive supranuclear palsy
    - Partial CN 3
    - Myasthenia
  - Treatment
    - Primary
      - Correct hypermetropia for asthenia symptoms
      - Pencil 'push-ups'
      - Avoid surgery
    - Uncorrected hypermetropia
- Spasm
  - Excess convergence

Decompensated Phoria
- Diagnosis of exclusion
  - Intermittent history, no other history
- Clinical
  - No limitation in any direction
  - Normal saccades
  - Comitant

Decompensated Childhood Strabismus
- Cause
  - Loss of motor control
    - Congenital CN 4 palsy, intermittent exotropia (XT)
  - Subtopic
    - Tired, alcohol

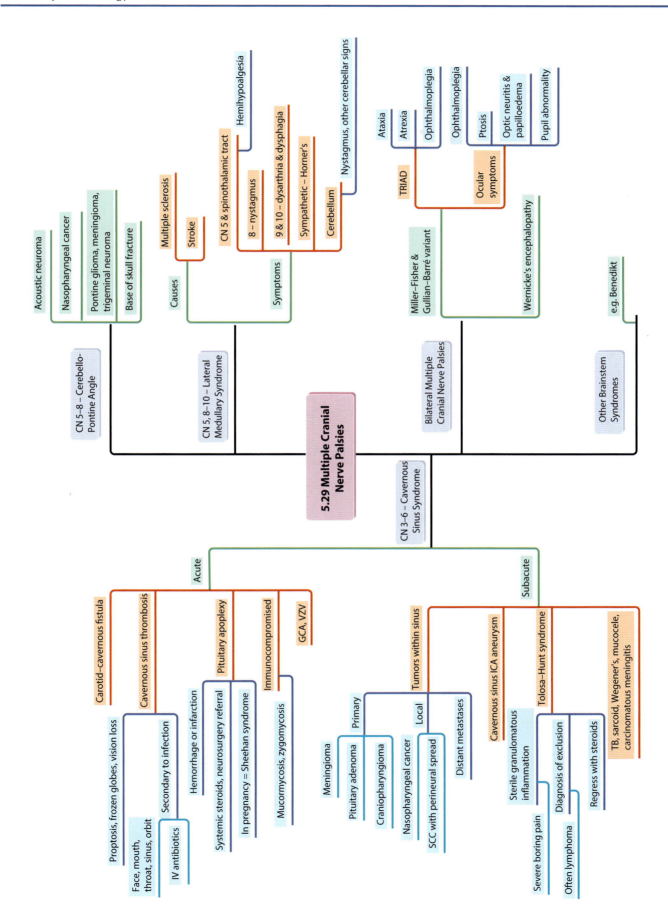

5.29 Multiple Cranial Nerve Palsies

CN 5–8 – Cerebello-Pontine Angle
- Acoustic neuroma
- Nasopharyngeal cancer
- Pontine glioma, meningioma, trigeminal neuroma
- Base of skull fracture

CN 5, 8–10 – Lateral Medullary Syndrome
- Causes
  - Multiple sclerosis
  - Stroke
- Symptoms
  - CN 5 & spinothalamic tract
    - Hemihypoalgesia
  - 8 – nystagmus
  - 9 & 10 – dysarthria & dysphagia
  - Sympathetic – Horner's
  - Cerebellum
    - Nystagmus, other cerebellar signs

Bilateral Multiple Cranial Nerve Palsies
- Miller–Fisher & Gullian–Barré variant
  - TRIAD
    - Ataxia
    - Atrexia
    - Ophthalmoplegia
- Wernicke's encephalopathy
  - Ocular symptoms
    - Ophthalmoplegia
    - Ptosis
    - Optic neuritis & papilloedema
    - Pupil abnormality

Other Brainstem Syndromes
- e.g. Benedikt

CN 3–6 – Cavernous Sinus Syndrome
- Acute
  - Carotid–cavernous fistula
    - Proptosis, frozen globes, vision loss
  - Cavernous sinus thrombosis
    - Face, mouth, throat, sinus, orbit
    - Secondary to infection
      - IV antibiotics
  - Pituitary apoplexy
    - Hemorrhage or infarction
    - Systemic steroids, neurosurgery referral
    - In pregnancy = Sheehan syndrome
  - Immunocompromised
    - Mucormycosis, zygomycosis
  - GCA, VZV
- Subacute
  - Tumors within sinus
    - Primary
      - Meningioma
      - Pituitary adenoma
      - Craniopharyngioma
    - Local
      - Nasopharyngeal cancer
      - SCC with perineural spread
    - Distant metastases
  - Cavernous sinus ICA aneurysm
  - Tolosa–Hunt syndrome
    - Sterile granulomatous inflammation
      - Severe boring pain
    - Diagnosis of exclusion
      - Often lymphoma
    - Regress with steroids
  - TB, sarcoid, Wegener's, mucocele, carcinomatous meningitis

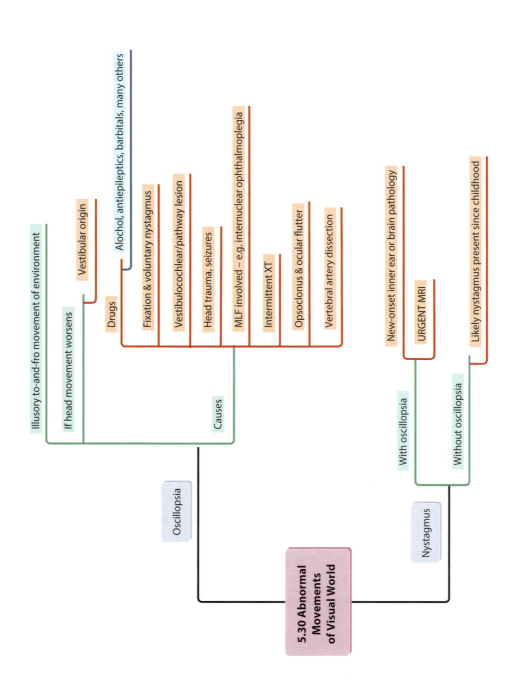

Oscillopsia

Illusory to-and-fro movement of environment

If head movement worsens

Vestibular origin

Drugs — Alochol, antiepileptics, barbitals, many others

Causes

Fixation & voluntary nystagmus

Vestibulocochlear/pathway lesion

Head trauma, seizures

MLF involved – e.g. internuclear ophthalmoplegia

Intermittent XT

Opsoclonus & ocular flutter

Vertebral artery dissection

5.30 Abnormal Movements of Visual World

Nystagmus

With oscillopsia

New-onset inner ear or brain pathology

URGENT MRI

Without oscillopsia

Likely nystagmus present since childhood

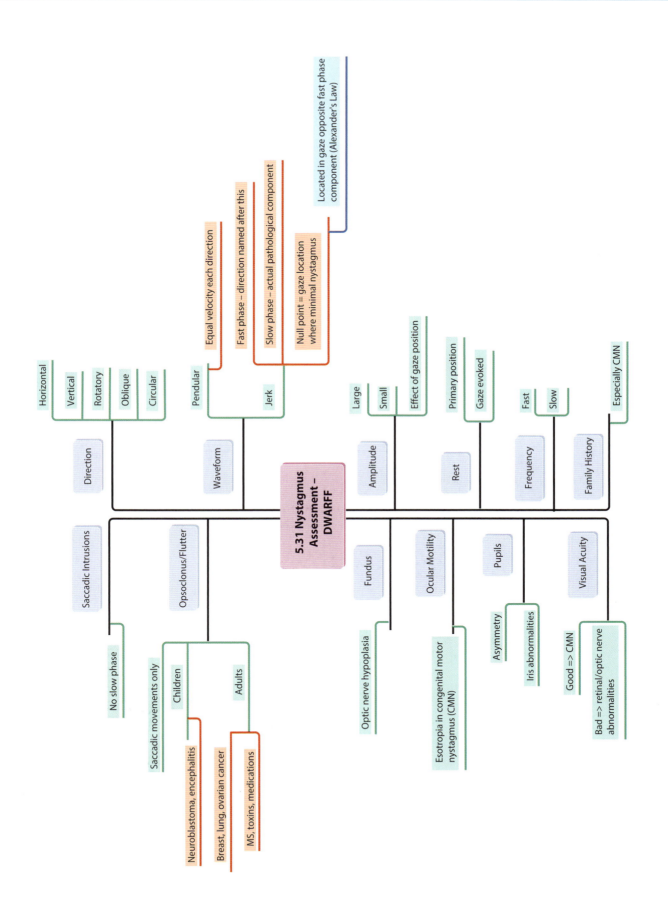

5.31 Nystagmus Assessment – DWARFF

Direction
- Horizontal
- Vertical
- Rotatory
- Oblique
- Circular

Waveform
- Pendular
  - Equal velocity each direction
- Jerk
  - Fast phase – direction named after this
  - Slow phase – actual pathological component
  - Null point = gaze location where minimal nystagmus
  - Located in gaze opposite fast phase component (Alexander's Law)

Amplitude
- Large
- Small
- Effect of gaze position

Rest
- Primary position
- Gaze evoked

Frequency
- Fast
- Slow

Family History
- Especially CMN

Saccadic Intrusions
- No slow phase

Opsoclonus/Flutter
- Saccadic movements only
  - Children
    - Neuroblastoma, encephalitis
  - Adults
    - Breast, lung, ovarian cancer
    - MS, toxins, medications

Fundus
- Optic nerve hypoplasia

Ocular Motility
- Esotropia in congenital motor nystagmus (CMN)

Pupils
- Asymmetry
- Iris abnormalities

Visual Acuity
- Good => CMN
- Bad => retinal/optic nerve abnormalities

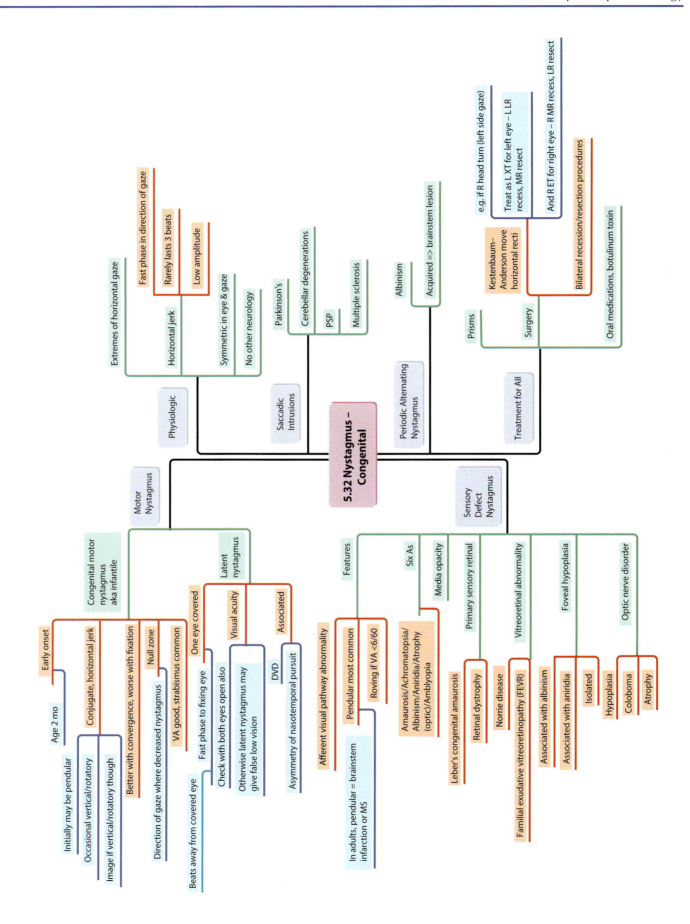

5.32 Nystagmus – Congenital

Physiologic
- Extremes of horizontal gaze
- Horizontal jerk
  - Fast phase in direction of gaze
  - Rarely lasts 3 beats
  - Low amplitude
- Symmetric in eye & gaze
- No other neurology

Saccadic Intrusions
- Parkinson's
- Cerebellar degenerations
- PSP
- Multiple sclerosis

Periodic Alternating Nystagmus
- Albinism
- Acquired => brainstem lesion

Treatment for All
- Prisms
- Surgery
  - Kestenbaum–Anderson move horizontal recti
    - e.g. if R head turn (left side gaze)
    - Treat as L XT for left eye – L LR recess, MR resect
    - And R ET for right eye – R MR recess, LR resect
  - Bilateral recession/resection procedures
- Oral medications, botulinum toxin

Motor Nystagmus
- Congenital motor nystagmus aka infantile
  - Early onset
    - Age 2 mo
    - Initially may be pendular
  - Conjugate, horizontal jerk
    - Occasional vertical/rotatory
    - Image if vertical/rotatory though
  - Better with convergence, worse with fixation
  - Null zone
    - Direction of gaze where decreased nystagmus
  - VA good, strabismus common
- Latent nystagmus
  - One eye covered
    - Fast phase to fixing eye
    - Beats away from covered eye
    - Check with both eyes open also
    - Otherwise latent nystagmus may give false low vision
  - Visual acuity
  - Associated
    - DVD
    - Asymmetry of nasotemporal pursuit

Sensory Defect Nystagmus
- Features
  - Afferent visual pathway abnormality
  - Pendular most common
    - In adults, pendular = brainstem infarction or MS
  - Roving if VA <6/60
- Six As
  - Amaurosis/Achromatopsia/Albinism/Aniridia/Atrophy (optic)/Amblyopia
- Media opacity
- Primary sensory retinal
  - Leber's congenital amaurosis
  - Retinal dystrophy
  - Norrie disease
- Vitreoretinal abnormality
  - Familial exudative vitreoretinopathy (FEVR)
- Foveal hypoplasia
  - Associated with albinism
  - Associated with aniridia
  - Isolated
- Optic nerve disorder
  - Hypoplasia
  - Coloboma
  - Atrophy

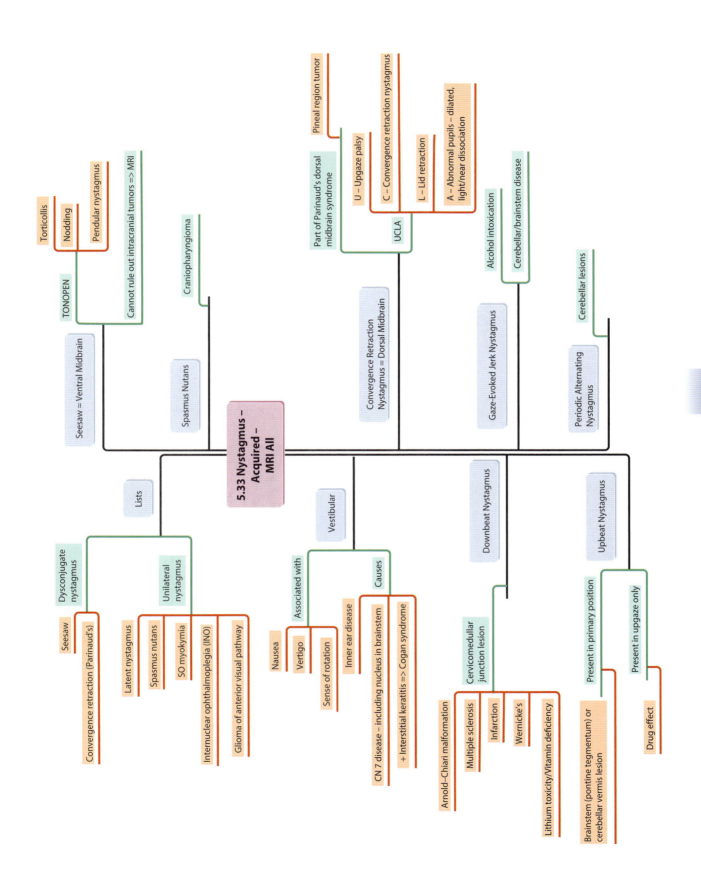

5.33 Nystagmus – Acquired – MRI All

Seesaw = Ventral Midbrain
- TONOPEN
  - Torticollis
  - Nodding
  - Pendular nystagmus
- Cannot rule out intracranial tumors => MRI

Spasmus Nutans
- Craniopharyngioma

Convergence Retraction Nystagmus = Dorsal Midbrain
- Part of Parinaud's dorsal midbrain syndrome
- UCLA
  - U – Upgaze palsy
  - C – Convergence retraction nystagmus
  - L – Lid retraction
  - A – Abnormal pupils – dilated, light/near dissociation
  - Pineal region tumor

Gaze-Evoked Jerk Nystagmus
- Alcohol intoxication
- Cerebellar/brainstem disease

Periodic Alternating Nystagmus
- Cerebellar lesions

Lists
- Dysconjugate nystagmus
  - Seesaw
  - Convergence retraction (Parinaud's)
- Unilateral nystagmus
  - Latent nystagmus
  - Spasmus nutans
  - SO myokymia
  - Internuclear ophthalmoplegia (INO)
  - Glioma of anterior visual pathway

Vestibular
- Associated with
  - Nausea
  - Vertigo
  - Sense of rotation
- Causes
  - Inner ear disease
  - CN 7 disease – including nucleus in brainstem
  - + Interstitial keratitis => Cogan syndrome

Downbeat Nystagmus
- Cervicomedullar junction lesion
  - Arnold–Chiari malformation
  - Multiple sclerosis
  - Infarction
  - Wernicke's
  - Lithium toxicity/Vitamin deficiency

Upbeat Nystagmus
- Present in primary position
  - Brainstem (pontine tegmentum) or cerebellar vermis lesion
- Present in upgaze only
  - Drug effect

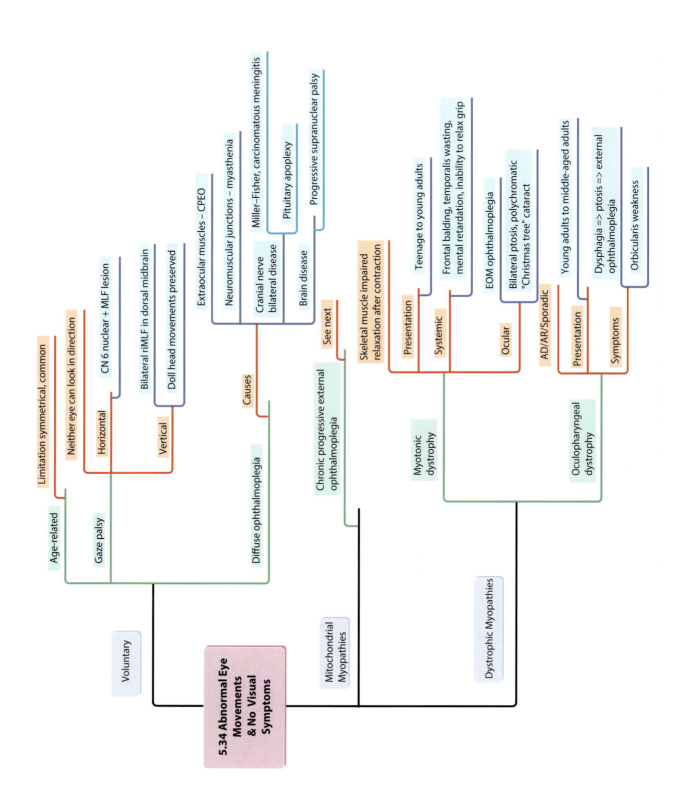

5.34 Abnormal Eye Movements & No Visual Symptoms

Voluntary

- Gaze palsy
  - Age-related — Limitation symmetrical, common
  - Neither eye can look in direction
    - Horizontal — CN 6 nuclear + MLF lesion
    - Vertical
      - Bilateral riMLF in dorsal midbrain
      - Doll head movements preserved

Diffuse ophthalmoplegia

- Causes
  - Extraocular muscles – CPEO
  - Neuromuscular junctions – myasthenia
  - Cranial nerve bilateral disease — Miller–Fisher, carcinomatous meningitis
  - Brain disease
    - Pituitary apoplexy
    - Progressive supranuclear palsy

Mitochondrial Myopathies

- Chronic progressive external ophthalmoplegia — See next

Dystrophic Myopathies

- Myotonic dystrophy — Skeletal muscle impaired relaxation after contraction
  - Presentation — Teenage to young adults
  - Systemic — Frontal balding, temporalis wasting, mental retardation, inability to relax grip
  - Ocular
    - EOM ophthalmoplegia
    - Bilateral ptosis, polychromatic "Christmas tree" cataract
- Oculopharyngeal dystrophy
  - AD/AR/Sporadic
  - Presentation — Young adults to middle-aged adults
  - Symptoms
    - Dysphagia => ptosis => external ophthalmoplegia
    - Orbicularis weakness

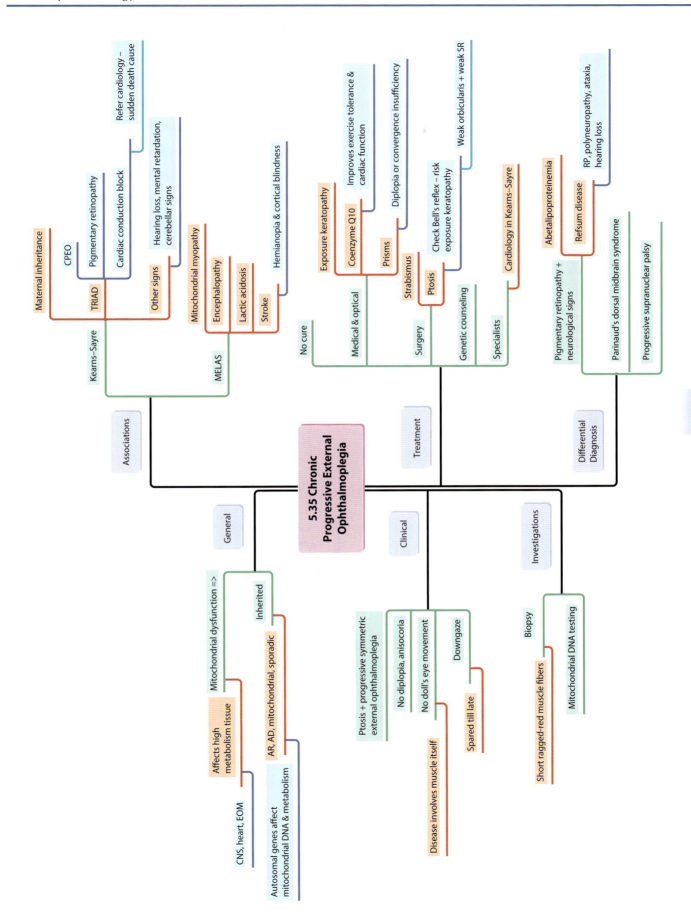

5.35 Chronic Progressive External Ophthalmoplegia

General

Mitochondrial dysfunction =>
- Affects high metabolism tissue
  - CNS, heart, EOM

Inherited
- AR, AD, mitochondrial, sporadic
  - Autosomal genes affect mitochondrial DNA & metabolism

Clinical

- Ptosis + progressive symmetric external ophthalmoplegia
- No diplopia, anisocoria
- No doll's eye movement
- Downgaze
  - Spared till late
- Disease involves muscle itself

Investigations

- Biopsy
  - Short ragged-red muscle fibers
- Mitochondrial DNA testing

Associations

Kearns–Sayre
- Maternal inheritance
- TRIAD
  - CPEO
  - Pigmentary retinopathy
  - Cardiac conduction block
    - Refer cardiology – sudden death cause
- Other signs
  - Hearing loss, mental retardation, cerebellar signs

MELAS
- Mitochondrial myopathy
- Encephalopathy
- Lactic acidosis
- Stroke
  - Hemianopia & cortical blindness

Treatment

No cure

Medical & optical
- Exposure keratopathy
- Coenzyme Q10
  - Improves exercise tolerance & cardiac function
- Prisms
  - Diplopia or convergence insufficiency

Surgery
- Strabismus
- Ptosis
  - Check Bell's reflex – risk exposure keratopathy
  - Weak orbicularis + weak SR

Genetic counseling

Specialists
- Cardiology in Kearns–Sayre

Differential Diagnosis

- Abetalipoproteinemia
- Refsum disease
  - RP, polyneuropathy, ataxia, hearing loss
- Pigmentary retinopathy + neurological signs
- Parinaud's dorsal midbrain syndrome
- Progressive supranuclear palsy

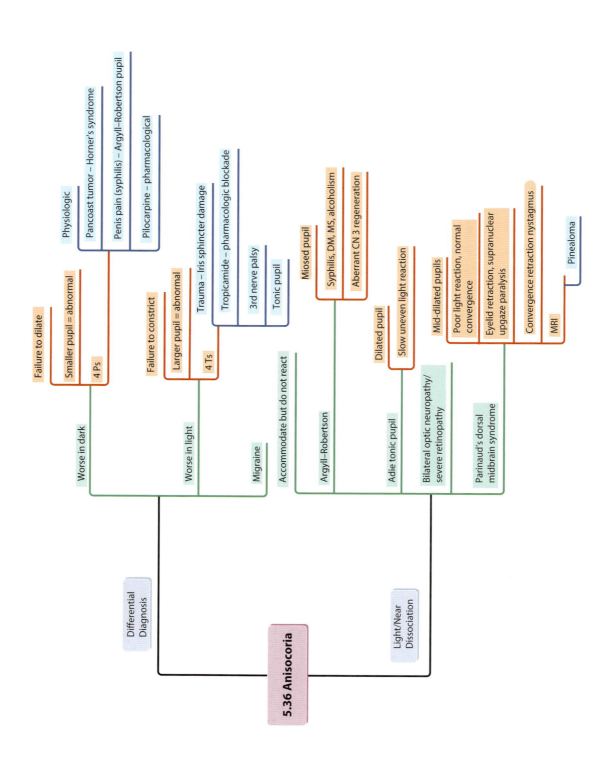

5.36 Anisocoria

Differential Diagnosis

- Worse in dark
  - Failure to dilate
    - Smaller pupil = abnormal
      - 4 Ps
        - Physiologic
        - Pancoast tumor – Horner's syndrome
        - Penis pain (syphilis) – Argyll–Robertson pupil
        - Pilocarpine – pharmacological
- Worse in light
  - Failure to constrict
    - Larger pupil = abnormal
      - 4 Ts
        - Trauma – Iris sphincter damage
        - Tropicamide – pharmacologic blockade
        - 3rd nerve palsy
        - Tonic pupil
- Migraine

Light/Near Dissociation

- Accommodate but do not react
- Argyll–Robertson
  - Miosed pupil
    - Syphilis, DM, MS, alcoholism
    - Aberrant CN 3 regeneration
- Adie tonic pupil
  - Dilated pupil
    - Slow uneven light reaction
- Bilateral optic neuropathy/ severe retinopathy
- Parinaud's dorsal midbrain syndrome
  - Mid-dilated pupils
    - Poor light reaction, normal convergence
    - Eyelid retraction, supranuclear upgaze paralysis
    - Convergence retraction nystagmus
    - MRI
      - Pinealoma

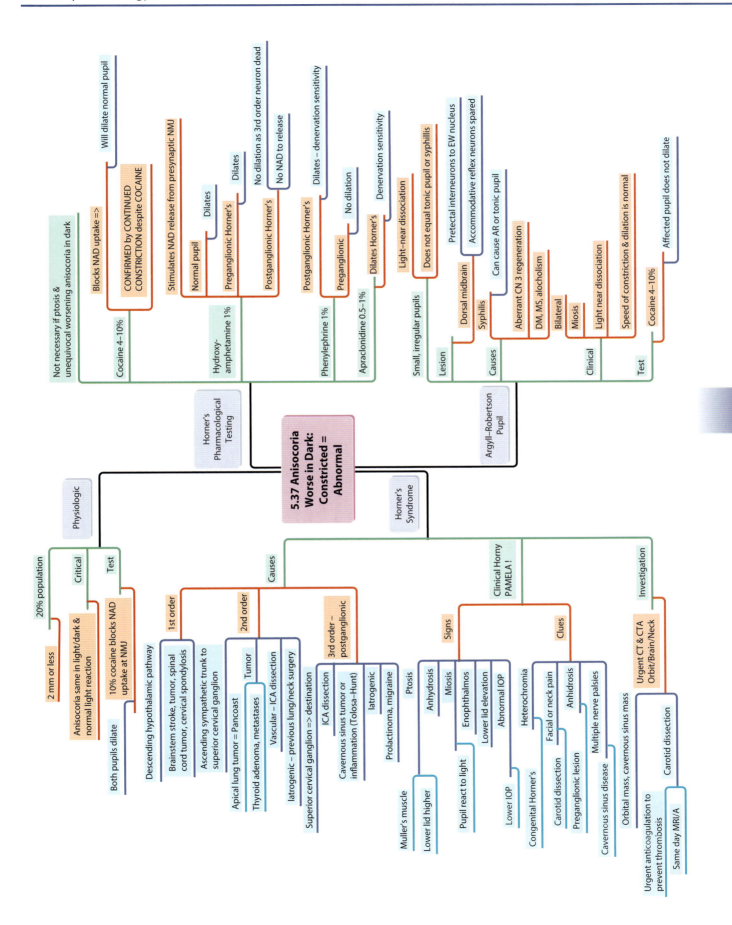

5.37 Anisocoria Worse in Dark: Constricted = Abnormal

Horner's Pharmacological Testing

- Cocaine 4–10%
  - Not necessary if ptosis & unequivocal worsening anisocoria in dark
  - Blocks NAD uptake =>
    - Will dilate normal pupil
  - CONFIRMED by CONTINUED CONSTRICTION despite COCAINE
- Hydroxy-amphetamine 1%
  - Stimulates NAD release from presynaptic NMJ
  - Normal pupil
    - Dilates
  - Preganglionic Horner's
    - Dilates
  - Postganglionic Horner's
    - No dilation as 3rd order neuron dead
    - No NAD to release
- Phenylephrine 1%
  - Postganglionic Horner's
    - Dilates – denervation sensitivity
  - Preganglionic
    - No dilation
- Apraclonidine 0.5–1%
  - Dilates Horner's
    - Denervation sensitivity

Argyll–Robertson Pupil

- Small, irregular pupils
  - Light–near dissociation
  - Does not equal tonic pupil or syphilis
- Lesion
  - Dorsal midbrain
    - Pretectal interneurons to EW nucleus
    - Accommodative reflex neurons spared
- Causes
  - Syphilis
    - Can cause AR or tonic pupil
  - Aberrant CN 3 regeneration
  - DM, MS, alcoholism
- Clinical
  - Bilateral
  - Miosis
  - Light near dissociation
  - Speed of constriction & dilation is normal
- Test
  - Cocaine 4–10%
    - Affected pupil does not dilate

Physiologic

- 20% population
- Critical
  - 2 mm or less
  - Anisocoria same in light/dark & normal light reaction
  - Both pupils dilate
- Test
  - 10% cocaine blocks NAD uptake at NMJ

Horner's Syndrome

- Causes
  - 1st order
    - Descending hypothalamic pathway
    - Brainstem stroke, tumor, spinal cord tumor, cervical spondylosis
  - 2nd order
    - Ascending sympathetic trunk to superior cervical ganglion
    - Apical lung tumor = Pancoast
    - Thyroid adenoma, metastases
      - Tumor
    - Vascular – ICA dissection
    - Iatrogenic – previous lung/neck surgery
  - 3rd order – postganglionic
    - Superior cervical ganglion => destination
    - ICA dissection
    - Cavernous sinus tumor or inflammation (Tolosa–Hunt)
    - Iatrogenic
    - Prolactinoma, migraine
- Clinical Horny PAMELA !
  - Signs
    - Ptosis
      - Muller's muscle
      - Lower lid higher
    - Anhydrosis
    - Miosis
      - Pupil react to light
      - Lower lid higher
    - Enophthalmos
    - Lower lid elevation
      - Lower IOP
    - Abnormal IOP
  - Clues
    - Heterochromia
      - Congenital Horner's
    - Facial or neck pain
      - Carotid dissection
    - Anhidrosis
      - Preganglionic lesion
    - Multiple nerve palsies
      - Cavernous sinus disease
      - Orbital mass, cavernous sinus mass
- Investigation
  - Urgent CT & CTA Orbit/Brain/Neck
  - Carotid dissection
    - Urgent anticoagulation to prevent thrombosis
    - Same day MRI/A

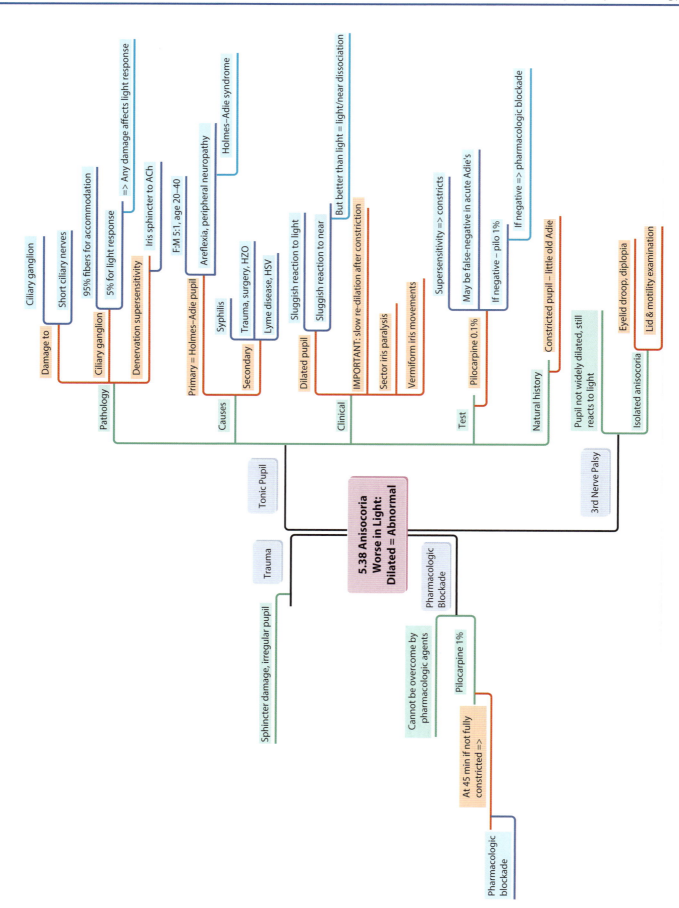

5.38 Anisocoria Worse in Light: Dilated = Abnormal

Tonic Pupil

Pathology
- Damage to
  - Ciliary ganglion
  - Short ciliary nerves
- Ciliary ganglion
  - 95% fibers for accommodation
  - 5% for light response
    => Any damage affects light response
- Denervation supersensitivity
  - Iris sphincter to ACh

Causes
- Primary = Holmes–Adie pupil
  - F:M 5:1, age 20–40
  - Areflexia, peripheral neuropathy
  - Holmes–Adie syndrome
- Secondary
  - Syphilis
  - Trauma, surgery, HZO
  - Lyme disease, HSV

Clinical
- Dilated pupil
  - Sluggish reaction to light
  - Sluggish reaction to near
  - But better than light = light/near dissociation
- IMPORTANT: slow re-dilation after constriction
- Sector iris paralysis
- Vermiform iris movements

Test
- Pilocarpine 0.1%
  - Supersensitivity => constricts
  - May be false-negative in acute Adie's
  - If negative – pilo 1%
    - If negative => pharmacologic blockade

Natural history
- Constricted pupil – little old Adie

Trauma
- Sphincter damage, irregular pupil

Pharmacologic Blockade
- Cannot be overcome by pharmacologic agents
- Pilocarpine 1%
  - At 45 min if not fully constricted =>
    - Pharmacologic blockade

3rd Nerve Palsy
- Pupil not widely dilated, still reacts to light
- Isolated anisocoria
  - Eyelid droop, diplopia
  - Lid & motility examination

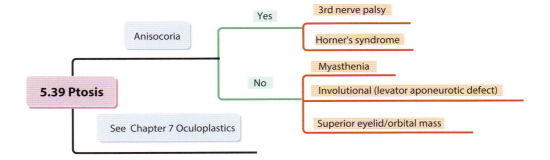

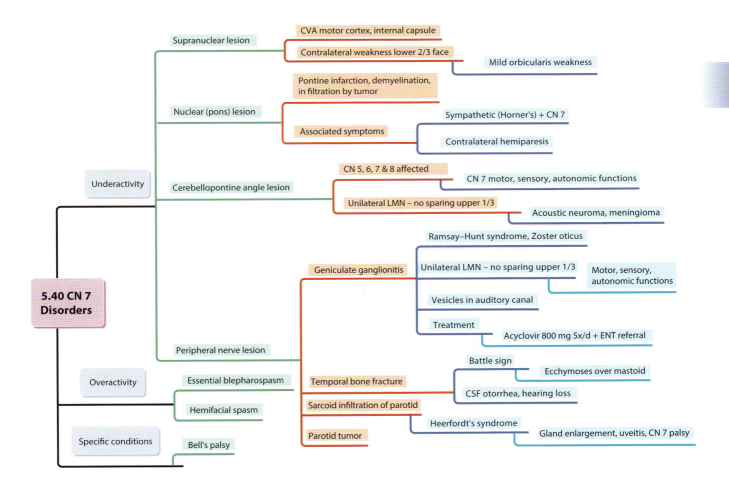

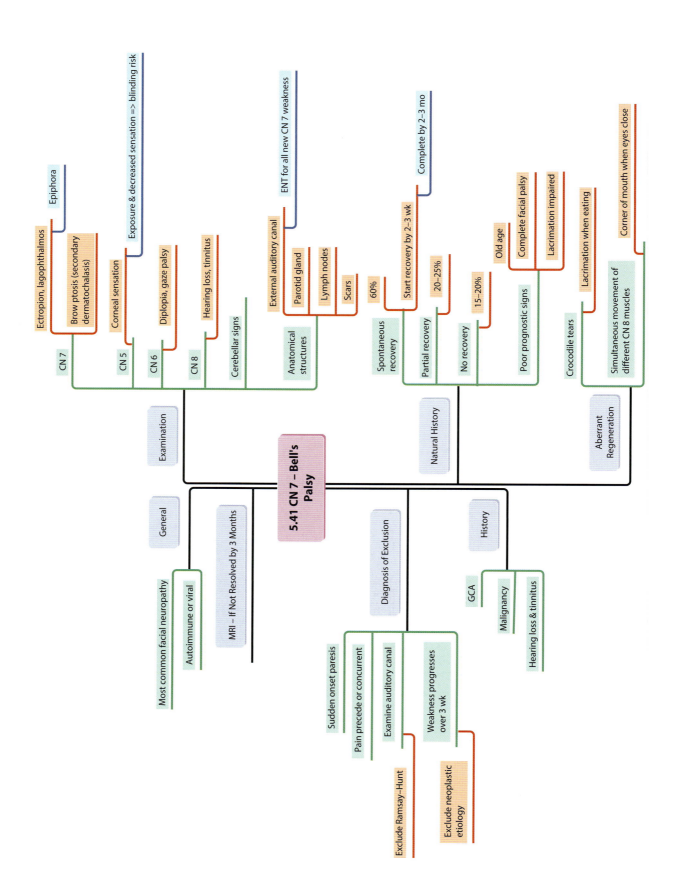

5.41 CN 7 – Bell's Palsy

Examination

CN 7
- Ectropion, lagophthalmos — Epiphora
- Brow ptosis (secondary dermatochalasis)

CN 5
- Corneal sensation — Exposure & decreased sensation => blinding risk

CN 6
- Diplopia, gaze palsy

CN 8
- Hearing loss, tinnitus

Cerebellar signs

Anatomical structures
- External auditory canal — ENT for all new CN 7 weakness
- Parotid gland
- Lymph nodes
- Scars

Natural History

Spontaneous recovery
- 60%

Partial recovery
- Start recovery by 2–3 wk — Complete by 2–3 mo
- 20–25%

No recovery
- 15–20%

Poor prognostic signs
- Old age
- Complete facial palsy
- Lacrimation impaired

Aberrant Regeneration

Crocodile tears
- Lacrimation when eating

Simultaneous movement of different CN 8 muscles
- Corner of mouth when eyes close

General
- Most common facial neuropathy
- Autoimmune or viral
- MRI – If Not Resolved by 3 Months

Diagnosis of Exclusion
- Sudden onset paresis
- Pain precede or concurrent
- Examine auditory canal — Exclude Ramsay–Hunt
- Weakness progresses over 3 wk — Exclude neoplastic etiology

History
- GCA
- Malignancy
- Hearing loss & tinnitus

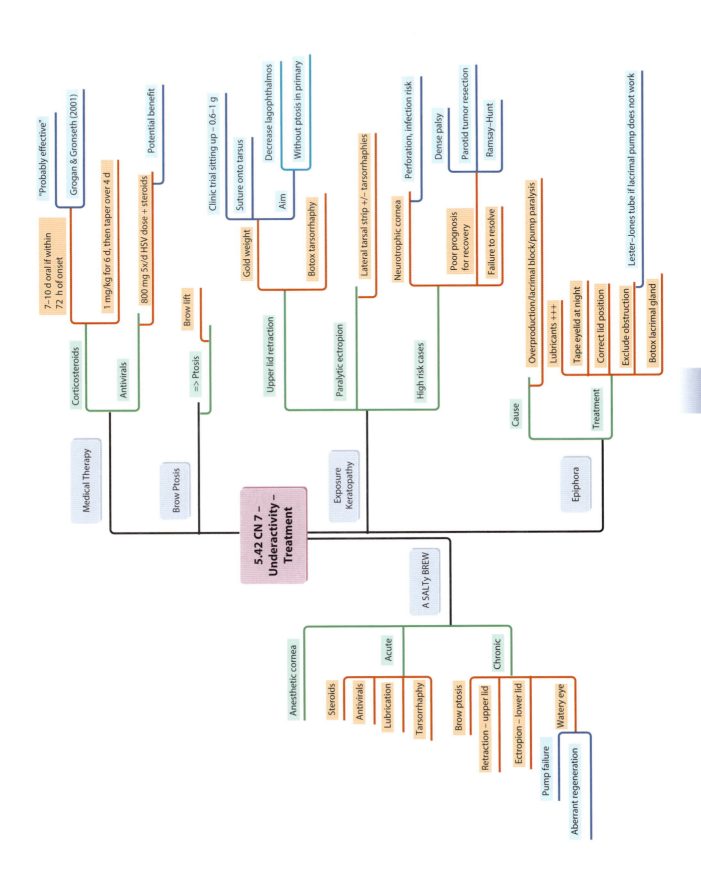

5.42 CN 7 – Underactivity – Treatment

Medical Therapy
- Corticosteroids
  - 7–10 d oral if within 72 h of onset
    - "Probably effective"
      - Grogan & Gronseth (2001)
    - 1 mg/kg for 6 d, then taper over 4 d
- Antivirals
  - 800 mg 5x/d HSV dose + steroids
    - Potential benefit

Brow Ptosis
- => Ptosis
  - Brow lift

Exposure Keratopathy
- Upper lid retraction
  - Gold weight
    - Clinic trial sitting up – 0.6–1 g
    - Suture onto tarsus
    - Aim
      - Decrease lagophthalmos
      - Without ptosis in primary
  - Botox tarsorrhaphy
- Paralytic ectropion
  - Lateral tarsal strip +/– tarsorrhaphies
- High risk cases
  - Neurotrophic cornea
    - Perforation, infection risk
  - Poor prognosis for recovery
    - Dense palsy
    - Parotid tumor resection
    - Ramsay–Hunt
  - Failure to resolve

Epiphora
- Cause
  - Overproduction/lacrimal block/pump paralysis
- Treatment
  - Lubricants +++
  - Tape eyelid at night
  - Correct lid position
  - Exclude obstruction
  - Botox lacrimal gland
  - Lester–Jones tube if lacrimal pump does not work

A SALTy BREW
- Acute
  - Anesthetic cornea
  - Steroids
  - Antivirals
  - Lubrication
  - Tarsorrhaphy
- Chronic
  - Brow ptosis
  - Retraction – upper lid
  - Ectropion – lower lid
  - Watery eye
    - Pump failure
    - Aberrant regeneration

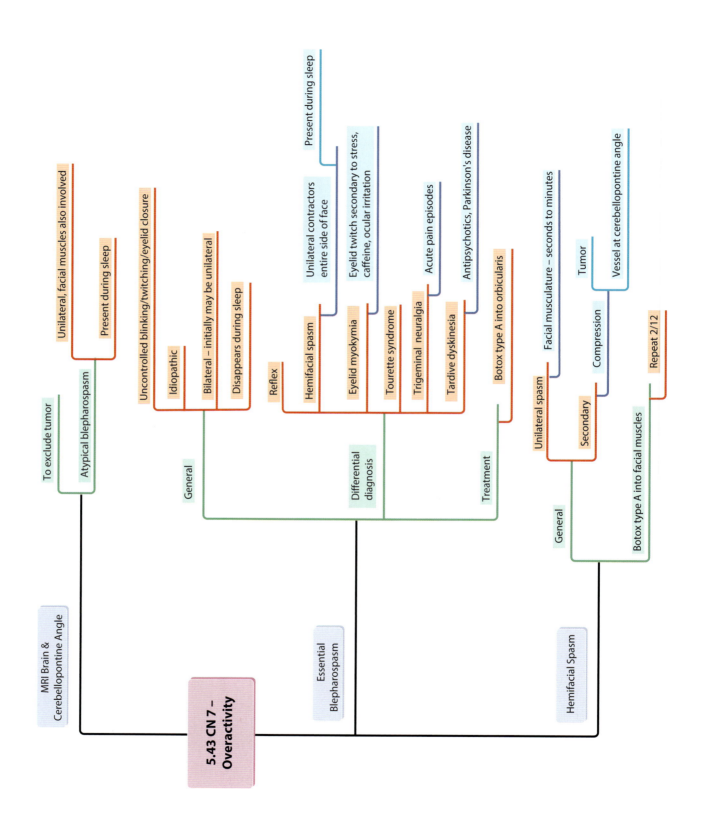

5.43 CN 7 – Overactivity

MRI Brain & Cerebellopontine Angle
- To exclude tumor
- Atypical blepharospasm
  - Unilateral, facial muscles also involved
  - Present during sleep

Essential Blepharospasm
- General
  - Uncontrolled blinking/twitching/eyelid closure
    - Idiopathic
    - Bilateral – initially may be unilateral
    - Disappears during sleep
      - Present during sleep
- Differential diagnosis
  - Reflex
  - Hemifacial spasm
    - Unilateral contractors entire side of face
  - Eyelid myokymia
    - Eyelid twitch secondary to stress, caffeine, ocular irritation
  - Tourette syndrome
  - Trigeminal neuralgia
    - Acute pain episodes
  - Tardive dyskinesia
    - Antipsychotics, Parkinson's disease
- Treatment
  - Botox type A into orbicularis

Hemifacial Spasm
- General
  - Unilateral spasm
    - Facial musculature – seconds to minutes
  - Secondary
    - Compression
      - Tumor
      - Vessel at cerebellopontine angle
- Botox type A into facial muscles
  - Repeat 2/12

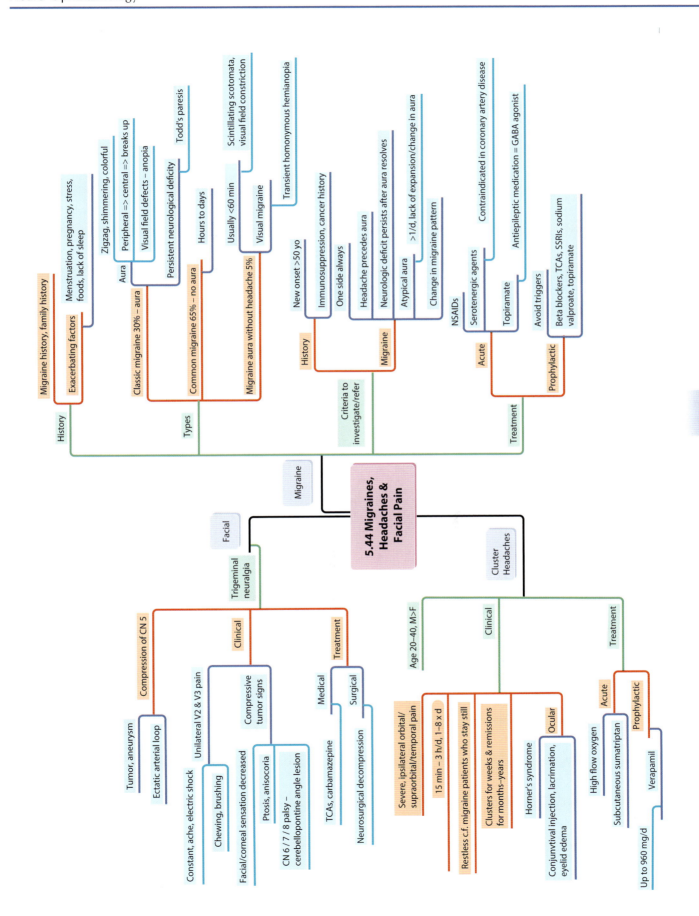

5.44 Migraines, Headaches & Facial Pain

Migraine

History
- Migraine history, family history
- Exacerbating factors
  - Menstruation, pregnancy, stress, foods, lack of sleep

Types
- Classic migraine 30% – aura
  - Aura
    - Zigzag, shimmering, colorful
    - Peripheral => central => breaks up
    - Visual field defects – anopia
    - Persistent neurological deficit
      - Todd's paresis
  - Hours to days
- Common migraine 65% – no aura
  - Usually <60 min
- Migraine aura without headache 5%
  - Visual migraine
    - Scintillating scotomata, visual field constriction
    - Transient homonymous hemianopia

Criteria to investigate/refer
- History
  - New onset >50 yo
  - Immunosuppression, cancer history
  - One side always
  - Headache precedes aura
  - Neurologic deficit persists after aura resolves
  - Atypical aura
  - >1/d, lack of expansion/change in aura
  - Change in migraine pattern

Treatment
- Acute
  - NSAIDs
  - Serotenergic agents
    - Contraindicated in coronary artery disease
  - Topiramate
- Prophylactic
  - Avoid triggers
  - Beta blockers, TCAs, SSRIs, sodium valproate, topiramate
    - Antiepileptic medication = GABA agonist

Facial

Trigeminal neuralgia
- Compression of CN 5
  - Tumor, aneurysm
  - Ectatic arterial loop
  - Constant, ache, electric shock
  - Unilateral V2 & V3 pain
    - Chewing, brushing
- Clinical
  - Compressive tumor signs
    - Facial/corneal sensation decreased
    - Ptosis, anisocoria
    - CN 6 / 7 / 8 palsy – cerebellopontine angle lesion
- Treatment
  - Medical
    - TCAs, carbamazepine
  - Surgical
    - Neurosurgical decompression

Cluster Headaches

- Age 20–40, M>F
- Clinical
  - Severe, ipsilateral orbital/supraorbital/temporal pain
  - 15 min – 3 h/d, 1–8 x d
  - Restless c.f. migraine patients who stay still
  - Clusters for weeks & remissions for months–years
  - Ocular
    - Horner's syndrome
    - Conjunvtival injection, lacrimation, eyelid edema
- Treatment
  - Acute
    - High flow oxygen
    - Subcutaneous sumatriptan
  - Prophylactic
    - Verapamil
      - Up to 960 mg/d

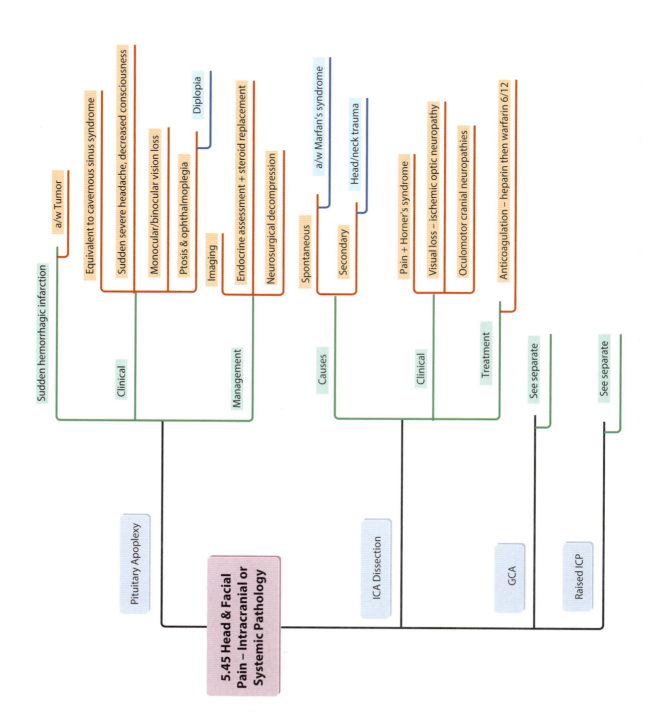

Sudden hemorrhagic infarction

a/w Tumor

Clinical
- Equivalent to cavernous sinus syndrome
- Sudden severe headache, decreased consciousness
- Monocular/binocular vision loss
- Ptosis & ophthalmoplegia
- Diplopia

Imaging

Management
- Endocrine assessment + steroid replacement
- Neurosurgical decompression

Pituitary Apoplexy

Causes
- Spontaneous
  - a/w Marfan's syndrome
- Secondary
  - Head/neck trauma

Clinical
- Pain + Horner's syndrome
- Visual loss – ischemic optic neuropathy
- Oculomotor cranial neuropathies

Treatment
- Anticoagulation – heparin then warfarin 6/12

ICA Dissection

See separate — GCA

See separate — Raised ICP

5.45 Head & Facial Pain – Intracranial or Systemic Pathology

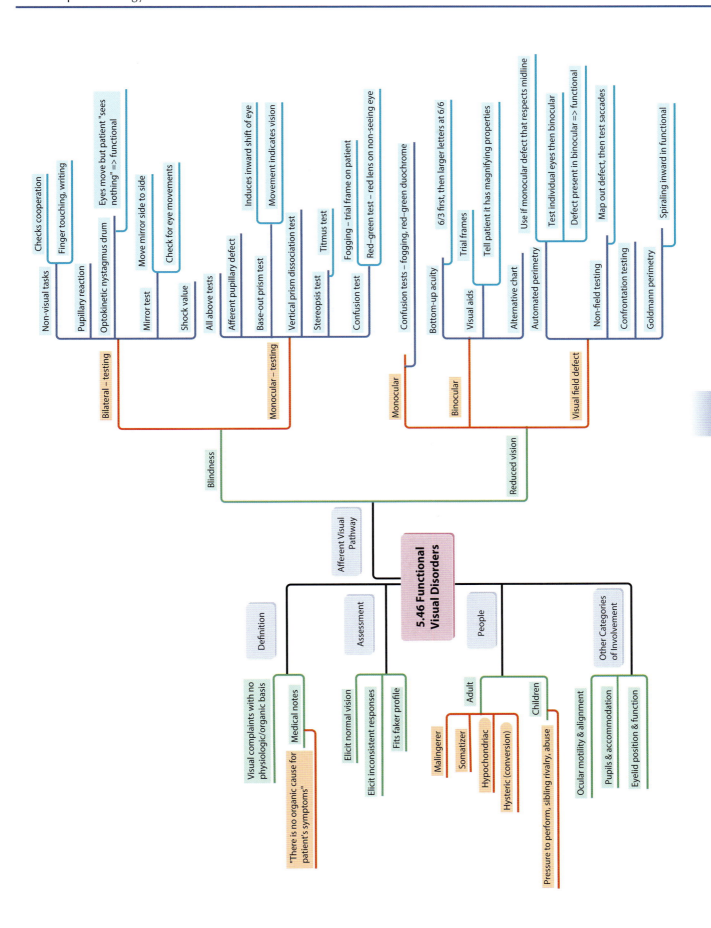

5.46 Functional Visual Disorders

Definition
- Visual complaints with no physiologic/organic basis
- Medical notes
  - "There is no organic cause for patient's symptoms"

Assessment
- Elicit normal vision
- Elicit inconsistent responses
- Fits faker profile

People
- Adult
  - Malingerer
  - Somatizer
  - Hypochondriac
  - Hysteric (conversion)
- Children
  - Pressure to perform, sibling rivalry, abuse

Other Categories of Involvement
- Ocular motility & alignment
- Pupils & accommodation
- Eyelid position & function

Afferent Visual Pathway
- Blindness
  - Bilateral – testing
    - Non-visual tasks
      - Checks cooperation
      - Finger touching, writing
    - Pupillary reaction
    - Optokinetic nystagmus drum
      - Eyes move but patient "sees nothing" => functional
    - Mirror test
      - Move mirror side to side
    - Shock value
      - Check for eye movements
  - Monocular – testing
    - All above tests
    - Afferent pupillary defect
    - Base-out prism test
      - Induces inward shift of eye
      - Movement indicates vision
    - Vertical prism dissociation test
    - Stereopsis test
      - Titmus test
    - Confusion test
      - Fogging – trial frame on patient
      - Red–green test – red lens on non-seeing eye
- Reduced vision
  - Monocular
    - Confusion tests – fogging, red–green duochrome
    - Bottom-up acuity
      - 6/3 first, then larger letters at 6/6
    - Visual aids
      - Trial frames
      - Tell patient it has magnifying properties
    - Alternative chart
  - Binocular
    - Automated perimetry
      - Use if monocular defect that respects midline
  - Visual field defect
    - Non-field testing
      - Test individual eyes then binocular
      - Defect present in binocular => functional
    - Confrontation testing
      - Map out defect, then test saccades
    - Goldmann perimetry
      - Spiraling inward in functional

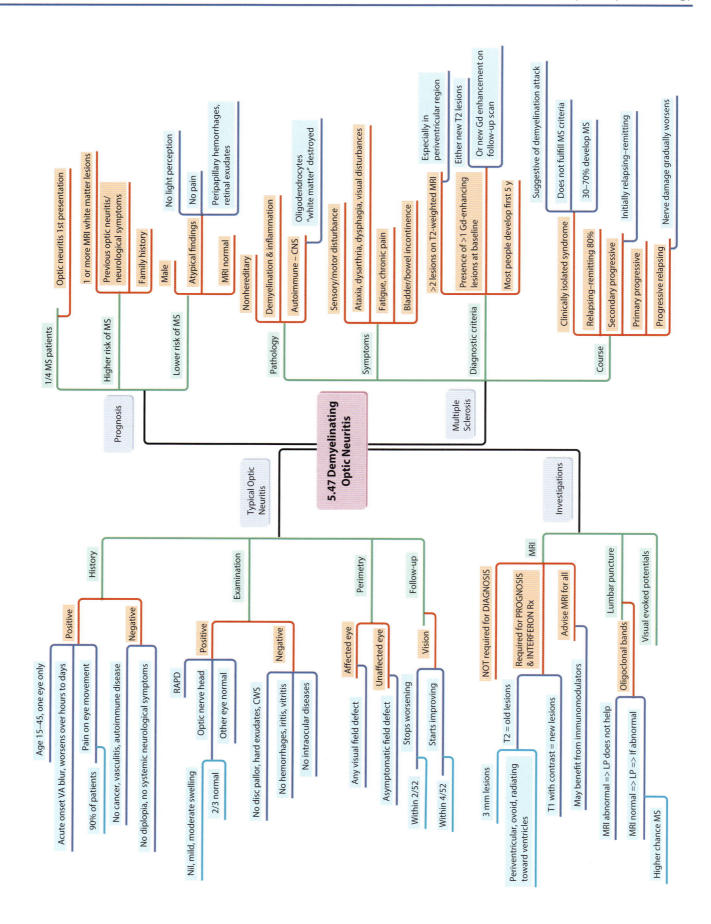

5.47 Demyelinating Optic Neuritis

Prognosis

- 1/4 MS patients
  - Optic neuritis 1st presentation
- Higher risk of MS
  - 1 or more MRI white matter lesions
  - Previous optic neuritis/neurological symptoms
  - Family history
- Lower risk of MS
  - Male
  - Atypical findings
    - No light perception
    - No pain
    - Peripapillary hemorrhages, retinal exudates
  - MRI normal

Multiple Sclerosis

- Pathology
  - Nonhereditary
  - Demyelination & inflammation
  - Autoimmune – CNS
    - Oligodendrocytes "white matter" destroyed
- Symptoms
  - Sensory/motor disturbance
  - Ataxia, dysarthria, dysphagia, visual disturbances
  - Fatigue, chronic pain
  - Bladder/bowel incontinence
- Diagnostic criteria
  - >2 lesions on T2-weighted MRI
    - Especially in periventricular region
  - Presence of >1 Gd-enhancing lesions at baseline
    - Either new T2 lesions
    - Or new Gd enhancement on follow-up scan
  - Most people develop first 5 y
- Course
  - Clinically isolated syndrome
    - Suggestive of demyelination attack
    - Does not fulfill MS criteria
    - 30–70% develop MS
  - Relapsing–remitting 80%
  - Secondary progressive
    - Initially relapsing–remitting
    - Nerve damage gradually worsens
  - Primary progressive
  - Progressive relapsing

Typical Optic Neuritis

- History
  - Positive
    - Age 15–45, one eye only
    - Acute onset VA blur, worsens over hours to days
    - Pain on eye movement
    - 90% of patients
  - Negative
    - No cancer, vasculitis, autoimmune disease
    - No diplopia, no systemic neurological symptoms
- Examination
  - Positive
    - RAPD
    - Optic nerve head
      - Nil, mild, moderate swelling
    - Other eye normal
      - 2/3 normal
  - Negative
    - No disc pallor, hard exudates, CWS
    - No hemorrhages, iritis, vitritis
    - No intraocular diseases
- Perimetry
  - Affected eye
    - Any visual field defect
  - Unaffected eye
    - Asymptomatic field defect
- Follow-up
  - Vision
    - Stops worsening
      - Within 2/52
    - Starts improving
      - Within 4/52

Investigations

- MRI
  - NOT required for DIAGNOSIS
  - Required for PROGNOSIS & INTERFERON Rx
  - Advise MRI for all
    - May benefit from immunomodulators
    - T1 with contrast = new lesions
    - T2 = old lesions
      - 3 mm lesions
      - Periventricular, ovoid, radiating toward ventricles
- Lumbar puncture
  - Oligoclonal bands
    - MRI abnormal => LP does not help
    - MRI normal => LP => If abnormal
      - Higher chance MS
- Visual evoked potentials

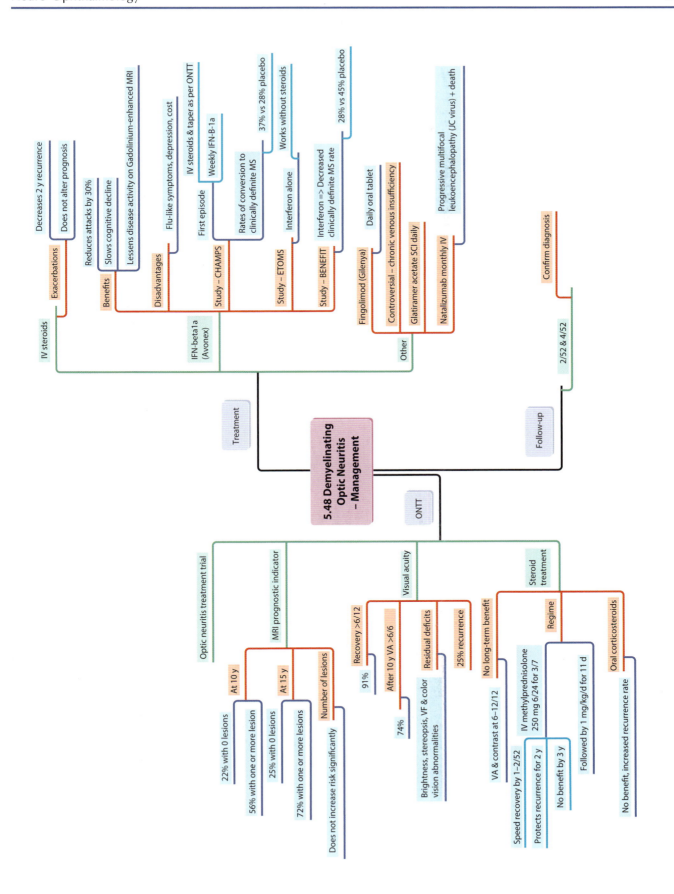

5.48 Demyelinating Optic Neuritis – Management

Treatment

IV steroids
- Exacerbations
  - Decreases 2 y recurrence
  - Does not alter prognosis

IFN-beta1a (Avonex)
- Benefits
  - Reduces attacks by 30%
  - Slows cognitive decline
  - Lessens disease activity on Gadolinium-enhanced MRI
- Disadvantages
  - Flu-like symptoms, depression, cost
  - IV steroids & taper as per ONTT
- Study – CHAMPS
  - First episode
  - Weekly IFN-B-1a
  - Rates of conversion to clinically definite MS — 37% vs 28% placebo
- Study – ETOMS
  - Interferon alone
  - Works without steroids
- Study – BENEFIT
  - Interferon => Decreased clinically definite MS rate — 28% vs 45% placebo

Other
- Fingolimod (Gilenya)
  - Daily oral tablet
- Controversial – chronic venous insufficiency
- Glatiramer acetate SCI daily
- Natalizumab monthly IV
  - Progressive multifocal leukoencephalopathy (JC virus) + death

Follow-up

2/52 & 4/52
- Confirm diagnosis

ONTT

Optic neuritis treatment trial

MRI prognostic indicator
- At 10 y
  - 22% with 0 lesions
  - 56% with one or more lesion
- At 15 y
  - 25% with 0 lesions
  - 72% with one or more lesions
- Number of lesions
  - Does not increase risk significantly

Visual acuity
- Recovery >6/12
  - 91%
- After 10 y VA >6/6
  - 74%
- Residual deficits
  - Brightness, stereopsis, VF & color vision abnormalities
- 25% recurrence

Steroid treatment
- No long-term benefit
  - VA & contrast at 6–12/12
- Regime
  - IV methylprednisolone 250 mg 6/24 for 3/7
    - Speed recovery by 1–2/52
    - Protects recurrence for 2 y
    - No benefit by 3 y
  - Followed by 1 mg/kg/d for 11 d
- Oral corticosteroids
  - No benefit, increased recurrence rate

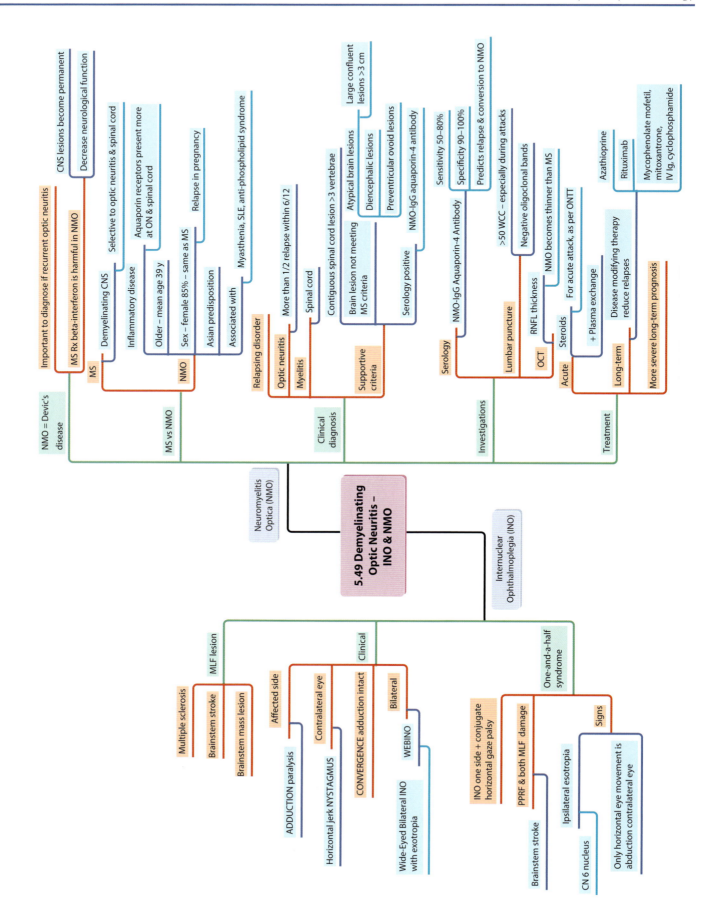

5.49 Demyelinating Optic Neuritis – INO & NMO

Neuromyelitis Optica (NMO)

NMO = Devic's disease

Important to diagnose if recurrent optic neuritis
- CNS lesions become permanent
- Decrease neurological function

MS Rx beta-interferon is harmful in NMO

MS
- Demyelinating CNS
- Inflammatory disease
- Selective to optic neuritis & spinal cord
- Aquaporin receptors present more at ON & spinal cord

NMO
- Older – mean age 39 y
- Sex – female 85% – same as MS
- Relapse in pregnancy
- Asian predisposition
- Associated with
  - Myasthenia, SLE, anti-phospholipid syndrome

MS vs NMO

Clinical diagnosis
- Relapsing disorder
  - Optic neuritis
  - Myelitis
    - More than 1/2 relapse within 6/12
    - Spinal cord
- Supportive criteria
  - Contiguous spinal cord lesion >3 vertebrae
  - Brain lesion not meeting MS criteria
    - Atypical brain lesions
      - Large confluent lesions >3 cm
    - Diencephalic lesions
    - Preventricular ovoid lesions
  - Serology positive
    - NMO-IgG aquaporin-4 antibody

Investigations
- Serology
  - NMO-IgG Aquaporin-4 Antibody
    - Sensitivity 50–80%
    - Specificity 90–100%
    - Predicts relapse & conversion to NMO
- Lumbar puncture
  - >50 WCC – especially during attacks
  - Negative oligoclonal bands
- OCT
  - RNFL thickness
    - NMO becomes thinner than MS

Treatment
- Acute
  - Steroids
    - For acute attack, as per ONTT
  - + Plasma exchange
- Long-term
  - Disease modifying therapy reduce relapses
    - Azathioprine
    - Rituximab
    - Mycophenolate mofetil, mitoxantrone, IV Ig, cyclophosphamide
- More severe long-term prognosis

Internuclear Ophthalmoplegia (INO)

Clinical
- MLF lesion
  - Multiple sclerosis
  - Brainstem stroke
  - Brainstem mass lesion
- Affected side
  - ADDUCTION paralysis
- Contralateral eye
  - Horizontal jerk NYSTAGMUS
- CONVERGENCE adduction intact
- Bilateral
  - WEBINO
    - Wide-Eyed Bilateral INO with exotropia

One-and-a-half syndrome
- INO one side + conjugate horizontal gaze palsy
- PPRF & both MLF damage
  - Brainstem stroke
- Signs
  - Ipsilateral esotropia
    - CN 6 nucleus
  - Only horizontal eye movement is abduction contralateral eye

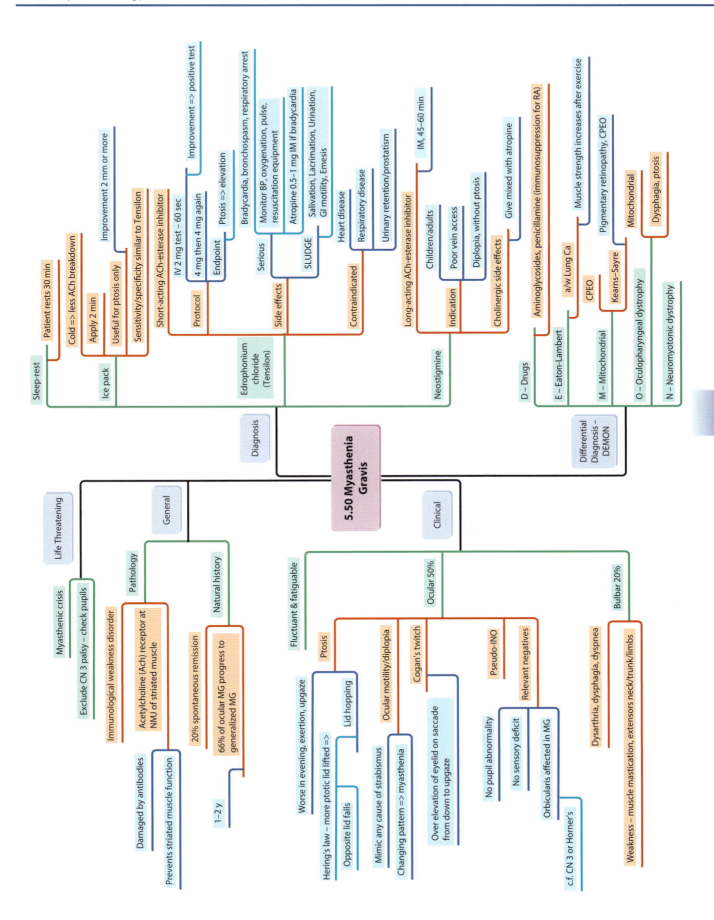

5.50 Myasthenia Gravis

Diagnosis

Sleep-rest
- Patient rests 30 min

Ice pack
- Cold => less ACh breakdown
- Apply 2 min
- Useful for ptosis only

Edrophonium chloride (Tensilon)
- Sensitivity/specificity similar to Tensilon
- Short-acting ACh-esterase inhibitor
- Improvement 2 mm or more
- Improvement => positive test
- Protocol
  - IV 2 mg test – 60 sec
  - 4 mg then 4 mg again
  - Endpoint
    - Ptosis => elevation
- Side effects
  - Serious
    - Bradycardia, bronchospasm, respiratory arrest
    - Monitor BP, oxygenation, pulse, resuscitation equipment
    - Atropine 0.5–1 mg IM if bradycardia
  - SLUDGE
    - Salivation, Lacrimation, Urination, GI motility, Emesis
- Contraindicated
  - Heart disease
  - Respiratory disease
  - Urinary retention/prostatism

Neostigmine
- Long-acting ACh-esterase inhibitor
  - IM, 45–60 min
- Indication
  - Children/adults
  - Poor vein access
  - Diplopia, without ptosis
- Cholinergic side effects
  - Give mixed with atropine

Differential Diagnosis – DEMON
- D – Drugs
  - Aminoglycosides, penicillamine (immunosuppression for RA)
- E – Eaton-Lambert
  - a/w Lung Ca
  - Muscle strength increases after exercise
- M – Mitochondrial
  - CPEO
    - Pigmentary retinopathy, CPEO
  - Kearns–Sayre
  - Mitochondrial
- O – Oculopharyngeal dystrophy
  - Dysphagia, ptosis
- N – Neuromyotonic dystrophy

Life Threatening
- Myasthenic crisis
- Exclude CN 3 palsy – check pupils

General

Pathology
- Immunological weakness disorder
- Acetylcholine (Ach) receptor at NMJ of striated muscle
  - Damaged by antibodies
  - Prevents striated muscle function

Natural history
- 20% spontaneous remission
- 66% of ocular MG progress to generalized MG
  - 1–2 y

Clinical

Ocular 50%
- Fluctuant & fatiguable
- Ptosis
  - Worse in evening, exertion, upgaze
  - Lid hopping
  - Hering's law – more ptotic lid lifted =>
    - Opposite lid falls
- Ocular motility/diplopia
  - Mimic any cause of strabismus
  - Changing pattern => myasthenia
- Cogan's twitch
  - Over elevation of eyelid on saccade from down to upgaze
- Pseudo-INO
- Relevant negatives
  - No pupil abnormality
  - No sensory deficit
  - Orbicularis affected in MG
    - c.f. CN 3 or Horner's

Bulbar 20%
- Dysarthria, dysphagia, dyspnea
- Weakness – muscle mastication, extensors neck/trunk/limbs

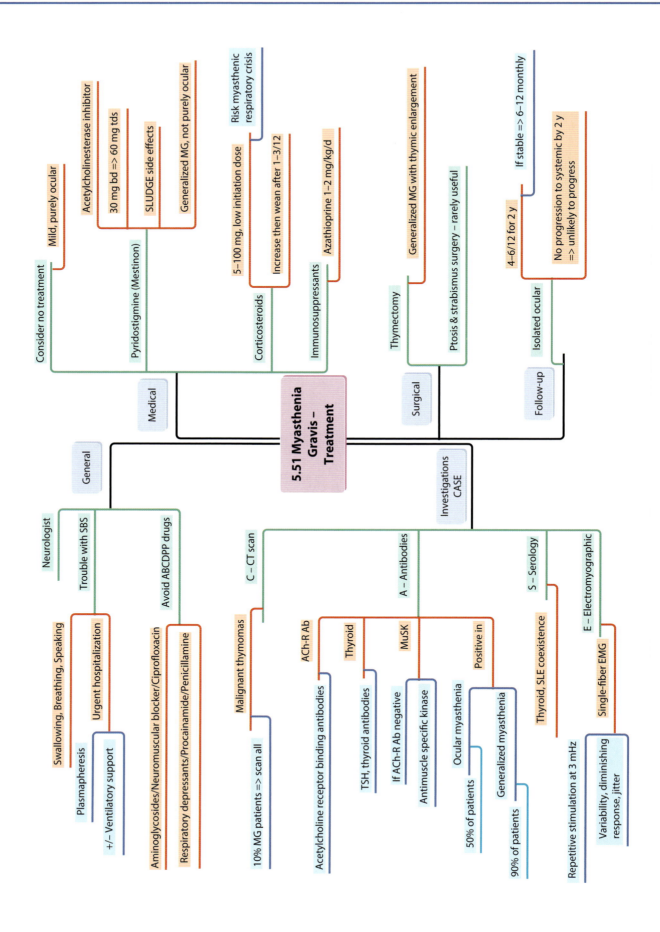

5.51 Myasthenia Gravis – Treatment

Medical

Consider no treatment
- Mild, purely ocular

Pyridostigmine (Mestinon)
- Acetylcholinesterase inhibitor
- 30 mg bd => 60 mg tds
- SLUDGE side effects
- Generalized MG, not purely ocular

Corticosteroids
- 5–100 mg, low initiation dose
- Increase then wean after 1–3/12
  - Risk myasthenic respiratory crisis

Immunosuppressants
- Azathioprine 1–2 mg/kg/d

Surgical

Thymectomy
- Generalized MG with thymic enlargement

Ptosis & strabismus surgery – rarely useful

Follow-up

Isolated ocular
- 4–6/12 for 2 y
- No progression to systemic by 2 y => unlikely to progress
- If stable => 6–12 monthly

General

Neurologist

Trouble with SBS
- Swallowing, Breathing, Speaking
- Urgent hospitalization
  - Plasmapheresis
  - +/– Ventilatory support

Avoid ABCDPP drugs
- Aminoglycosides/Neuromuscular blocker/Ciprofloxacin
- Respiratory depressants/Procainamide/Penicillamine

Investigations CASE

C – CT scan
- Malignant thymomas
- 10% MG patients => scan all

A – Antibodies
- ACh-R Ab
  - Acetylcholine receptor binding antibodies
- Thyroid
  - TSH, thyroid antibodies
- MuSK
  - If ACh-R Ab negative
  - Antimuscle specific kinase
  - Muscle specific kinase
- Positive in
  - Ocular myasthenia – 50% of patients
  - Generalized myasthenia – 90% of patients

S – Serology
- Thyroid, SLE coexistence

E – Electromyographic
- Single-fiber EMG
- Repetitive stimulation at 3 mHz
- Variability, diminishing response, jitter

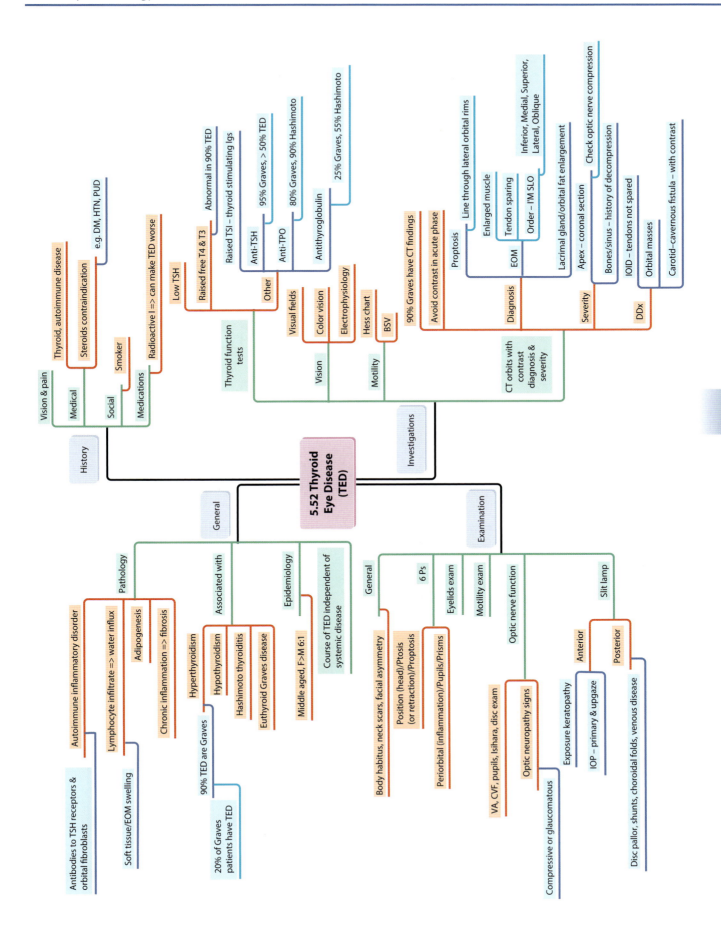

5.52 Thyroid Eye Disease (TED)

History

Vision & pain

Medical
- Thyroid, autoimmune disease
- Steroids contraindication — e.g. DM, HTN, PUD

Social
- Smoker

Medications
- Radioactive I => can make TED worse

Thyroid function tests
- Low TSH
- Raised free T4 & T3 — Abnormal in 90% TED
- Raised TSI – thyroid stimulating Igs
- Other
  - Anti-TSH — 95% Graves, > 50% TED
  - Anti-TPO — 80% Graves, 90% Hashimoto
  - Antithyroglobulin — 25% Graves, 55% Hashimoto

Investigations

Vision
- Visual fields
- Color vision
- Electrophysiology

Motility
- Hess chart
- BSV

CT orbits with contrast diagnosis & severity
- 90% Graves have CT findings
- Avoid contrast in acute phase
- **Diagnosis**
  - Proptosis — Line through lateral orbital rims
  - Enlarged muscle
  - EOM
    - Tendon sparing
    - Order – I'M SLO — Inferior, Medial, Superior, Lateral, Oblique
  - Lacrimal gland/orbital fat enlargement
  - Apex – coronal section — Check optic nerve compression
- **Severity**
  - Bones/sinus – history of decompression
  - IOID – tendons not spared
- **DDx**
  - Orbital masses
  - Carotid–cavernous fistula – with contrast

General

Pathology
- Autoimmune inflammatory disorder — Antibodies to TSH receptors & orbital fibroblasts
- Lymphocyte infiltrate => water influx — Soft tissue/EOM swelling
- Adipogenesis
- Chronic inflammation => fibrosis

Associated with
- Hyperthyroidism — 90% TED are Graves
- Hypothyroidism
- Hashimoto thyroiditis
- Euthyroid Graves disease — 20% of Graves patients have TED

Epidemiology
- Middle aged, F>M 6:1
- Course of TED independent of systemic disease

Examination

General
- Body habitus, neck scars, facial asymmetry

6 Ps
- Position (head)/Ptosis (or retraction)/Proptosis
- Periorbital (inflammation)/Pupils/Prisms

Eyelids exam

Motility exam

Optic nerve function
- VA, CVF, pupils, Isihara, disc exam
- Optic neuropathy signs — Compressive or glaucomatous

Slit lamp
- Anterior — Exposure keratopathy
  - IOP – primary & upgaze
- Posterior — Disc pallor, shunts, choroidal folds, venous disease

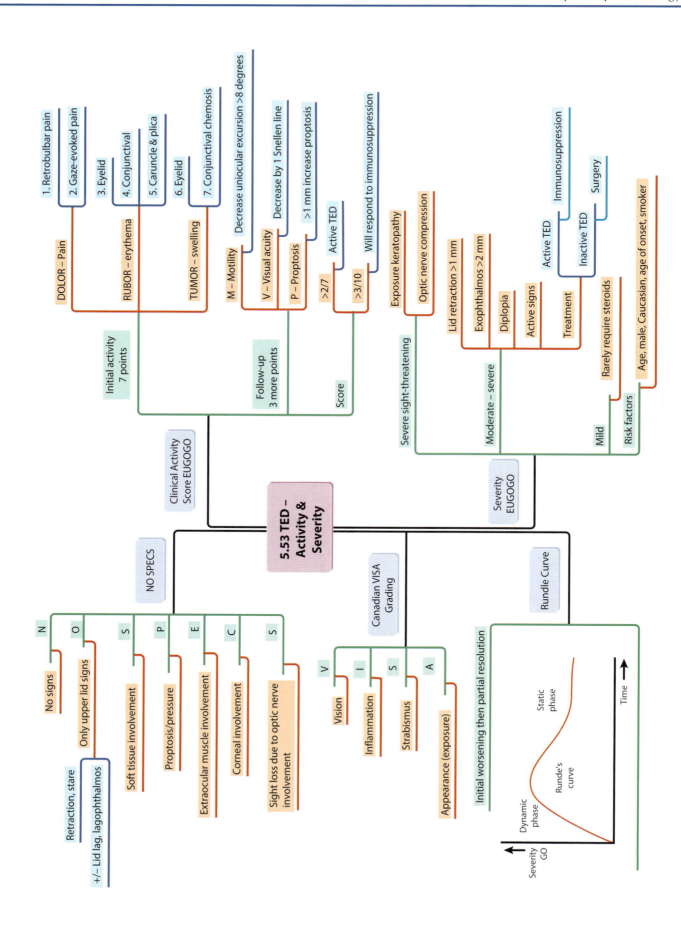

5.53 TED – Activity & Severity

Clinical Activity Score EUGOGO

Initial activity 7 points
- DOLOR – Pain
  - 1. Retrobulbar pain
  - 2. Gaze-evoked pain
- RUBOR – erythema
  - 3. Eyelid
  - 4. Conjunctival
- TUMOR – swelling
  - 5. Caruncle & plica
  - 6. Eyelid
  - 7. Conjunctival chemosis

Follow-up 3 more points
- M – Motility — Decrease uniocular excursion >8 degrees
- V – Visual acuity — Decrease by 1 Snellen line
- P – Proptosis — >1 mm increase proptosis

Score
- >2/7 — Active TED
- >3/10 — Will respond to immunosuppression

Severity EUGOGO

- Severe sight-threatening
  - Exposure keratopathy
  - Optic nerve compression
- Moderate – severe
  - Lid retraction >1 mm
  - Exophthalmos >2 mm
  - Diplopia
  - Active signs
  - Treatment
    - Active TED — Immunosuppression
    - Inactive TED — Surgery
- Mild
  - Rarely require steroids
- Risk factors
  - Age, male, Caucasian, age of onset, smoker

NO SPECS
- N — No signs
- O — Only upper lid signs
  - Retraction, stare
  - +/– Lid lag, lagophthalmos
- S — Soft tissue involvement
- P — Proptosis/pressure
- E — Extraocular muscle involvement
- C — Corneal involvement
- S — Sight loss due to optic nerve involvement

Canadian VISA Grading
- V — Vision
- I — Inflammation
- S — Strabismus
- A — Appearance (exposure)

Rundle Curve
- Initial worsening then partial resolution

Severity GO — Dynamic phase — Runde's curve — Static phase — Time

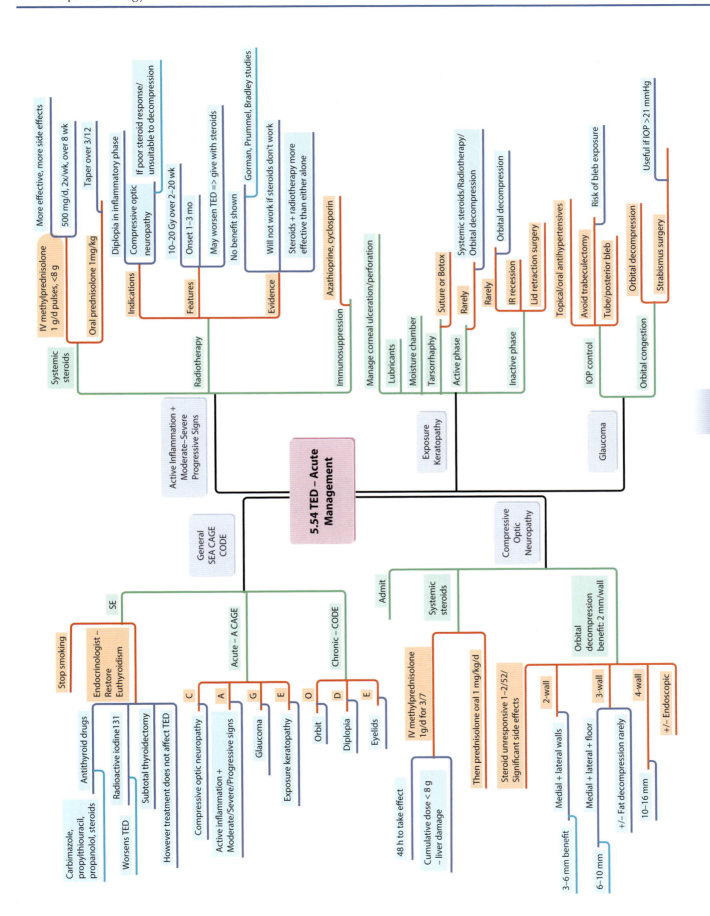

5.54 TED – Acute Management

Active Inflammation + Moderate–Severe Progressive Signs

Systemic steroids
- IV methylprednisolone 1 g/d pulses, <8 g
  - More effective, more side effects
  - 500 mg/d, 2x/wk, over 8 wk
  - Taper over 3/12
- Oral prednisolone 1mg/kg

Radiotherapy
- Indications
  - Diplopia in inflammatory phase
  - Compressive optic neuropathy
    - If poor steroid response/unsuitable to decompression
- Features
  - 10–20 Gy over 2–20 wk
  - Onset 1–3 mo
  - May worsen TED => give with steroids
  - No benefit shown
- Evidence
  - Will not work if steroids don't work
  - Gorman, Prummel, Bradley studies
  - Steroids + radiotherapy more effective than either alone

Immunosuppression
- Azathioprine, cyclosporin

Exposure Keratopathy
- Manage corneal ulceration/perforation
- Lubricants
- Moisture chamber
- Tarsorrhaphy
- Active phase
  - Suture or Botox
  - Systemic steroids/Radiotherapy/Orbital decompression
  - Rarely
- Inactive phase
  - Rarely: Orbital decompression
  - IR recession
  - Lid retraction surgery

Glaucoma
- IOP control
  - Topical/oral antihypertensives
  - Avoid trabeculectomy
    - Risk of bleb exposure
    - Tube/posterior bleb
- Orbital congestion
  - Orbital decompression
  - Strabismus surgery
  - Useful if IOP >21 mmHg

General SEA CAGE CODE
- SE
  - Stop smoking
  - Endocrinologist – Restore Euthyroidism
    - Antithyroid drugs
      - Carbimazole, propylthiouracil, propanolol, steroids
    - Radioactive iodine131
      - Worsens TED
    - Subtotal thyroidectomy
      - However treatment does not affect TED
- Acute – A CAGE
  - C: Compressive optic neuropathy
  - A: Active inflammation + Moderate/Severe/Progressive signs
  - G: Glaucoma
  - E: Exposure keratopathy
- Chronic – CODE
  - O: Orbit
  - D: Diplopia
  - E: Eyelids

Compressive Optic Neuropathy
- Admit
- Systemic steroids
  - IV methylprednisolone 1g/d for 3/7
    - 48 h to take effect
    - Cumulative dose < 8 g – liver damage
  - Then prednisolone oral 1 mg/kg/d
  - Steroid unresponsive 1–2/52/Significant side effects
- Orbital decompression benefit: 2 mm/wall
  - 2-wall
    - Medial + lateral walls
      - 3–6 mm benefit
  - 3-wall
    - Medial + lateral + floor
      - 6–10 mm
  - 4-wall
    - +/- Fat decompression rarely
    - 10–16 mm
  - +/- Endoscopic

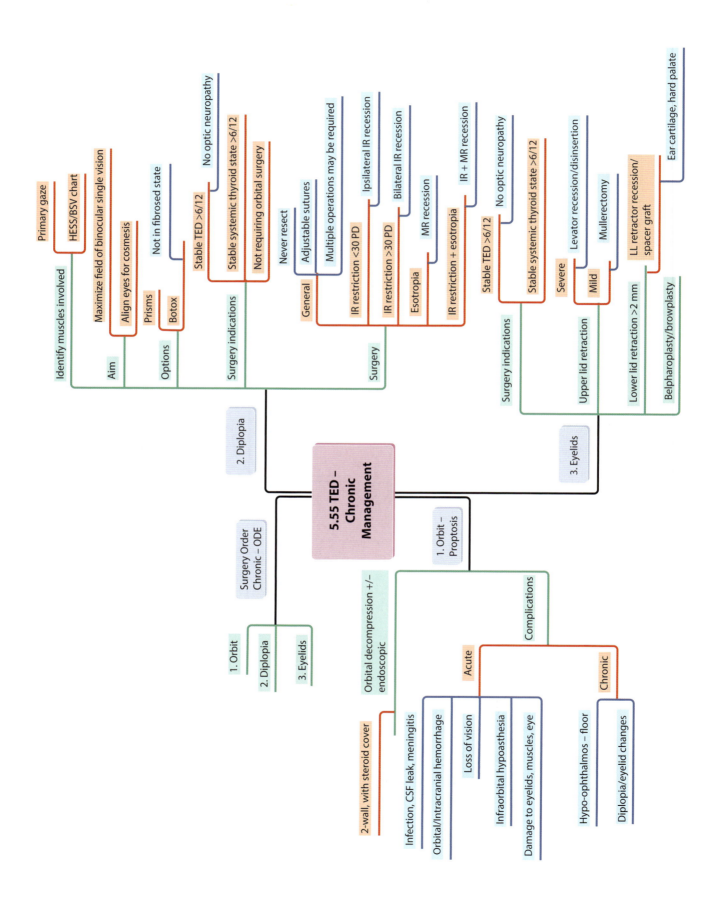

5.55 TED – Chronic Management

Surgery Order Chronic – ODE
- 1. Orbit
- 2. Diplopia
- 3. Eyelids

1. Orbit – Proptosis

Orbital decompression +/− endoscopic
- 2-wall, with steroid cover

Complications
- Acute
  - Infection, CSF leak, meningitis
  - Orbital/Intracranial hemorrhage
  - Loss of vision
  - Infraorbital hypoasthesia
  - Damage to eyelids, muscles, eye
- Chronic
  - Hypo-ophthalmos – floor
  - Diplopia/eyelid changes

2. Diplopia

Identify muscles involved
- Primary gaze
- HESS/BSV chart

Aim
- Maximize field of binocular single vision
- Align eyes for cosmesis

Options
- Prisms
- Botox
  - Not in fibrosed state

Surgery indications
- Stable TED >6/12
- Stable systemic thyroid state >6/12
- Not requiring orbital surgery
  - No optic neuropathy

Surgery
- General
  - Never resect
  - Adjustable sutures
  - Multiple operations may be required
- IR restriction <30 PD
  - Ipsilateral IR recession
- IR restriction >30 PD
  - Bilateral IR recession
- Esotropia
  - MR recession
- IR restriction + esotropia
  - IR + MR recession

3. Eyelids

Surgery indications
- Stable TED >6/12
- Stable systemic thyroid state >6/12
  - No optic neuropathy

Upper lid retraction
- Severe
  - Levator recession/disinsertion
- Mild
  - Mullerectomy

Lower lid retraction >2 mm
- LL retractor recession/spacer graft
  - Ear cartilage, hard palate

Belpharoplasty/browplasty

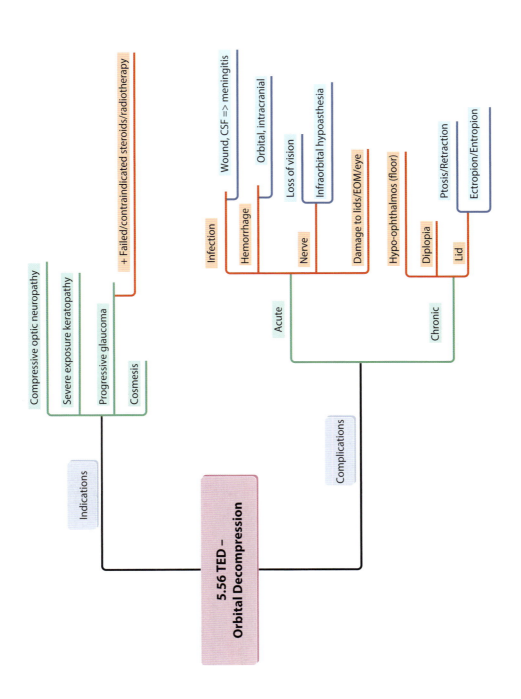

5.56 TED – Orbital Decompression

Indications

- Compressive optic neuropathy
- Severe exposure keratopathy
- Progressive glaucoma
- Cosmesis
  - + Failed/contraindicated steroids/radiotherapy

Complications

- Acute
  - Infection
    - Wound, CSF => meningitis
  - Hemorrhage
    - Orbital, intracranial
  - Nerve
    - Loss of vision
    - Infraorbital hypoasthesia
  - Damage to lids/EOM/eye
- Chronic
  - Hypo-ophthalmos (floor)
  - Diplopia
  - Lid
    - Ptosis/Retraction
    - Ectropion/Entropion

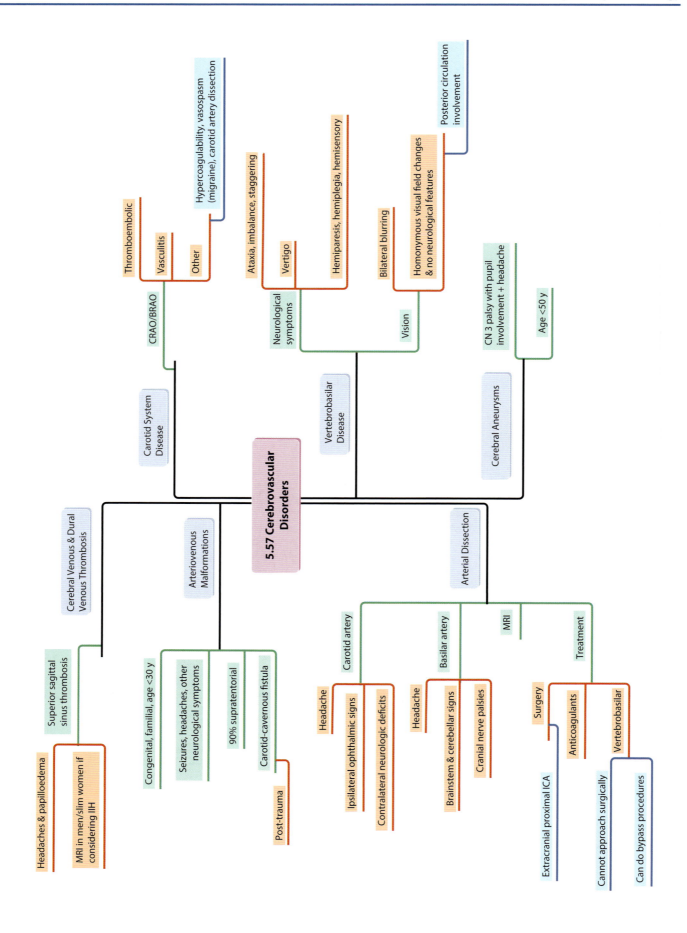

5.57 Cerebrovascular Disorders

Carotid System Disease
- CRAO/BRAO
  - Thromboembolic
  - Vasculitis
  - Other
    - Hypercoagulability, vasospasm (migraine), carotid artery dissection

Vertebrobasilar Disease
- Neurological symptoms
  - Ataxia, imbalance, staggering
  - Vertigo
  - Hemiparesis, hemiplegia, hemisensory
- Vision
  - Bilateral blurring
  - Homonymous visual field changes & no neurological features
    - Posterior circulation involvement

Cerebral Aneurysms
- CN 3 palsy with pupil involvement + headache
- Age <50 y

Cerebral Venous & Dural Venous Thrombosis
- Superior sagittal sinus thrombosis
  - Headaches & papilloedema
  - MRI in men/slim women if considering IIH

Arteriovenous Malformations
- Congenital, familial, age <30 y
- Seizures, headaches, other neurological symptoms
- 90% supratentorial
- Carotid-cavernous fistula
  - Post-trauma

Arterial Dissection
- Carotid artery
  - Headache
  - Ipsilateral ophthalmic signs
  - Contralateral neurologic deficits
- Basilar artery
  - Headache
  - Brainstem & cerebellar signs
  - Cranial nerve palsies
- MRI
- Treatment
  - Surgery
    - Extracranial proximal ICA
  - Anticoagulants
  - Vertebrobasilar
    - Cannot approach surgically
    - Can do bypass procedures

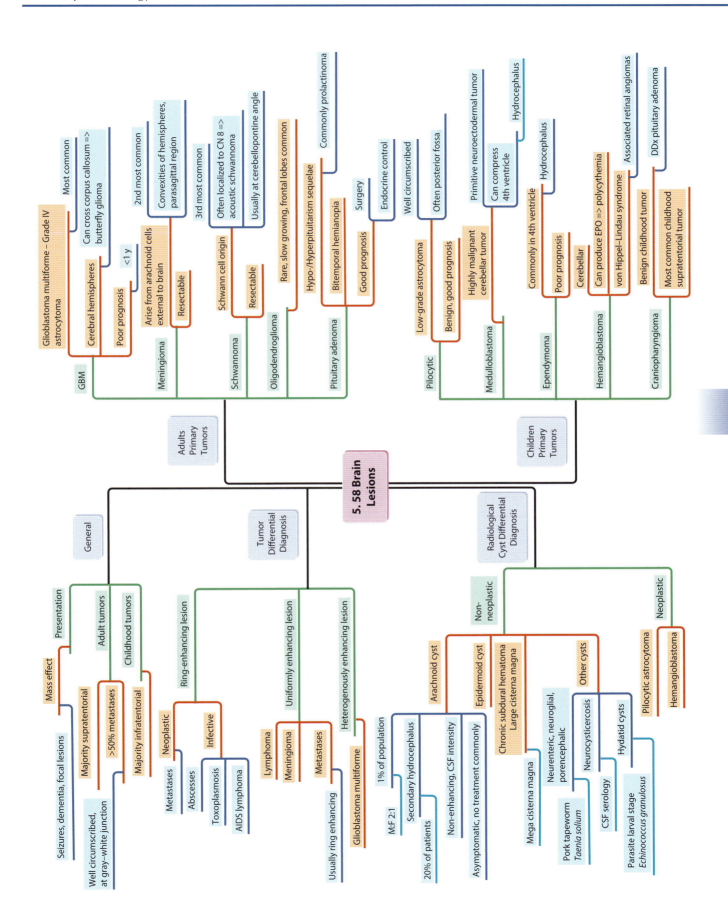

5. 58 Brain Lesions

Adults Primary Tumors

GBM
- Glioblastoma multiforme – Grade IV astrocytoma
  - Most common
  - Can cross corpus callosum => butterfly glioma
- Cerebral hemispheres
- Poor prognosis
  - <1 y

Meningioma
- Arise from arachnoid cells external to brain
- 2nd most common
- Convexities of hemispheres, parasagittal region
- Resectable

Schwannoma
- Schwann cell origin
- 3rd most common
- Often localized to CN 8 => acoustic schwannoma
- Usually at cerebellopontine angle
- Resectable

Oligodendroglioma
- Rare, slow growing, frontal lobes common

Pituitary adenoma
- Hypo-/Hyperpituitarism sequelae
- Bitemporal hemianopia
- Good prognosis
- Surgery
- Endocrine control
- Commonly prolactinoma

Children Primary Tumors

Pilocytic
- Low-grade astrocytoma
- Well circumscribed
- Benign, good prognosis
- Often posterior fossa

Medulloblastoma
- Primitive neuroectodermal tumor
- Highly malignant cerebellar tumor
- Can compress 4th ventricle
- Hydrocephalus

Ependymoma
- Commonly in 4th ventricle
- Poor prognosis
- Hydrocephalus

Hemangioblastoma
- Cerebellar
- Can produce EPO => polycythemia
- von Hippel–Lindau syndrome
- Associated retinal angiomas

Craniopharyngioma
- Benign childhood tumor
- Most common childhood supratentorial tumor
- DDx pituitary adenoma

General

Presentation
- Mass effect
- Seizures, dementia, focal lesions

Adult tumors
- Majority supratentorial
- >50% metastases

Childhood tumors
- Majority infratentorial

Tumor Differential Diagnosis

Ring-enhancing lesion
- Neoplastic
  - Metastases
- Infective
  - Abscesses
  - Toxoplasmosis
  - AIDS lymphoma
- Well circumscribed, at gray–white junction

Uniformly enhancing lesion
- Lymphoma
- Meningioma
- Usually ring enhancing

Heterogenously enhancing lesion
- Metastases
- Glioblastoma multiforme

Radiological Cyst Differential Diagnosis

Non-neoplastic
- Arachnoid cyst
  - 1% of population
  - M:F 2:1
  - Secondary hydrocephalus
  - 20% of patients
- Epidermoid cyst
  - Non-enhancing, CSF intensity
  - Asymptomatic, no treatment commonly
- Chronic subdural hematoma
- Large cisterna magna
  - Mega cisterna magna
- Other cysts
  - Neurenteric, neuroglial, porencephalic
  - Neurocysticercosis
    - Pork tapeworm
    - Taenia solium
    - CSF serology
  - Hydatid cysts
    - Parasite larval stage
    - Echinococcus granulosus

Neoplastic
- Pilocytic astrocytoma
- Hemangioblastoma

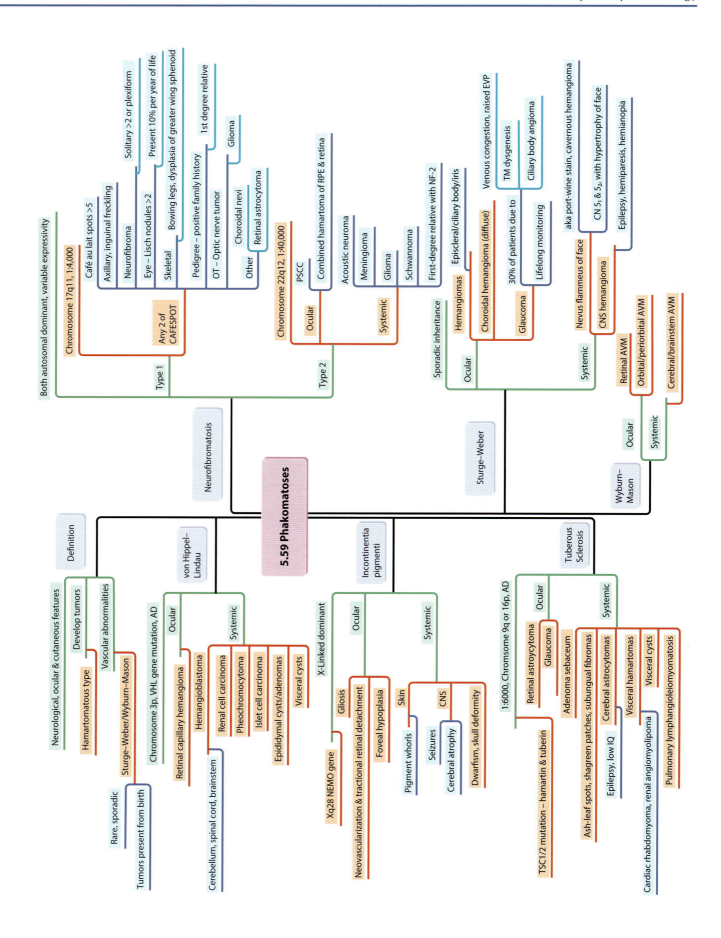

5.59 Phakomatoses

Neurofibromatosis

Type 1
- Both autosomal dominant, variable expressivity
- Chromosome 17q11, 1:4,000
- Any 2 of CAFESPOT
  - Café au lait spots >5
  - Axillary, inguinal freckling
  - Neurofibroma
    - Solitary >2 or plexiform
  - Eye – Lisch nodules >2
    - Present 10% per year of life
  - Skeletal
    - Bowing legs, dysplasia of greater wing sphenoid
  - Pedigree – positive family history
    - 1st degree relative
  - OT – Optic nerve tumor
    - Glioma
  - Other
    - Choroidal nevi
    - Retinal astrocytoma

Type 2
- Chromosome 22q12, 1:40,000
- Ocular
  - PSCC
  - Combined hamartoma of RPE & retina
- Systemic
  - Acoustic neuroma
  - Meningioma
  - Glioma
  - Schwannoma
  - First-degree relative with NF-2

Sturge–Weber
- Sporadic inheritance
- Ocular
  - Episcleral/ciliary body/iris
  - Hemangiomas
  - Choroidal hemangioma (diffuse)
  - Glaucoma
    - 30% of patients due to
      - Venous congestion, raised EVP
      - TM dysgenesis
      - Ciliary body angioma
    - Lifelong monitoring
- Systemic
  - Nevus flammeus of face
    - aka port-wine stain, cavernous hemangioma
  - CNS hemangioma
    - CN 5₁ & 5₂, with hypertrophy of face
    - Epilepsy, hemiparesis, hemianopia

Wyburn–Mason
- Ocular
  - Retinal AVM
- Systemic
  - Orbital/periorbital AVM
  - Cerebral/brainstem AVM

Definition
- Neurological, ocular & cutaneous features
- Develop tumors
  - Hamartomatous type
- Vascular abnormalities
  - Sturge–Weber/Wyburn–Mason
    - Rare, sporadic
    - Tumors present from birth

von Hippel–Lindau
- Chromosome 3p, VHL gene mutation, AD
- Ocular
  - Retinal capillary hemangioma
- Systemic
  - Hemangioblastoma
    - Cerebellum, spinal cord, brainstem
  - Renal cell carcinoma
  - Pheochromocytoma
  - Islet cell carcinoma
  - Epididymal cysts/adenomas
  - Visceral cysts

Incontinentia pigmenti
- X-Linked dominant
  - Xq28 NEMO gene
- Ocular
  - Gliosis
  - Neovascularization & tractional retinal detachment
  - Foveal hypoplasia
- Systemic
  - Skin
    - Pigment whorls
  - CNS
    - Seizures
    - Cerebral atrophy
    - Dwarfism, skull deformity

Tuberous Sclerosis
- 1:6000, Chromosome 9q or 16p, AD
  - TSC1/2 mutation – hamartin & tuberin
- Ocular
  - Retinal astrocytoma
  - Glaucoma
- Systemic
  - Adenoma sebaceum
    - Ash-leaf spots, shagreen patches, subungual fibromas
  - Cerebral astrocytoma
    - Epilepsy, low IQ
  - Visceral hamartomas
    - Cardiac rhabdomyoma, renal angiomyolipoma
  - Visceral cysts
  - Pulmonary lymphangioleiomyomatosis

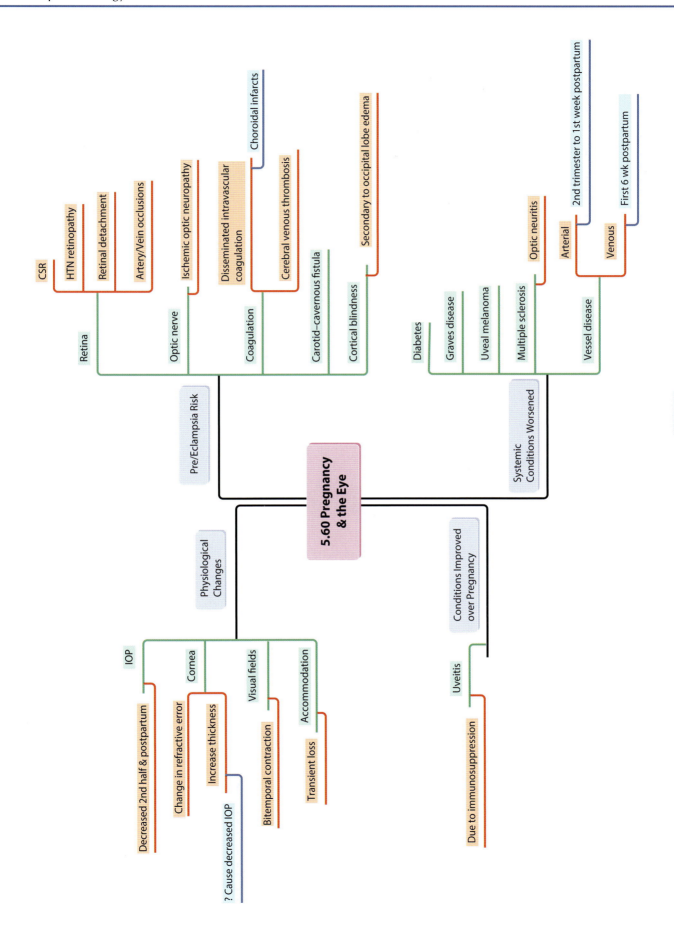

5.60 Pregnancy & the Eye

Pre/Eclampsia Risk

Retina
- CSR
- HTN retinopathy
- Retinal detachment
- Artery/Vein occlusions

Optic nerve
- Ischemic optic neuropathy

Coagulation
- Disseminated intravascular coagulation — Choroidal infarcts
- Cerebral venous thrombosis

Carotid–cavernous fistula

Cortical blindness — Secondary to occipital lobe edema

Systemic Conditions Worsened

Diabetes

Graves disease

Uveal melanoma

Multiple sclerosis — Optic neuritis

Vessel disease
- Arterial — 2nd trimester to 1st week postpartum
- Venous — First 6 wk postpartum

Physiological Changes

IOP
- Decreased 2nd half & postpartum
- ? Cause decreased IOP

Cornea
- Change in refractive error
- Increase thickness

Visual fields
- Bitemporal contraction

Accommodation
- Transient loss

Conditions Improved over Pregnancy

Uveitis — Due to immunosuppression

6 Oncology

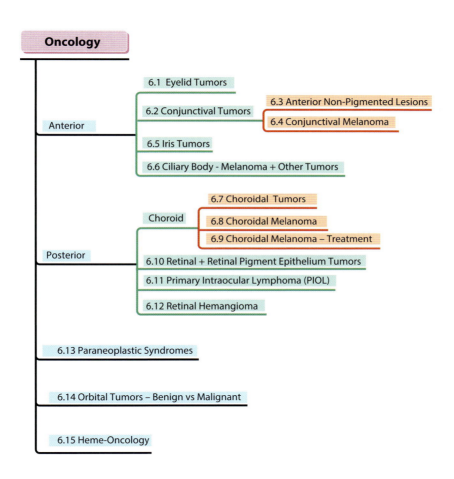

Oncology

- **Anterior**
  - 6.1 Eyelid Tumors
  - 6.2 Conjunctival Tumors
    - 6.3 Anterior Non-Pigmented Lesions
    - 6.4 Conjunctival Melanoma
  - 6.5 Iris Tumors
  - 6.6 Ciliary Body - Melanoma + Other Tumors
- **Posterior**
  - Choroid
    - 6.7 Choroidal Tumors
    - 6.8 Choroidal Melanoma
    - 6.9 Choroidal Melanoma – Treatment
  - 6.10 Retinal + Retinal Pigment Epithelium Tumors
  - 6.11 Primary Intraocular Lymphoma (PIOL)
  - 6.12 Retinal Hemangioma
- 6.13 Paraneoplastic Syndromes
- 6.14 Orbital Tumors – Benign vs Malignant
- 6.15 Heme-Oncology

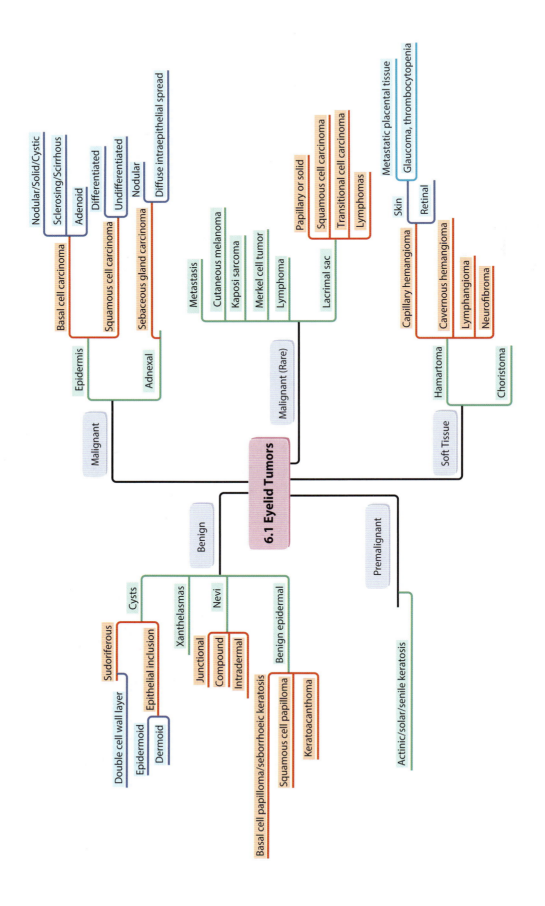

6.1 Eyelid Tumors

Malignant

- Epidermis
  - Basal cell carcinoma
    - Nodular/Solid/Cystic
    - Sclerosing/Scirrhous
    - Adenoid
  - Squamous cell carcinoma
    - Differentiated
    - Undifferentiated
- Adnexal
  - Sebaceous gland carcinoma
    - Nodular
    - Diffuse intraepithelial spread

Malignant (Rare)

- Metastasis
- Cutaneous melanoma
- Kaposi sarcoma
- Merkel cell tumor
- Lymphoma
- Lacrimal sac
  - Papillary or solid
  - Squamous cell carcinoma
  - Transitional cell carcinoma
  - Lymphomas

Soft Tissue

- Hamartoma
  - Capillary hemangioma
    - Skin
    - Retinal
      - Metastatic placental tissue
      - Glaucoma, thrombocytopenia
  - Cavernous hemangioma
  - Lymphangioma
  - Neurofibroma
- Choristoma

Benign

- Cysts
  - Sudoriferous
  - Epithelial inclusion
    - Double cell wall layer
    - Epidermoid
    - Dermoid
- Xanthelasmas
- Nevi
  - Junctional
  - Compound
  - Intradermal
- Benign epidermal
  - Basal cell papilloma/seborrhoeic keratosis
  - Squamous cell papilloma
  - Keratoacanthoma

Premalignant

- Actinic/solar/senile keratosis

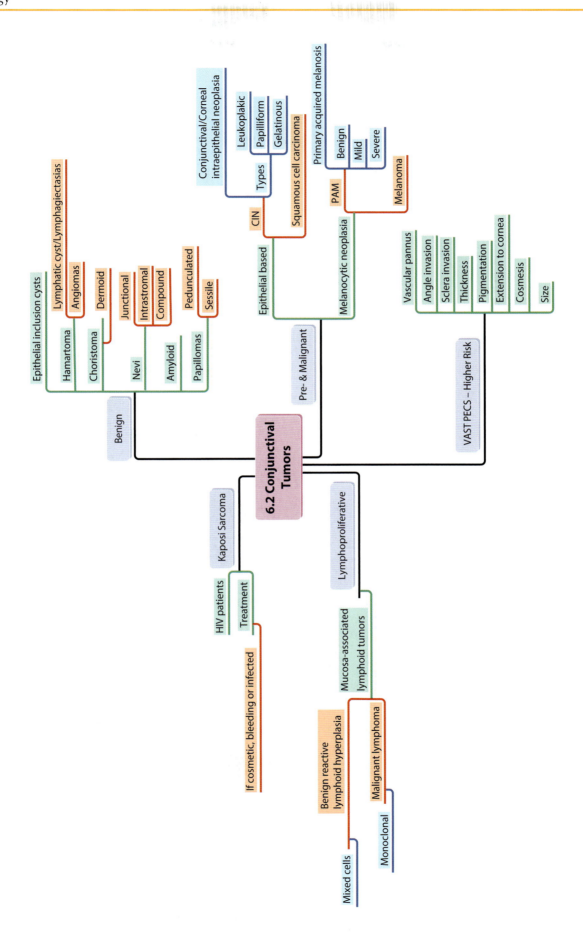

6.2 Conjunctival Tumors

Benign

- Epithelial inclusion cysts
- Hamartoma
- Choristoma
- Nevi
  - Lymphatic cyst/Lymphagiectasias
  - Angiomas
  - Dermoid
  - Junctional
  - Intrastromal
  - Compound
- Amyloid
- Papillomas
  - Pedunculated
  - Sessile

Pre- & Malignant

- Epithelial based
  - CIN — Conjunctival/Corneal intraepithelial neoplasia
    - Types
      - Leukoplakic
      - Papilliform
      - Gelatinous
  - Squamous cell carcinoma
- Melanocytic neoplasia
  - PAM — Primary acquired melanosis
    - Benign
    - Mild
    - Severe
  - Melanoma

VAST PECS – Higher Risk
- Vascular pannus
- Angle invasion
- Sclera invasion
- Thickness
- Pigmentation
- Extension to cornea
- Cosmesis
- Size

Kaposi Sarcoma
- HIV patients
- Treatment
  - If cosmetic, bleeding or infected

Lymphoproliferative
- Mucosa-associated lymphoid tumors
  - Benign reactive lymphoid hyperplasia
  - Malignant lymphoma
    - Mixed cells
    - Monoclonal

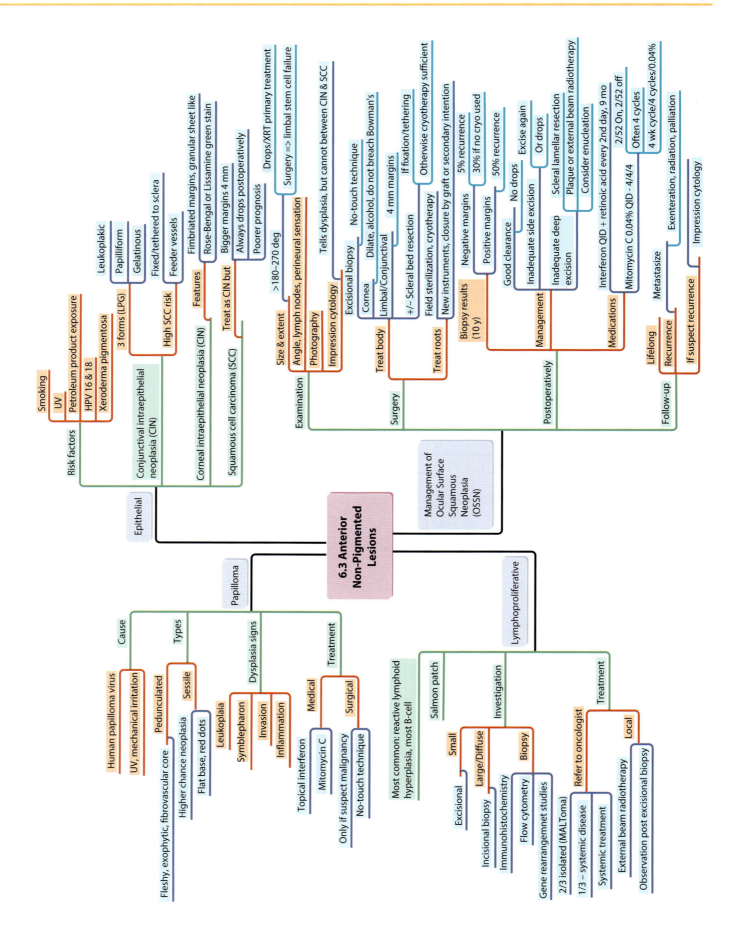

6.3 Anterior Non-Pigmented Lesions

Management of Ocular Surface Squamous Neoplasia (OSSN)

Epithelial

Risk factors
- Smoking
- UV
- Petroleum product exposure
- HPV 16 & 18
- Xeroderma pigmentosa

Conjunctival intraepithelial neoplasia (CIN)
- 3 forms (LPG)
  - Leukoplakic
  - Papilliform
  - Gelatinous
- High SCC risk

Corneal intraepithelial neoplasia (CIN)
- Features
  - Fixed/tethered to sclera
  - Feeder vessels
  - Fimbriated margins, granular sheet like
  - Rose-Bengal or Lissamine green stain
- Treat as CIN but
  - Bigger margins 4 mm
  - Always drops postoperatively
  - Poorer prognosis

Squamous cell carcinoma (SCC)
- Drops/XRT primary treatment
- Surgery => limbal stem cell failure

Examination
- Size & extent
  - >180–270 deg
  - Tells dysplasia, but cannot between CIN & SCC
- Angle, lymph nodes, perineural sensation
- Photography
- Impression cytology

Surgery
- Treat body
  - Excisional biopsy
  - No-touch technique
  - Cornea
    - Dilate, alcohol, do not breach Bowman's
  - Limbal/Conjunctival
    - 4 mm margins
    - If fixation/tethering
    - +/- Scleral bed resection
    - Otherwise cryotherapy sufficient
- Treat roots
  - Field sterilization, cryotherapy
  - New instruments, closure by graft or secondary intention

Biopsy results (10 y)
- Negative margins
  - 5% recurrence
  - 30% if no cryo used
- Positive margins
  - 50% recurrence

Postoperatively
- Management
  - Good clearance
    - No drops
    - Or drops
  - Inadequate side excision
    - Excise again
  - Inadequate deep excision
    - Scleral lamellar resection
    - Plaque or external beam radiotherapy
    - Consider enucleation
- Medications
  - Interferon QID + retinoic acid every 2nd day, 9 mo
  - Mitomycin C 0.04% QID – 4/4/4
    - 2/52 On, 2/52 off
    - Often 4 cycles
    - 4 wk cycle/4 cycles/0.04%

Follow-up
- Lifelong
- Recurrence
  - Metastasize
    - Exenteration, radiation, palliation
- If suspect recurrence
  - Impression cytology

Papilloma

Cause
- Human papilloma virus
- UV, mechanical irritation

Types
- Pedunculated
  - Fleshy, exophytic, fibrovascular core
  - Higher chance neoplasia
- Sessile
  - Flat base, red dots

Dysplasia signs
- Leukoplaia
- Symblepharon
- Invasion
- Inflammation

Treatment
- Medical
  - Topical interferon
  - Mitomycin C
- Surgical
  - Only if suspect malignancy
  - No-touch technique

Lymphoproliferative

Most common: reactive lymphoid hyperplasia, most B-cell
- Salmon patch

Investigation
- Small
  - Excisional
- Large/Diffuse
  - Incisional biopsy
- Biopsy
  - Immunohistochemistry
  - Flow cytometry
  - Gene rearrangemnet studies
- 2/3 isolated (MALToma)
- 1/3 – systemic disease

Treatment
- Refer to oncologist
  - Systemic treatment
- Local
  - External beam radiotherapy
  - Observation post excisional biopsy

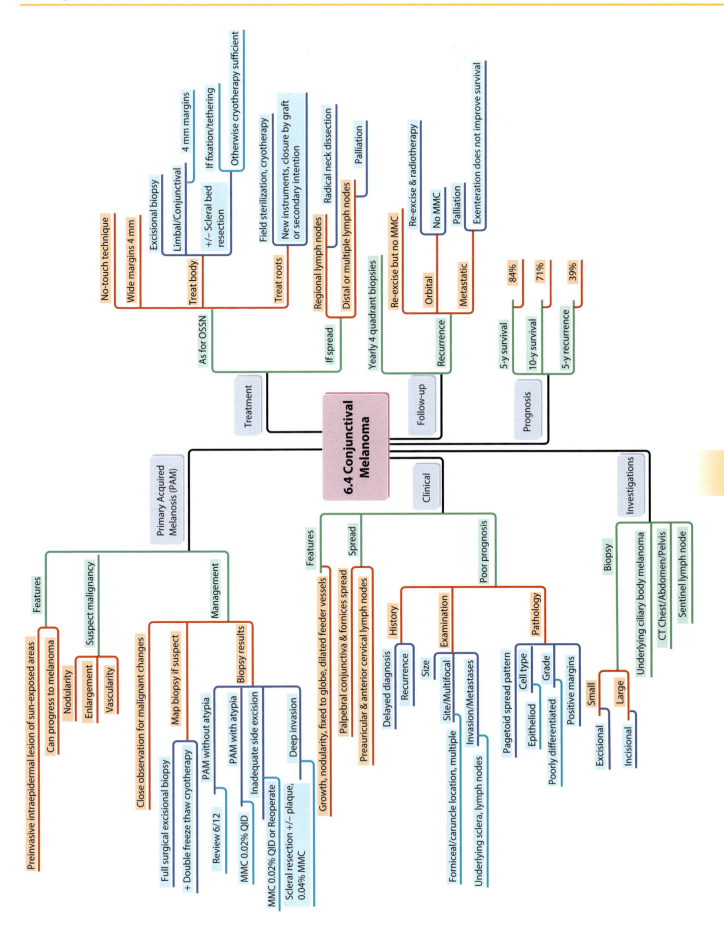

6.4 Conjunctival Melanoma

Treatment

As for OSSN
- Treat body
  - No-touch technique
  - Wide margins 4 mm
  - Excisional biopsy
  - Limbal/Conjunctival
    - 4 mm margins
  - +/- Scleral bed resection
    - If fixation/tethering
    - Otherwise cryotherapy sufficient
- Treat roots
  - Field sterilization, cryotherapy
  - New instruments, closure by graft or secondary intention

If spread
- Regional lymph nodes
  - Radical neck dissection
- Distal or multiple lymph nodes
  - Palliation

Follow-up

Yearly 4 quadrant biopsies
Recurrence
- Re-excise but no MMC
  - Re-excise & radiotherapy
  - No MMC
- Orbital
  - Palliation
- Metastatic
  - Exenteration does not improve survival

Prognosis
- 5-y survival — 84%
- 10-y survival — 71%
- 5-y recurrence — 39%

Primary Acquired Melanosis (PAM)

Features
- Preinvasive intraepidermal lesion of sun-exposed areas
- Can progress to melanoma
- Suspect malignancy
  - Nodularity
  - Enlargement
  - Vascularity

Management
- Close observation for malignant changes
  - Full surgical excisional biopsy
  - + Double freeze thaw cryotherapy
- Map biopsy if suspect
- Biopsy results
  - PAM without atypia
    - Review 6/12
  - PAM with atypia
    - MMC 0.02% QID
  - Inadequate side excision
    - MMC 0.02% QID or Reoperate
  - Deep invasion
    - Scleral resection +/- plaque, 0.04% MMC

Clinical

Features
- Growth, nodularity, fixed to globe, dilated feeder vessels
- Palpebral conjunctiva & fornices spread

Spread
- Preauricular & anterior cervical lymph nodes

Poor prognosis
- History
  - Delayed diagnosis
  - Recurrence
- Examination
  - Size
  - Site/Multifocal
    - Forniceal/caruncle location, multiple
  - Invasion/Metastases
    - Underlying sclera, lymph nodes
- Pathology
  - Pagetoid spread pattern
  - Cell type
    - Epitheliod
  - Grade
    - Poorly differentiated
  - Positive margins

Investigations

Biopsy
- Small
  - Excisional
- Large
  - Incisional
- Underlying ciliary body melanoma
- CT Chest/Abdomen/Pelvis
- Sentinel lymph node

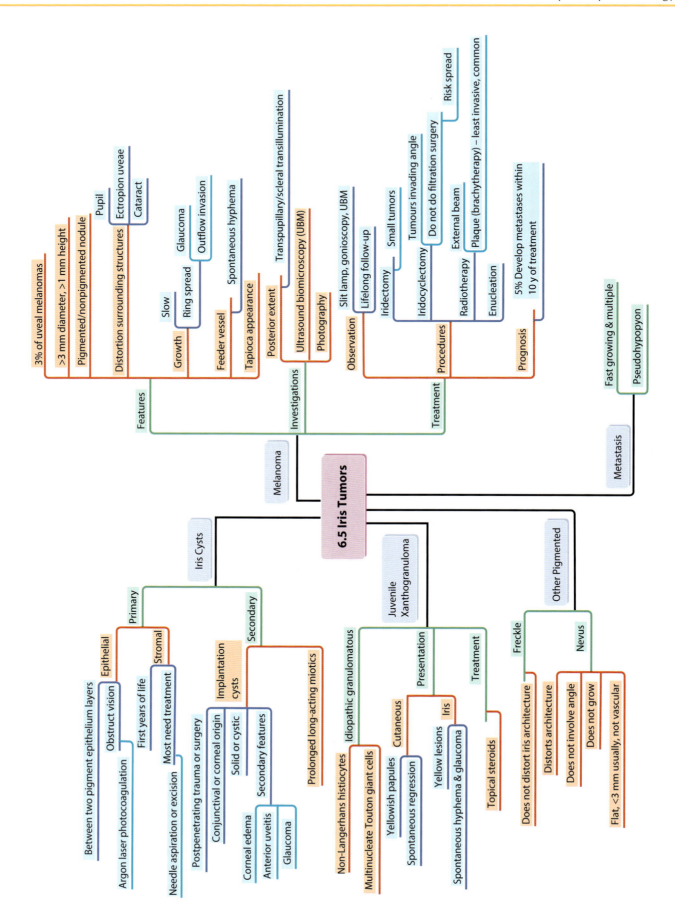

6.5 Iris Tumors

Melanoma

Features
- 3% of uveal melanomas
- >3 mm diameter, >1 mm height
- Pigmented/nonpigmented nodule
- Distortion surrounding structures
  - Pupil
  - Ectropion uveae
  - Cataract
- Growth
  - Slow
  - Ring spread
    - Glaucoma
    - Outflow invasion
- Feeder vessel
  - Spontaneous hyphema
- Tapioca appearance

Investigations
- Posterior extent
  - Transpupillary/scleral transillumination
- Ultrasound biomicroscopy (UBM)
- Photography
- Slit lamp, gonioscopy, UBM

Treatment
- Observation
  - Lifelong follow-up
- Procedures
  - Iridectomy
  - Small tumors
  - Iridocyclectomy
    - Tumours invading angle
    - Do not do filtration surgery
  - Radiotherapy
    - External beam
    - Plaque (brachytherapy) – least invasive, common
      - Risk spread
  - Enucleation
- Prognosis
  - 5% Develop metastases within 10 y of treatment

Metastasis
- Fast growing & multiple
- Pseudohypopyon

Iris Cysts
- Primary
  - Epithelial
    - Between two pigment epithelium layers
    - Obstruct vision
      - Argon laser photocoagulation
    - First years of life
    - Most need treatment
      - Needle aspiration or excision
  - Stromal
- Secondary
  - Implantation cysts
    - Postpenetrating trauma or surgery
    - Conjunctival or corneal origin
    - Solid or cystic
    - Secondary features
      - Corneal edema
      - Anterior uveitis
      - Glaucoma
  - Prolonged long-acting miotics

Juvenile Xanthogranuloma
- Non-Langerhans histiocytes
- Idiopathic granulomatous
- Multinucleate Touton giant cells
- Presentation
  - Cutaneous
    - Yellowish papules
    - Spontaneous regression
  - Iris
    - Yellow lesions
    - Spontaneous hyphema & glaucoma
- Treatment
  - Topical steroids

Other Pigmented
- Freckle
  - Does not distort iris architecture
- Nevus
  - Distorts architecture
  - Does not involve angle
  - Does not grow
  - Flat, <3 mm usually, not vascular

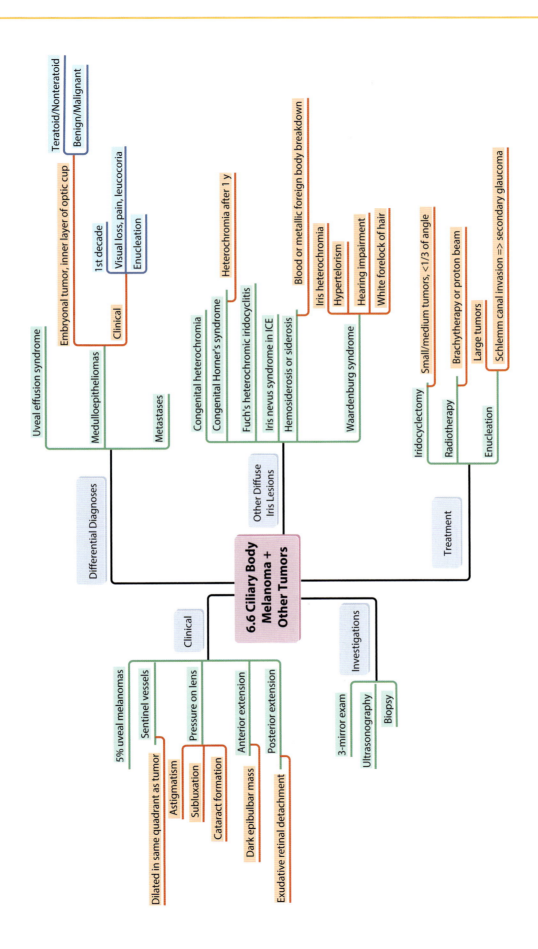

6.6 Ciliary Body Melanoma + Other Tumors

Differential Diagnoses

- Uveal effusion syndrome
- Medulloepitheliomas
  - Embryonal tumor, inner layer of optic cup
    - Teratoid/Nonteratoid
    - Benign/Malignant
  - Clinical
    - 1st decade
    - Visual loss, pain, leucocoria
    - Enucleation
- Metastases

Other Diffuse Iris Lesions

- Congenital heterochromia
- Congenital Horner's syndrome
- Fuch's heterochromic iridocyclitis
  - Heterochromia after 1 y
- Iris nevus syndrome in ICE
- Hemosiderosis or siderosis
  - Blood or metallic foreign body breakdown
- Waardenburg syndrome
  - Iris heterochromia
  - Hypertelorism
  - Hearing impairment
  - White forelock of hair

Treatment

- Iridocyclectomy
  - Small/medium tumors, <1/3 of angle
- Radiotherapy
  - Brachytherapy or proton beam
- Enucleation
  - Large tumors
  - Schlemm canal invasion => secondary glaucoma

Clinical

- 5% uveal melanomas
- Sentinel vessels
  - Dilated in same quadrant as tumor
- Pressure on lens
  - Astigmatism
  - Subluxation
  - Cataract formation
- Anterior extension
  - Dark epibulbar mass
- Posterior extension
  - Exudative retinal detachment

Investigations

- 3-mirror exam
- Ultrasonography
- Biopsy

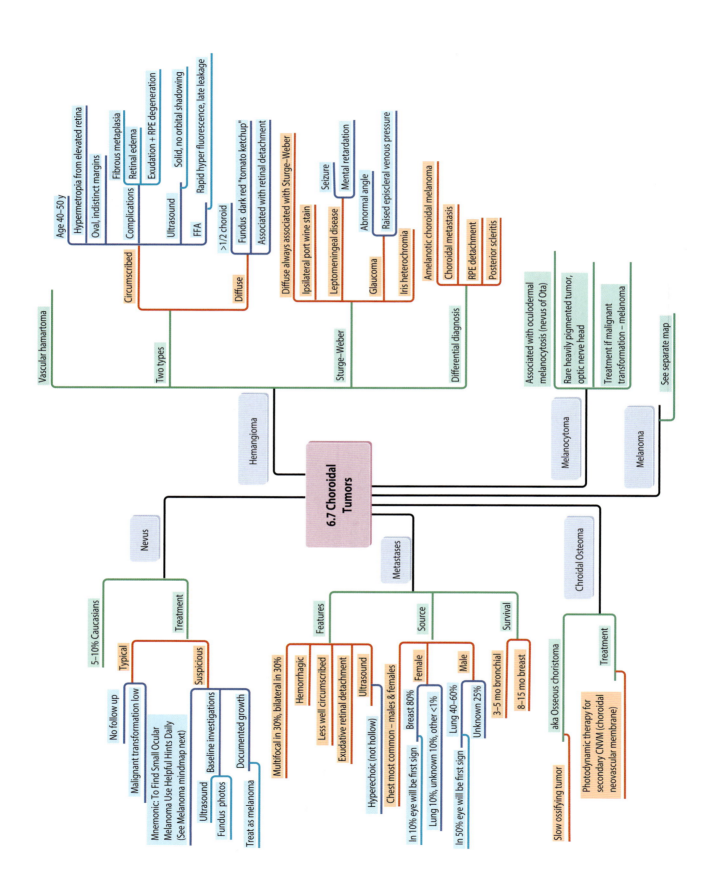

6.7 Choroidal Tumors

Hemangioma

Vascular hamartoma

Two types
- Circumscribed
  - Age 40–50 y
  - Hypermetropia from elevated retina
  - Oval, indistinct margins
  - Complications
    - Fibrous metaplasia
    - Retinal edema
    - Exudation + RPE degeneration
  - Ultrasound — Solid, no orbital shadowing
  - FFA — Rapid hyper fluorescence, late leakage
- Diffuse
  - >1/2 choroid
  - Fundus dark red "tomato ketchup"
  - Associated with retinal detachment

Sturge–Weber
- Diffuse always associated with Sturge–Weber
- Ipsilateral port wine stain
- Leptomeningeal disease
  - Seizure
  - Mental retardation
- Glaucoma
  - Abnormal angle
  - Raised episcleral venous pressure
- Iris heterochromia

Differential diagnosis
- Amelanotic choroidal melanoma
- Choroidal metastasis
- RPE detachment
- Posterior scleritis

Melanocytoma
- Associated with oculodermal melanocytosis (nevus of Ota)
- Rare heavily pigmented tumor, optic nerve head
- Treatment if malignant transformation – melanoma

Melanoma
- See separate map

Nevus
- 5–10% Caucasians
- Treatment
  - Typical
    - No follow up
    - Malignant transformation low
    - Mnemonic: To Find Small Ocular Melanoma Use Helpful Hints Daily (See Melanoma mindmap next)
  - Suspicious
    - Baseline investigations
      - Ultrasound
      - Fundus photos
    - Documented growth
    - Treat as melanoma

Metastases
- Features
  - Multifocal in 30%, bilateral in 30%
  - Hemorrhagic
  - Less well circumscribed
  - Exudative retinal detachment
  - Ultrasound
    - Hyperechoic (not hollow)
- Source
  - Chest most common – males & females
    - Breast 80%
    - In 10% eye will be first sign
    - Lung 10%, unknown 10%, other <1%
  - Female
  - Male
    - Lung 40–60%
    - In 50% eye will be first sign
    - Unknown 25%
- Survival
  - 3–5 mo bronchial
  - 8–15 mo breast

Choroidal Osteoma
- aka Osseous choristoma
- Slow ossifying tumor
- Treatment
  - Photodynamic therapy for secondary CNVM (choroidal neovascular membrane)

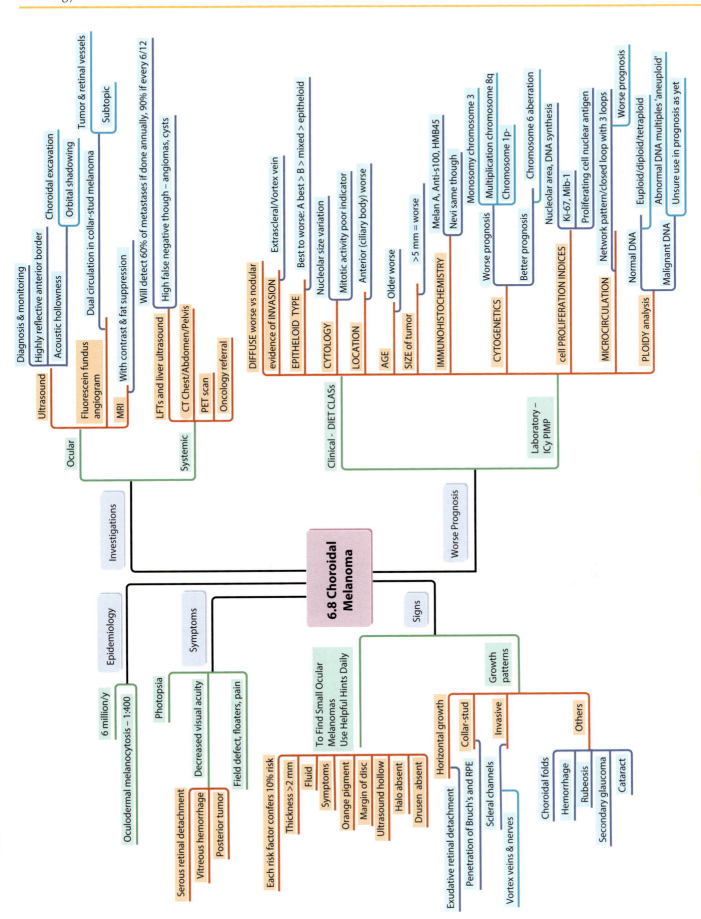

6.8 Choroidal Melanoma

Investigations

Ocular

- Ultrasound
  - Diagnosis & monitoring
  - Highly reflective anterior border
  - Acoustic hollowness
  - Choroidal excavation
  - Orbital shadowing
  - Subtopic
    - Tumor & retinal vessels
- Fluorescein fundus angiogram
  - Dual circulation in collar-stud melanoma
- MRI
  - With contrast & fat suppression

Systemic

- LFTs and liver ultrasound
  - Will detect 60% of metastases if done annually, 90% if every 6/12
  - High false negative though – angiomas, cysts
- CT Chest/Abdomen/Pelvis
- PET scan
- Oncology referral

Worse Prognosis

Clinical - DIET CLASs

- DIFFUSE worse vs nodular
  - evidence of INVASION
    - Extrascleral/Vortex vein
- EPITHELOID TYPE
  - Best to worse: A best > B > mixed > epitheloid
- CYTOLOGY
  - Nucleolar size variation
  - Mitotic activity poor indicator
- LOCATION
  - Anterior (ciliary body) worse
- AGE
  - Older worse
- SIZE of tumor
  - >5 mm = worse

Laboratory – ICy PIMP

- IMMUNOHISTOCHEMISTRY
  - Melan A, Anti-s100, HMB45
  - Nevi same though
- CYTOGENETICS
  - Worse prognosis
    - Monosomy chromosome 3
    - Multiplication chromosome 8q
    - Chromosome 1p
  - Better prognosis
    - Chromosome 6 aberration
- cell PROLIFERATION INDICES
  - Nucleolar area, DNA synthesis
  - Ki-67, Mib-1
  - Proliferating cell nuclear antigen
- MICROCIRCULATION
  - Network pattern/closed loop with 3 loops
    - Worse prognosis
- PLOIDY analysis
  - Normal DNA
    - Euploid/diploid/tetraploid
  - Malignant DNA
    - Abnormal DNA multiples 'aneuploid'
    - Unsure use in prognosis as yet

Epidemiology

- 6 million/y
- Oculodermal melanocytosis – 1:400

Symptoms

- Photopsia
- Decreased visual acuity
- Field defect, floaters, pain
- Serous retinal detachment
- Vitreous hemorrhage
- Posterior tumor

Signs

To Find Small Ocular Melanomas Use Helpful Hints Daily

- Each risk factor confers 10% risk
- Thickness >2 mm
- Fluid
- Symptoms
- Orange pigment
- Margin of disc
- Ultrasound hollow
- Halo absent
- Drusen absent

Growth patterns

- Horizontal growth
  - Exudative retinal detachment
  - Penetration of Bruch's and RPE
- Collar-stud
  - Scleral channels
  - Vortex veins & nerves
- Invasive
- Others
  - Choroidal folds
  - Hemorrhage
  - Rubeosis
  - Secondary glaucoma
  - Cataract

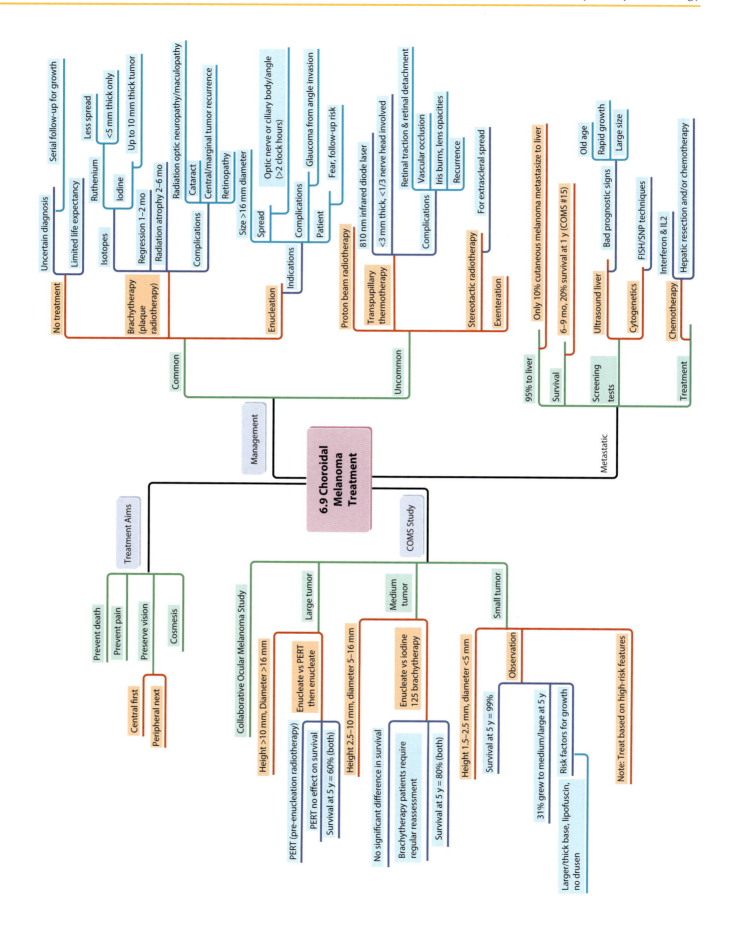

6.9 Choroidal Melanoma Treatment

Management

Common

No treatment
- Uncertain diagnosis
- Limited life expectancy
- Serial follow-up for growth

Brachytherapy (plaque radiotherapy)
- Isotopes
  - Ruthenium
    - Less spread
    - <5 mm thick only
  - Iodine
    - Up to 10 mm thick tumor
- Regression 1–2 mo
- Radiation atrophy 2–6 mo
- Complications
  - Radiation optic neuropathy/maculopathy
  - Cataract
  - Central/marginal tumor recurrence
  - Retinopathy

Enucleation
- Indications
  - Size >16 mm diameter
  - Spread
    - Optic nerve or ciliary body/angle (>2 clock hours)
    - Glaucoma from angle invasion
  - Complications
  - Patient
    - Fear, follow-up risk

Uncommon

Proton beam radiotherapy

Transpupillary thermotherapy
- 810 nm infrared diode laser
- <3 mm thick, <1/3 nerve head involved
- Complications
  - Retinal traction & retinal detachment
  - Vascular occlusion
  - Iris burns, lens opacities
  - Recurrence

Stereotactic radiotherapy
- For extrascleral spread

Exenteration

Metastatic

95% to liver
- Only 10% cutaneous melanoma metastasize to liver

Survival
- 6–9 mo, 20% survival at 1 y (COMS #15)

Screening tests
- Ultrasound liver
- Cytogenetics
  - FISH/SNP techniques
- Bad prognostic signs
  - Old age
  - Rapid growth
  - Large size

Treatment
- Chemotherapy
  - Interferon & IL2
  - Hepatic resection and/or chemotherapy

Treatment Aims
- Prevent death
- Prevent pain
- Preserve vision
  - Central first
  - Peripheral next
- Cosmesis

COMS Study

Collaborative Ocular Melanoma Study

Large tumor
- Height >10 mm, Diameter >16 mm
- Enucleate vs PERT then enucleate
  - PERT (pre-enucleation radiotherapy)
  - PERT no effect on survival
  - Survival at 5 y = 60% (both)

Medium tumor
- Height 2.5–10 mm, diameter 5–16 mm
- Enucleate vs iodine 125 brachytherapy
  - No significant difference in survival
  - Brachytherapy patients require regular reassessment
  - Survival at 5 y = 80% (both)

Small tumor
- Height 1.5–2.5 mm, diameter <5 mm
- Observation
  - Survival at 5 y = 99%
  - 31% grew to medium/large at 5 y
  - Risk factors for growth
    - Larger/thick base, lipofuscin, no drusen
  - Note: Treat based on high-risk features

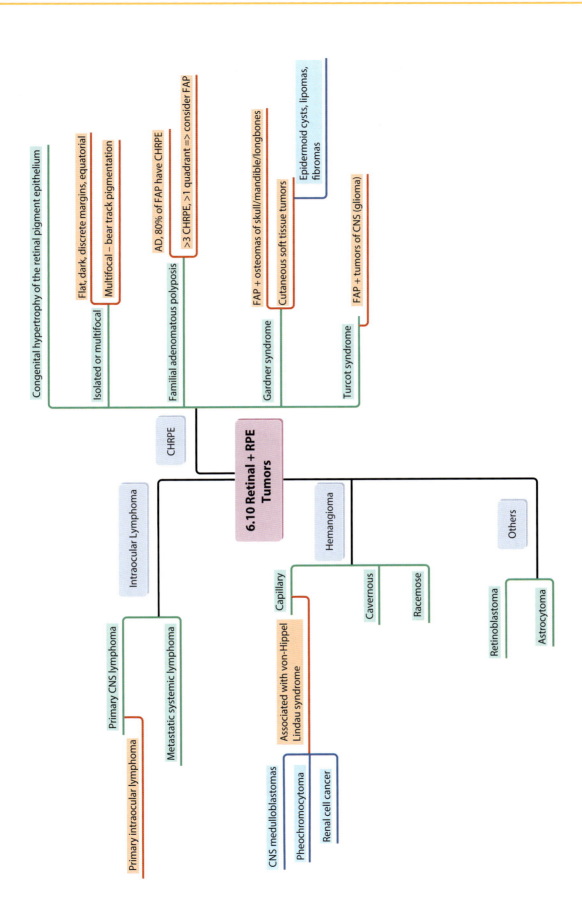

Congenital hypertrophy of the retinal pigment epithelium

Flat, dark, discrete margins, equatorial

Multifocal – bear track pigmentation

Isolated or multifocal

AD, 80% of FAP have CHRPE

>3 CHRPE, >1 quadrant => consider FAP

Familial adenomatous polyposis

FAP + osteomas of skull/mandible/longbones

Cutaneous soft tissue tumors

Epidermoid cysts, lipomas, fibromas

Gardner syndrome

FAP + tumors of CNS (glioma)

Turcot syndrome

CHRPE

6.10 Retinal + RPE Tumors

Intraocular Lymphoma

Primary CNS lymphoma

Primary intraocular lymphoma

Metastatic systemic lymphoma

Hemangioma

Capillary

Associated with von-Hippel Lindau syndrome

CNS medulloblastomas

Pheochromocytoma

Renal cell cancer

Cavernous

Racemose

Others

Retinoblastoma

Astrocytoma

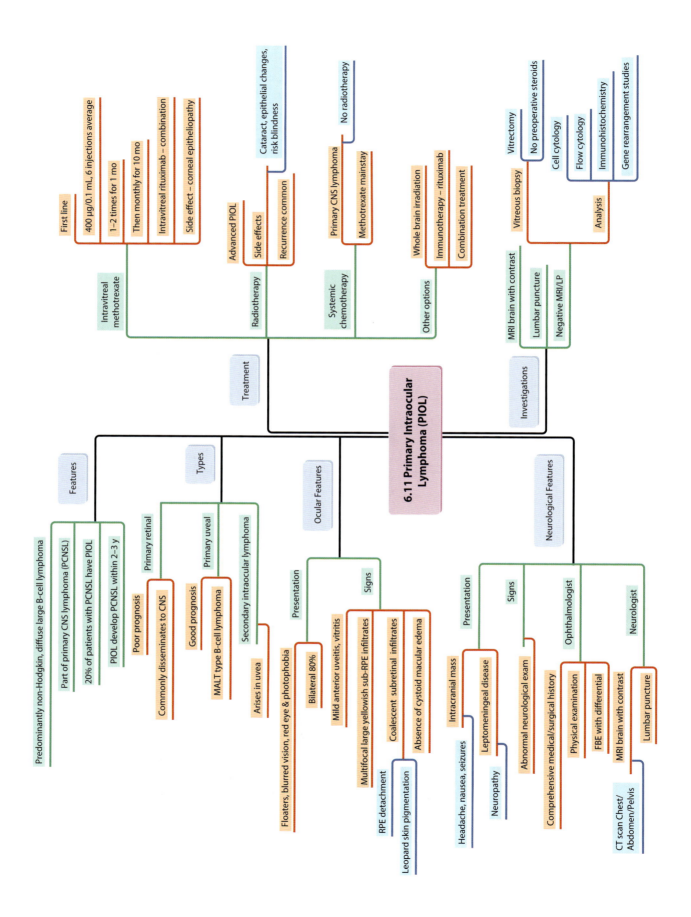

6.11 Primary Intraocular Lymphoma (PIOL)

Treatment

Intravitreal methotrexate
- First line
- 400 µg/0.1 mL, 6 injections average
- 1–2 times for 1 mo
- Then monthly for 10 mo
- Intravitreal rituximab – combination
- Side effect – corneal epitheliopathy

Radiotherapy
- Cataract, epithelial changes, risk blindness
- Advanced PIOL
- Side effects
- Recurrence common

Systemic chemotherapy
- Primary CNS lymphoma
- No radiotherapy
- Methotrexate mainstay

Other options
- Whole brain irradiation
- Immunotherapy – rituximab
- Combination treatment

Investigations

- Vitreous biopsy
  - Vitrectomy
  - No preoperative steroids
  - Analysis
    - Cell cytology
    - Flow cytology
    - Immunohistochemistry
    - Gene rearrangement studies
- MRI brain with contrast
- Lumbar puncture
- Negative MRI/LP

Features
- Predominantly non-Hodgkin, diffuse large B-cell lymphoma
- Part of primary CNS lymphoma (PCNSL)
- 20% of patients with PCNSL have PIOL
- PIOL develop PCNSL within 2–3 y

Types
- Primary retinal
  - Poor prognosis
  - Commonly disseminates to CNS
- Primary uveal
  - Good prognosis
  - MALT type B-cell lymphoma
- Secondary intraocular lymphoma
  - Arises in uvea

Ocular Features
- Presentation
  - Floaters, blurred vision, red eye & photophobia
  - Bilateral 80%
- Signs
  - Mild anterior uveitis, vitritis
  - Multifocal large yellowish sub-RPE infiltrates
  - Coalescent subretinal infiltrates
  - Absence of cystoid macular edema
  - RPE detachment
  - Leopard skin pigmentation

Neurological Features
- Presentation
  - Intracranial mass
  - Headache, nausea, seizures
  - Leptomeningeal disease
  - Neuropathy
- Signs
  - Abnormal neurological exam
- Ophthalmologist
  - Comprehensive medical/surgical history
  - Physical examination
  - FBE with differential
  - MRI brain with contrast
  - Lumbar puncture
- Neurologist
  - CT scan Chest/Abdomen/Pelvis

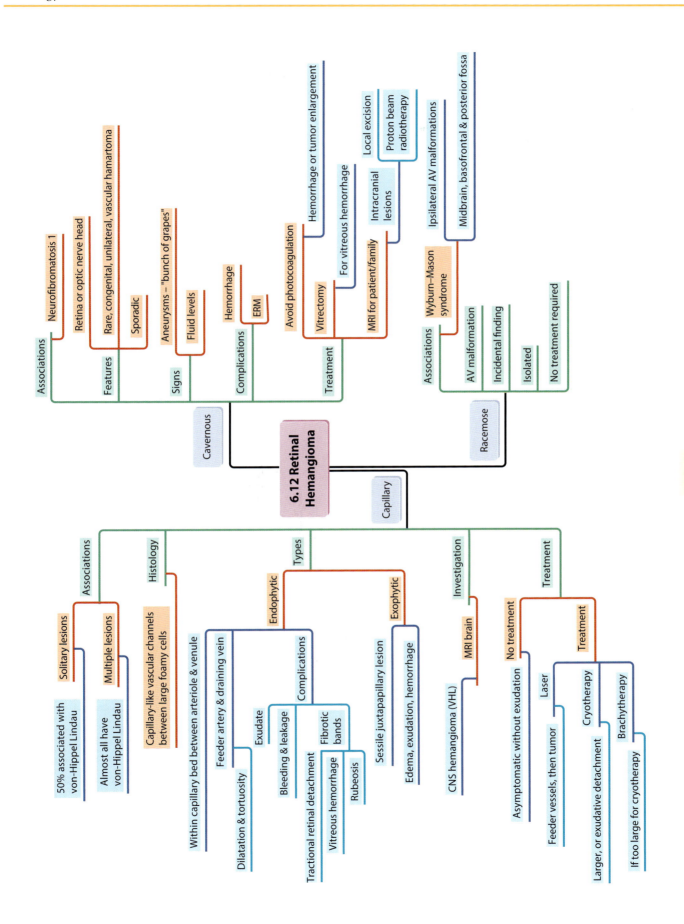

6.12 Retinal Hemangioma

Cavernous

- Associations
  - Neurofibromatosis 1
- Features
  - Retina or optic nerve head
  - Rare, congenital, unilateral, vascular hamartoma
  - Sporadic
- Signs
  - Aneurysms – "bunch of grapes"
  - Fluid levels
- Complications
  - Hemorrhage
  - ERM
- Treatment
  - Avoid photocoagulation
  - Vitrectomy
    - Hemorrhage or tumor enlargement
    - For vitreous hemorrhage
  - MRI for patient/family
    - Intracranial lesions
      - Local excision
      - Proton beam radiotherapy

Racemose

- Associations
  - Wyburn–Mason syndrome
    - Ipsilateral AV malformations
    - Midbrain, basofrontal & posterior fossa
- AV malformation
- Incidental finding
- Isolated
- No treatment required

Capillary

- Associations
  - Solitary lesions
    - 50% associated with von-Hippel Lindau
  - Multiple lesions
    - Almost all have von-Hippel Lindau
- Histology
  - Capillary-like vascular channels between large foamy cells
- Types
  - Endophytic
    - Within capillary bed between arteriole & venule
    - Feeder artery & draining vein
      - Dilatation & tortuosity
    - Exudate
    - Complications
      - Bleeding & leakage
      - Tractional retinal detachment
      - Fibrotic bands
      - Vitreous hemorrhage
      - Rubeosis
  - Exophytic
    - Sessile juxtapapillary lesion
    - Edema, exudation, hemorrhage
- Investigation
  - MRI brain
    - CNS hemangioma (VHL)
- Treatment
  - No treatment
    - Asymptomatic without exudation
  - Treatment
    - Laser
      - Feeder vessels, then tumor
    - Cryotherapy
      - Larger, or exudative detachment
    - Brachytherapy
      - If too large for cryotherapy

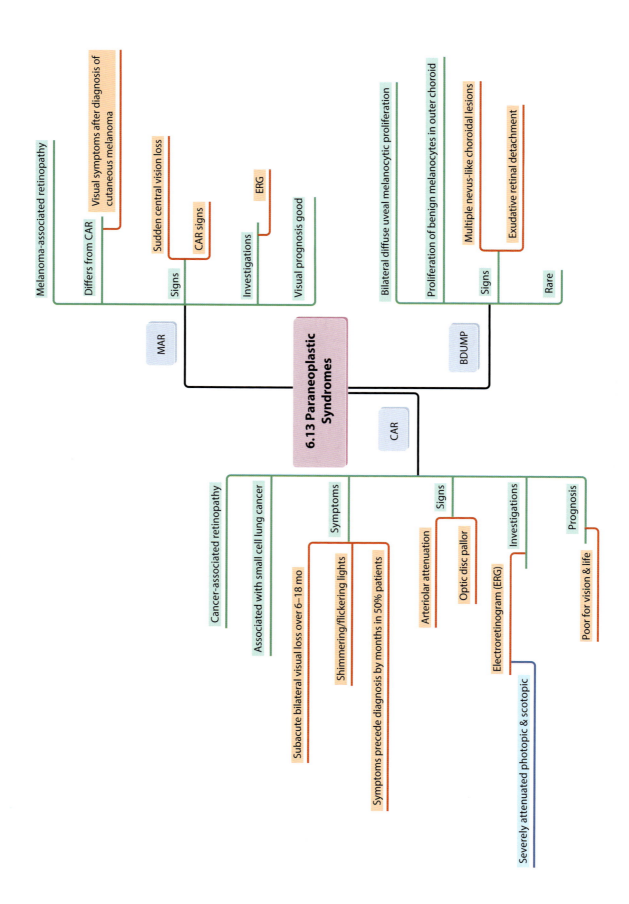

6.13 Paraneoplastic Syndromes

MAR
- Melanoma-associated retinopathy
- Differs from CAR
  - Visual symptoms after diagnosis of cutaneous melanoma
- Signs
  - Sudden central vision loss
  - CAR signs
- Investigations
  - ERG
- Visual prognosis good

BDUMP
- Bilateral diffuse uveal melanocytic proliferation
- Proliferation of benign melanocytes in outer choroid
- Signs
  - Multiple nevus-like choroidal lesions
  - Exudative retinal detachment
- Rare

CAR
- Cancer-associated retinopathy
- Associated with small cell lung cancer
- Symptoms
  - Subacute bilateral visual loss over 6–18 mo
  - Shimmering/flickering lights
  - Symptoms precede diagnosis by months in 50% patients
- Signs
  - Arteriolar attenuation
  - Optic disc pallor
- Investigations
  - Electroretinogram (ERG)
    - Severely attenuated photopic & scotopic
- Prognosis
  - Poor for vision & life

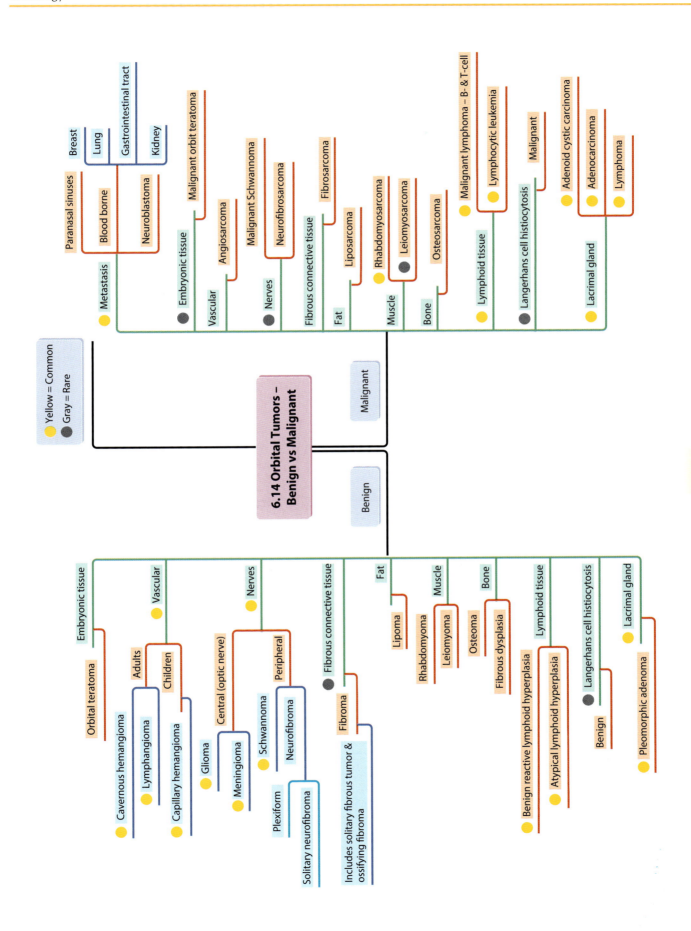

6.14 Orbital Tumors – Benign vs Malignant

Yellow = Common
Gray = Rare

Malignant

Metastasis
- Paranasal sinuses
- Blood borne
  - Breast
  - Lung
  - Gastrointestinal tract
  - Kidney
- Neuroblastoma

Embryonic tissue
- Malignant orbit teratoma

Vascular
- Angiosarcoma

Nerves
- Malignant Schwannoma
- Neurofibrosarcoma

Fibrous connective tissue
- Fibrosarcoma

Fat
- Liposarcoma

Muscle
- Rhabdomyosarcoma
- Leiomyosarcoma

Bone
- Osteosarcoma

Lymphoid tissue
- Malignant lymphoma – B- & T-cell
- Lymphocytic leukemia

Langerhans cell histiocytosis
- Malignant

Lacrimal gland
- Adenoid cystic carcinoma
- Adenocarcinoma
- Lymphoma

Benign

Embryonic tissue
- Orbital teratoma

Vascular
- Adults
  - Cavernous hemangioma
  - Lymphangioma
- Children
  - Capillary hemangioma

Nerves
- Central (optic nerve)
  - Glioma
  - Meningioma
- Peripheral
  - Schwannoma
  - Neurofibroma
    - Plexiform
    - Solitary neurofibroma

Fibrous connective tissue
- Fibroma
  - Includes solitary fibrous tumor & ossifying fibroma

Fat
- Lipoma

Muscle
- Rhabdomyoma
- Leiomyoma

Bone
- Osteoma
- Fibrous dysplasia

Lymphoid tissue
- Benign reactive lymphoid hyperplasia
- Atypical lymphoid hyperplasia

Langerhans cell histiocytosis
- Benign

Lacrimal gland
- Pleomorphic adenoma

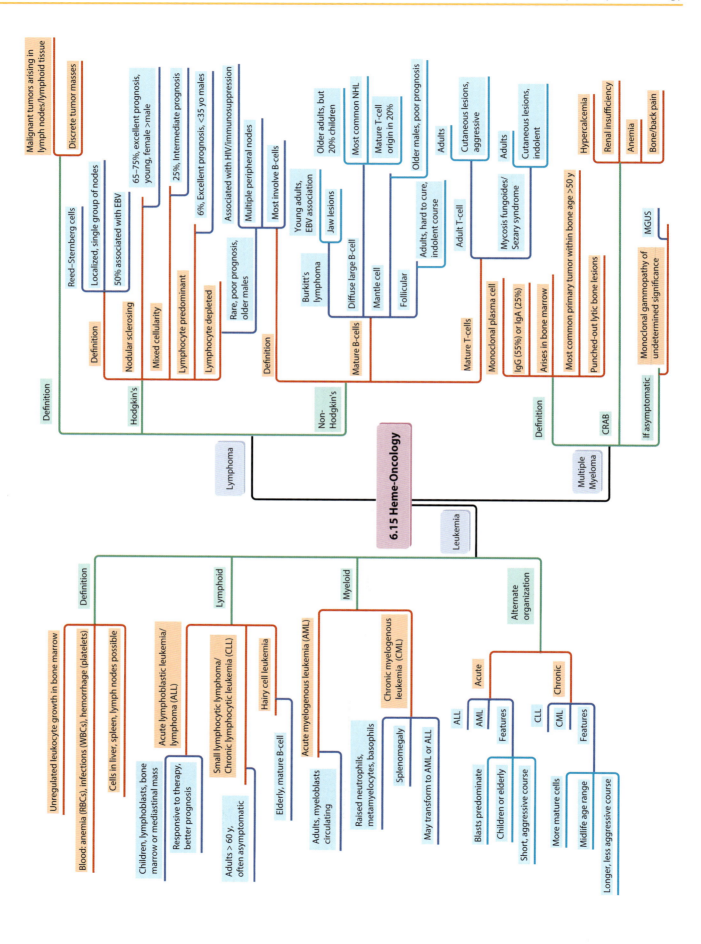

6.15 Heme-Oncology

Lymphoma

Definition
- Malignant tumors arising in lymph nodes/lymphoid tissue
- Discrete tumor masses

Hodgkin's
- Definition
  - Reed–Sternberg cells
  - Localized, single group of nodes
  - 50% associated with EBV
- Nodular sclerosing — 65–75%, excellent prognosis, young, female >male
- Mixed cellularity — 25%, Intermediate prognosis
- Lymphocyte predominant — 6%, Excellent prognosis, <35 yo males
- Lymphocyte depleted — Rare, poor prognosis, older males

Non-Hodgkin's
- Definition
  - Associated with HIV/immunosuppression
  - Multiple peripheral nodes
  - Most involve B-cells
- Mature B-cells
  - Burkitt's lymphoma — Young adults, EBV association; Jaw lesions
  - Diffuse large B-cell — Older adults, but 20% children; Most common NHL
  - Mantle cell — Mature T-cell origin in 20%; Older males, poor prognosis
  - Follicular — Adults, hard to cure, indolent course
- Mature T-cells
  - Adult T-cell — Adults; Cutaneous lesions, aggressive
  - Mycosis fungoides/Sezary syndrome — Adults; Cutaneous lesions, indolent

Multiple Myeloma

Definition
- Monoclonal plasma cell
- IgG (55%) or IgA (25%)
- Arises in bone marrow
- Most common primary tumor within bone age >50 y
- Punched-out lytic bone lesions

CRAB
- Hypercalcemia
- Renal insufficiency
- Anemia
- Bone/back pain

If asymptomatic
- Monoclonal gammopathy of undetermined significance — MGUS

Leukemia

Definition
- Unregulated leukocyte growth in bone marrow
- Blood: anemia (RBCs), infections (WBCs), hemorrhage (platelets)
- Cells in liver, spleen, lymph nodes possible

Lymphoid
- Acute lymphoblastic leukemia/lymphoma (ALL) — Children, lymphoblasts, bone marrow or mediastinal mass; Responsive to therapy, better prognosis
- Small lymphocytic lymphoma/Chronic lymphocytic leukemia (CLL) — Adults > 60 y, often asymptomatic
- Hairy cell leukemia — Elderly, mature B-cell

Myeloid
- Acute myelogenous leukemia (AML) — Adults, myeloblasts circulating
- Chronic myelogenous leukemia (CML) — Raised neutrophils, metamyelocytes, basophils; Splenomegaly; May transform to AML or ALL

Alternate organization
- Acute
  - ALL
  - AML
  - Features — Blasts predominate; Children or elderly; Short, aggressive course
- Chronic
  - CLL
  - CML
  - Features — More mature cells; Midlife age range; Longer, less aggressive course

7 Orbit, Oculoplastics, and Lacrimal System

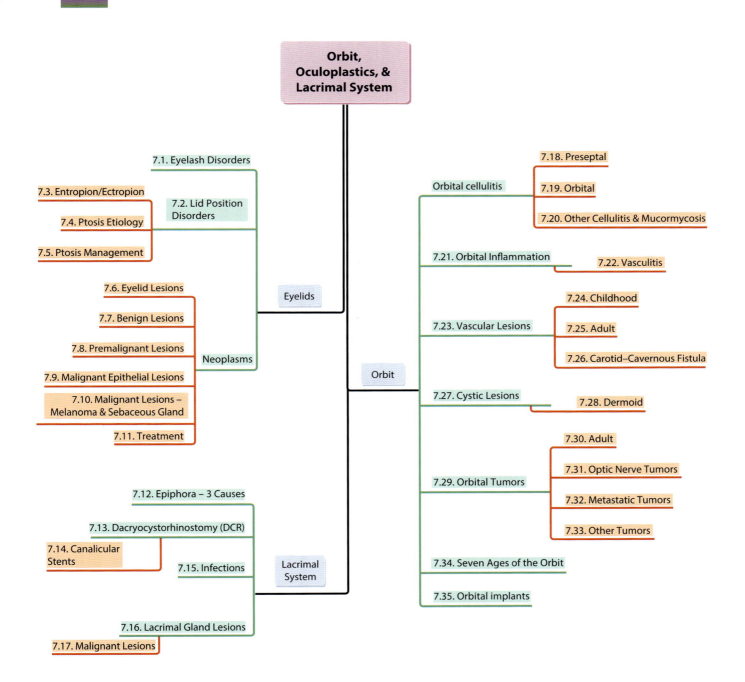

Orbit, Oculoplastics, & Lacrimal System

Eyelids

- 7.1. Eyelash Disorders
- 7.2. Lid Position Disorders
  - 7.3. Entropion/Ectropion
  - 7.4. Ptosis Etiology
  - 7.5. Ptosis Management
- Neoplasms
  - 7.6. Eyelid Lesions
  - 7.7. Benign Lesions
  - 7.8. Premalignant Lesions
  - 7.9. Malignant Epithelial Lesions
  - 7.10. Malignant Lesions – Melanoma & Sebaceous Gland
  - 7.11. Treatment

Lacrimal System

- 7.12. Epiphora – 3 Causes
- 7.13. Dacryocystorhinostomy (DCR)
  - 7.14. Canalicular Stents
  - 7.15. Infections
- 7.16. Lacrimal Gland Lesions
  - 7.17. Malignant Lesions

Orbit

- Orbital cellulitis
  - 7.18. Preseptal
  - 7.19. Orbital
  - 7.20. Other Cellulitis & Mucormycosis
- 7.21. Orbital Inflammation
  - 7.22. Vasculitis
- 7.23. Vascular Lesions
  - 7.24. Childhood
  - 7.25. Adult
  - 7.26. Carotid–Cavernous Fistula
- 7.27. Cystic Lesions
  - 7.28. Dermoid
- 7.29. Orbital Tumors
  - 7.30. Adult
  - 7.31. Optic Nerve Tumors
  - 7.32. Metastatic Tumors
  - 7.33. Other Tumors
- 7.34. Seven Ages of the Orbit
- 7.35. Orbital implants

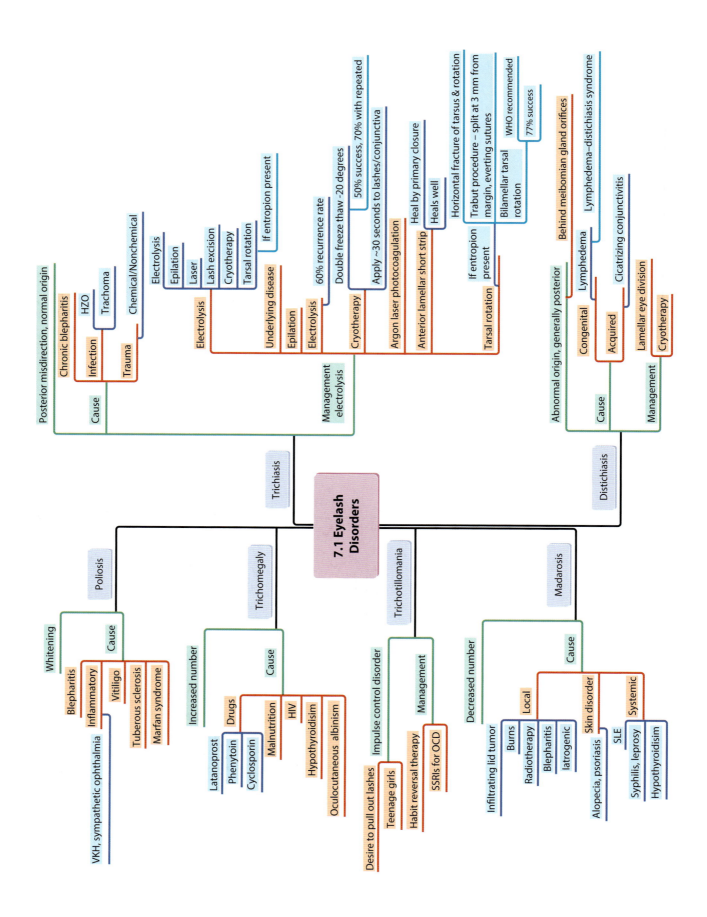

7.1 Eyelash Disorders

Trichiasis

Cause
- Posterior misdirection, normal origin
- Chronic blepharitis
- HZO
- Infection — Trachoma
- Trauma — Chemical/Nonchemical

Management electrolysis
- Electrolysis
  - Electrolysis
  - Epilation
  - Laser
  - Lash excision
  - Cryotherapy
  - Tarsal rotation — If entropion present
- Underlying disease
- Epilation — 60% recurrence rate
- Electrolysis
- Cryotherapy
  - Double freeze thaw -20 degrees
  - 50% success, 70% with repeated
  - Apply ~30 seconds to lashes/conjunctiva
- Argon laser photocoagulation
- Anterior lamellar short strip
  - Heal by primary closure
  - Heals well
- Tarsal rotation
  - Horizontal fracture of tarsus & rotation
  - Trabut procedure – split at 3 mm from margin, everting sutures
  - Bilamellar tarsal rotation — WHO recommended — 77% success
  - If entropion present

Distichiasis

- Abnormal origin, generally posterior
  - Behind meibomian gland orifices
  - Lymphedema–distichiasis syndrome
- Cause
  - Congenital — Lymphedema
  - Acquired — Cicatrizing conjunctivitis
- Management
  - Lamellar eye division
  - Cryotherapy

Poliosis

- Whitening
- Cause
  - Blepharitis
  - Inflammatory — VKH, sympathetic ophthalmia
  - Vitiligo
  - Tuberous sclerosis
  - Marfan syndrome

Trichomegaly

- Increased number
- Cause
  - Drugs
    - Latanoprost
    - Phenytoin
    - Cyclosporin
  - Malnutrition
  - HIV
  - Hypothyroidism
  - Oculocutaneous albinism

Trichotillomania

- Impulse control disorder
  - Desire to pull out lashes
  - Teenage girls
- Management
  - Habit reversal therapy
  - SSRIs for OCD

Madarosis

- Decreased number
- Cause
  - Local
    - Infiltrating lid tumor
    - Burns
    - Radiotherapy
    - Blepharitis
    - Iatrogenic
  - Skin disorder
    - Alopecia, psoriasis
  - Systemic
    - SLE
    - Syphilis, leprosy
    - Hypothyroidism

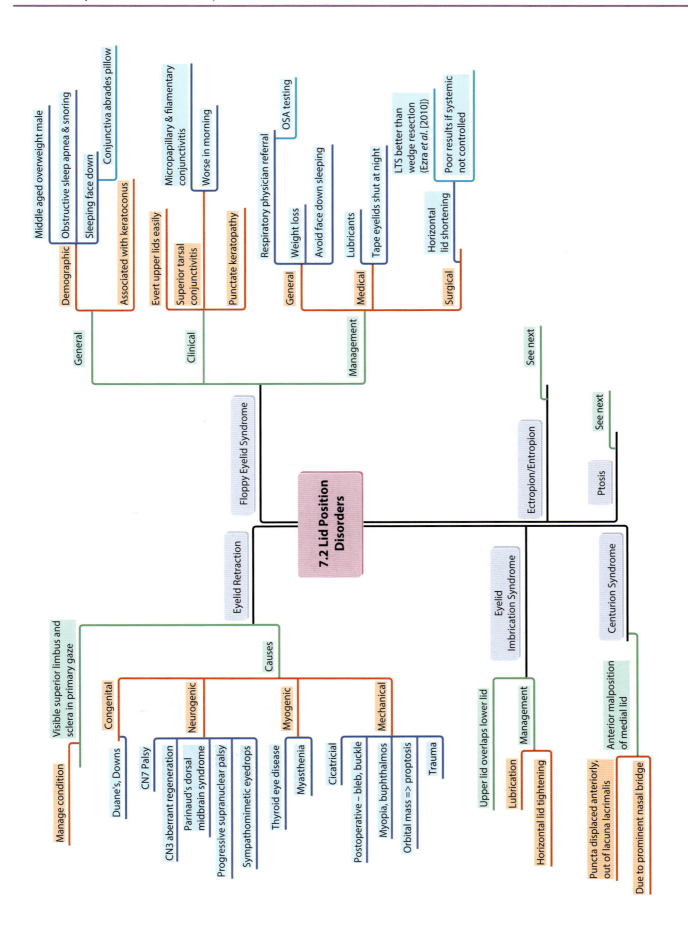

7.2 Lid Position Disorders

Floppy Eyelid Syndrome

- General
  - Demographic
    - Middle aged overweight male
    - Obstructive sleep apnea & snoring
    - Sleeping face down
    - Conjunctiva abrades pillow
  - Associated with keratoconus
- Clinical
  - Evert upper lids easily
  - Superior tarsal conjunctivitis
    - Micropapillary & filamentary conjunctivitis
    - Worse in morning
  - Punctate keratopathy
- Management
  - General
    - Respiratory physician referral
      - OSA testing
    - Weight loss
    - Avoid face down sleeping
  - Medical
    - Lubricants
    - Tape eyelids shut at night
  - Surgical
    - Horizontal lid shortening
      - LTS better than wedge resection (Ezra et al. [2010])
      - Poor results if systemic not controlled

Eyelid Retraction

- Visible superior limbus and sclera in primary gaze
- Causes
  - Congenital
    - Manage condition
    - Duane's, Downs
  - Neurogenic
    - CN7 Palsy
    - CN3 aberrant regeneration
    - Parinaud's dorsal midbrain syndrome
    - Progressive supranuclear palsy
    - Sympathomimetic eyedrops
  - Myogenic
    - Thyroid eye disease
    - Myasthenia
  - Mechanical
    - Cicatricial
    - Postoperative – bleb, buckle
    - Myopia, buphthalmos
    - Orbital mass => proptosis
    - Trauma

Ectropion/Entropion
- See next

Ptosis
- See next

Eyelid Imbrication Syndrome
- Upper lid overlaps lower lid
- Management
  - Lubrication
  - Horizontal lid tightening

Centurion Syndrome
- Anterior malposition of medial lid
- Puncta displaced anteriorly, out of lacuna lacrimalis
- Due to prominent nasal bridge

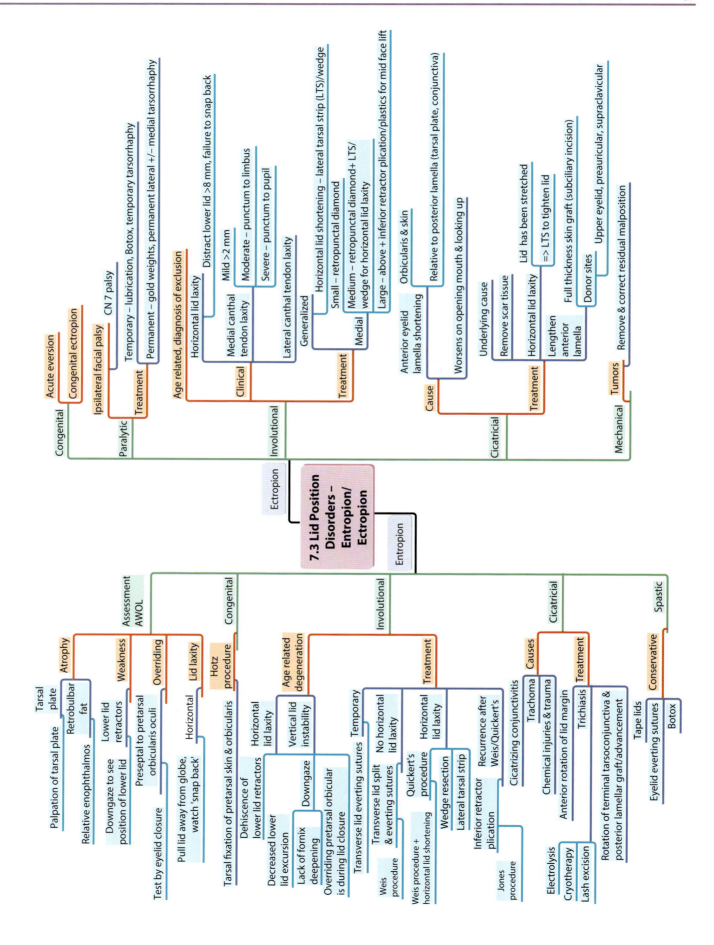

7.3 Lid Position Disorders – Entropion/Ectropion

Ectropion

- Congenital
  - Acute eversion
  - Congenital ectropion
- Paralytic
  - Ipsilateral facial palsy
    - CN 7 palsy
  - Treatment
    - Temporary – lubrication, Botox, temporary tarsorrhaphy
    - Permanent – gold weights, permanent lateral +/– medial tarsorrhaphy
- Involutional
  - Age related, diagnosis of exclusion
  - Clinical
    - Horizontal lid laxity
      - Distract lower lid >8 mm, failure to snap back
    - Medial canthal tendon laxity
      - Mild >2 mm
      - Moderate – punctum to limbus
      - Severe – punctum to pupil
    - Lateral canthal tendon laxity
  - Treatment
    - Generalized
      - Horizontal lid shortening – lateral tarsal strip (LTS)/wedge
    - Medial
      - Small – retropunctal diamond
      - Medium – retropunctal diamond+ LTS/ wedge for horizontal lid laxity
      - Large – above + inferior retractor plication/plastics for mid face lift
- Cicatricial
  - Cause
    - Anterior eyelid lamella shortening
      - Orbicularis & skin
      - Relative to posterior lamella (tarsal plate, conjunctiva)
    - Worsens on opening mouth & looking up
  - Treatment
    - Underlying cause
      - Remove scar tissue
    - Horizontal lid laxity
      - Lid has been stretched
        - => LTS to tighten lid
    - Lengthen anterior lamella
      - Full thickness skin graft (subciliary incision)
      - Donor sites
        - Upper eyelid, preauricular, supraclavicular
- Mechanical
  - Tumors
    - Remove & correct residual malposition

Entropion

- Congenital
  - Assessment
  - AWOL
  - Atrophy
    - Tarsal plate
    - Retrobulbar fat
  - Weakness
    - Lower lid retractors
  - Overriding
    - Preseptal to pretarsal orbicularis oculi
  - Lid laxity
    - Horizontal
    - Pull lid away from globe, watch 'snap back'
  - Hotz procedure
    - Palpation of tarsal plate
    - Relative enophthalmos
    - Downgaze to see position of lower lid
    - Test by eyelid closure
- Involutional
  - Age related degeneration
    - Tarsal fixation of pretarsal skin & orbicularis
    - Dehiscence of lower lid retractors
      - Horizontal lid laxity
      - Decreased lower lid excursion
    - Vertical lid instability
      - Downgaze
      - Lack of fornix deepening
    - Overriding pretarsal orbicular is during lid closure
  - Treatment
    - Temporary
      - Transverse lid everting sutures
      - Transverse lid split & everting sutures
    - No horizontal lid laxity
      - Weis procedure
      - Quickert's procedure
      - Weis procedure + horizontal lid shortening
    - Horizontal lid laxity
      - Wedge resection
      - Lateral tarsal strip
      - Inferior retractor plication
      - Jones procedure
    - Recurrence after Weis/Quickert's
- Cicatricial
  - Causes
    - Cicatrizing conjunctivitis
    - Trachoma
    - Chemical injuries & trauma
    - Anterior rotation of lid margin
    - Trichiasis
      - Electrolysis
      - Cryotherapy
      - Lash excision
  - Treatment
    - Rotation of terminal tarsoconjunctiva & posterior lamellar graft/advancement
- Spastic
  - Conservative
    - Tape lids
    - Eyelid everting sutures
    - Botox

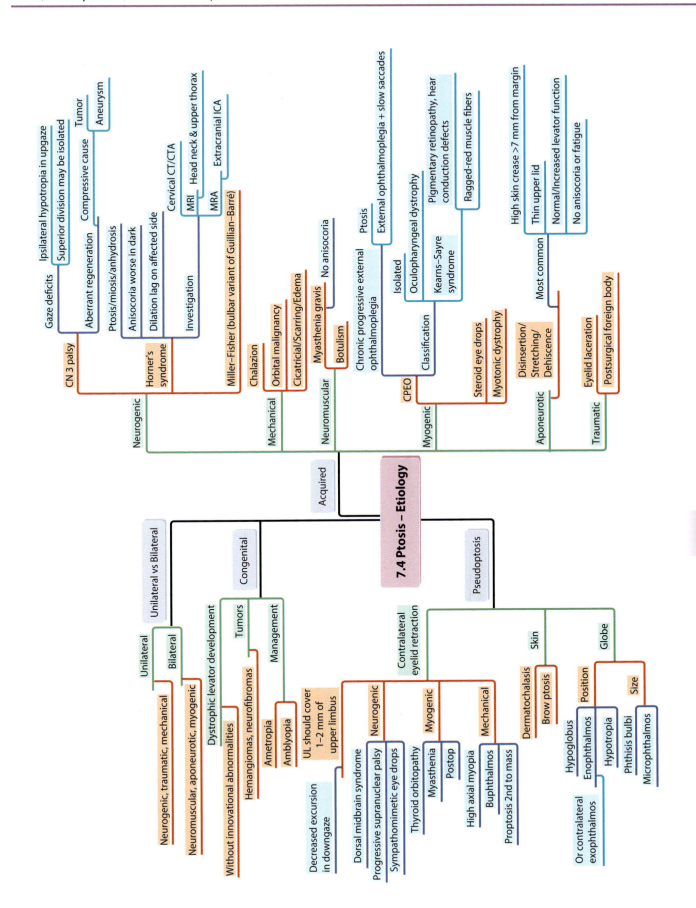

7.4 Ptosis – Etiology

Acquired

Neurogenic
- CN 3 palsy
  - Gaze deficits
    - Ipsilateral hypotropia in upgaze
    - Superior division may be isolated
  - Aberrant regeneration
  - Compressive cause
    - Tumor
    - Aneurysm
- Horner's syndrome
  - Ptosis/miosis/anhydrosis
  - Anisocoria worse in dark
  - Dilation lag on affected side
  - Investigation
    - Cervical CT/CTA
    - MRI — Head neck & upper thorax
    - MRA — Extracranial ICA
- Miller–Fisher (bulbar variant of Guillian–Barré)

Mechanical
- Chalazion
- Orbital malignancy
- Cicatricial/Scarring/Edema

Neuromuscular
- Myasthenia gravis
  - No anisocoria
- Botulism

Myogenic
- CPEO
  - Chronic progressive external ophthalmoplegia
    - Ptosis
    - External ophthalmoplegia + slow saccades
  - Classification
    - Isolated
    - Oculopharyngeal dystrophy
    - Kearns–Sayre syndrome
      - Pigmentary retinopathy, hear conduction defects
      - Ragged-red muscle fibers
- Steroid eye drops
- Myotonic dystrophy

Aponeurotic
- Disinsertion/Stretching/Dehiscence
  - Most common
    - High skin crease >7 mm from margin
    - Thin upper lid
    - Normal/Increased levator function
    - No anisocoria or fatigue

Traumatic
- Eyelid laceration
- Postsurgical foreign body

Unilateral vs Bilateral
- Unilateral
  - Neurogenic, traumatic, mechanical
- Bilateral
  - Neuromuscular, aponeurotic, myogenic

Congenital
- Dystrophic levator development
  - Without innovational abnormalities
    - Decreased excursion in downgaze
- Tumors
  - Hemangiomas, neurofibromas
- Management
  - Ametropia
  - Amblyopia
  - UL should cover 1–2 mm of upper limbus

Pseudoptosis
- Contralateral eyelid retraction
  - Neurogenic
    - Dorsal midbrain syndrome
    - Progressive supranuclear palsy
    - Sympathomimetic eye drops
  - Myogenic
    - Thyroid orbitopathy
    - Myasthenia
    - Postop
  - Mechanical
    - High axial myopia
    - Buphthalmos
    - Proptosis 2nd to mass
- Skin
  - Dermatochalasis
  - Brow ptosis
- Globe
  - Position
    - Hypoglobus
    - Enophthalmos
      - Or contralateral exophthalmos
    - Hypotropia
  - Size
    - Phthisis bulbi
    - Microphthalmos

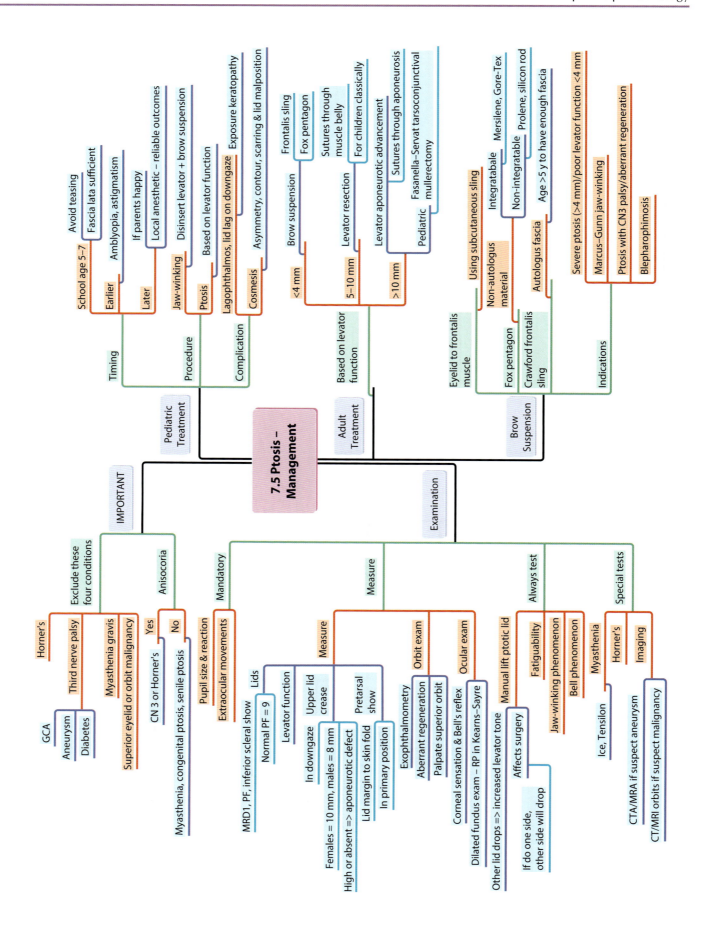

7.5 Ptosis – Management

Pediatric Treatment

Timing
- School age 5–7
- Earlier
  - Avoid teasing
  - Fascia lata sufficient
  - Amblyopia, astigmatism
- Later
  - If parents happy
  - Local anesthetic – reliable outcomes

Procedure
- Jaw-winking
  - Disinsert levator + brow suspension
- Ptosis
  - Based on levator function

Complication
- Lagophthalmos, lid lag on downgaze
  - Exposure keratopathy
- Cosmesis
  - Asymmetry, contour, scarring & lid malposition

Adult Treatment

Based on levator function
- <4 mm
  - Brow suspension
    - Frontalis sling
    - Fox pentagon
- 5–10 mm
  - Levator resection
    - Sutures through muscle belly
    - For children classically
- >10 mm
  - Levator aponeurotic advancement
    - Sutures through aponeurosis
  - Pediatric
    - Fasanella–Servat tarsoconjunctival mullerectomy

Brow Suspension
- Eyelid to frontalis muscle
  - Using subcutaneous sling
    - Non-autologus material
      - Integratable
        - Mersilene, Gore-Tex
      - Non-integratable
        - Prolene, silicon rod
    - Autologus fascia
      - Age >5 y to have enough fascia
  - Fox pentagon
  - Crawford frontalis sling
- Indications
  - Severe ptosis (>4 mm)/poor levator function <4 mm
  - Marcus–Gunn jaw-winking
  - Ptosis with CN3 palsy/aberrant regeneration
  - Blepharophimosis

IMPORTANT

Exclude these four conditions
- Horner's
  - GCA
- Third nerve palsy
  - Aneurysm
  - Diabetes
- Myasthenia gravis
- Superior eyelid or orbit malignancy

Anisocoria
- Yes
  - CN 3 or Horner's
- No
  - Myasthenia, congenital ptosis, senile ptosis

Examination

Mandatory
- Pupil size & reaction
- Extraocular movements

Measure
- Lids
  - MRD1, PF, inferior scleral show
  - Normal PF = 9
    - Females = 10 mm, males = 8 mm
  - Levator function
    - In downgaze
  - Upper lid crease
    - High or absent => aponeurotic defect
  - Pretarsal show
    - Lid margin to skin fold
    - In primary position
- Orbit exam
  - Exophthalmometry
  - Aberrant regeneration
  - Palpate superior orbit
- Ocular exam
  - Corneal sensation & Bell's reflex
  - Dilated fundus exam – RP in Kearns–Sayre

Always test
- Manual lift ptotic lid
  - Other lid drops => increased levator tone
  - Affects surgery
  - If do one side, other side will drop
- Fatiguability
- Jaw-winking phenomenon
- Bell phenomenon

Special tests
- Myasthenia
  - Ice, Tensilon
- Horner's
- Imaging
  - CTA/MRA if suspect aneurysm
  - CT/MRI orbits if suspect malignancy

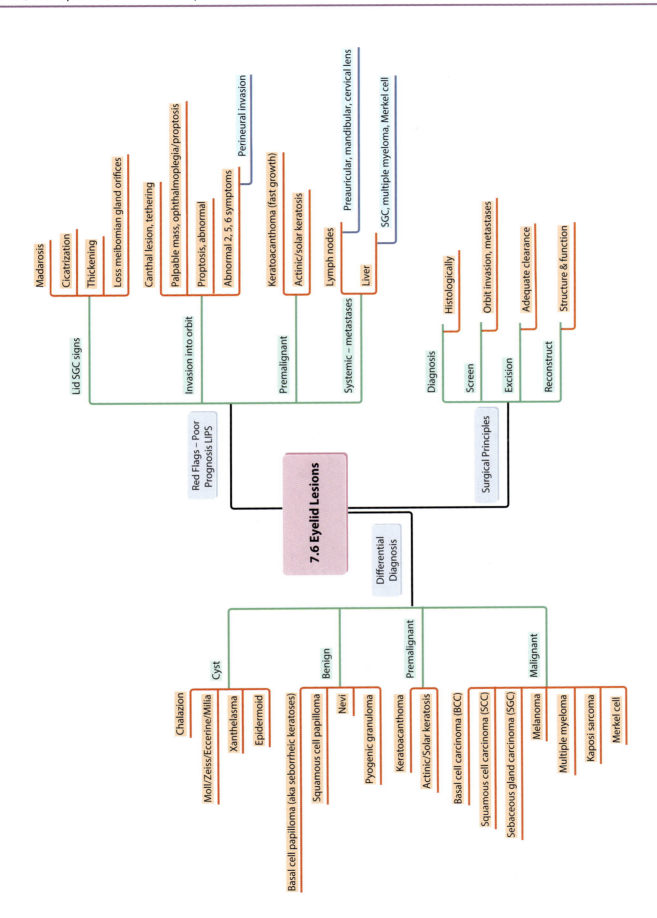

7.6 Eyelid Lesions

Red Flags – Poor Prognosis LIPS

Lid SGC signs
- Madarosis
- Cicatrization
- Thickening
- Loss meibomian gland orifices

Invasion into orbit
- Canthal lesion, tethering
- Palpable mass, ophthalmoplegia/proptosis
- Proptosis, abnormal
- Abnormal 2, 5, 6 symptoms
  - Perineural invasion

Premalignant
- Keratoacanthoma (fast growth)
- Actinic/solar keratosis

Systemic – metastases
- Lymph nodes
  - Preauricular, mandibular, cervical lens
- Liver
  - SGC, multiple myeloma, Merkel cell

Surgical Principles
- Diagnosis
  - Histologically
- Screen
  - Orbit invasion, metastases
- Excision
  - Adequate clearance
- Reconstruct
  - Structure & function

Differential Diagnosis

Cyst
- Chalazion
- Moll/Zeiss/Eccerine/Milia
- Xanthelasma
- Epidermoid

Benign
- Basal cell papilloma (aka seborrheic keratoses)
- Squamous cell papilloma
- Nevi
- Pyogenic granuloma

Premalignant
- Keratoacanthoma
- Actinic/Solar keratosis

Malignant
- Basal cell carcinoma (BCC)
- Squamous cell carcinoma (SCC)
- Sebaceous gland carcinoma (SGC)
- Melanoma
- Multiple myeloma
- Kaposi sarcoma
- Merkel cell

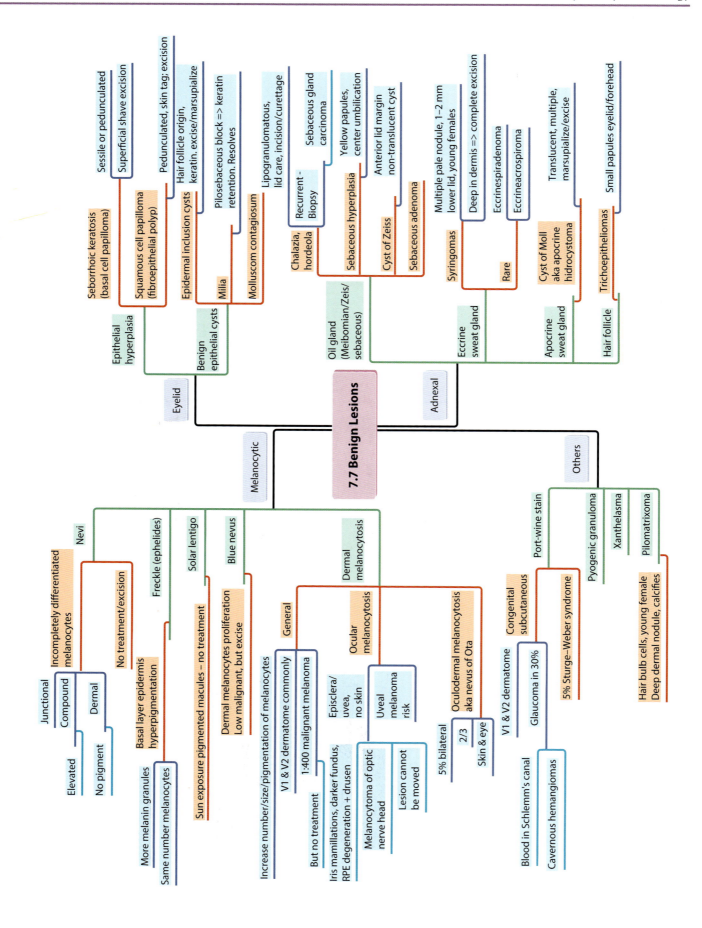

7.7 Benign Lesions

Eyelid

Epithelial hyperplasia
- Seborrhoic keratosis (basal cell papilloma)
  - Sessile or pedunculated
  - Superficial shave excision
- Squamous cell papilloma (fibroepithelial polyp)
  - Pedunculated, skin tag; excision

Benign epithelial cysts
- Epidermal inclusion cysts
  - Hair follicle origin, keratin. excise/marsupialize
- Milia
  - Pilosebaceous block => keratin retention. Resolves
- Molluscum contagiosum

Adnexal

Oil gland (Meibomian/Zeis/sebaceous)
- Chalazia, hordeola
  - Lipogranulomatous, lid care, incision/curettage
  - Recurrent - Biopsy
- Sebaceous hyperplasia
  - Sebaceous gland carcinoma
- Cyst of Zeiss
  - Yellow papules, center umbilication
- Sebaceous adenoma
  - Anterior lid margin non-translucent cyst

Eccrine sweat gland
- Syringomas
  - Multiple pale nodule, 1–2 mm lower lid, young females
- Rare
  - Deep in dermis => complete excision
  - Eccrinespiradenoma
  - Eccrineacrospiroma

Apocrine sweat gland
- Cyst of Moll aka apocrine hidrocystoma
  - Translucent, multiple, marsupialize/excise

Hair follicle
- Trichoepitheliomas
  - Small papules eyelid/forehead

Melanocytic

Nevi
- Incompletely differentiated melanocytes
- No treatment/excision
  - Junctional
    - Elevated
    - No pigment
  - Compound
  - Dermal
    - More melanin granules
    - Same number melanocytes
- Basal layer epidermis hyperpigmentation

Freckle (ephelides)
- Sun exposure pigmented macules – no treatment

Solar lentigo
- Dermal melanocytes proliferation. Low malignant, but excise
- Increase number/size/pigmentation of melanocytes

Blue nevus

Dermal melanocytosis
- General
  - V1 & V2 dermatome commonly
  - But no treatment
  - 1:400 malignant melanoma
  - Iris mamillations, darker fundus, RPE degeneration + drusen
  - Melanocytoma of optic nerve head
- Ocular melanocytosis
  - Episclera/uvea, no skin
  - Uveal melanoma risk
  - Lesion cannot be moved
- Oculodermal melanocytosis aka nevus of Ota
  - 5% bilateral
  - 2/3
  - Skin & eye
  - V1 & V2 dermatome
  - Glaucoma in 30%

Others

- Port-wine stain
  - Congenital subcutaneous
  - 5% Sturge–Weber syndrome
  - Blood in Schlemm's canal
  - Cavernous hemangiomas
- Pyogenic granuloma
- Xanthelasma
- Pilomatrixoma
  - Hair bulb cells, young female Deep dermal nodule, calcifies

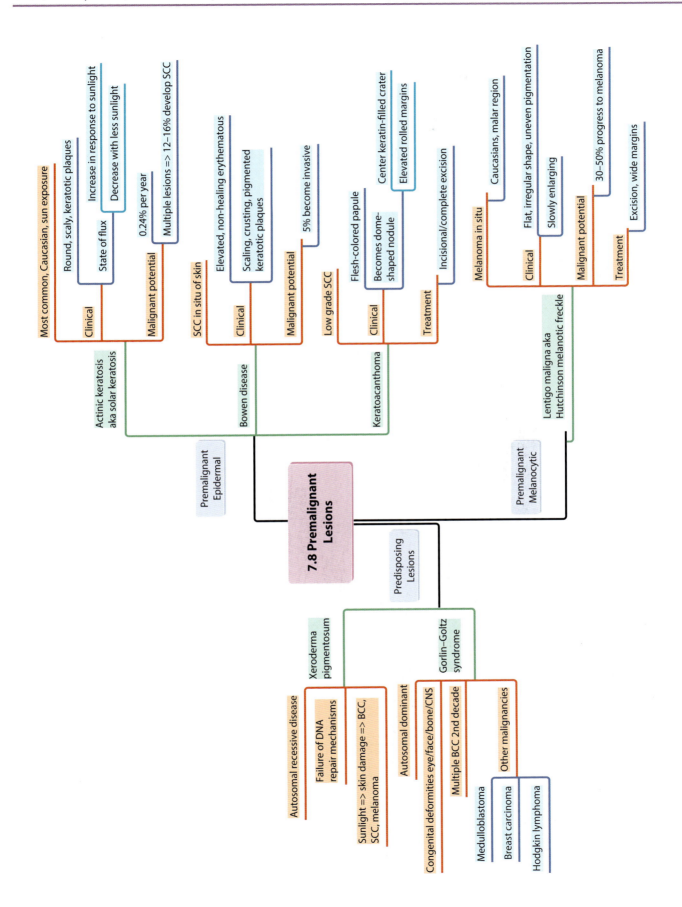

7.8 Premalignant Lesions

Premalignant Epidermal

Actinic keratosis aka solar keratosis
- Clinical
  - Most common, Caucasian, sun exposure
  - Round, scaly, keratotic plaques
  - State of flux
    - Increase in response to sunlight
    - Decrease with less sunlight
- Malignant potential
  - 0.24% per year
  - Multiple lesions => 12–16% develop SCC

Bowen disease
- SCC in situ of skin
- Clinical
  - Elevated, non-healing erythematous
  - Scaling, crusting, pigmented keratotic plaques
- Malignant potential
  - 5% become invasive

Keratoacanthoma
- Low grade SCC
- Clinical
  - Flesh-colored papule
  - Becomes dome-shaped nodule
    - Center keratin-filled crater
    - Elevated rolled margins
- Treatment
  - Incisional/complete excision

Premalignant Melanocytic

Lentigo maligna aka Hutchinson melanotic freckle
- Melanoma in situ
- Clinical
  - Caucasians, malar region
  - Flat, irregular shape, uneven pigmentation
  - Slowly enlarging
- Malignant potential
  - 30–50% progress to melanoma
- Treatment
  - Excision, wide margins

Predisposing Lesions

Xeroderma pigmentosum
- Autosomal recessive disease
- Failure of DNA repair mechanisms
- Sunlight => skin damage => BCC, SCC, melanoma

Gorlin–Goltz syndrome
- Autosomal dominant
- Congenital deformities eye/face/bone/CNS
- Multiple BCC 2nd decade
- Other malignancies
  - Medulloblastoma
  - Breast carcinoma
  - Hodgkin lymphoma

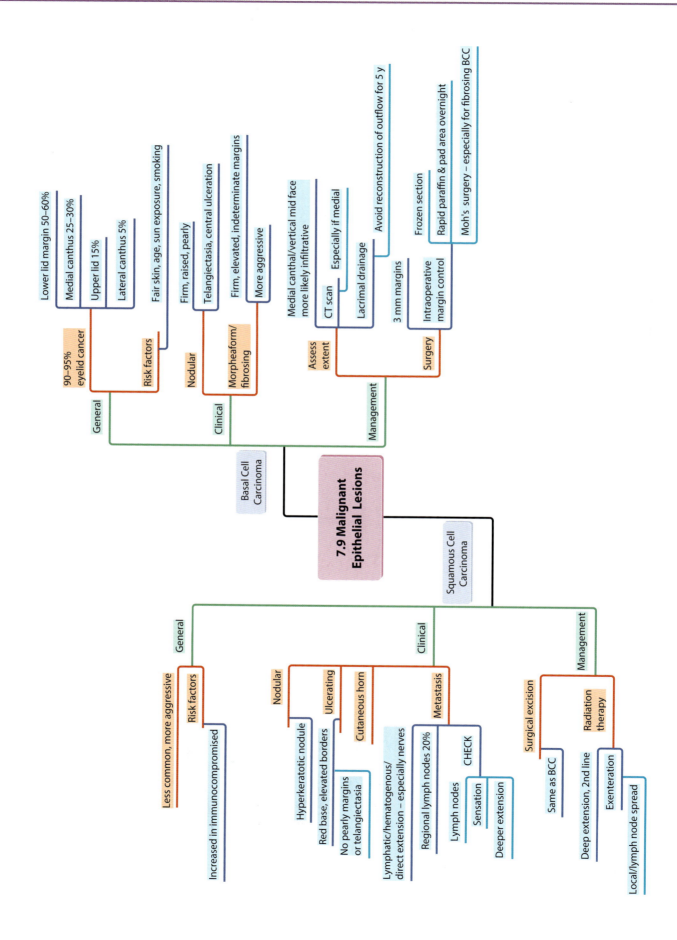

7.9 Malignant Epithelial Lesions

Basal Cell Carcinoma

General
- 90–95% eyelid cancer
  - Lower lid margin 50–60%
  - Medial canthus 25–30%
  - Upper lid 15%
  - Lateral canthus 5%
- Risk factors
  - Fair skin, age, sun exposure, smoking

Clinical
- Nodular
  - Firm, raised, pearly
  - Telangiectasia, central ulceration
- Morpheaform/fibrosing
  - Firm, elevated, indeterminate margins
  - More aggressive

Management
- Assess extent
  - Medial canthal/vertical mid face more likely infiltrative
  - CT scan
    - Especially if medial
  - Lacrimal drainage
    - Avoid reconstruction of outflow for 5 y
- Surgery
  - 3 mm margins
  - Intraoperative margin control
    - Frozen section
    - Rapid paraffin & pad area overnight
    - Moh's surgery – especially for fibrosing BCC

Squamous Cell Carcinoma

General
- Less common, more aggressive
- Risk factors
  - Increased in immunocompromised

Clinical
- Nodular
  - Hyperkeratotic nodule
  - Red base, elevated borders
  - No pearly margins or telangiectasia
- Ulcerating
- Cutaneous horn
- Metastasis
  - Lymphatic/hematogenous/direct extension – especially nerves
  - Regional lymph nodes 20%
  - CHECK
    - Lymph nodes
    - Sensation
    - Deeper extension

Management
- Surgical excision
  - Same as BCC
  - Deep extension, 2nd line
    - Exenteration
- Radiation therapy
  - Local/lymph node spread

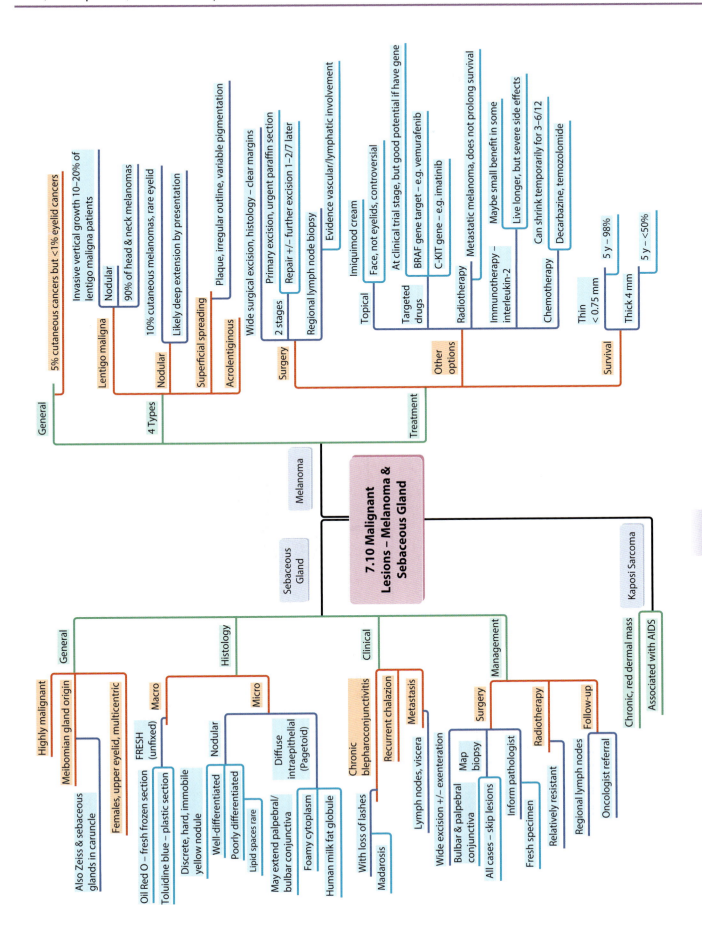

7.10 Malignant Lesions – Melanoma & Sebaceous Gland

Melanoma

General

4 Types

- 5% cutaneous cancers but <1% eyelid cancers
- Lentigo maligna
  - Invasive vertical growth 10–20% of lentigo maligna patients
  - Nodular
  - 90% of head & neck melanomas
- Nodular
  - 10% cutaneous melanomas, rare eyelid
  - Likely deep extension by presentation
- Superficial spreading
  - Plaque, irregular outline, variable pigmentation
- Acrolentiginous

Treatment

- Surgery
  - Wide surgical excision, histology – clear margins
  - 2 stages
    - Primary excision, urgent paraffin section
    - Repair +/– further excision 1–2/7 later
  - Regional lymph node biopsy
    - Evidence vascular/lymphatic involvement
- Other options
  - Topical
    - Imiquimod cream
    - Face, not eyelids, controversial
  - Targeted drugs
    - At clinical trial stage, but good potential if have gene
    - BRAF gene target – e.g. vemurafenib
    - C-KIT gene – e.g. imatinib
  - Radiotherapy
    - Metastatic melanoma, does not prolong survival
  - Immunotherapy – interleukin-2
    - Maybe small benefit in some
    - Live longer, but severe side effects
  - Chemotherapy
    - Can shrink temporarily for 3–6/12
    - Decarbazine, temozolomide
- Survival
  - Thin <0.75 mm
    - 5 y – 98%
  - Thick 4 mm
    - 5 y – <50%

Sebaceous Gland

General

- Highly malignant
- Meibomian gland origin
  - Also Zeiss & sebaceous glands in caruncle
- Females, upper eyelid, multicentric

Histology

- Macro
  - FRESH (unfixed)
    - Oil Red O – fresh frozen section
    - Toluidine blue – plastic section
  - Discrete, hard, immobile yellow nodule
- Micro
  - Nodular
    - Well-differentiated
    - Poorly differentiated
    - Lipid spaces rare
  - Diffuse intraepithelial (Pagetoid)
    - May extend palpebral/bulbar conjunctiva
    - Foamy cytoplasm
    - Human milk fat globule

Clinical

- Chronic blepharoconjunctivitis
  - With loss of lashes
  - Madarosis
- Recurrent chalazion
- Metastasis
  - Lymph nodes, viscera

Management

- Surgery
  - Wide excision +/– exenteration
    - Bulbar & palpebral conjunctiva
    - All cases – skip lesions
  - Map biopsy
    - Inform pathologist
    - Fresh specimen
- Radiotherapy
  - Relatively resistant
- Follow-up
  - Regional lymph nodes
  - Oncologist referral

Kaposi Sarcoma

- Chronic, red dermal mass
- Associated with AIDS

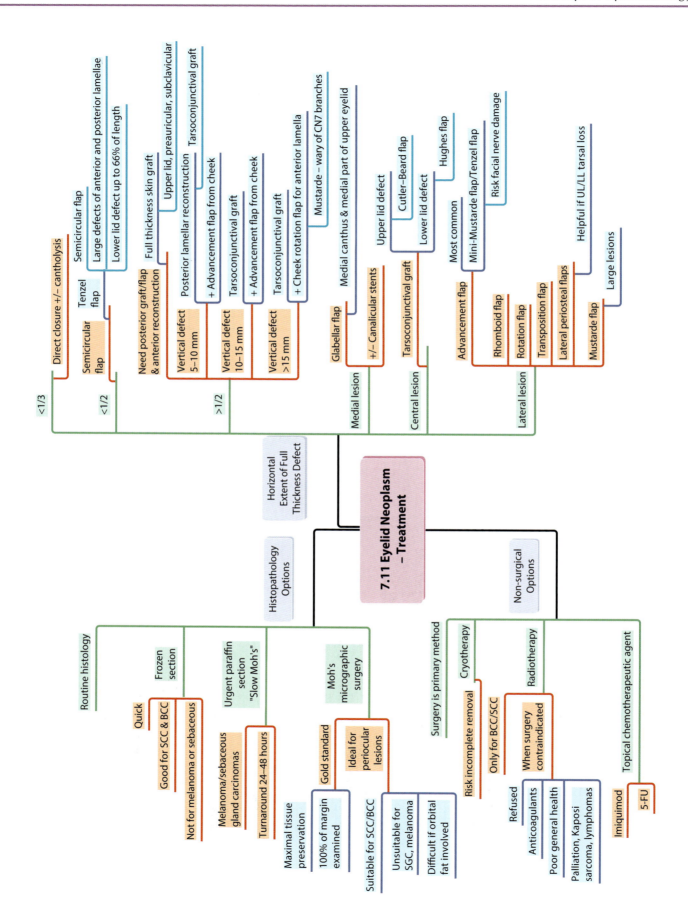

7.11 Eyelid Neoplasm – Treatment

Horizontal Extent of Full Thickness Defect

<1/3
- Direct closure +/– cantholysis

<1/2
- Semicircular flap
  - Tenzel flap
    - Semicircular flap
    - Large defects of anterior and posterior lamellae
    - Lower lid defect up to 66% of length

>1/2
- Need posterior graft/flap & anterior reconstruction
  - Vertical defect 5–10 mm
    - Full thickness skin graft
    - Posterior lamellar reconstruction
      - Upper lid, preauricular, subclavicular
      - Tarsoconjunctival graft
  - Vertical defect 10–15 mm
    - Tarsoconjunctival graft
    - + Advancement flap from cheek
  - Vertical defect >15 mm
    - Tarsoconjunctival graft
    - + Advancement flap from cheek
    - + Cheek rotation flap for anterior lamella
    - Mustarde – wary of CN7 branches

Medial lesion
- Glabellar flap
- +/– Canalicular stents
- Medial canthus & medial part of upper eyelid

Central lesion
- Tarsoconjunctival graft
  - Upper lid defect
    - Cutler–Beard flap
  - Lower lid defect
    - Hughes flap

Lateral lesion
- Advancement flap
  - Most common
- Rhomboid flap
- Rotation flap
  - Mini-Mustarde flap/Tenzel flap
  - Risk facial nerve damage
- Transposition flap
- Lateral periosteal flaps
  - Helpful if UL/LL tarsal loss
- Mustarde flap
  - Large lesions

Histopathology Options

- Routine histology
- Frozen section
  - Quick
    - Good for SCC & BCC
    - Not for melanoma or sebaceous
- Urgent paraffin section "Slow Moh's"
  - Melanoma/sebaceous gland carcinomas
  - Turnaround 24–48 hours
- Moh's micrographic surgery
  - Gold standard
    - Maximal tissue preservation
    - 100% of margin examined
  - Ideal for periocular lesions
    - Suitable for SCC/BCC
    - Unsuitable for SGC, melanoma
    - Difficult if orbital fat involved

Non-surgical Options

- Surgery is primary method
- Cryotherapy
  - Risk incomplete removal
  - Only for BCC/SCC
- Radiotherapy
  - When surgery contraindicated
    - Refused
    - Anticoagulants
    - Poor general health
    - Palliation, Kaposi sarcoma, lymphomas
- Topical chemotherapeutic agent
  - Imiquimod
  - 5-FU

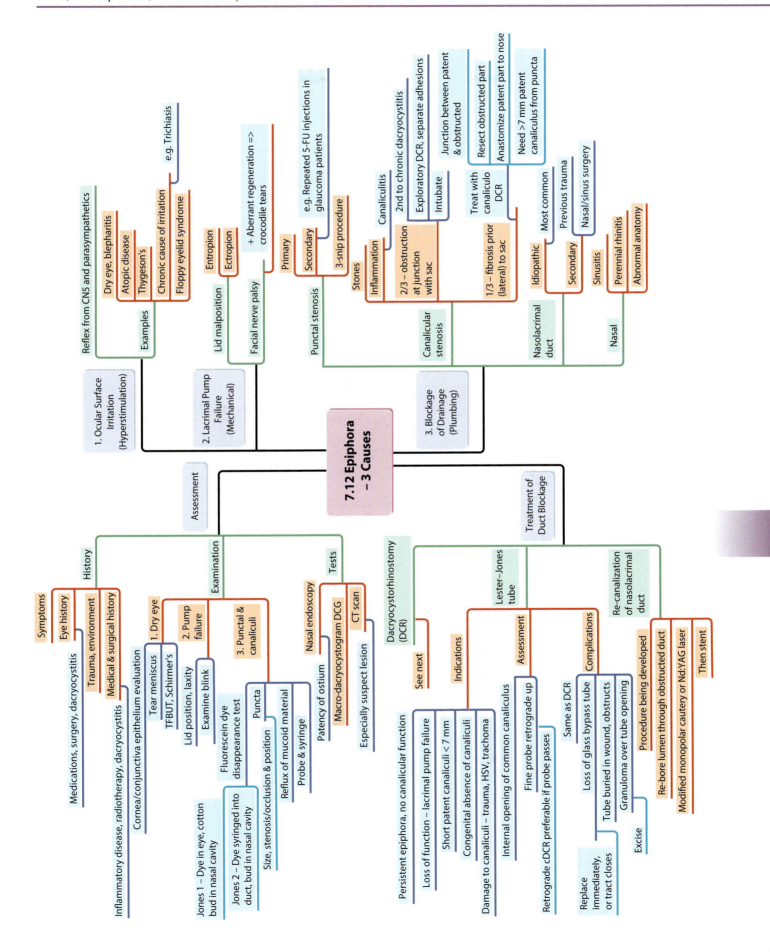

7.12 Epiphora – 3 Causes

1. Ocular Surface Irritation (Hyperstimulation)
- Reflex from CN5 and parasympathetics
- Examples
  - Dry eye, blepharitis
  - Atopic disease
  - Thygeson's
  - Chronic cause of irritation — e.g. Trichiasis
  - Floppy eyelid syndrome

2. Lacrimal Pump Failure (Mechanical)
- Lid malposition
  - Entropion
  - Ectropion
- Facial nerve palsy
  - + Aberrant regeneration => crocodile tears

3. Blockage of Drainage (Plumbing)
- Punctal stenosis
  - Primary
  - Secondary — 3-snip procedure
- Canalicular stenosis
  - Stones
  - Inflammation
    - Canaliculitis
    - 2nd to chronic dacryocystitis — Exploratory DCR, separate adhesions — Junction between patent & obstructed
    - Intubate
  - 2/3 – obstruction at junction with sac — Treat with canaliculo DCR
  - 1/3 – fibrosis prior (lateral) to sac
    - Resect obstructed part
    - Anastomize patent part to nose — Need >7 mm patent canaliculus from puncta
  - e.g. Repeated 5-FU injections in glaucoma patients
- Nasolacrimal duct
  - Idiopathic — Most common
  - Secondary
    - Previous trauma
    - Nasal/sinus surgery
- Nasal
  - Sinusitis
  - Perennial rhinitis
  - Abnormal anatomy

Assessment
- History
  - Symptoms
  - Eye history — Medications, surgery, dacryocystitis
  - Trauma, environment — Inflammatory disease, radiotherapy, dacryocystitis
  - Medical & surgical history
- Examination
  - Cornea/conjunctiva epithelium evaluation
  - 1. Dry eye
    - Tear meniscus
    - TFBUT, Schirmer's
  - 2. Pump failure
    - Lid position, laxity
    - Examine blink
  - 3. Punctal & canaliculi
    - Puncta
      - Size, stenosis/occlusion & position
      - Reflux of mucoid material
    - Fluorescein dye disappearance test
    - Probe & syringe
      - Jones 1 – Dye in eye, cotton bud in nasal cavity
      - Jones 2 – Dye syringed into duct, bud in nasal cavity
- Tests
  - Nasal endoscopy
    - Patency of ostium
  - Macro-dacryocystogram DCG
  - CT scan — Especially suspect lesion

Treatment of Duct Blockage
- Dacryocystorhinostomy (DCR) — See next
- Lester–Jones tube
  - Indications
    - Persistent epiphora, no canalicular function
    - Loss of function – lacrimal pump failure
    - Short patent canaliculi < 7 mm
    - Congenital absence of canaliculi
    - Damage to canaliculi – trauma, HSV, trachoma
    - Internal opening of common canaliculus
    - Retrograde cDCR preferable if probe passes
  - Assessment
    - Fine probe retrograde up
    - Same as DCR
  - Complications
    - Loss of glass bypass tube — Replace immediately, or tract closes
    - Tube buried in wound, obstructs — Excise
    - Granuloma over tube opening
- Re-canalization of nasolacrimal duct
  - Procedure being developed
  - Re-bore lumen through obstructed duct
  - Modified monopolar cautery or Nd:YAG laser
  - Then stent

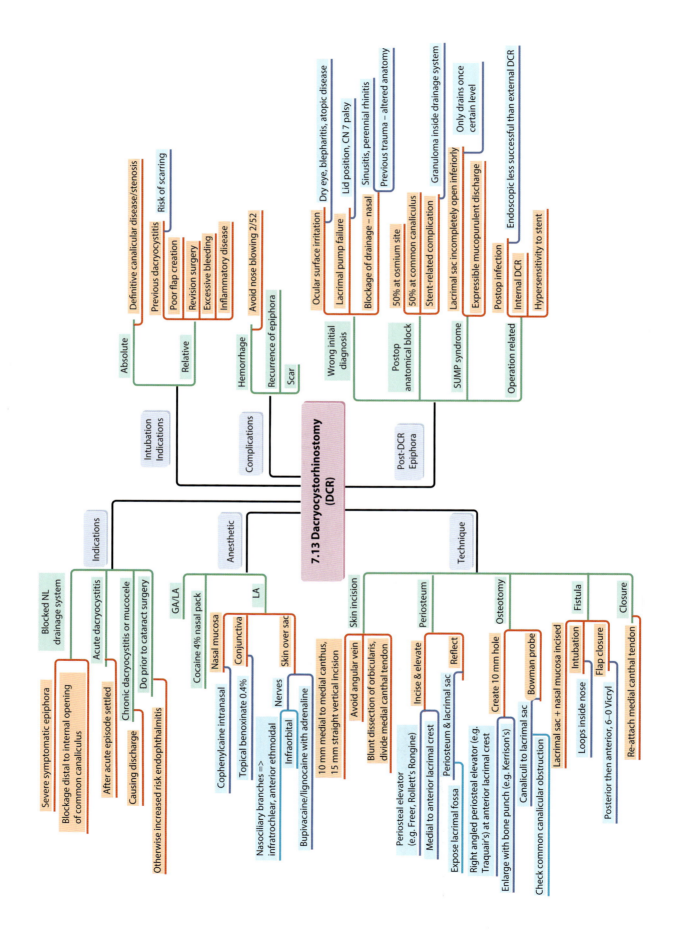

7.13 Dacryocystorhinostomy (DCR)

Intubation Indications

Absolute
- Definitive canalicular disease/stenosis

Relative
- Previous dacryocystitis
- Risk of scarring
- Poor flap creation
- Revision surgery
- Excessive bleeding
- Inflammatory disease

Complications

Hemorrhage
- Avoid nose blowing 2/52

Recurrence of epiphora

Scar

Post-DCR Epiphora

Wrong initial diagnosis
- Ocular surface irritation
  - Dry eye, blepharitis, atopic disease
- Lacrimal pump failure
  - Lid position, CN 7 palsy
- Blockage of drainage — nasal
  - Sinusitis, perennial rhinitis
  - Previous trauma – altered anatomy

Postop anatomical block
- 50% at osmium site
- 50% at common caniculus
- Stent-related complication
  - Granuloma inside drainage system

SUMP syndrome
- Lacrimal sac incompletely open inferiorly
  - Only drains once certain level
- Expressible mucopurulent discharge

Operation related
- Postop infection
- Internal DCR
  - Endoscopic less successful than external DCR
- Hypersensitivity to stent

Indications

Blocked NL drainage system
- Severe symptomatic epiphora
- Blockage distal to internal opening of common caniculus

Acute dacryocystitis
- After acute episode settled

Chronic dacryocystitis or mucocele
- Causing discharge

Do prior to cataract surgery
- Otherwise increased risk endophthalmitis

Anesthetic

GA/LA
- Cocaine 4% nasal pack

LA
- Nasal mucosa
  - Cophenylcaine intranasal
  - Topical benoxinate 0.4%
- Conjunctiva
- Nerves
  - Nasociliary branches => infratrochlear, anterior ethmoidal
  - Infraorbital
- Skin over sac
  - Bupivacaine/lignocaine with adrenaline

Technique

Skin incision
- 10 mm medial to medial canthus, 15 mm straight vertical incision
- Avoid angular vein
- Blunt dissection of orbicularis, divide medial canthal tendon

Periosteum
- Incise & elevate
  - Periosteal elevator (e.g. Freer, Rollett's Rongine)
  - Medial to anterior lacrimal crest
- Reflect
  - Expose lacrimal fossa
  - Right angled periosteal elevator (e.g. Traquair's) at anterior lacrimal crest

Periosteum & lacrimal sac

Osteotomy
- Create 10 mm hole
  - Enlarge with bone punch (e.g. Kerrison's)
- Bowman probe
  - Canaliculi to lacrimal sac
  - Check common canalicular obstruction

Fistula
- Lacrimal sac + nasal mucosa incised
- Intubation
  - Loops inside nose
- Flap closure
  - Posterior then anterior, 6–0 Vicryl

Closure
- Re-attach medial canthal tendon

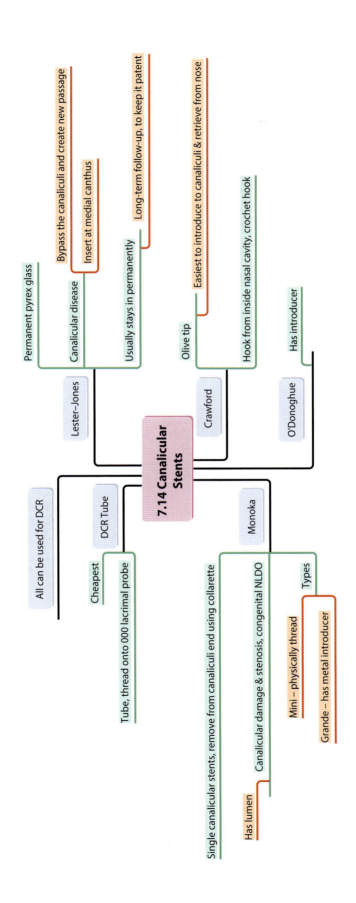

7.14 Canalicular Stents

Lester–Jones
- Permanent pyrex glass
- Canalicular disease
  - Bypass the canaliculi and create new passage
  - Insert at medial canthus
- Usually stays in permanently
  - Long-term follow-up, to keep it patent

Crawford
- Olive tip
  - Easiest to introduce to canaliculi & retrieve from nose
- Hook from inside nasal cavity, crochet hook

O'Donoghue
- Has introducer

DCR Tube
- All can be used for DCR
- Cheapest
- Tube, thread onto 000 lacrimal probe

Monoka
- Single canalicular stents, remove from canaliculi end using collarette
- Canalicular damage & stenosis, congenital NLDO
- Has lumen
- Types
  - Mini – physically thread
  - Grande – has metal introducer

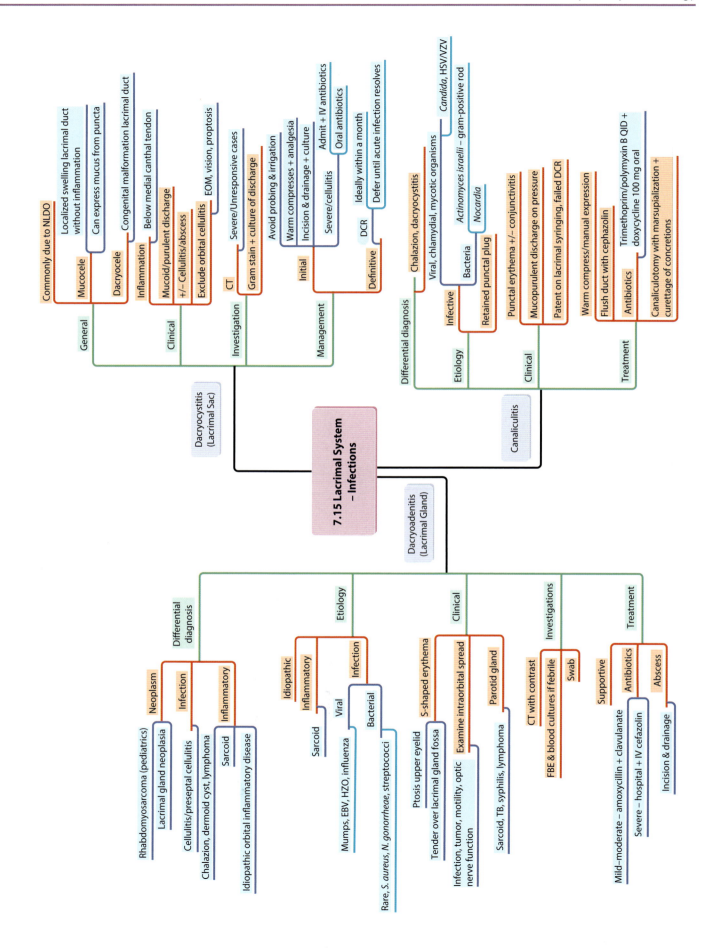

7.15 Lacrimal System – Infections

Dacryocystitis (Lacrimal Sac)

General
- Commonly due to NLDO
- Mucocele
  - Localized swelling lacrimal duct without inflammation
  - Can express mucus from puncta
- Dacryocele
  - Congenital malformation lacrimal duct
  - Below medial canthal tendon

Clinical
- Inflammation
- Mucoid/purulent discharge
- +/– Cellulitis/abscess
- Exclude orbital cellulitis
- EOM, vision, proptosis

Investigation
- CT
  - Severe/Unresponsive cases
- Gram stain + culture of discharge

Management
- Initial
  - Avoid probing & irrigation
  - Warm compresses + analgesia
  - Incision & drainage + culture
  - Severe/cellulitis
    - Admit + IV antibiotics
    - Oral antibiotics
- Definitive
  - DCR
    - Ideally within a month
    - Defer until acute infection resolves

Canaliculitis

Differential diagnosis
- Chalazion, dacryocystitis
- Viral, chlamydial, mycotic organisms

Etiology
- Infective
  - Bacteria
    - Actinomyces israelii – gram-positive rod
    - Nocardia
  - Candida, HSV/VZV
- Retained punctal plug

Clinical
- Punctal erythema +/– conjunctivitis
- Mucopurulent discharge on pressure
- Patent on lacrimal syringing, failed DCR

Treatment
- Warm compress/manual expression
- Flush duct with cephazolin
- Antibiotics
  - Trimethoprim/polymyxin B QID + doxycycline 100 mg oral
- Canaliculotomy with marsupialization + curettage of concretions

Dacryoadenitis (Lacrimal Gland)

Differential diagnosis
- Neoplasm
  - Rhabdomyosarcoma (pediatrics)
  - Lacrimal gland neoplasia
- Infection
  - Cellulitis/preseptal cellulitis
- Inflammatory
  - Chalazion, dermoid cyst, lymphoma
  - Sarcoid
  - Idiopathic orbital inflammatory disease

Etiology
- Idiopathic
- Inflammatory
  - Sarcoid
- Infection
  - Viral
    - Mumps, EBV, HZO, influenza
  - Bacterial
    - Rare, S. aureus, N. gonorrheae, streptococci

Clinical
- S-shaped erythema
  - Ptosis upper eyelid
- Tender over lacrimal gland fossa
- Examine intraorbital spread
  - Infection, tumor, motility, optic nerve function
- Parotid gland
  - Sarcoid, TB, syphilis, lymphoma

Investigations
- CT with contrast
- FBE & blood cultures if febrile
- Swab

Treatment
- Supportive
- Antibiotics
  - Mild-moderate – amoxycillin + clavulanate
  - Severe – hospital + IV cefazolin
- Abscess
  - Incision & drainage

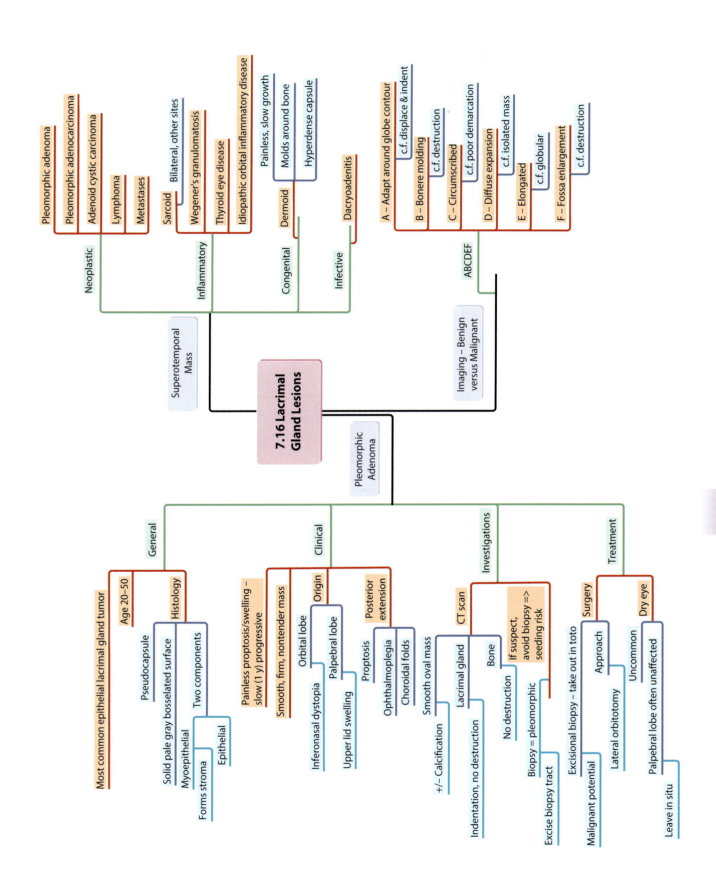

7.16 Lacrimal Gland Lesions

Superotemporal Mass

Neoplastic
- Pleomorphic adenoma
- Pleomorphic adenocarcinoma
- Adenoid cystic carcinoma
- Lymphoma
- Metastases

Inflammatory
- Sarcoid — Bilateral, other sites
- Wegener's granulomatosis
- Thyroid eye disease
- Idiopathic orbital inflammatory disease

Congenital
- Dermoid
  - Painless, slow growth
  - Molds around bone
  - Hyperdense capsule

Infective
- Dacryoadenitis

Imaging – Benign versus Malignant

ABCDEF
- A – Adapt around globe contour
  - c.f. displace & indent
- B – Bone molding
  - c.f. destruction
- C – Circumscribed
  - c.f. poor demarcation
- D – Diffuse expansion
  - c.f. isolated mass
- E – Elongated
  - c.f. globular
- F – Fossa enlargement
  - c.f. destruction

Pleomorphic Adenoma

General
- Most common epithelial lacrimal gland tumor
- Age 20–50
- Histology
  - Pseudocapsule
  - Solid pale gray bosselated surface
  - Two components
    - Myoepithelial
      - Forms stroma
    - Epithelial

Clinical
- Painless proptosis/swelling – slow (1 y) progressive
- Smooth, firm, nontender mass
- Origin
  - Orbital lobe
    - Inferonasal dystopia
  - Palpebral lobe
    - Upper lid swelling
- Posterior extension
  - Proptosis
  - Ophthalmoplegia
  - Choroidal folds
- Smooth oval mass

Investigations
- CT scan
  - Lacrimal gland
    - +/– Calcification
  - Bone
    - Indentation, no destruction
    - No destruction
- If suspect, avoid biopsy => seeding risk
  - Biopsy = pleomorphic
    - Excise biopsy tract

Treatment
- Surgery
  - Excisional biopsy – take out in toto
    - Malignant potential
  - Approach
    - Lateral orbitotomy
- Dry eye
  - Uncommon
  - Palpebral lobe often unaffected
    - Leave in situ

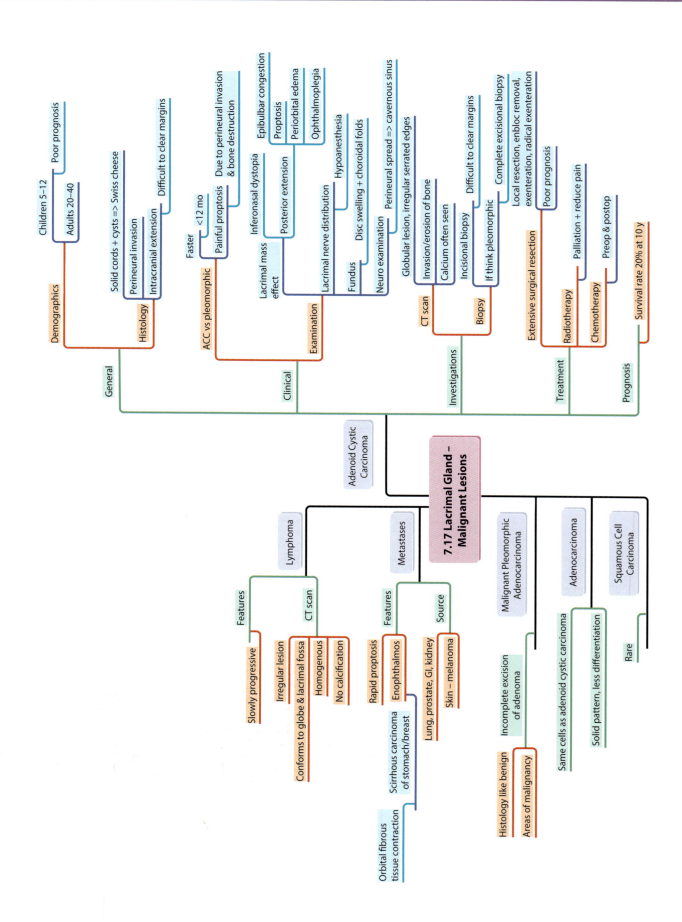

7.17 Lacrimal Gland – Malignant Lesions

Adenoid Cystic Carcinoma

General
- Demographics
  - Children 5–12
  - Adults 20–40
    - Poor prognosis
- Histology
  - Solid cords + cysts => Swiss cheese
  - Perineural invasion
  - Intracranial extension
    - Difficult to clear margins

Clinical
- ACC vs pleomorphic
  - Faster
    - <12 mo
  - Painful proptosis
    - Due to perineural invasion & bone destruction
- Examination
  - Lacrimal mass effect
    - Inferonasal dystopia
    - Posterior extension
      - Epibulbar congestion
      - Proptosis
      - Periorbital edema
      - Ophthalmoplegia
  - Lacrimal nerve distribution
    - Hypoanesthesia
  - Fundus
    - Disc swelling + choroidal folds
  - Neuro examination
    - Perineural spread => cavernous sinus

Investigations
- CT scan
  - Globular lesion, irregular serrated edges
  - Invasion/erosion of bone
  - Calcium often seen
- Biopsy
  - Incisional biopsy
    - Difficult to clear margins
  - If think pleomorphic
    - Complete excisional biopsy

Treatment
- Extensive surgical resection
  - Local resection, enbloc removal, exenteration, radical exenteration
- Radiotherapy
  - Poor prognosis
- Chemotherapy
  - Palliation + reduce pain
  - Preop & postop

Prognosis
- Survival rate 20% at 10 y

Lymphoma
- Features
  - Slowly progressive
  - Irregular lesion
  - Conforms to globe & lacrimal fossa
- CT scan
  - Homogenous
  - No calcification

Metastases
- Features
  - Rapid proptosis
  - Enophthalmos
    - Scirrhous carcinoma of stomach/breast
    - Orbital fibrous tissue contraction
- Source
  - Lung, prostate, GI, kidney
  - Skin – melanoma

Malignant Pleomorphic Adenocarcinoma
- Incomplete excision of adenoma
  - Histology like benign
  - Areas of malignancy

Adenocarcinoma
- Same cells as adenoid cystic carcinoma
- Solid pattern, less differentiation

Squamous Cell Carcinoma
- Rare

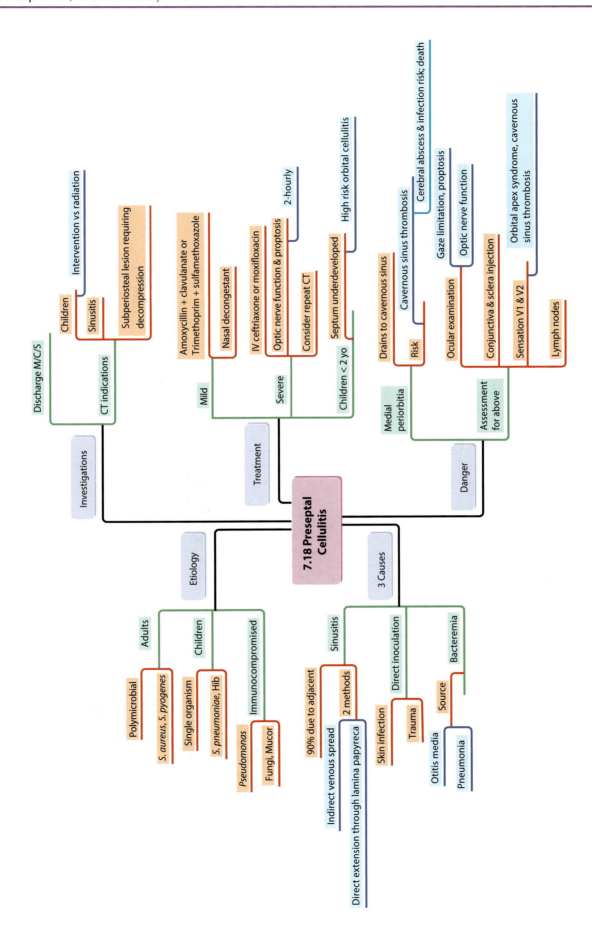

7.18 Preseptal Cellulitis

Investigations
- Discharge M/C/S
- CT indications
  - Children
  - Sinusitis
    - Intervention vs radiation
  - Subperiosteal lesion requiring decompression

Treatment
- Mild
  - Amoxycillin + clavulanate or Trimethoprim + sulfamethoxazole
  - Nasal decongestant
- Severe
  - IV ceftriaxone or moxifloxacin
  - Optic nerve function & proptosis
    - 2-hourly
  - Consider repeat CT
- Children < 2 yo
  - Septum underdeveloped
    - High risk orbital cellulitis

Danger
- Medial periorbitia
  - Drains to cavernous sinus
  - Risk
    - Cavernous sinus thrombosis
      - Cerebral abscess & infection risk; death
- Assessment for above
  - Ocular examination
    - Gaze limitation, proptosis
    - Optic nerve function
  - Conjunctiva & sclera injection
  - Sensation V1 & V2
    - Orbital apex syndrome, cavernous sinus thrombosis
  - Lymph nodes

Etiology
- Adults
  - Polymicrobial
  - S. aureus, S. pyogenes
- Children
  - Single organism
  - S. pneumoniae, Hib
- Immunocompromised
  - Pseudomonas
  - Fungi, Mucor

3 Causes
- Sinusitis
  - 90% due to adjacent
  - 2 methods
    - Indirect venous spread
    - Direct extension through lamina papyreca
- Direct inoculation
  - Skin infection
  - Trauma
- Bacteremia
  - Source
    - Otitis media
    - Pneumonia

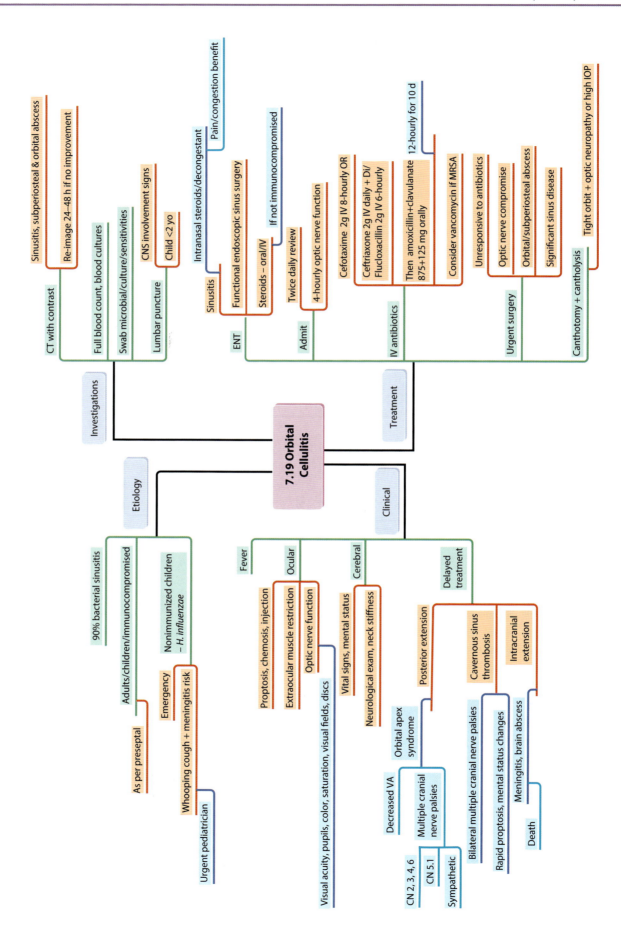

7.19 Orbital Cellulitis

Investigations

CT with contrast
- Sinusitis, subperiosteal & orbital abscess
- Re-image 24–48 h if no improvement

Full blood count, blood cultures

Swab microbial/culture/sensitivities

Lumbar puncture
- CNS involvement signs
- Child <2 yo

Treatment

ENT
- Sinusitis
  - Intranasal steroids/decongestant
  - Pain/congestion benefit
- Functional endoscopic sinus surgery

Admit
- Steroids – oral/IV
  - If not immunocompromised
- Twice daily review
- 4-hourly optic nerve function

IV antibiotics
- Cefotaxime 2g IV 8-hourly OR
- Ceftriaxone 2g IV daily + Di/ Flucloxacillin 2g IV 6-hourly
- Then amoxicillin+clavulanate 875+125 mg orally 12-hourly for 10 d
- Consider vancomycin if MRSA

Urgent surgery
- Unresponsive to antibiotics
- Optic nerve compromise
- Orbital/subperiosteal abscess
- Significant sinus disease

Canthotomy + cantholysis
- Tight orbit + optic neuropathy or high IOP

Etiology

As per preseptal
- 90% bacterial sinusitis
- Adults/children/immunocompromised

Emergency
- Nonimmunized children – H. influenzae

Whooping cough + meningitis risk
- Urgent pediatrician

Clinical

Fever

Ocular
- Proptosis, chemosis, injection
- Extraocular muscle restriction
- Optic nerve function
  - Visual acuity, pupils, color, saturation, visual fields, discs

Cerebral
- Vital signs, mental status
- Neurological exam, neck stiffness

Delayed treatment
- Posterior extension
  - Orbital apex syndrome
    - Decreased VA
    - Multiple cranial nerve palsies
      - CN 2, 3, 4, 6
      - CN 5.1
      - Sympathetic
- Cavernous sinus thrombosis
  - Bilateral multiple cranial nerve palsies
  - Rapid proptosis, mental status changes
- Intracranial extension
  - Meningitis, brain abscess
  - Death

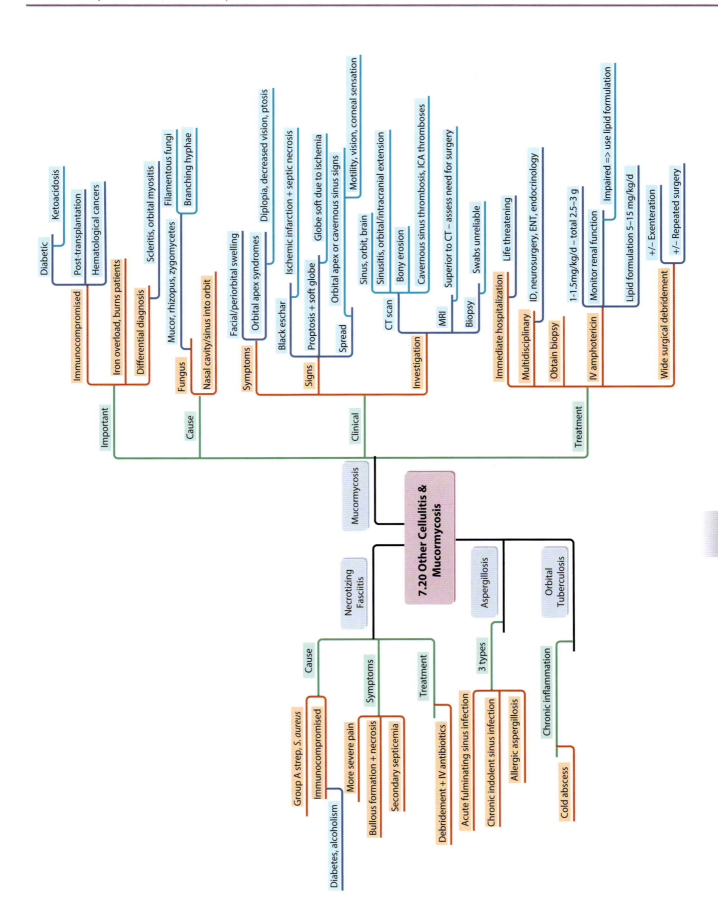

7.20 Other Cellulitis & Mucormycosis

Mucormycosis

Important
- Immunocompromised
  - Diabetic — Ketoacidosis
  - Post-transplantation
  - Hematological cancers
- Iron overload, burns patients
- Differential diagnosis
  - Scleritis, orbital myositis

Cause
- Fungus
  - Mucor, rhizopus, zygomycetes
  - Filamentous fungi
  - Branching hyphae
- Nasal cavity/sinus into orbit

Clinical
- Symptoms
  - Facial/periorbital swelling
  - Orbital apex syndromes — Diplopia, decreased vision, ptosis
- Signs
  - Black eschar — Ischemic infarction + septic necrosis
  - Proptosis + soft globe — Globe soft due to ischemia
  - Spread — Orbital apex or cavernous sinus signs — Motility, vision, corneal sensation
- Investigation
  - CT scan
    - Sinus, orbit, brain
    - Sinusitis, orbital/intracranial extension
    - Bony erosion
    - Cavernous sinus thrombosis, ICA thromboses
  - MRI — Superior to CT – assess need for surgery
  - Biopsy — Swabs unreliable

Treatment
- Immediate hospitalization — Life threatening
- Multidisciplinary — ID, neurosurgery, ENT, endocrinology
- Obtain biopsy
- IV amphotericin
  - 1-1.5mg/kg/d – total 2.5–3 g
  - Monitor renal function — Impaired => use lipid formulation
  - Lipid formulation 5–15 mg/kg/d
- Wide surgical debridement
  - +/– Exenteration
  - +/– Repeated surgery

Necrotizing Fasciitis

Cause
- Group A strep, S. aureus
- Immunocompromised — Diabetes, alcoholism

Symptoms
- More severe pain
- Bullous formation + necrosis
- Secondary septicemia

Treatment
- Debridement + IV antibiotics

Aspergillosis

3 types
- Acute fulminating sinus infection
- Chronic indolent sinus infection
- Allergic aspergillosis

Orbital Tuberculosis

- Chronic inflammation
- Cold abscess

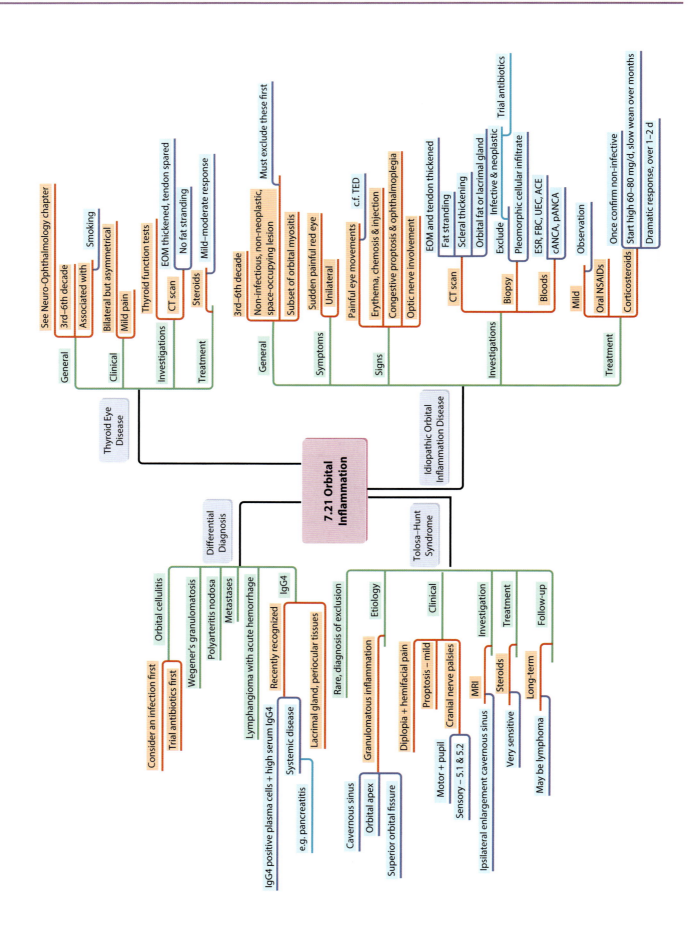

7.21 Orbital Inflammation

Thyroid Eye Disease

General
- See Neuro-Ophthalmology chapter
- 3rd–6th decade
- Associated with
  - Smoking

Clinical
- Bilateral but asymmetrical
- Mild pain

Investigations
- Thyroid function tests
- CT scan
  - EOM thickened, tendon spared
  - No fat stranding

Treatment
- Steroids
  - Mild–moderate response

Idiopathic Orbital Inflammation Disease

General
- 3rd–6th decade
- Non-infectious, non-neoplastic, space-occupying lesion
  - Must exclude these first
- Subset of orbital myositis

Symptoms
- Sudden painful red eye
- Unilateral

Signs
- Painful eye movements
  - c.f. TED
- Erythema, chemosis & injection
- Congestive proptosis & ophthalmoplegia
- Optic nerve involvement

Investigations
- CT scan
  - EOM and tendon thickened
  - Fat stranding
  - Scleral thickening
  - Orbital fat or lacrimal gland
- Biopsy
  - Exclude
    - Infective & neoplastic
      - Trial antibiotics
  - Pleomorphic cellular infiltrate
- Bloods
  - ESR, FBC, UEC, ACE
  - cANCA, pANCA

Treatment
- Mild
  - Observation
  - Oral NSAIDs
- Corticosteroids
  - Once confirm non-infective
  - Start high 60–80 mg/d, slow wean over months
  - Dramatic response, over 1–2 d

Differential Diagnosis
- Orbital cellulitis
  - Consider an infection first
  - Trial antibiotics first
- Wegener's granulomatosis
- Polyarteritis nodosa
- Metastases
- Lymphangioma with acute hemorrhage
- IgG4
  - Recently recognized
  - IgG4 positive plasma cells + high serum IgG4
  - Systemic disease
    - e.g. pancreatitis
  - Lacrimal gland, periocular tissues

Tolosa–Hunt Syndrome

Etiology
- Rare, diagnosis of exclusion
- Granulomatous inflammation
  - Cavernous sinus
  - Orbital apex
  - Superior orbital fissure

Clinical
- Diplopia + hemifacial pain
- Proptosis – mild
- Cranial nerve palsies
  - Motor + pupil
  - Sensory – 5.1 & 5.2

Investigation
- MRI
  - Ipsilateral enlargement cavernous sinus

Treatment
- Steroids
  - Very sensitive

Follow-up
- Long-term
  - May be lymphoma

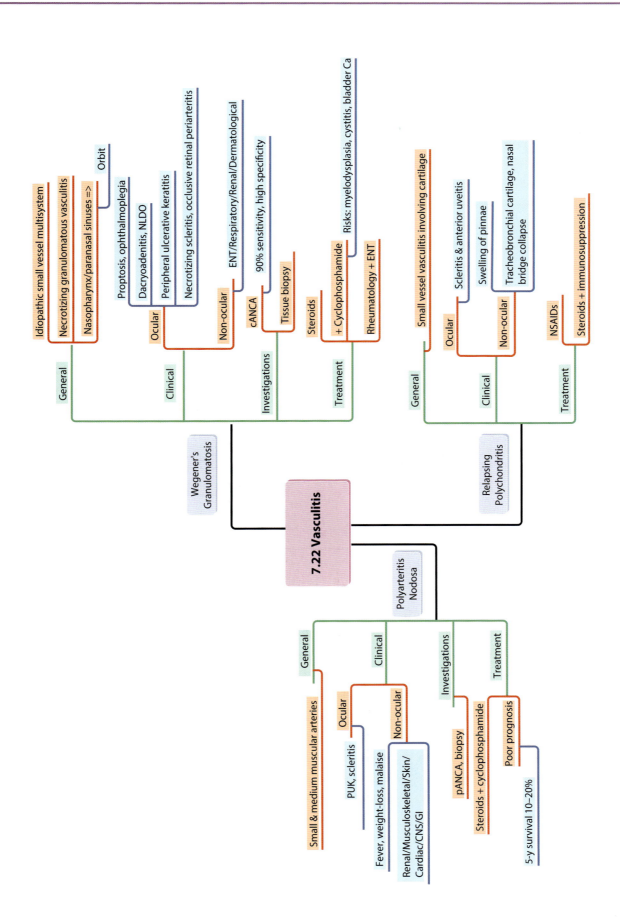

Wegener's Granulomatosis

General
- Idiopathic small vessel multisystem
- Necrotizing granulomatous vasculitis
- Nasopharynx/paranasal sinuses => Orbit

Clinical
- Ocular
  - Proptosis, ophthalmoplegia
  - Dacryoadenitis, NLDO
  - Peripheral ulcerative keratitis
  - Necrotizing scleritis, occlusive retinal periarteritis
- Non-ocular
  - ENT/Respiratory/Renal/Dermatological

Investigations
- cANCA
  - 90% sensitivity, high specificity
- Tissue biopsy

Treatment
- Steroids
- + Cyclophosphamide
  - Risks: myelodysplasia, cystitis, bladder Ca
- Rheumatology + ENT

Relapsing Polychondritis

General
- Small vessel vasculitis involving cartilage

Clinical
- Ocular
  - Scleritis & anterior uveitis
  - Swelling of pinnae
- Non-ocular
  - Tracheobronchial cartilage, nasal bridge collapse

Treatment
- NSAIDs
- Steroids + immunosuppression

7.22 Vasculitis

Polyarteritis Nodosa

General
- Small & medium muscular arteries

Clinical
- Ocular
  - PUK, scleritis
- Non-ocular
  - Fever, weight-loss, malaise
  - Renal/Musculoskeletal/Skin/Cardiac/CNS/GI

Investigations
- pANCA, biopsy

Treatment
- Steroids + cyclophosphamide
- Poor prognosis
  - 5-y survival 10–20%

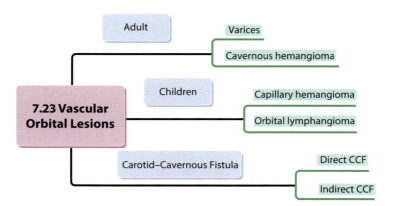

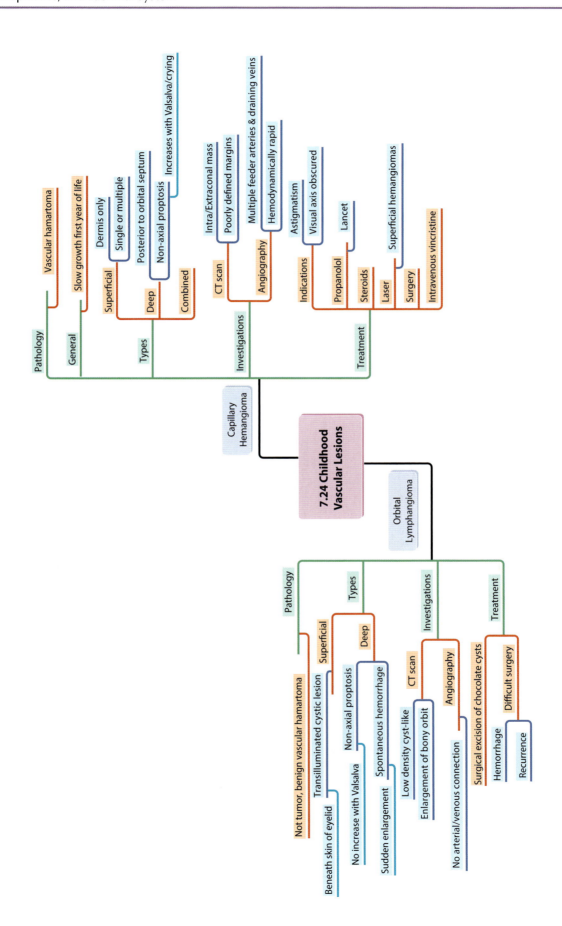

7.24 Childhood Vascular Lesions

Capillary Hemangioma

Pathology
- Vascular hamartoma

General
- Slow growth first year of life

Types
- Superficial
  - Dermis only
  - Single or multiple
- Deep
  - Posterior to orbital septum
  - Non-axial proptosis
  - Increases with Valsalva/crying
- Combined

Investigations
- CT scan
  - Intra/Extraconal mass
  - Poorly defined margins
- Angiography
  - Multiple feeder arteries & draining veins
  - Hemodynamically rapid

Treatment
- Indications
  - Astigmatism
  - Visual axis obscured
- Propanolol
- Steroids
  - Lancet
- Laser
  - Superficial hemangiomas
- Surgery
- Intravenous vincristine

Orbital Lymphangioma

Pathology
- Not tumor, benign vascular hamartoma
- Transilluminated cystic lesion
- Beneath skin of eyelid
- No increase with Valsalva

Types
- Superficial
- Deep
  - Non-axial proptosis
  - Spontaneous hemorrhage
  - Sudden enlargement

Investigations
- CT scan
  - Low density cyst-like
  - Enlargement of bony orbit
- Angiography
  - No arterial/venous connection

Treatment
- Surgical excision of chocolate cysts
- Difficult surgery
  - Hemorrhage
  - Recurrence

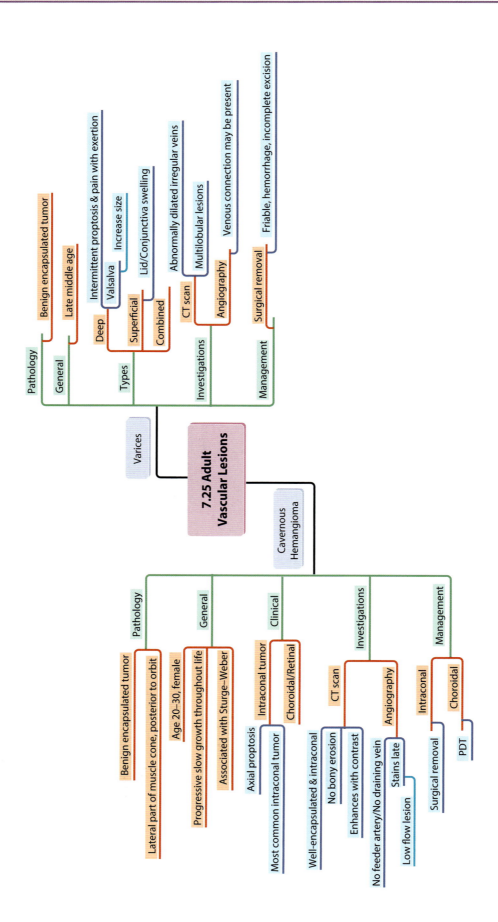

7.25 Adult Vascular Lesions

Varices

- Pathology
  - Benign encapsulated tumor
- General
  - Late middle age
- Types
  - Deep
    - Intermittent proptosis & pain with exertion
    - Valsalva
      - Increase size
  - Superficial
    - Lid/Conjunctiva swelling
  - Combined
- Investigations
  - CT scan
    - Abnormally dilated irregular veins
    - Multilobular lesions
  - Angiography
    - Venous connection may be present
- Management
  - Surgical removal
    - Friable, hemorrhage, incomplete excision

Cavernous Hemangioma

- Pathology
  - Benign encapsulated tumor
  - Lateral part of muscle cone, posterior to orbit
- General
  - Age 20–30, female
  - Progressive slow growth throughout life
  - Associated with Sturge–Weber
- Clinical
  - Intraconal tumor
    - Axial proptosis
    - Most common intraconal tumor
  - Choroidal/Retinal
- Investigations
  - CT scan
    - Well-encapsulated & intraconal
    - No bony erosion
    - Enhances with contrast
  - Angiography
    - No feeder artery/No draining vein
    - Stains late
    - Low flow lesion
- Management
  - Intraconal
    - Surgical removal
  - Choroidal
    - PDT

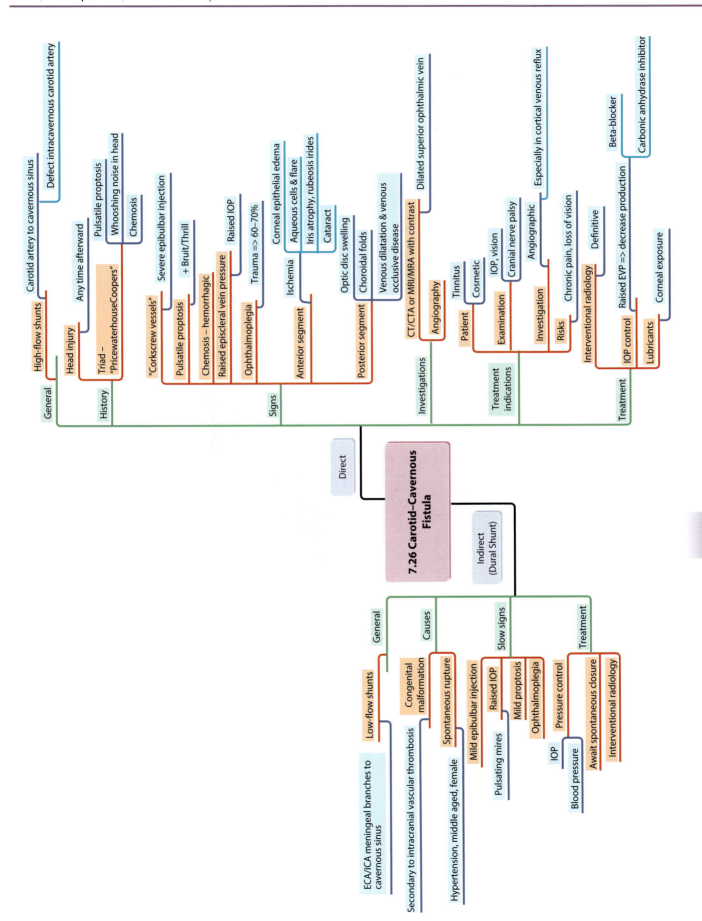

7.26 Carotid–Cavernous Fistula

Direct

General
- High-flow shunts
  - Carotid artery to cavernous sinus
  - Defect intracavernous carotid artery

History
- Head injury
  - Any time afterward
- Triad – "PricewaterhouseCoopers"
  - Pulsatile proptosis
  - Whooshing noise in head
  - Chemosis

Signs
- "Corkscrew vessels"
  - Severe epibulbar injection
- Pulsatile proptosis
  - + Bruit/Thrill
- Chemosis – hemorrhagic
- Raised episcleral vein pressure
  - Raised IOP
- Ophthalmoplegia
  - Trauma => 60–70%
- Anterior segment
  - Ischemia
  - Corneal epithelial edema
  - Aqueous cells & flare
  - Iris atrophy, rubeosis irides
  - Cataract
- Posterior segment
  - Optic disc swelling
  - Choroidal folds
  - Venous dilatation & venous occlusive disease

Investigations
- CT/CTA or MRI/MRA with contrast
  - Dilated superior ophthalmic vein
- Angiography

Treatment indications
- Patient
  - Tinnitus
  - Cosmetic
- Examination
  - IOP, vision
  - Cranial nerve palsy
- Investigation
  - Angiographic
    - Especially in cortical venous reflux
- Risks
  - Chronic pain, loss of vision

Treatment
- Interventional radiology
  - Definitive
- IOP control
  - Raised EVP => decrease production
    - Beta-blocker
    - Carbonic anhydrase inhibitor
- Lubricants
  - Corneal exposure

Indirect (Dural Shunt)

General
- Low-flow shunts
  - ECA/ICA meningeal branches to cavernous sinus

Causes
- Congenital malformation
- Spontaneous rupture
  - Secondary to intracranial vascular thrombosis
  - Hypertension, middle aged, female

Slow signs
- Mild epibulbar injection
- Raised IOP
  - Pulsating mires
- Mild proptosis
- Ophthalmoplegia

Treatment
- Pressure control
  - IOP
  - Blood pressure
- Await spontaneous closure
- Interventional radiology

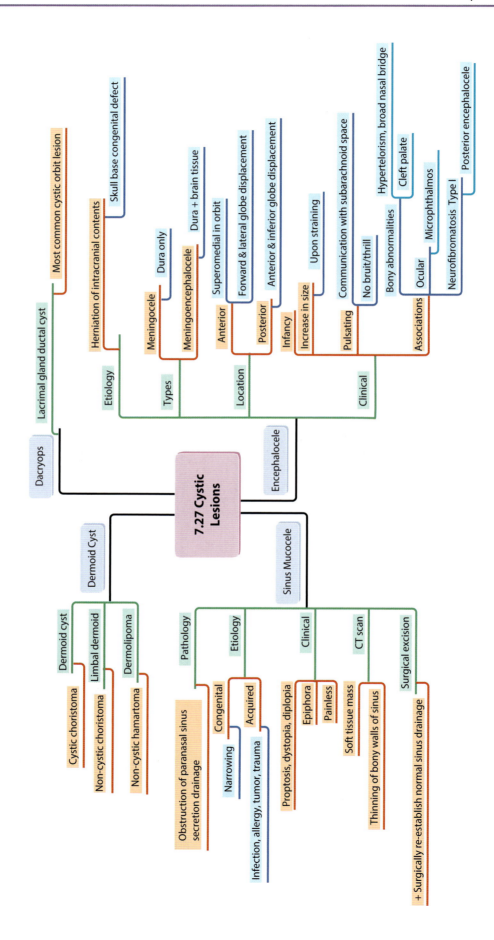

7.27 Cystic Lesions

Dacryops
- Lacrimal gland ductal cyst
  - Most common cystic orbit lesion

Encephalocele
- Etiology
  - Herniation of intracranial contents
    - Skull base congenital defect
- Types
  - Meningocele
    - Dura only
  - Meningoencephalocele
    - Dura + brain tissue
- Location
  - Anterior
    - Superomedial in orbit
    - Forward & lateral globe displacement
  - Posterior
    - Anterior & inferior globe displacement
- Clinical
  - Infancy
  - Increase in size
    - Upon straining
  - Pulsating
    - Communication with subarachnoid space
    - No bruit/thrill
  - Associations
    - Bony abnormalities
      - Hypertelorism, broad nasal bridge
      - Cleft palate
    - Ocular
      - Microphthalmos
    - Neurofibromatosis Type I
      - Posterior encephalocele

Dermoid Cyst
- Dermoid cyst
  - Cystic choristoma
- Limbal dermoid
  - Non-cystic choristoma
- Dermolipoma
  - Non-cystic hamartoma

Sinus Mucocele
- Pathology
  - Obstruction of paranasal sinus secretion drainage
- Etiology
  - Congenital
    - Narrowing
  - Acquired
    - Infection, allergy, tumor, trauma
- Clinical
  - Proptosis, dystopia, diplopia
  - Epiphora
  - Painless
- CT scan
  - Soft tissue mass
  - Thinning of bony walls of sinus
- Surgical excision
  - + Surgically re-establish normal sinus drainage

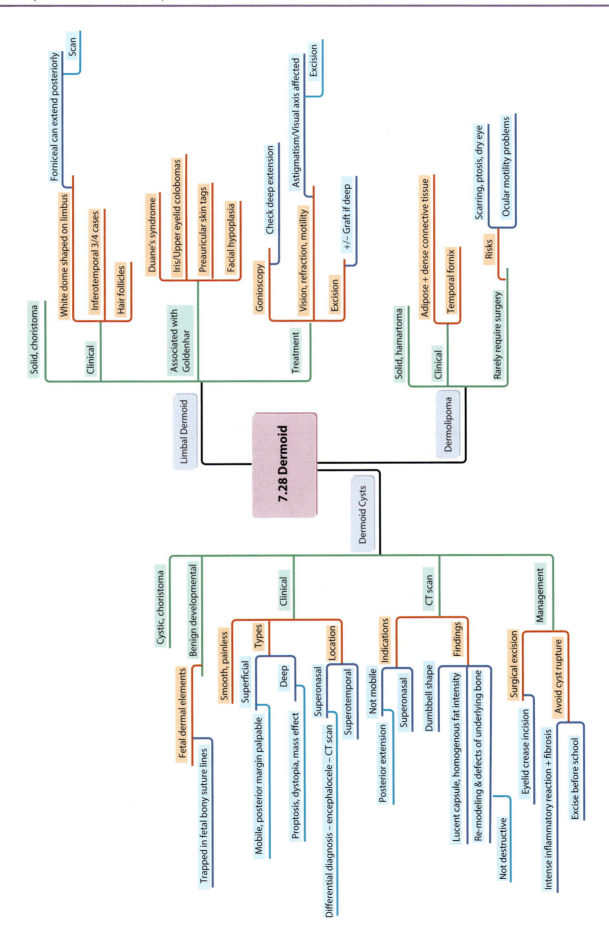

7.28 Dermoid

Limbal Dermoid

Solid, choristoma

Clinical
- White dome shaped on limbus
  - Forniceal can extend posteriorly
    - Scan
- Inferotemporal 3/4 cases
- Hair follicles

Associated with Goldenhar
- Duane's syndrome
- Iris/Upper eyelid colobomas
- Preauricular skin tags
- Facial hypoplasia

Treatment
- Gonioscopy
  - Check deep extension
  - Astigmatism/Visual axis affected
    - Excision
- Vision, refraction, motility
- Excision
  - +/- Graft if deep

Dermolipoma

Solid, hamartoma

Clinical
- Adipose + dense connective tissue
- Temporal fornix

Rarely require surgery
- Risks
  - Scarring, ptosis, dry eye
  - Ocular motility problems

Dermoid Cysts

Cystic, choristoma

Benign developmental
- Fetal dermal elements
  - Trapped in fetal bony suture lines

Clinical
- Smooth, painless
- Types
  - Superficial
    - Mobile, posterior margin palpable
  - Deep
    - Proptosis, dystopia, mass effect
    - Differential diagnosis – encephalocele – CT scan
- Location
  - Superonasal
  - Superotemporal

CT scan
- Indications
  - Not mobile
    - Posterior extension
  - Superonasal
  - Dumbbell shape
- Findings
  - Lucent capsule, homogenous fat intensity
  - Re-modeling & defects of underlying bone
    - Not destructive

Management
- Surgical excision
  - Eyelid crease incision
  - Intense inflammatory reaction + fibrosis
    - Excise before school
- Avoid cyst rupture

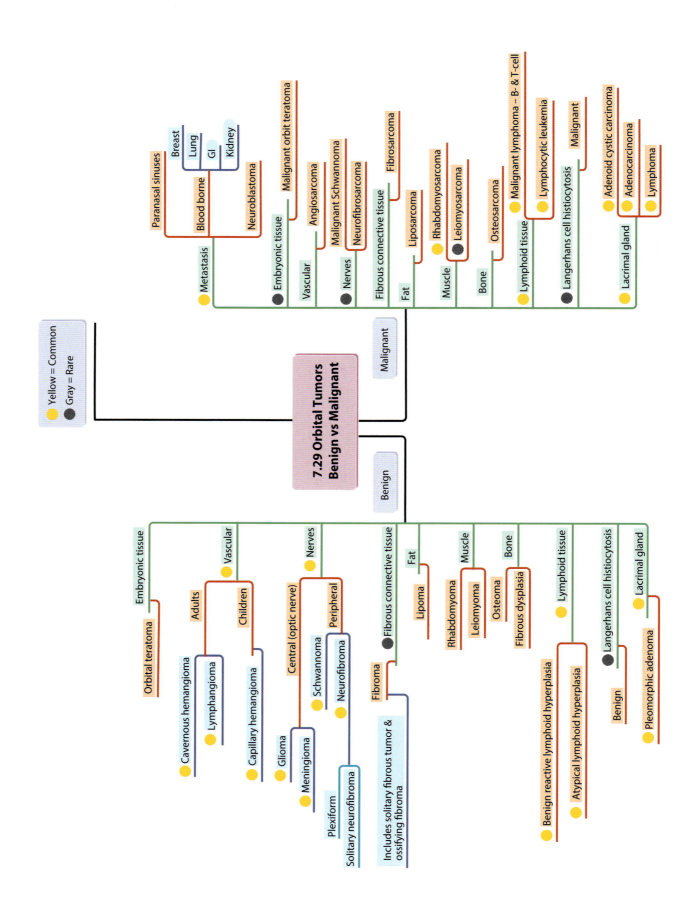

7.29 Orbital Tumors Benign vs Malignant

Yellow = Common
Gray = Rare

Malignant

Metastasis
- Paranasal sinuses
- Blood borne
  - Breast
  - Lung
  - GI
  - Kidney
- Neuroblastoma

Embryonic tissue
- Malignant orbit teratoma

Vascular
- Angiosarcoma

Nerves
- Malignant Schwannoma
- Neurofibrosarcoma

Fibrous connective tissue
- Fibrosarcoma

Fat
- Liposarcoma

Muscle
- Rhabdomyosarcoma
- Leiomyosarcoma

Bone
- Osteosarcoma

Lymphoid tissue
- Malignant lymphoma – B- & T-cell
- Lymphocytic leukemia

Langerhans cell histiocytosis
- Malignant

Lacrimal gland
- Adenoid cystic carcinoma
- Adenocarcinoma
- Lymphoma

Benign

Embryonic tissue
- Orbital teratoma

Vascular
- Adults
  - Cavernous hemangioma
  - Lymphangioma
- Children
  - Capillary hemangioma

Nerves
- Central (optic nerve)
  - Glioma
  - Meningioma
- Peripheral
  - Schwannoma
  - Neurofibroma
    - Plexiform
    - Solitary neurofibroma

Fibrous connective tissue
- Fibroma
  - Includes solitary fibrous tumor & ossifying fibroma

Fat
- Lipoma

Muscle
- Rhabdomyoma
- Leiomyoma

Bone
- Osteoma
- Fibrous dysplasia

Lymphoid tissue
- Benign reactive lymphoid hyperplasia
- Atypical lymphoid hyperplasia

Langerhans cell histiocytosis
- Benign

Lacrimal gland
- Pleomorphic adenoma

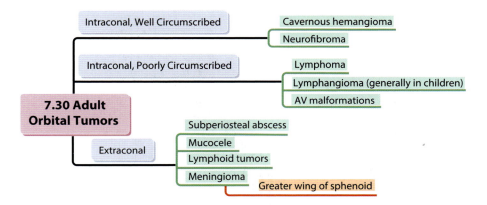

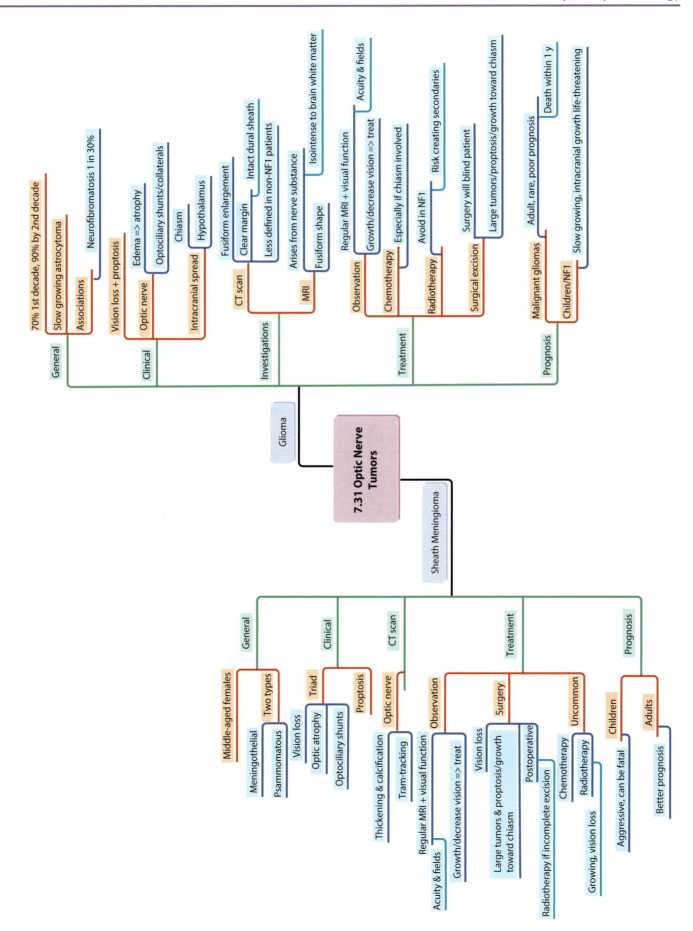

7.31 Optic Nerve Tumors

Glioma

General
- 70% 1st decade, 90% by 2nd decade
- Slow growing astrocytoma
- Associations
  - Neurofibromatosis 1 in 30%

Clinical
- Vision loss + proptosis
- Optic nerve
  - Edema => atrophy
  - Optociliary shunts/collaterals
- Intracranial spread
  - Chiasm
  - Hypothalamus

Investigations
- CT scan
  - Fusiform enlargement
  - Clear margin
    - Intact dural sheath
  - Less defined in non-NF1 patients
- MRI
  - Arises from nerve substance
  - Fusiform shape
    - Isointense to brain white matter

Treatment
- Observation
  - Regular MRI + visual function
    - Acuity & fields
  - Growth/decrease vision => treat
- Chemotherapy
  - Especially if chiasm involved
- Radiotherapy
  - Avoid in NF1
    - Risk creating secondaries
- Surgical excision
  - Surgery will blind patient
  - Large tumors/proptosis/growth toward chiasm

Prognosis
- Malignant gliomas
  - Adult, rare, poor prognosis
    - Death within 1 y
- Children/NF1
  - Slow growing, intracranial growth life-threatening

Sheath Meningioma

General
- Middle-aged females
- Two types
  - Meningothelial
  - Psammomatous

Clinical
- Triad
  - Vision loss
  - Optic atrophy
  - Optociliary shunts
- Proptosis

CT scan
- Optic nerve
  - Thickening & calcification
  - Tram-tracking

Treatment
- Observation
  - Regular MRI + visual function
    - Acuity & fields
  - Growth/decrease vision => treat
    - Vision loss
- Surgery
  - Large tumors & proptosis/growth toward chiasm
  - Postoperative
    - Radiotherapy if incomplete excision
- Uncommon
  - Chemotherapy
  - Radiotherapy
    - Growing, vision loss

Prognosis
- Children
  - Aggressive, can be fatal
- Adults
  - Better prognosis

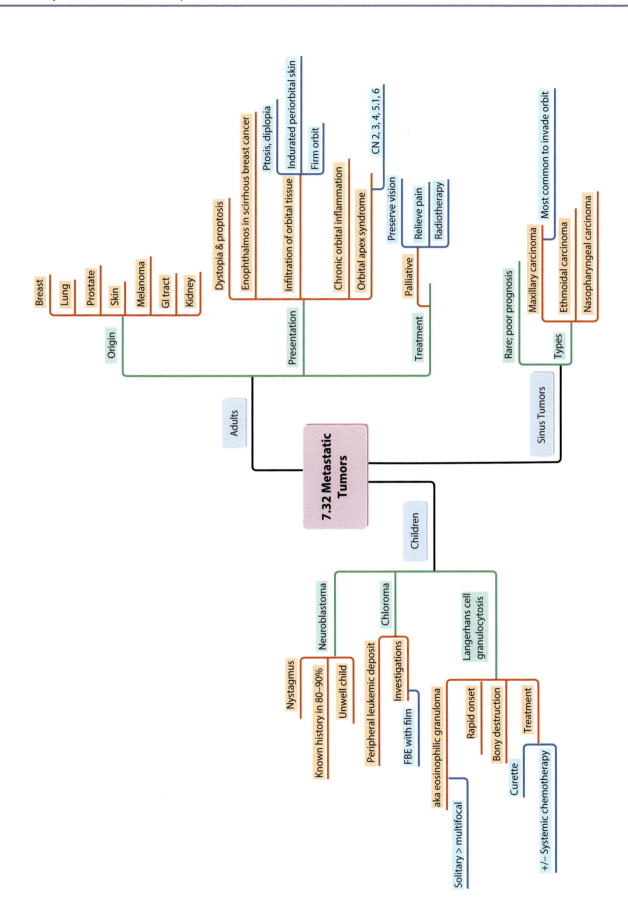

7.32 Metastatic Tumors

Adults
- Origin
  - Breast
  - Lung
  - Prostate
  - Skin
  - Melanoma
  - GI tract
  - Kidney
- Presentation
  - Dystopia & proptosis
  - Enophthalmos in scirrhous breast cancer
    - Ptosis, diplopia
    - Indurated periorbital skin
    - Firm orbit
  - Infiltration of orbital tissue
  - Chronic orbital inflammation
  - Orbital apex syndrome
    - CN 2, 3, 4, 5.1, 6
- Treatment
  - Palliative
    - Preserve vision
    - Relieve pain
    - Radiotherapy

Sinus Tumors
- Rare; poor prognosis
- Types
  - Maxillary carcinoma
    - Most common to invade orbit
  - Ethmoidal carcinoma
  - Nasopharyngeal carcinoma

Children
- Neuroblastoma
  - Nystagmus
  - Known history in 80–90%
  - Unwell child
- Chloroma
  - Peripheral leukemic deposit
  - Investigations
    - FBE with film
- Langerhans cell granulocytosis
  - aka eosinophilic granuloma
    - Solitary > multifocal
  - Rapid onset
  - Bony destruction
  - Treatment
    - Curette
    - +/– Systemic chemotherapy

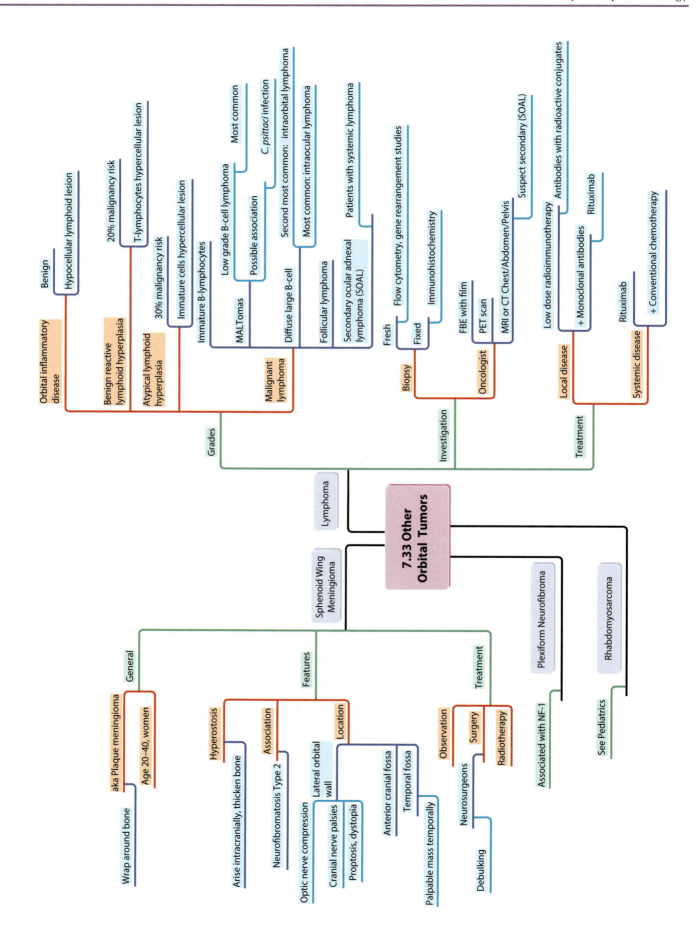

7.33 Other Orbital Tumors

Lymphoma

Grades
- Orbital inflammatory disease
  - Benign
    - Hypocellular lymphoid lesion
- Benign reactive lymphoid hyperplasia
  - 20% malignancy risk
- Atypical lymphoid hyperplasia
  - T-lymphocytes hypercellular lesion
  - 30% malignancy risk
  - Immature cells hypercellular lesion
- Malignant lymphoma
  - Immature B-lymphocytes
  - MALTomas
    - Low grade B-cell lymphoma
    - Most common
    - Possible association
      - C. psittaci infection
  - Diffuse large B-cell
    - Second most common: intraorbital lymphoma
  - Follicular lymphoma
    - Most common: intraocular lymphoma
  - Secondary ocular adnexal lymphoma (SOAL)
    - Patients with systemic lymphoma

Investigation
- Biopsy
  - Fresh
    - Flow cytometry, gene rearrangement studies
  - Fixed
    - Immunohistochemistry
- Oncologist
  - FBE with film
  - PET scan
  - MRI or CT Chest/Abdomen/Pelvis
    - Suspect secondary (SOAL)

Treatment
- Local disease
  - Low dose radioimmunotherapy
    - Antibodies with radioactive conjugates
  - + Monoclonal antibodies
    - Rituximab
- Systemic disease
  - Rituximab
  - + Conventional chemotherapy

Sphenoid Wing Meningioma

General
- aka Plaque meningioma
  - Wrap around bone
- Age 20–40, women

Features
- Hyperostosis
  - Arise intracranially, thicken bone
- Association
  - Neurofibromatosis Type 2
- Location
  - Lateral orbital wall
    - Optic nerve compression
    - Cranial nerve palsies
    - Proptosis, dystopia
  - Anterior cranial fossa
  - Temporal fossa
    - Palpable mass temporally

Treatment
- Observation
- Surgery
  - Neurosurgeons
  - Debulking
- Radiotherapy

Plexiform Neurofibroma
- Associated with NF-1

Rhabdomyosarcoma
- See Pediatrics

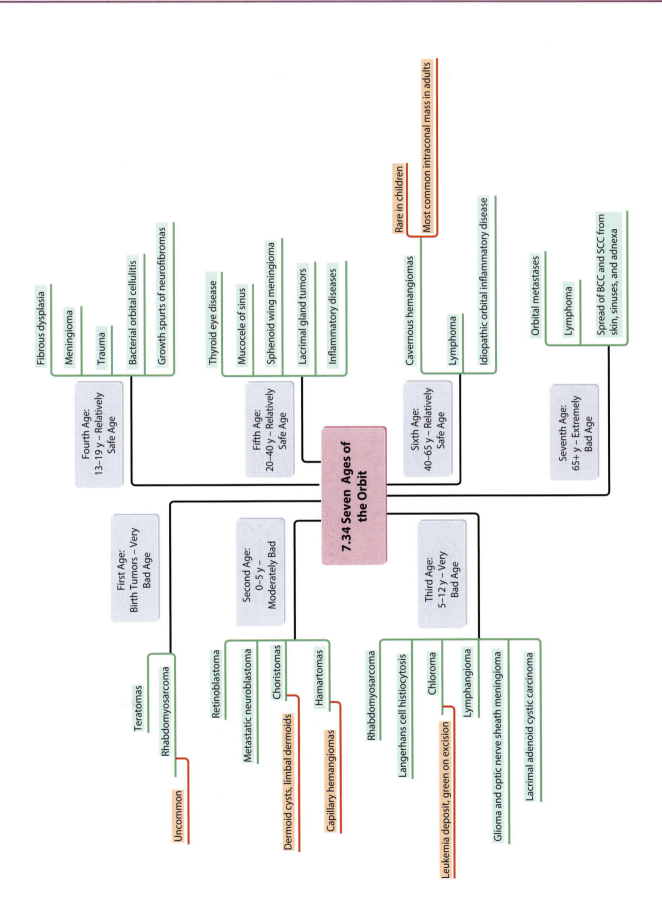

7.34 Seven Ages of the Orbit

First Age: Birth Tumors – Very Bad Age
- Teratomas
- Rhabdomyosarcoma
  - Uncommon

Second Age: 0–5 y – Moderately Bad
- Retinoblastoma
- Metastatic neuroblastoma
- Choristomas
  - Dermoid cysts, limbal dermoids
- Hamartomas
  - Capillary hemangiomas

Third Age: 5–12 y – Very Bad Age
- Rhabdomyosarcoma
- Langerhans cell histiocytosis
- Chloroma
  - Leukemia deposit, green on excision
- Lymphangioma
- Glioma and optic nerve sheath meningioma
- Lacrimal adenoid cystic carcinoma

Fourth Age: 13–19 y – Relatively Safe Age
- Fibrous dysplasia
- Meningioma
- Trauma
- Bacterial orbital cellulitis
- Growth spurts of neurofibromas

Fifth Age: 20–40 y – Relatively Safe Age
- Thyroid eye disease
- Mucocele of sinus
- Sphenoid wing meningioma
- Lacrimal gland tumors
- Inflammatory diseases

Sixth Age: 40–65 y – Relatively Safe Age
- Cavernous hemangiomas
  - Rare in children
  - Most common intraconal mass in adults
- Lymphoma
- Idiopathic orbital inflammatory disease

Seventh Age: 65+ y – Extremely Bad Age
- Orbital metastases
- Lymphoma
- Spread of BCC and SCC from skin, sinuses, and adnexa

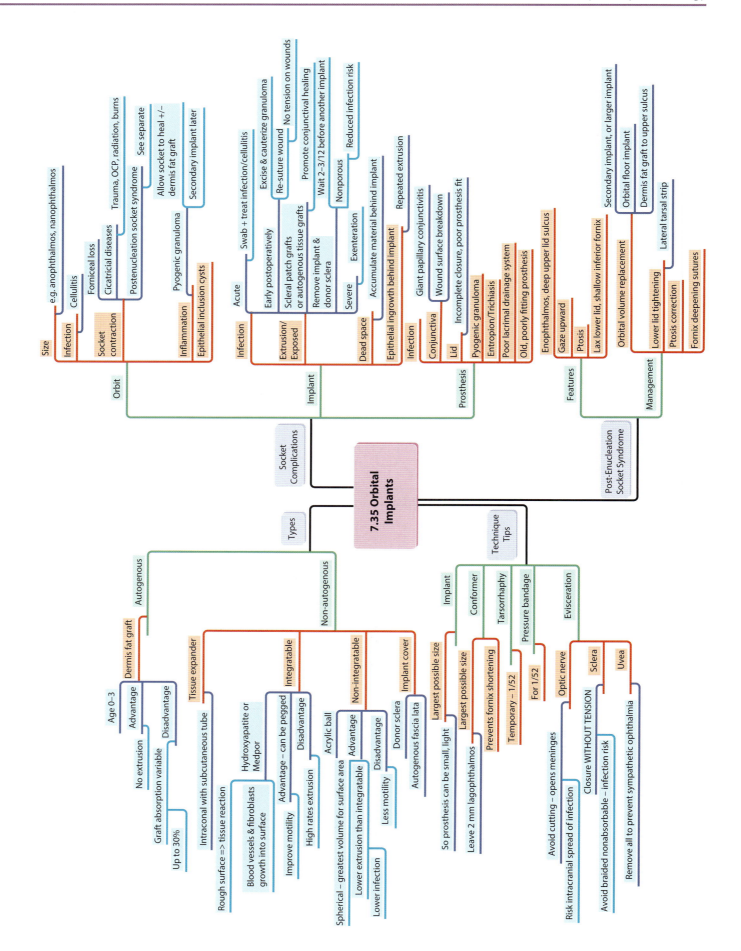

7.35 Orbital Implants

Socket Complications

Orbit

- Size
  - e.g. anophthalmos, nanophthalmos
- Infection
  - Cellulitis
- Socket contraction
  - Forniceal loss
  - Cicatricial diseases
    - Trauma, OCP, radiation, burns
  - Postenucleation socket syndrome
    - See separate
    - Allow socket to heal +/– dermis fat graft
    - Secondary implant later
- Inflammation
  - Pyogenic granuloma
- Epithelial inclusion cysts

Implant

- Infection
  - Acute
    - Swab + treat infection/cellulitis
  - Early postoperatively
    - Excise & cauterize granuloma
    - Re-suture wound
    - No tension on wounds
  - Scleral patch grafts or autogenous tissue grafts
    - Promote conjunctival healing
  - Remove implant & donor sclera
    - Wait 2–3/12 before another implant
  - Severe
    - Nonporous
      - Reduced infection risk
    - Exenteration
- Extrusion/Exposed
  - Dead space
    - Accumulate material behind implant
  - Epithelial ingrowth behind implant
    - Repeated extrusion

Prosthesis

- Infection
  - Conjunctiva
    - Giant papillary conjunctivitis
  - Lid
    - Wound surface breakdown
    - Incomplete closure, poor prosthesis fit
  - Pyogenic granuloma
  - Entropion/Trichiasis
  - Poor lacrimal drainage system
  - Old, poorly fitting prosthesis

Post-Enucleation Socket Syndrome

- Features
  - Enophthalmos, deep upper lid sulcus
  - Gaze upward
  - Ptosis
  - Lax lower lid, shallow inferior fornix
- Management
  - Orbital volume replacement
    - Secondary implant, or larger implant
    - Orbital floor implant
    - Dermis fat graft to upper sulcus
  - Lower lid tightening
    - Lateral tarsal strip
  - Ptosis correction
  - Fornix deepening sutures

Types

- Autogenous
  - Dermis fat graft
    - Age 0–3
    - Advantage
      - No extrusion
    - Disadvantage
      - Graft absorption variable
      - Up to 30%
  - Tissue expander
    - Intraconal with subcutaneous tube
- Non-autogenous
  - Integratable
    - Rough surface => tissue reaction
      - Blood vessels & fibroblasts growth into surface
    - Hydroxyapatite or Medpor
    - Improve motility
    - Advantage – can be pegged
    - Disadvantage
      - High rates extrusion
  - Non-integratable
    - Acrylic ball
    - Advantage
      - Lower extrusion than integratable
      - Lower infection
    - Disadvantage
      - Less motility
  - Implant cover
    - Donor sclera
    - Autogenous fascia lata
  - Spherical – greatest volume for surface area

Technique Tips

- Implant
  - Largest possible size
- Conformer
  - Largest possible size
    - So prosthesis can be small, light
  - Prevents fornix shortening
- Tarsorrhaphy
  - Temporary – 1/52
  - Leave 2 mm lagophthalmos
- Pressure bandage
  - For 1/52
- Evisceration
  - Optic nerve
    - Avoid cutting – opens meninges
    - Risk intracranial spread of infection
  - Sclera
    - Closure WITHOUT TENSION
    - Avoid braided nonabsorbable – infection risk
  - Uvea
    - Remove all to prevent sympathetic ophthalmia

8 Pediatric Ophthalmology

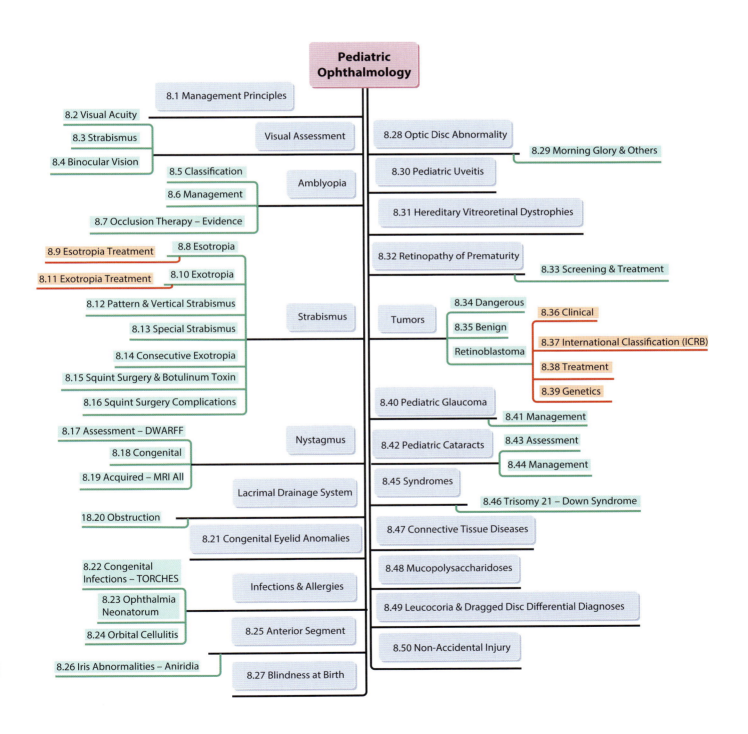

Pediatric Ophthalmology

8.1 Management Principles

8.2 Visual Acuity

8.3 Strabismus

8.4 Binocular Vision

Visual Assessment

8.5 Classification

8.6 Management

Amblyopia

8.7 Occlusion Therapy – Evidence

8.9 Esotropia Treatment

8.8 Esotropia

8.11 Exotropia Treatment

8.10 Exotropia

8.12 Pattern & Vertical Strabismus

8.13 Special Strabismus

Strabismus

8.14 Consecutive Exotropia

8.15 Squint Surgery & Botulinum Toxin

8.16 Squint Surgery Complications

8.17 Assessment – DWARFF

Nystagmus

8.18 Congenital

8.19 Acquired – MRI All

Lacrimal Drainage System

18.20 Obstruction

8.21 Congenital Eyelid Anomalies

8.22 Congenital Infections – TORCHES

Infections & Allergies

8.23 Ophthalmia Neonatorum

8.24 Orbital Cellulitis

8.25 Anterior Segment

8.26 Iris Abnormalities – Aniridia

8.27 Blindness at Birth

8.28 Optic Disc Abnormality

8.29 Morning Glory & Others

8.30 Pediatric Uveitis

8.31 Hereditary Vitreoretinal Dystrophies

8.32 Retinopathy of Prematurity

8.33 Screening & Treatment

Tumors

8.34 Dangerous

8.35 Benign

Retinoblastoma

8.36 Clinical

8.37 International Classification (ICRB)

8.38 Treatment

8.39 Genetics

8.40 Pediatric Glaucoma

8.41 Management

8.42 Pediatric Cataracts

8.43 Assessment

8.44 Management

8.45 Syndromes

8.46 Trisomy 21 – Down Syndrome

8.47 Connective Tissue Diseases

8.48 Mucopolysaccharidoses

8.49 Leucocoria & Dragged Disc Differential Diagnoses

8.50 Non-Accidental Injury

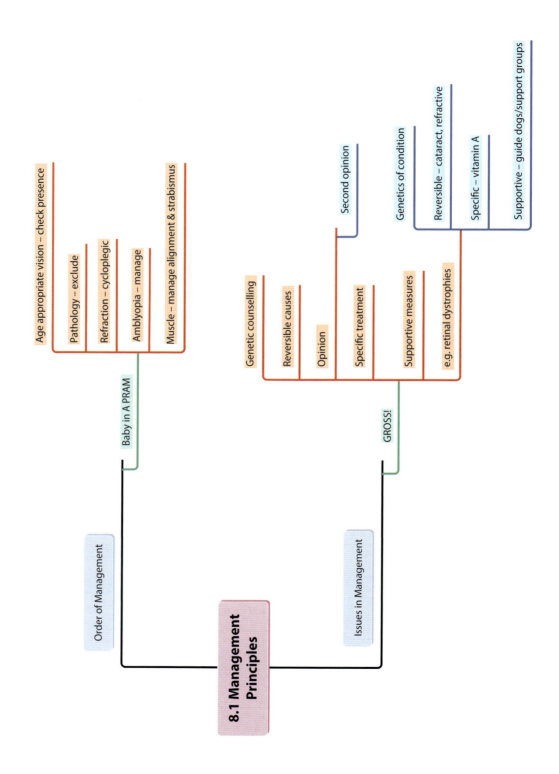

Order of Management

Baby in A PRAM

- Age appropriate vision – check presence
- Pathology – exclude
- Refraction – cycloplegic
- Amblyopia – manage
- Muscle – manage alignment & strabismus

8.1 Management Principles

Issues in Management

GROSS!

- Genetic counselling
- Reversible causes
- Opinion
  - Second opinion
- Specific treatment
- Supportive measures
- e.g. retinal dystrophies
  - Genetics of condition
  - Reversible – cataract, refractive
  - Specific – vitamin A
  - Supportive – guide dogs/support groups

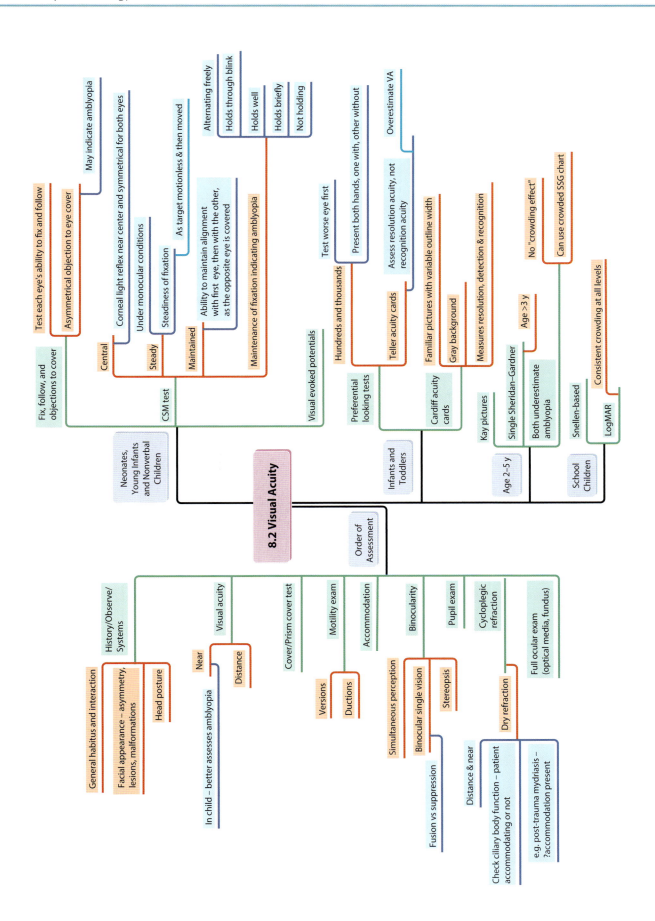

8.2 Visual Acuity

Neonates, Young Infants and Nonverbal Children

- Fix, follow, and objections to cover
  - Test each eye's ability to fix and follow
  - Asymmetrical objection to eye cover
    - May indicate amblyopia
- CSM test
  - Central
    - Corneal light reflex near center and symmetrical for both eyes
    - Under monocular conditions
  - Steady
    - Steadiness of fixation
    - As target motionless & then moved
  - Maintained
    - Ability to maintain alignment with first eye, then with the other, as the opposite eye is covered
    - Maintenance of fixation indicating amblyopia
      - Alternating freely
      - Holds through blink
      - Holds well
      - Holds briefly
      - Not holding
- Visual evoked potentials

Infants and Toddlers

- Preferential looking tests
  - Test worse eye first
  - Present both hands, one with, other without
  - Hundreds and thousands
  - Teller acuity cards
    - Assess resolution acuity, not recognition acuity
    - Overestimate VA
- Cardiff acuity cards
  - Familiar pictures with variable outline width
  - Gray background
  - Measures resolution, detection & recognition

Age 2–5 y

- Kay pictures
- Single Sheridan–Gardner
  - Age >3 y
  - No "crowding effect"
  - Can use crowded SSG chart
- Both underestimate amblyopia

School Children

- Snellen-based
- LogMAR
  - Consistent crowding at all levels

Order of Assessment

- History/Observe/Systems
  - General habitus and interaction
  - Facial appearance – asymmetry, lesions, malformations
  - Head posture
- Visual acuity
  - Near
  - Distance
  - In child – better assesses amblyopia
- Cover/Prism cover test
- Motility exam
  - Versions
  - Ductions
- Accommodation
- Binocularity
  - Simultaneous perception
  - Binocular single vision
  - Stereopsis
    - Fusion vs suppression
    - Distance & near
- Pupil exam
- Cycloplegic refraction
  - Dry refraction
    - Check ciliary body function – patient accommodating or not
    - e.g. post-trauma mydriasis – ?accommodation present
- Full ocular exam (optical media, fundus)

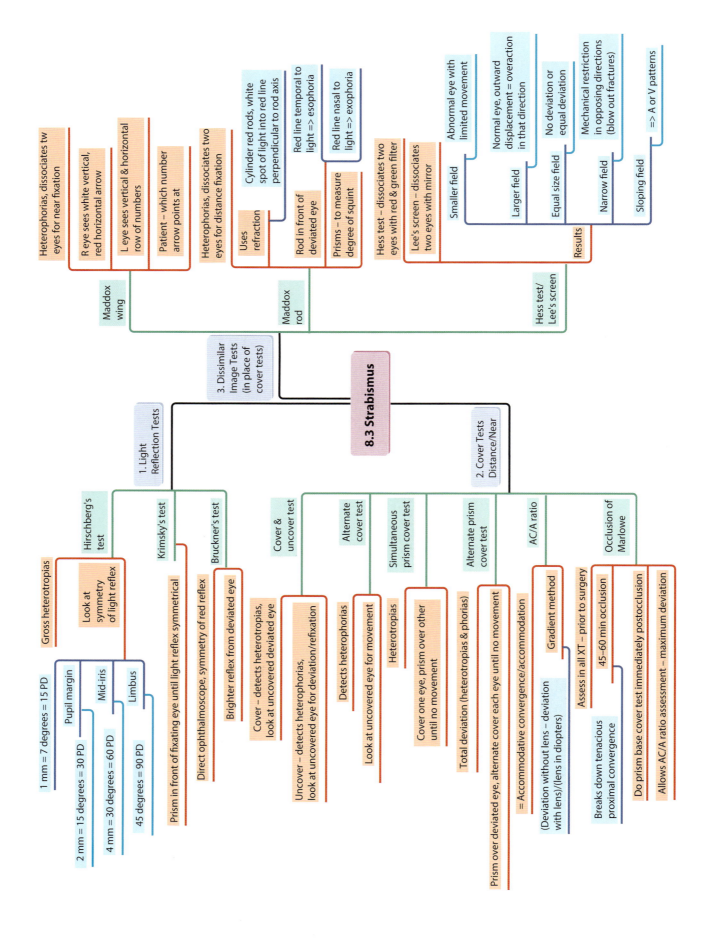

8.3 Strabismus

1. Light Reflection Tests

Hirschberg's test
- Gross heterotropias
- Look at symmetry of light reflex
  - 1 mm = 7 degrees = 15 PD
  - Pupil margin
    - 2 mm = 15 degrees = 30 PD
  - Mid-iris
    - 4 mm = 30 degrees = 60 PD
  - Limbus
    - 45 degrees = 90 PD

Krimsky's test
- Prism in front of fixating eye until light reflex symmetrical

Bruckner's test
- Direct ophthalmoscope, symmetry of red reflex
- Brighter reflex from deviated eye

2. Cover Tests Distance/Near

Cover & uncover test
- Cover – detects heterotropias; look at uncovered deviated eye
- Uncover – detects heterophorias, look at uncovered eye for deviation/refixation

Alternate cover test
- Detects heterophorias
- Look at uncovered eye for movement

Simultaneous prism cover test
- Heterotropias

Alternate prism cover test
- Cover one eye, prism over other until no movement
- Total deviation (heterotropias & phorias)
- Prism over deviated eye, alternate cover each eye until no movement

AC/A ratio
- = Accommodative convergence/accommodation
- Gradient method
  - (Deviation without lens – deviation with lens)/(lens in diopters)
  - Breaks down tenacious proximal convergence
- Assess in all XT – prior to surgery
  - 45–60 min occlusion

Occlusion of Marlowe
- Do prism base cover test immediately postocclusion
- Allows AC/A ratio assessment – maximum deviation

3. Dissimilar Image Tests (in place of cover tests)

Maddox wing
- Heterophorias, dissociates tw eyes for near fixation
- R eye sees white vertical, red horizontal arrow
- L eye sees vertical & horizontal row of numbers
- Patient – which number arrow points at

Maddox rod
- Heterophorias, dissociates two eyes for distance fixation
- Uses refraction
  - Cylinder red rods, white spot of light into red line perpendicular to rod axis
  - Red line temporal to light => esophoria
  - Red line nasal to light => exophoria
- Rod in front of deviated eye
- Prisms – to measure degree of squint

Hess test/Lee's screen
- Hess test – dissociates two eyes with red & green filter
- Lee's screen – dissociates two eyes with mirror
- Results
  - Smaller field
    - Abnormal eye with limited movement
  - Larger field
    - Normal eye, outward displacement = overaction in that direction
  - Equal size field
    - No deviation or equal deviation
  - Narrow field
    - Mechanical restriction in opposing directions (blow out fractures)
  - Sloping field
    - => A or V patterns

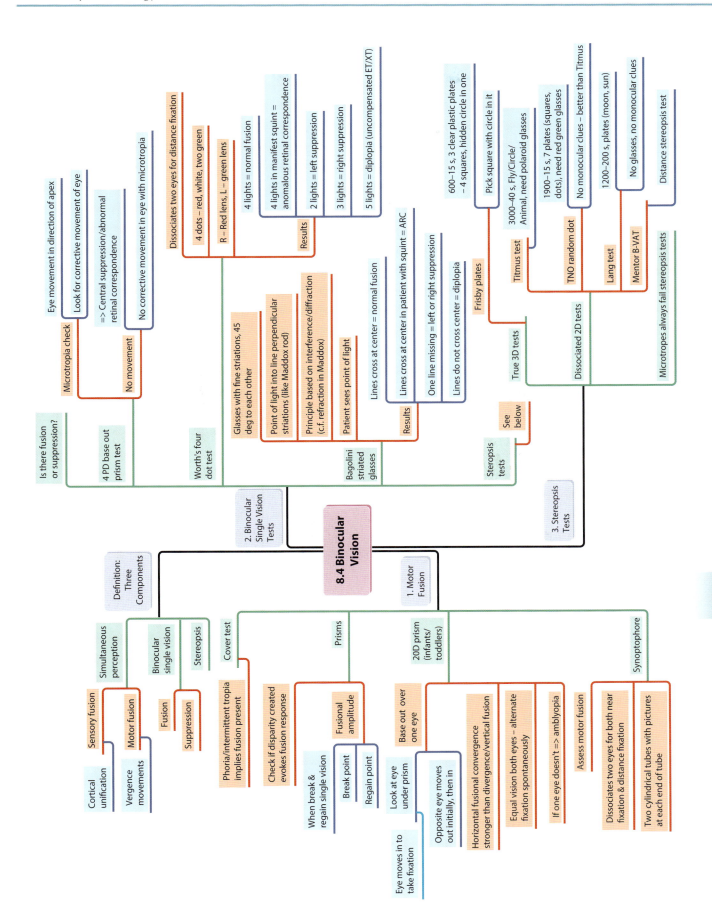

8.4 Binocular Vision

Definition: Three Components

- Simultaneous perception
  - Sensory fusion
    - Cortical unification
  - Motor fusion
    - Vergence movements
- Binocular single vision
  - Fusion
  - Suppression
- Stereopsis

1. Motor Fusion

- Cover test
  - Phoria/intermittent tropia implies fusion present
  - Check if disparity created evokes fusion response
- Prisms
  - Fusional amplitude
    - When break & regain single vision
      - Break point
      - Regain point
  - Base out over one eye
    - Look at eye under prism
      - Eye moves in to take fixation
    - Opposite eye moves out initially, then in
  - Horizontal fusional convergence stronger than divergence/vertical fusion
- 20D prism (infants/toddlers)
  - Equal vision both eyes – alternate fixation spontaneously
  - If one eye doesn't => amplyopia
  - Assess motor fusion
- Synoptophore
  - Dissociates two eyes for both near fixation & distance fixation
  - Two cylindrical tubes with pictures at each end of tube

2. Binocular Single Vision Tests

- Is there fusion or suppression?
  - Microtropia check
    - Eye movement in direction of apex
    - Look for corrective movement of eye
    - => Central suppression/abnormal retinal correspondence
    - No corrective movement in eye with microtropia
  - No movement
- 4 PD base out prism test
- Worth's four dot test
  - Dissociates two eyes for distance fixation
  - 4 dots – red, white, two green
  - R – Red lens, L – green lens
  - Results
    - 4 lights = normal fusion
    - 4 lights in manifest squint = anomalous retinal correspondence
    - 2 lights = left suppression
    - 3 lights = right suppression
    - 5 lights = diplopia (uncompensated ET/XT)
- Bagolini striated glasses
  - Glasses with fine striations, 45 deg to each other
  - Point of light into line perpendicular striations (like Maddox rod)
  - Principle based on interference/diffraction (c.f. refraction in Maddox)
  - Patient sees point of light
  - Results
    - Lines cross at center = normal fusion
    - Lines cross at center in patient with squint = ARC
    - One line missing = left or right suppression
    - Lines do not cross center = diplopia
- Stereopsis tests
  - See below

3. Stereopsis Tests

- True 3D tests
  - Frisby plates
    - 600–15 s, 3 clear plastic plates – 4 squares, hidden circle in one
    - Pick square with circle in it
- Dissociated 2D tests
  - Titmus test
    - 3000–40 s, Fly/Circle/Animal, need polaroid glasses
    - 1900–15 s, 7 plates (squares, dots), need red green glasses
  - TNO random dot
    - No monocular clues – better than Titmus
  - Lang test
    - 1200–200 s, plates (moon, sun)
    - No glasses, no monocular clues
  - Mentor B-VAT
    - Distance stereopsis test
  - Microtropes always fail stereopsis tests

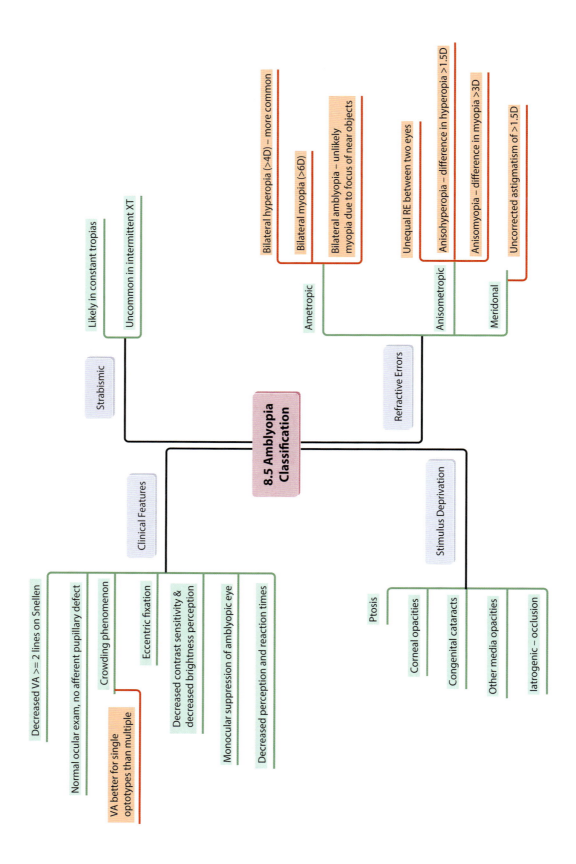

8.5 Amblyopia Classification

Strabismic
- Likely in constant tropias
- Uncommon in intermittent XT

Refractive Errors
- Ametropic
  - Bilateral hyperopia (>4D) – more common
  - Bilateral myopia (>6D)
  - Bilateral amblyopia – unlikely myopia due to focus of near objects
- Anisometropic
  - Unequal RE between two eyes
  - Anisohyperopia – difference in hyperopia >1.5D
  - Anisomyopia – difference in myopia >3D
- Meridonal
  - Uncorrected astigmatism of >1.5D

Clinical Features
- Decreased VA >= 2 lines on Snellen
- Normal ocular exam, no afferent pupillary defect
- Crowding phenomenon
  - VA better for single optotypes than multiple
- Eccentric fixation
- Decreased contrast sensitivity & decreased brightness perception
- Monocular suppression of amblyopic eye
- Decreased perception and reaction times

Stimulus Deprivation
- Ptosis
- Corneal opacities
- Congenital cataracts
- Other media opacities
- Iatrogenic – occlusion

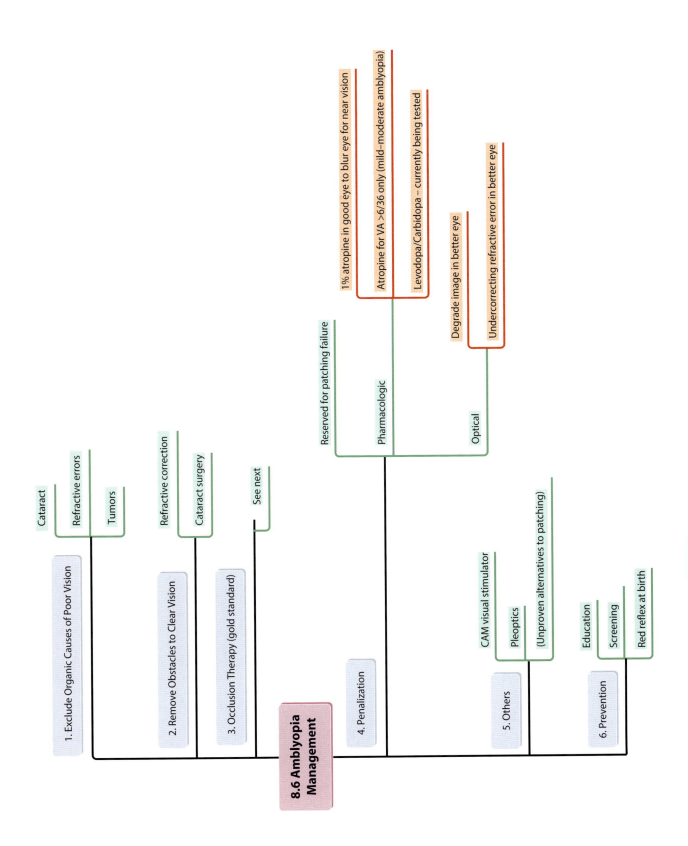

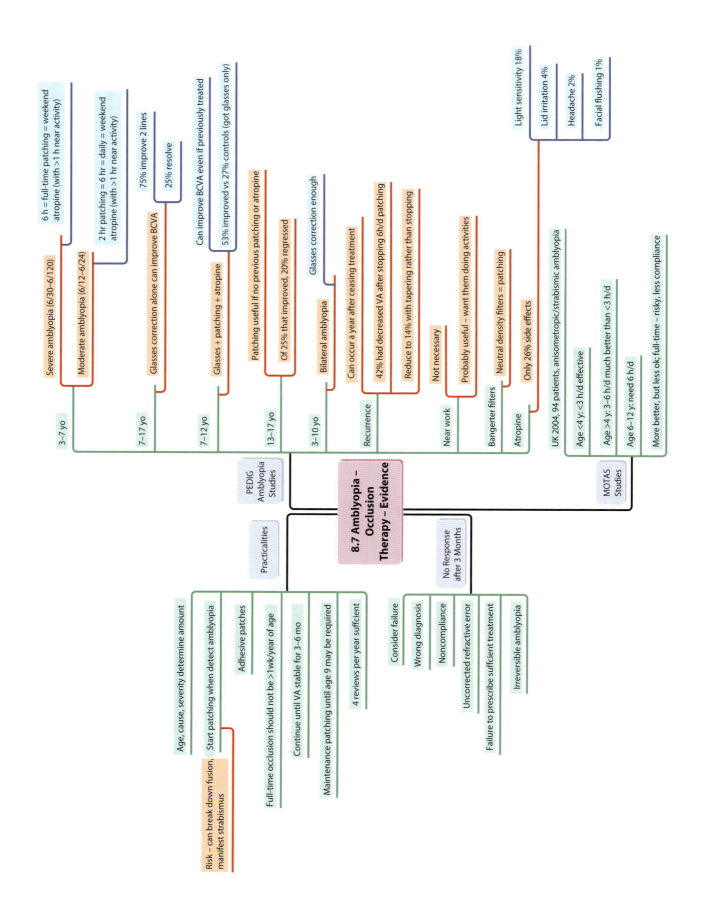

8.7 Amblyopia – Occlusion Therapy – Evidence

PEDIG Amblyopia Studies

- 3–7 yo
  - Severe amblyopia (6/30–6/120)
  - Moderate amblyopia (6/12–6/24)
    - 6 h = full-time patching = weekend atropine (with >1 h near activity)
    - 2 hr patching = 6 hr = daily = weekend atropine (with >1 hr near activity)
- 7–17 yo
  - Glasses correction alone can improve BCVA
    - 75% improve 2 lines
    - 25% resolve
- 7–12 yo
  - Glasses + patching + atropine
    - Can improve BCVA even if previously treated
    - 53% improved vs 27% controls (got glasses only)
- 13–17 yo
  - Patching useful if no previous patching or atropine
    - Of 25% that improved, 20% regressed
- 3–10 yo
  - Bilateral amblyopia
    - Glasses correction enough
- Recurrence
  - Can occur a year after ceasing treatment
  - 42% had decreased VA after stopping 6h/d patching
  - Reduce to 14% with tapering rather than stopping
- Near work
  - Not necessary
  - Probably useful – want them doing activities
- Bangerter filters
  - Neutral density filters = patching
- Atropine
  - Only 26% side effects
    - Light sensitivity 18%
    - Lid irritation 4%
    - Headache 2%
    - Facial flushing 1%

MOTAS Studies

- UK 2004, 94 patients, anisometropic/strabismic amblyopia
- Age <4 y: <3 h/d effective
- Age >4 y: 3–6 h/d much better than <3 h/d
- Age 6–12 y: need 6 h/d
- More better, but less ok; full-time – risky, less compliance

Practicalities

- Age, cause, severity determine amount
- Start patching when detect amblyopia
  - Risk – can break down fusion, manifest strabismus
- Adhesive patches
- Full-time occlusion should not be >1wk/year of age
- Continue until VA stable for 3–6 mo
- Maintenance patching until age 9 may be required
- 4 reviews per year sufficient

No Response after 3 Months

- Consider failure
- Wrong diagnosis
- Noncompliance
- Uncorrected refractive error
- Failure to prescribe sufficient treatment
- Irreversible amblyopia

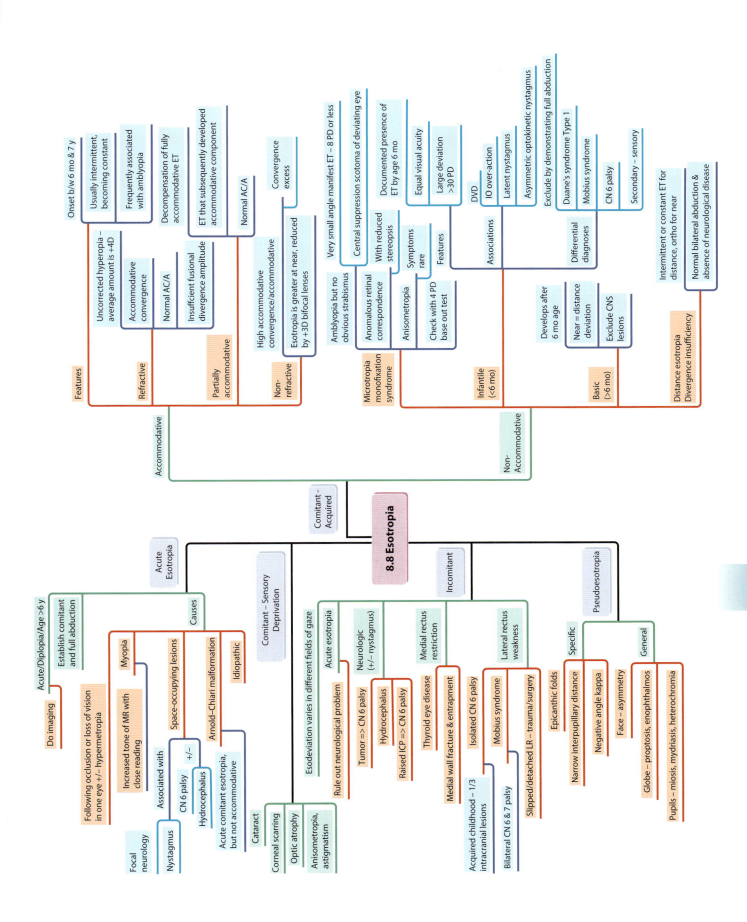

8.8 Esotropia

Comitant - Acquired

Accommodative

Refractive
- Features
  - Onset b/w 6 mo & 7 y
  - Usually intermittent, becoming constant
  - Frequently associated with amblyopia
- Uncorrected hyperopia – average amount is +4D
  - Accommodative convergence
  - Normal AC/A
  - Insufficient fusional divergence amplitude

Partially accommodative
- Decompensation of fully accommodative ET
- ET that subsequently developed accommodative component

Non-refractive
- Normal AC/A
  - Convergence excess
  - High accommodative convergence/accommodative
  - Esotropia is greater at near, reduced by +3D bifocal lenses

Non-Accommodative

Microtropia monofixation syndrome
- Very small angle manifest ET – 8 PD or less
- Central suppression scotoma of deviating eye
- With reduced stereopsis
- Symptoms rare
- Amblyopia but no obvious strabismus
- Anomalous retinal correspondence
- Anisometropia
- Check with 4 PD base out test

Infantile (<6 mo)
- Features
  - Documented presence of ET by age 6 mo
  - Equal visual acuity
  - Large deviation >30 PD
- Associations
  - DVD
  - IO over-action
  - Latent nystagmus
  - Asymmetric optokinetic nystagmus
  - Exclude by demonstrating full abduction
- Differential diagnoses
  - Duane's syndrome Type 1
  - Mobius syndrome
  - CN 6 palsy
  - Secondary – sensory

Basic (>6 mo)
- Develops after 6 mo age
- Near = distance deviation
- Exclude CNS lesions

Distance esotropia Divergence insufficiency
- Intermittent or constant ET for distance, ortho for near
- Normal bilateral abduction & absence of neurological disease

Acute Esotropia
- Acute/Diplopia/Age >6 y
  - Establish comitant and full abduction
  - Do imaging
- Causes
  - Myopia
    - Following occlusion or loss of vision in one eye +/- hypermetropia
    - Increased tone of MR with close reading
  - Space-occupying lesions
    - Associated with
      - Focal neurology
      - Nystagmus
      - CN 6 palsy
      - Hydrocephalus
      +/-
  - Arnold–Chiari malformation
  - Idiopathic
    - Acute comitant esotropia, but not accommodative

Comitant – Sensory Deprivation
- Cataract
- Corneal scarring
- Optic atrophy
- Anisometropia, astigmatism

Incomitant
- Esodeviation varies in different fields of gaze
- Acute esotropia
  - Rule out neurological problem
- Neurologic (+/- nystagmus)
  - Tumor => CN 6 palsy
  - Hydrocephalus
  - Raised ICP => CN 6 palsy
- Medial rectus restriction
  - Thyroid eye disease
  - Medial wall fracture & entrapment
- Lateral rectus weakness
  - Isolated CN 6 palsy
  - Mobius syndrome
    - Acquired childhood – 1/3 intracranial lesions
    - Bilateral CN 6 & 7 palsy
  - Slipped/detached LR – trauma/surgery

Pseudoesotropia
- Specific
  - Epicanthic folds
  - Narrow interpupillary distance
  - Negative angle kappa
- General
  - Face – asymmetry
  - Globe – proptosis, enophthalmos
  - Pupils – miosis, mydriasis, heterochromia

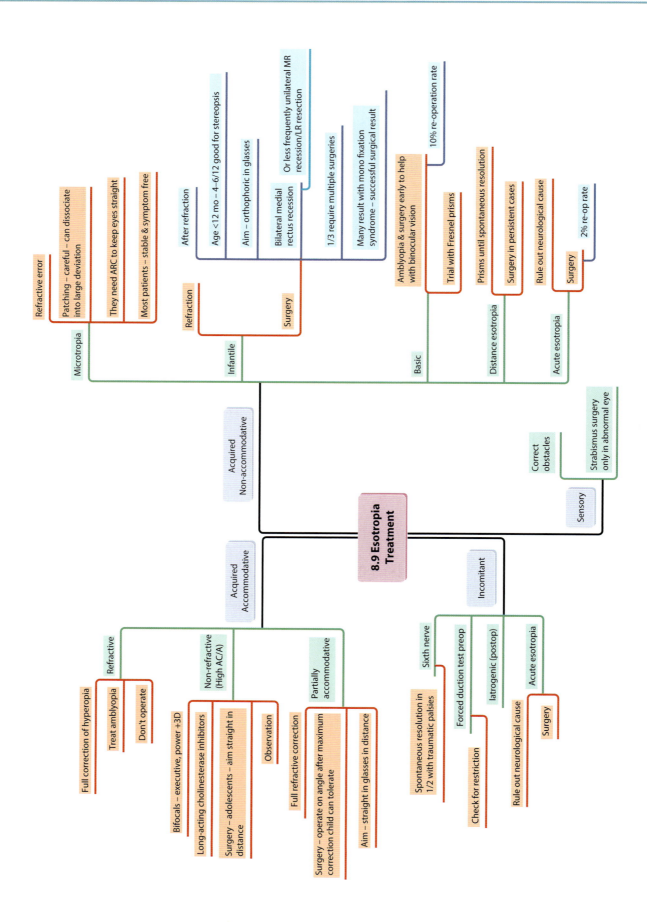

8.9 Esotropia Treatment

Acquired Non-accommodative

- **Microtropia**
  - Refractive error
  - Patching – careful – can dissociate into large deviation
  - They need ARC to keep eyes straight
  - Most patients – stable & symptom free

- **Infantile**
  - Refraction
    - After refraction
  - Surgery
    - Age <12 mo – 4–6/12 good for stereopsis
    - Aim – orthophoric in glasses
    - Bilateral medial rectus recession
    - Or less frequently unilateral MR recession/LR resection
    - 1/3 require multiple surgeries
    - Many result with mono fixation syndrome – successful surgical result

- **Basic**
  - Amblyopia & surgery early to help with binocular vision
    - 10% re-operation rate

- **Distance esotropia**
  - Trial with Fresnel prisms
  - Prisms until spontaneous resolution
  - Surgery in persistent cases

- **Acute esotropia**
  - Rule out neurological cause
  - Surgery
    - 2% re-op rate

Sensory
- Correct obstacles
- Strabismus surgery only in abnormal eye

Acquired Accommodative

- **Refractive**
  - Full correction of hyperopia
  - Treat amblyopia
  - Don't operate

- **Non-refractive (High AC/A)**
  - Bifocals – executive, power +3D
  - Long-acting cholinesterase inhibitors
  - Surgery – adolescents – aim straight in distance
  - Observation

- **Partially accommodative**
  - Full refractive correction
  - Surgery – operate on angle after maximum correction child can tolerate
  - Aim – straight in glasses in distance

Incomitant

- **Sixth nerve**
  - Spontaneous resolution in 1/2 with traumatic palsies
  - Forced duction test preop
  - Check for restriction
  - Iatrogenic (postop)

- **Acute esotropia**
  - Rule out neurological cause
  - Surgery

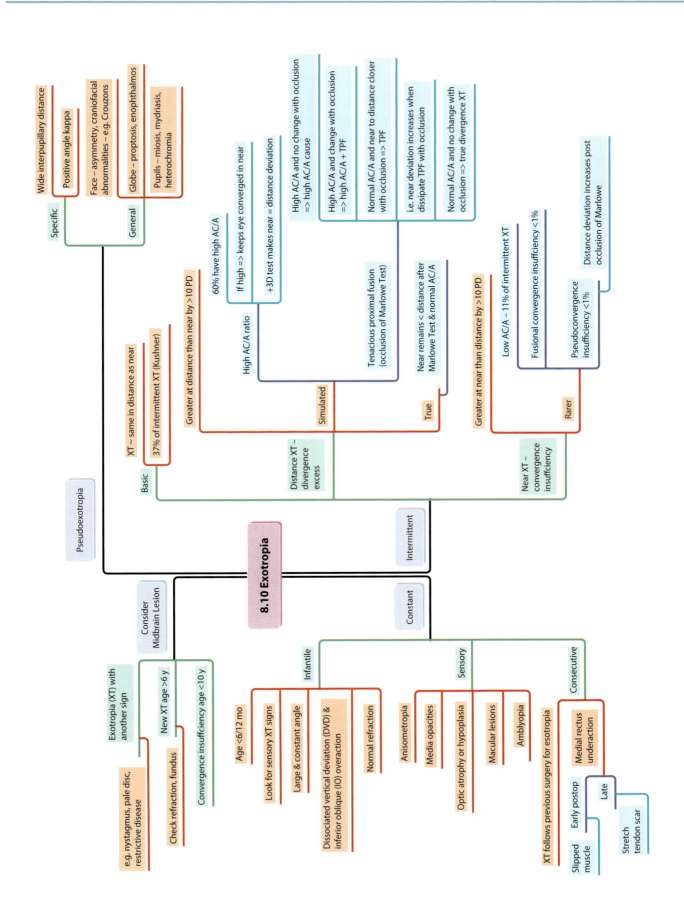

8.10 Exotropia

Pseudoexotropia

Specific
- Wide interpupillary distance
- Positive angle kappa

General
- Face – asymmetry, craniofacial abnormalities – e.g. Crouzons
- Globe – proptosis, enophthalmos
- Pupils – miosis, mydriasis, heterochromia

Consider Midbrain Lesion
- Exotropia (XT) with another sign
  - e.g. nystagmus, pale disc, restrictive disease
- New XT age >6 y
  - Check refraction, fundus
- Convergence insuffciency age <10 y

Intermittent

Basic
- XT ~ same in distance as near
- 37% of intermittent XT (Kushner)

Distance XT – divergence excess
- Greater at distance than near by >10 PD
  - Simulated
    - High AC/A ratio
      - 60% have high high AC/A
      - If high => keeps eye converged in near
      - +3D test makes near = distance deviation
        - High AC/A and no change with occlusion => high AC/A cause
        - High AC/A and change with occlusion => high AC/A + TPF
        - Normal AC/A and near to distance closer with occlusion => TPF
    - Tenacious proximal fusion (occlusion of Marlowe Test)
      - i.e. near deviation increases when dissipate TPF with occlusion
  - True
    - Near remains < distance after Marlowe Test & normal AC/A
      - Normal AC/A and no change with occlusion => true divergence XT

Near XT – convergence insuffciency
- Greater at near than distance by >10 PD
  - Rarer
    - Low AC/A – 11% of intermittent XT
    - Fusional convergence insuffciency <1%
    - Pseudoconvergence insufficiency <1%
      - Distance deviation increases post occlusion of Marlowe

Constant

Infantile
- Age <6/12 mo
- Look for sensory XT signs
- Large & constant angle
- Dissociated vertical deviation (DVD) & inferior oblique (IO) overaction
- Normal refraction

Sensory
- Anisometropia
- Media opacities
- Optic atrophy or hypoplasia
- Macular lesions
- Amblyopia

Consecutive
- XT follows previous surgery for esotropia
- Medial rectus underaction
  - Early postop
    - Slipped muscle
  - Late
    - Stretch tendon scar

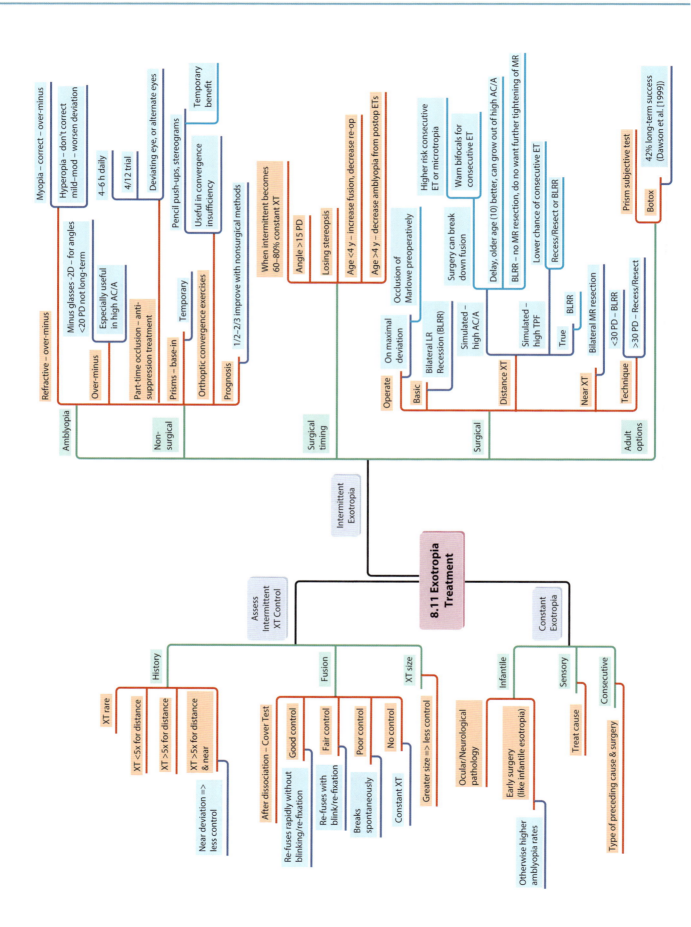

8.11 Exotropia Treatment

Intermittent Exotropia

Amblyopia
- Refractive – over-minus
  - Myopia – correct – over-minus
  - Hyperopia – don't correct mild–mod – worsen deviation
- Over-minus
  - Minus glasses -2D – for angles <20 PD not long-term
  - Especially useful in high AC/A
- Part-time occlusion – anti-suppression treatment
  - 4–6 h daily
  - 4/12 trial
  - Deviating eye, or alternate eyes
- Prisms – base-in
  - Temporary
  - Pencil push-ups, stereograms
  - Useful in convergence insufficiency
  - Temporary benefit

Non-surgical
- Orthoptic convergence exercises
- Prognosis
  - 1/2–2/3 improve with nonsurgical methods

Surgical timing
- When intermittent becomes 60–80% constant XT
- Angle >15 PD
- Losing stereopsis
- Age <4 y – increase fusion, decrease re-op
- Age >4 y – decrease amblyopia from postop ETs

Surgical
- Operate
  - On maximal deviation
  - Occlusion of Marlowe preoperatively
- Basic
  - Bilateral LR Recession (BLRR)
  - Simulated – high AC/A
- Distance XT
  - Simulated – high TPF
  - True
    - BLRR
  - Surgery can break down fusion
  - Delay, older age (10) better, can grow out of high AC/A
  - BLRR – no MR resection, do no want further tightening of MR
  - Higher risk consecutive ET or microtropia
  - Warn bifocals for consecutive ET
  - Lower chance of consecutive ET
  - Recess/Resect or BLRR
- Near XT
  - Bilateral MR resection
- Technique
  - <30 PD – BLRR
  - >30 PD – Recess/Resect

Adult options
- Prism subjective test
- Botox
  - 42% long-term success (Dawson et al. [1999])

Assess Intermittent XT Control
- History
  - XT rare
  - XT <5x for distance
  - XT >5x for distance
  - XT >5x for distance & near
    - Near deviation => less control
- Fusion
  - After dissociation – Cover Test
  - Good control
    - Re-fuses rapidly without blinking/re-fixation
  - Fair control
    - Re-fuses with blink/re-fixation
  - Poor control
    - Breaks spontaneously
  - No control
    - Constant XT
- XT size
  - Greater size => less control

Constant Exotropia
- Infantile
  - Ocular/Neurological pathology
  - Early surgery (like infantile esotropia)
    - Otherwise higher amblyopia rates
- Sensory
  - Treat cause
- Consecutive
  - Type of preceding cause & surgery

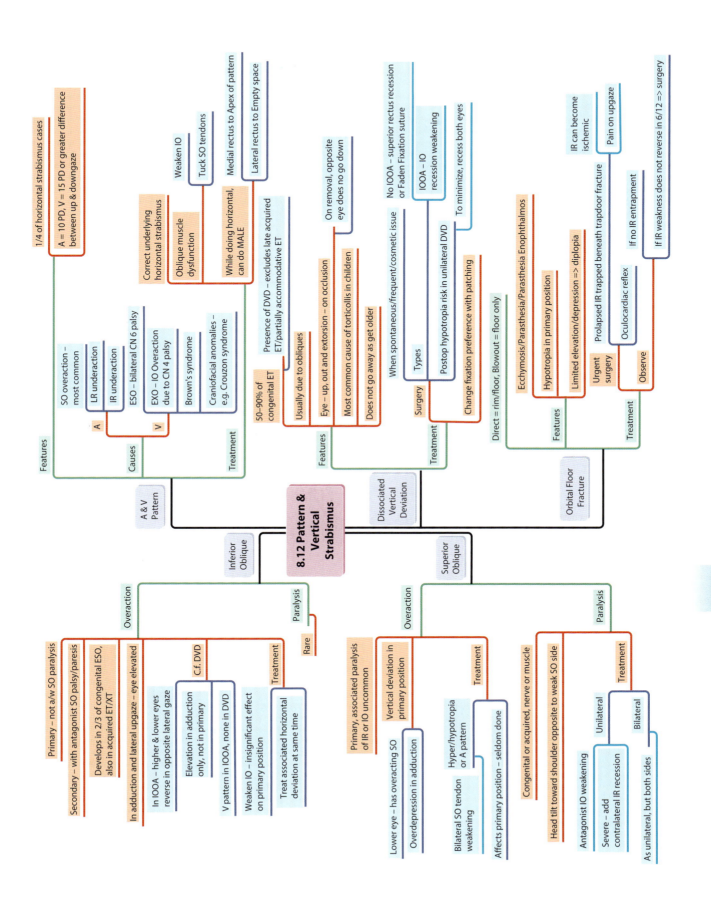

8.12 Pattern & Vertical Strabismus

A & V Pattern

Features
- 1/4 of horizontal strabismus cases
- A = 10 PD, V = 15 PD or greater difference between up & downgaze

Causes
- A
  - SO overaction – most common
  - LR underaction
  - IR underaction
  - ESO – bilateral CN 6 palsy
- V
  - EXO – IO Overaction due to CN 4 palsy
  - Brown's syndrome
  - Craniofacial anomalies – e.g. Crouzon syndrome

Treatment
- Correct underlying horizontal strabismus
- Oblique muscle dysfunction
  - Weaken IO
  - Tuck SO tendons
- While doing horizontal, can do MALE
  - Medial rectus to Apex of pattern
  - Lateral rectus to Empty space

Dissociated Vertical Deviation

Features
- Presence of DVD – excludes late acquired ET/partially accommodative ET
- 50–90% of congenital ET
- Usually due to obliques
- On removal, opposite eye does no go down
- Eye – up, out and extorsion – on occlusion
- Most common cause of torticollis in children
- Does not go away as get older
- When spontaneous/frequent/cosmetic issue
- Types
- Postop hypotropia risk in unilateral DVD

Surgery
- No IOOA – superior rectus recession or Faden Fixation suture
- IOOA – IO recession weakening
- To minimize, recess both eyes

Treatment
- Change fixation preference with patching

Orbital Floor Fracture

- Direct = rim/floor, Blowout = floor only

Features
- Ecchymosis/Parasthesia/Parasthesia Enophthalmos
- Hypotropia in primary position
- Limited elevation/depression => diplopia
- Prolapsed IR trapped beneath trapdoor fracture
- Oculocardiac reflex
  - IR can become ischemic
  - Pain on upgaze

Urgent surgery
- If no IR entrapment

Treatment
- Observe
  - If IR weakness does not reverse in 6/12 => surgery

Inferior Oblique

Overaction
- Primary – not a/w SO paralysis
- Secondary – with antagonist SO palsy/paresis
- Develops in 2/3 of congenital ESO, also in acquired ET/XT
- In adduction and lateral upgaze – eye elevated
- In IOOA – higher & lower eyes reverse in opposite lateral gaze
- Elevation in adduction only, not in primary
  - C.f. DVD
  - V pattern in IOOA, none in DVD

Treatment
- Weaken IO – insignificant effect on primary position
- Treat associated horizontal deviation at same time

Paralysis
- Rare

Superior Oblique

Overaction
- Primary, associated paralysis of IR or IO uncommon
- Vertical deviation in primary position
- Lower eye – has overacting SO
- Overdepression in adduction

Treatment
- Bilateral SO tendon weakening
- Hyper/hypotropia or A pattern
- Affects primary position – seldom done

Paralysis
- Congenital or acquired, nerve or muscle
- Head tilt toward shoulder opposite to weak SO side

Treatment
- Unilateral
  - Antagonist IO weakening
  - Severe – add contralateral IR recession
- Bilateral
  - As unilateral, but both sides

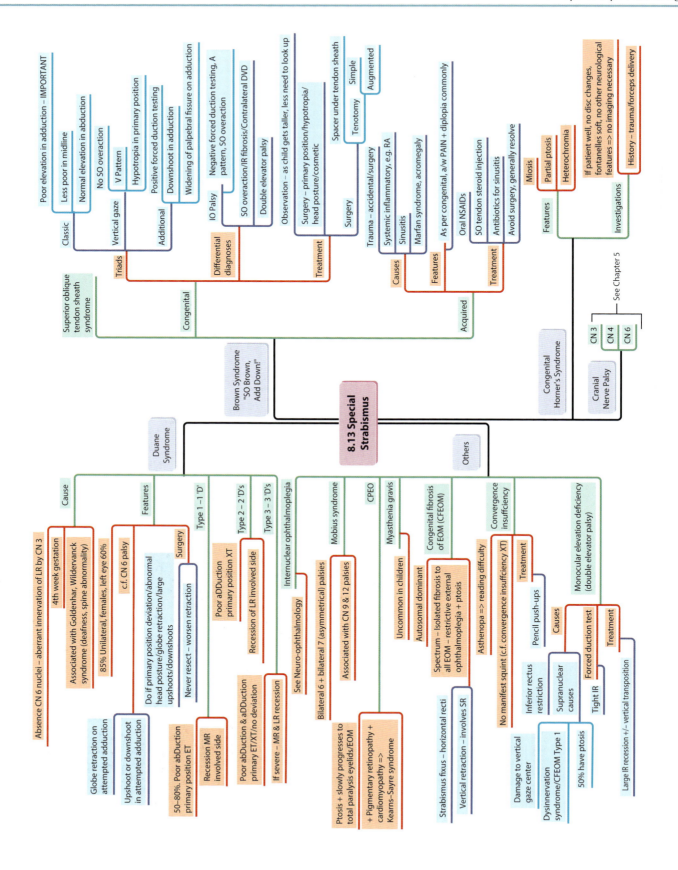

8.13 Special Strabismus

Brown Syndrome "SO Brown, Add Down!!"

Congenital

Triads
- Classic
  - Poor elevation in adduction – IMPORTANT
  - Less poor in midline
  - Normal elevation in abduction
- Vertical gaze
  - No SO overaction
  - V Pattern
- Additional
  - Hypotropia in primary position
  - Positive forced duction testing
  - Downshoot in adduction
  - Widening of palpebral fissure on adduction

Differential diagnoses
- IO Palsy
  - Negative forced duction testing, A pattern, SO overaction
- SO overaction/IR fibrosis/Contralateral DVD
- Double elevator palsy

Treatment
- Observation – as child gets taller, less need to look up
- Surgery – primary position/hypotropia/head posture/cosmetic
- Spacer under tendon sheath
- Surgery
  - Tenotomy
    - Simple
    - Augmented

Acquired

Causes
- Trauma – accidental/surgery
- Systemic inflammatory, e.g. RA
- Sinusitis
- Marfan syndrome, acromegaly

Features
- As per congenital, a/w PAIN + diplopia commonly

Treatment
- Oral NSAIDs
- SO tendon steroid injection
- Antibiotics for sinusitis
- Avoid surgery, generally resolve

Congenital Horner's Syndrome

Features
- Miosis
- Partial ptosis
- Heterochromia

Investigations
- If patient well, no disc changes, fontanelles soft, no other neurological features => no imaging necessary
- History – trauma/forceps delivery

Cranial Nerve Palsy
- CN 3
- CN 4
- CN 6

See Chapter 5

Duane Syndrome

Cause
- Absence CN 6 nuclei – aberrant innervation of LR by CN 3
- 4th week gestation
- Associated with Goldenhar, Wildervanck syndrome (deafness, spine abnormality)
- 85% Unilateral, females, left eye 60%
- c.f. CN 6 palsy

Features
- Globe retraction on attempted adduction
- Upshoot or downshoot in attempted adduction
- Type 1 – 1 'D'
  - 50–80%, Poor abDuction primary position ET
- Type 2 – 2 'D's
  - Poor abDuction primary position XT
- Type 3 – 3 'D's
  - Poor abDuction & aDDuction primary ET/XT/no deviation

Surgery
- Do if primary position deviation/abnormal head posture/globe retraction/large upshoots/downshoots
- Never resect – worsen retraction
- Recession MR involved side
- Recession of LR involved side
- If severe – MR & LR recession

Others

- Internuclear ophthalmoplegia
  - See Neuro-ophthalmology
- Mobius syndrome
  - Bilateral 6 + bilateral 7 (asymmetrical) palsies
  - Associated with CN 9 & 12 palsies
- CPEO
  - Ptosis + slowly progresses to total paralysis eyelids/EOM
  - + Pigmentary retinopathy + cardiomyopathy => Kearns–Sayre syndrome
- Myasthenia gravis
  - Uncommon in children
- Congenital fibrosis of EOM (CFEOM)
  - Autosomal dominant
  - Spectrum – Isolated fibrosis to all EOM – restrictive external ophthalmoplegia + ptosis
  - Strabismus fixus – horizontal recti
  - Vertical retraction – involves SR
- Convergence insufficiency
  - Asthenopa => reading difficulty
  - No manifest squint (c.f. convergence insufficiency XT)
  - **Treatment**
    - Pencil push-ups
- Monocular elevation deficiency (double elevator palsy)
  - **Causes**
    - Inferior rectus restriction
    - Supranuclear causes
      - Damage to vertical gaze center
      - Dysinnervation syndrome/CFEOM Type 1
      - 50% have ptosis
  - **Forced duction test**
    - Tight IR
  - **Treatment**
    - Large IR recession +/– vertical transposition

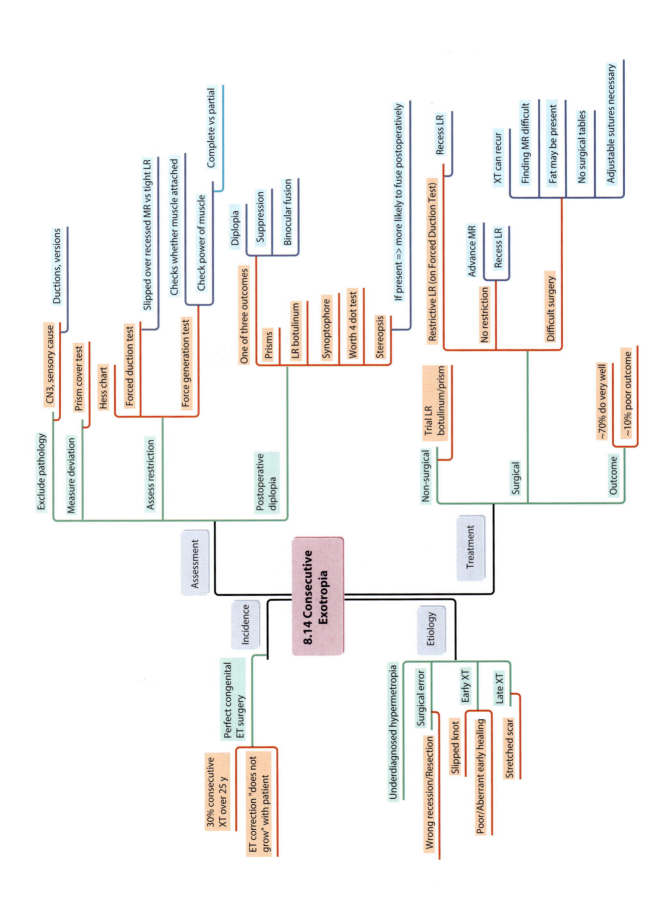

8.14 Consecutive Exotropia

Assessment
- Exclude pathology
  - CN3, sensory cause
    - Ductions, versions
- Measure deviation
  - Prism cover test
- Assess restriction
  - Hess chart
  - Forced duction test
    - Slipped over recessed MR vs tight LR
    - Checks whether muscle attached
  - Force generation test
    - Check power of muscle
      - Complete vs partial
- Postoperative diplopia
  - One of three outcomes
    - Diplopia
    - Suppression
    - Binocular fusion
  - Prisms
  - LR botulinum
  - Synoptophore
  - Worth 4 dot test
  - Stereopsis
    - If present => more likely to fuse postoperatively

Incidence
- Perfect congenital ET surgery
  - 30% consecutive XT over 25 y
  - ET correction "does not grow" with patient

Etiology
- Underdiagnosed hypermetropia
- Surgical error
  - Wrong recession/Resection
  - Slipped knot
  - Poor/Aberrant early healing
- Early XT
- Late XT
  - Stretched scar

Treatment
- Non-surgical
  - Trial LR botulinum/prism
- Surgical
  - Restrictive LR (on Forced Duction Test)
    - Recess LR
  - No restriction
    - Advance MR
    - Recess LR
  - Difficult surgery
    - XT can recur
    - Finding MR difficult
    - Fat may be present
    - No surgical tables
    - Adjustable sutures necessary
- Outcome
  - ~70% do very well
  - ~10% poor outcome

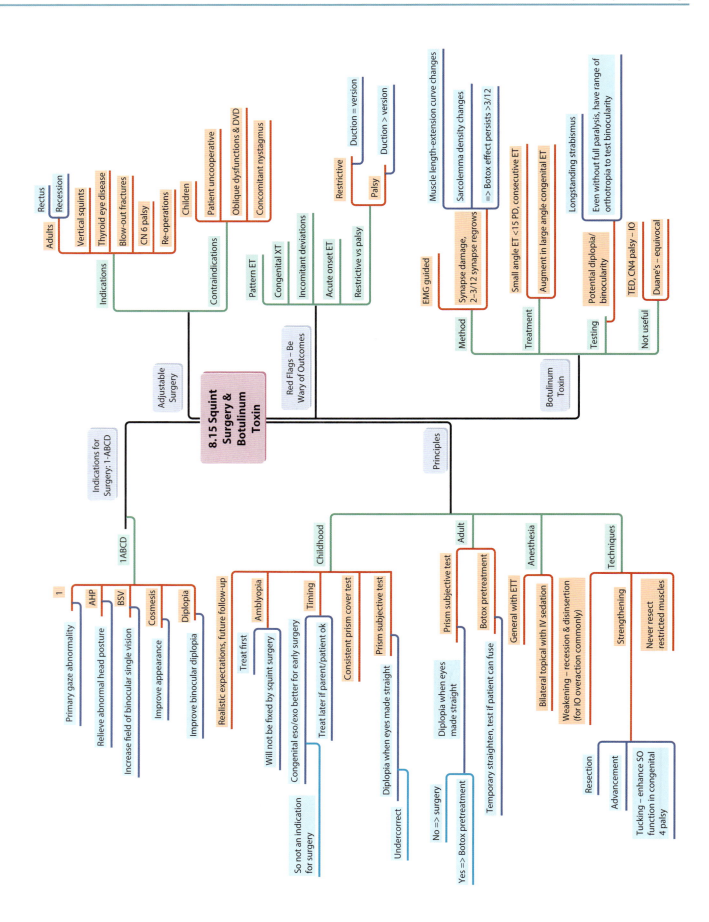

8.15 Squint Surgery & Botulinum Toxin

Adjustable Surgery
- Indications
  - Adults
    - Rectus
    - Recession
  - Vertical squints
  - Thyroid eye disease
  - Blow-out fractures
  - CN 6 palsy
  - Re-operations
- Contraindications
  - Children
  - Patient uncooperative
  - Oblique dysfunctions & DVD
  - Concomitant nystagmus

Red Flags – Be Wary of Outcomes
- Pattern ET
- Congenital XT
- Incomitant deviations
- Acute onset ET
- Restrictive vs palsy
  - Restrictive
    - Duction = version
  - Palsy
    - Duction > version

Botulinum Toxin
- Method
  - EMG guided
  - Muscle length-extension curve changes
  - Sarcolemma density changes
  - => Botox effect persists >3/12
  - Synapse damage, 2–3/12 synapse regrows
- Treatment
  - Small angle ET <15 PD, consecutive ET
  - Augment in large angle congenital ET
- Testing
  - Longstanding strabismus
  - Even without full paralysis, have range of orthotropia to test binocularity
  - Potential diplopia/binocularity
- Not useful
  - TED, CN4 palsy – IO
  - Duane's – equivocal

Indications for Surgery: 1-ABCD
- 1ABCD
  - 1
    - Primary gaze abnormality
  - AHP
    - Relieve abnormal head posture
  - BSV
    - Increase field of binocular single vision
  - Cosmesis
    - Improve appearance
  - Diplopia
    - Improve binocular diplopia

Principles
- Childhood
  - Realistic expectations, future follow-up
  - Amblyopia
    - Treat first
    - Will not be fixed by squint surgery
  - Timing
    - Congenital eso/exo better for early surgery
    - Treat later if parent/patient ok
  - Consistent prism cover test
  - Prism subjective test
    - Diplopia when eyes made straight
      - Undercorrect
      - So not an indication for surgery
- Adult
  - Prism subjective test
    - Diplopia when eyes made straight
      - No => surgery
      - Yes => Botox pretreatment
  - Botox pretreatment
    - Temporary straighten, test if patient can fuse
- Anesthesia
  - General with ETT
  - Bilateral topical with IV sedation
- Techniques
  - Weakening – recession & disinsertion (for IO overaction commonly)
  - Strengthening
    - Resection
    - Advancement
    - Tucking – enhance SO function in congenital 4 palsy
  - Never resect restricted muscles

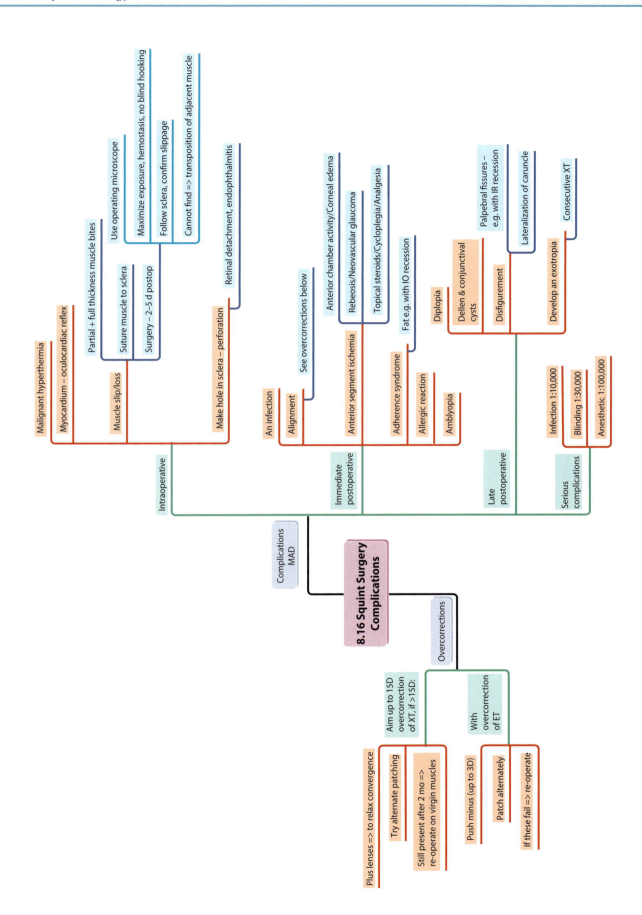

8.16 Squint Surgery Complications

Complications MAD

Intraoperative
- Malignant hyperthermia
- Myocardium – oculocardiac reflex
- Muscle slip/loss
  - Partial + full thickness muscle bites
  - Suture muscle to sclera
    - Use operating microscope
  - Surgery – 2–5 d postop
    - Maximize exposure, hemostasis, no blind hooking
    - Follow sclera, confirm slippage
    - Cannot find => transposition of adjacent muscle
- Make hole in sclera – perforation
  - Retinal detachment, endophthalmitis

Immediate postoperative
- An infection
- Alignment
  - See overcorrections below
- Anterior segment ischemia
  - Anterior chamber activity/Corneal edema
  - Rebeosis/Neovascular glaucoma
  - Topical steroids/Cycloplegia/Analgesia
- Adherence syndrome
  - Fat e.g. with IO recession
- Allergic reaction
- Amblyopia

Late postoperative
- Diplopia
- Dellen & conjunctival cysts
- Disfigurement
  - Palpebral fissures – e.g. with IR recession
  - Lateralization of caruncle
- Develop an exotropia
  - Consecutive XT

Serious complications
- Infection 1:10,000
- Blinding 1:30,000
- Anesthetic 1:100,000

Overcorrections
- Aim up to 15D overcorrection of XT, if >15D:
  - Plus lenses => to relax convergence
  - Try alternate patching
  - Still present after 2 mo => re-operate on virgin muscles
- With overcorrection of ET
  - Push minus (up to 3D)
  - Patch alternately
  - If these fail => re-operate

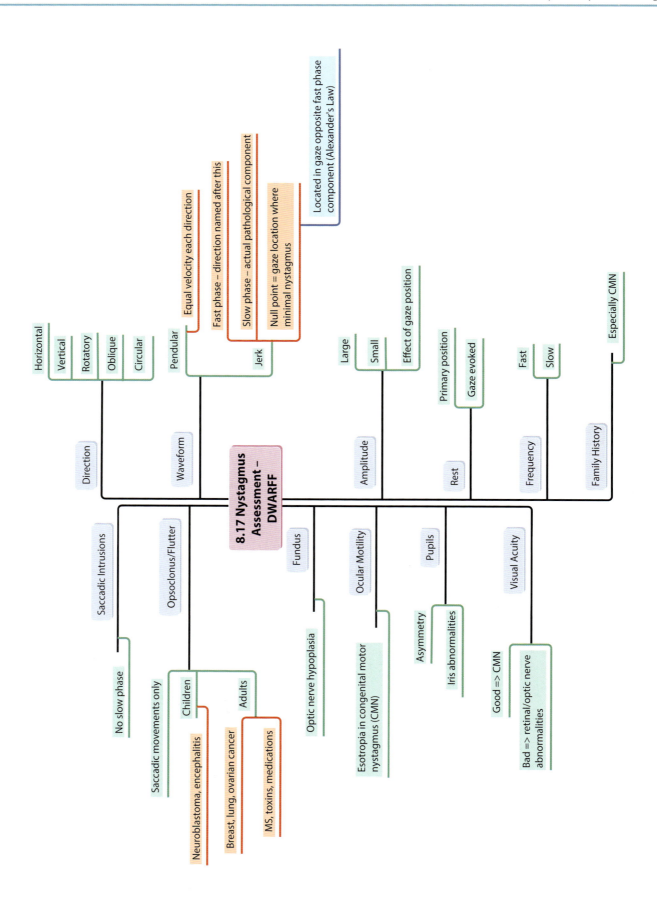

8.17 Nystagmus Assessment – DWARFF

Direction
- Horizontal
- Vertical
- Rotatory
- Oblique
- Circular

Waveform
- Pendular
  - Equal velocity each direction
- Jerk
  - Fast phase – direction named after this
  - Slow phase – actual pathological component
  - Null point = gaze location where minimal nystagmus
    - Located in gaze opposite fast phase component (Alexander's Law)

Amplitude
- Large
- Small
- Effect of gaze position

Rest
- Primary position
- Gaze evoked

Frequency
- Fast
- Slow

Family History
- Especially CMN

Saccadic Intrusions
- No slow phase
- Saccadic movements only

Opsoclonus/Flutter
- Children
  - Neuroblastoma, encephalitis
- Adults
  - Breast, lung, ovarian cancer
  - MS, toxins, medications

Fundus
- Optic nerve hypoplasia

Ocular Motility
- Esotropia in congenital motor nystagmus (CMN)

Pupils
- Asymmetry
- Iris abnormalities

Visual Acuity
- Good => CMN
- Bad => retinal/optic nerve abnormalities

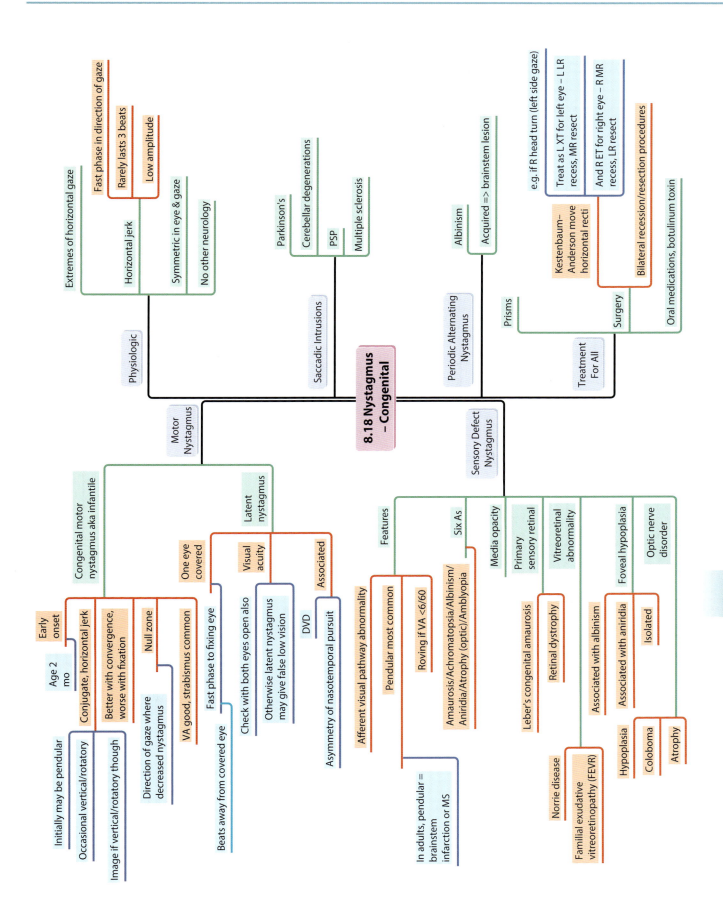

8.18 Nystagmus – Congenital

Physiologic
- Extremes of horizontal gaze
  - Fast phase in direction of gaze
    - Rarely lasts 3 beats
    - Low amplitude
  - Horizontal jerk
  - Symmetric in eye & gaze
  - No other neurology

Saccadic Intrusions
- Parkinson's
- Cerebellar degenerations
- PSP
- Multiple sclerosis

Periodic Alternating Nystagmus
- Albinism
- Acquired => brainstem lesion

Treatment For All
- Prisms
- Surgery
  - e.g. if R head turn (left side gaze)
    - Treat as L XT for left eye – L LR recess, MR resect
    - And R ET for right eye – R MR recess, LR resect
  - Kestenbaum–Anderson move horizontal recti
  - Bilateral recession/resection procedures
- Oral medications, botulinum toxin

Motor Nystagmus
- Congenital motor nystagmus aka infantile
  - Early onset
    - Age 2 mo
  - Conjugate, horizontal jerk
    - Initially may be pendular
    - Occasional vertical/rotatory
    - Image if vertical/rotatory though
  - Better with convergence, worse with fixation
  - Null zone
    - Direction of gaze where decreased nystagmus
- Latent nystagmus
  - One eye covered
    - Fast phase to fixing eye
    - VA good, strabismus common
    - Beats away from covered eye
  - Visual acuity
    - Check with both eyes open also
    - Otherwise latent nystagmus may give false low vision
  - Associated
    - DVD
    - Asymmetry of nasotemporal pursuit

Sensory Defect Nystagmus
- Features
  - Afferent visual pathway abnormality
    - Pendular most common
    - Roving if VA <6/60
    - In adults, pendular = brainstem infarction or MS
  - Six As
    - Amaurosis/Achromatopsia/Albinism/Aniridia/Atrophy (optic)/Amblyopia
  - Media opacity
  - Primary sensory retinal
    - Leber's congenital amaurosis
    - Retinal dystrophy
  - Vitreoretinal abnormality
    - Norrie disease
    - Familial exudative vitreoretinopathy (FEVR)
  - Foveal hypoplasia
    - Associated with albinism
    - Associated with aniridia
    - Isolated
  - Optic nerve disorder
    - Hypoplasia
    - Coloboma
    - Atrophy

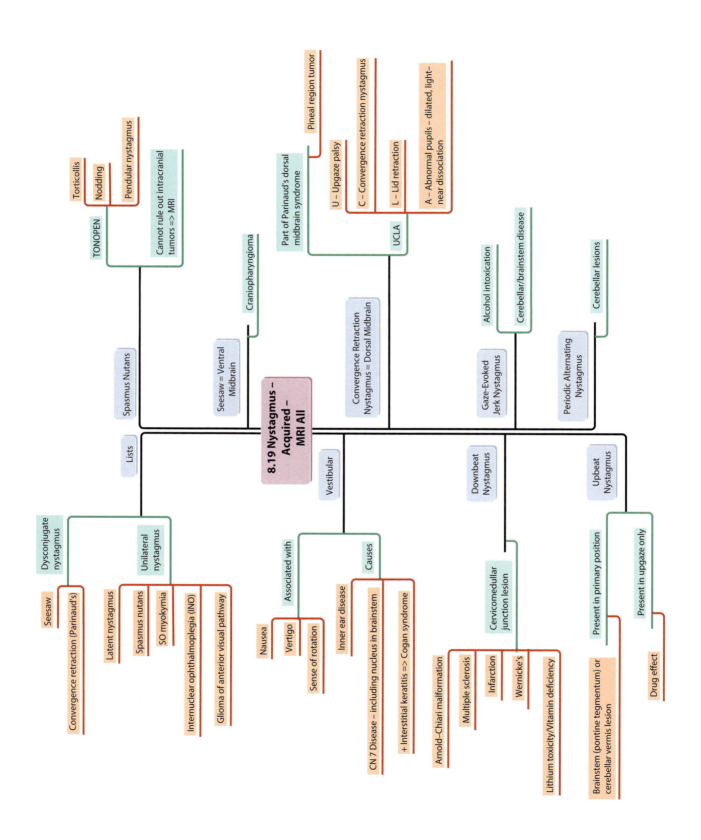

8.19 Nystagmus – Acquired – MRI All

Lists

Spasmus Nutans
- TONOPEN
  - Torticollis
  - Nodding
  - Pendular nystagmus
- Cannot rule out intracranial tumors => MRI

Seesaw = Ventral Midbrain
- Craniopharyngioma

Convergence Retraction Nystagmus = Dorsal Midbrain
- Part of Parinaud's dorsal midbrain syndrome
  - Pineal region tumor
- UCLA
  - U – Upgaze palsy
  - C – Convergence retraction nystagmus
  - L – Lid retraction
  - A – Abnormal pupils – dilated, light–near dissociation

Gaze-Evoked Jerk Nystagmus
- Alcohol intoxication
- Cerebellar/brainstem disease

Periodic Alternating Nystagmus
- Cerebellar lesions

Vestibular
- Associated with
  - Nausea
  - Vertigo
  - Sense of rotation
- Causes
  - Inner ear disease
  - CN 7 Disease – including nucleus in brainstem
  - + Interstitial keratitis => Cogan syndrome

Downbeat Nystagmus
- Cervicomedullar junction lesion
  - Arnold–Chiari malformation
  - Multiple sclerosis
  - Infarction
  - Wernicke's
  - Lithium toxicity/Vitamin deficiency

Upbeat Nystagmus
- Present in primary position
  - Brainstem (pontine tegmentum) or cerebellar vermis lesion
- Present in upgaze only
  - Drug effect

Dysconjugate nystagmus
- Seesaw
- Convergence retraction (Parinaud's)

Unilateral nystagmus
- Latent nystagmus
- Spasmus nutans
- SO myokymia
- Internuclear ophthalmoplegia (INO)
- Glioma of anterior visual pathway

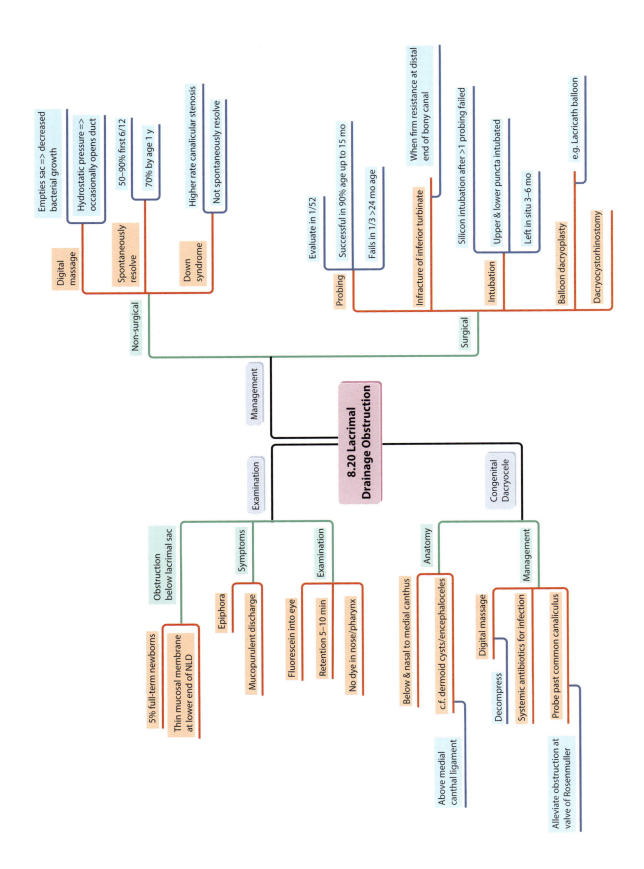

8.20 Lacrimal Drainage Obstruction

Management

Non-surgical
- Digital massage
  - Empties sac => decreased bacterial growth
  - Hydrostatic pressure => occasionally opens duct
- Spontaneously resolve
  - 50–90% first 6/12
  - 70% by age 1 y
- Down syndrome
  - Higher rate canalicular stenosis
  - Not spontaneously resolve

Surgical
- Probing
  - Evaluate in 1/52
  - Successful in 90% age up to 15 mo
  - Fails in 1/3 >24 mo age
- Infracture of inferior turbinate
  - When firm resistance at distal end of bony canal
- Intubation
  - Silicon intubation after >1 probing failed
  - Upper & lower puncta intubated
  - Left in situ 3–6 mo
- Balloon dacryoplasty
  - e.g. Lacricath balloon
- Dacryocystorhinostomy

Examination

Obstruction below lacrimal sac
- 5% full-term newborns
- Thin mucosal membrane at lower end of NLD

Symptoms
- Epiphora
- Mucopurulent discharge

Examination
- Fluorescein into eye
- Retention 5–10 min
- No dye in nose/pharynx

Congenital Dacryocele

Anatomy
- Below & nasal to medial canthus
- c.f. dermoid cysts/encephaloceles
- Above medial canthal ligament

Management
- Digital massage
- Decompress
- Systemic antibiotics for infection
- Probe past common canaliculus
- Alleviate obstruction at valve of Rosenmuller

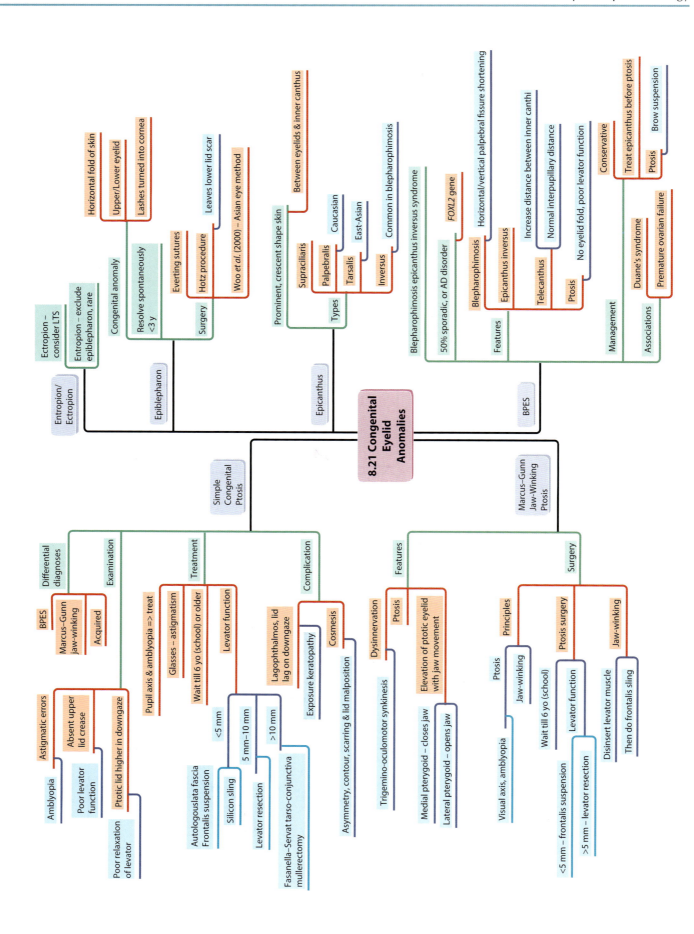

8.21 Congenital Eyelid Anomalies

Entropion/Ectropion
- Ectropion – consider LTS
- Entropion – exclude epiblepharon, rare

Epiblepharon
- Horizontal fold of skin
- Upper/Lower eyelid
- Lashes turned into cornea
- Congenital anomaly
- Resolve spontaneously <3 y
- Surgery
  - Everting sutures
  - Hotz procedure – Leaves lower lid scar
  - Woo et al. (2000) – Asian eye method

Epicanthus
- Prominent, crescent shape skin
- Between eyelids & inner canthus
- Types
  - Supraciliaris
  - Palpebralis – Caucasian
  - Tarsalis – East-Asian
  - Inversus – Common in blepharophimosis

BPES
- Blepharophimosis epicanthus inversus syndrome
- 50% sporadic, or AD disorder
  - FOXL2 gene
- Features
  - Blepharophimosis – Horizontal/vertical palpebral fissure shortening
  - Epicanthus inversus
  - Telecanthus – Increase distance between inner canthi / Normal interpupillary distance
  - Ptosis – No eyelid fold, poor levator function
- Management
  - Conservative
  - Treat epicanthus before ptosis
  - Ptosis – Brow suspension
- Associations
  - Duane's syndrome
  - Premature ovarian failure

Simple Congenital Ptosis
- Differential diagnoses
  - BPES
  - Marcus–Gunn jaw-winking
  - Acquired
- Examination
  - Ptotic lid higher in downgaze
  - Absent upper lid crease – Poor relaxation of levator
  - Poor levator function
  - Astigmatic errors
  - Amblyopia
- Treatment
  - Pupil axis & amblyopia => treat
  - Glasses – astigmatism
  - Wait till 6 yo (school) or older
  - Levator function
    - <5 mm – Autologouslata fascia Frontalis suspension / Silicon sling
    - 5 mm–10 mm – Levator resection
    - >10 mm – Fasanella–Servat tarso-conjunctiva mullerectomy
- Complication
  - Lagophthalmos, lid lag on downgaze – Exposure keratopathy
  - Cosmesis – Asymmetry, contour, scarring & lid malposition

Marcus–Gunn Jaw-Winking Ptosis
- Features
  - Dysinnervation – Trigemino-oculomotor synkinesis
  - Ptosis – Elevation of ptotic eyelid with jaw movement
    - Medial pterygoid – closes jaw
    - Lateral pterygoid – opens jaw
- Surgery
  - Principles
    - Ptosis – Visual axis, amblyopia
    - Jaw-winking
    - Wait till 6 yo (school)
    - Levator function
      - <5 mm – frontalis suspension
      - >5 mm – levator resection
  - Ptosis surgery
  - Jaw-winking – Disinsert levator muscle / Then do frontalis sling

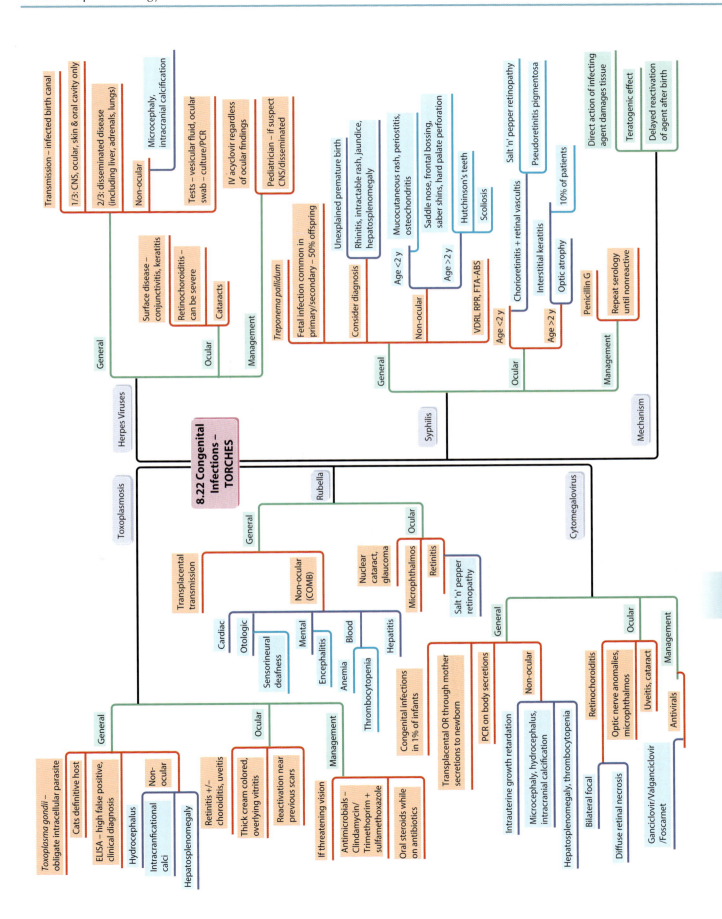

8.22 Congenital Infections – TORCHES

Herpes Viruses

General
- Transmission – infected birth canal
  - 1/3: CNS, ocular, skin & oral cavity only
  - 2/3: disseminated disease (including liver, adrenals, lungs)
  - Non-ocular
    - Microcephaly, intracranial calcification

Ocular
- Surface disease – conjunctivitis, keratitis
- Retinochoroiditis – can be severe
- Cataracts

Management
- Tests – vesicular fluid, ocular swab – culture/PCR
- IV acyclovir regardless of ocular findings
- Pediatrician – if suspect CNS/disseminated

Syphilis

Treponema pallidum

General
- Fetal infection common in primary/secondary – 50% offspring
- Consider diagnosis
  - Unexplained premature birth
  - Rhinitis, intractable rash, jaundice, hepatosplenomegaly
  - Age <2 y
    - Mucocutaneous rash, periostitis, osteochonditis
  - Age >2 y
    - Saddle nose, frontal bossing, saber shins, hard palate perforation
    - Hutchinson's teeth
    - Scoliosis
- Non-ocular

Ocular
- VDRL RPR, FTA-ABS
- Chorioretinitis + retinal vasculitis
- Interstitial keratitis
- Optic atrophy
- Salt 'n' pepper retinopathy
- Pseudoretinitis pigmentosa
- 10% of patients

Management
- Age <2 y
  - Penicillin G
- Age >2 y
  - Repeat serology until nonreactive

Mechanism
- Direct action of infecting agent damages tissue
- Teratogenic effect
- Delayed reactivation of agent after birth

Toxoplasmosis

General
- *Toxoplasma gondii* – obligate intracellular parasite
- Cats definitive host
- ELISA – high false positive, clinical diagnosis
- Hydrocephalus
- Intracranficational calci
- Non-ocular
  - Hepatosplenomegaly

Ocular
- Retinitis +/- choroiditis, uveitis
- Thick cream colored, overlying vitritis
- Reactivation near previous scars

Management
- If threatening vision
- Antimicrobials – Clindamycin/Trimethoprim + sulfamethoxazole
- Oral steroids while on antibiotics

Rubella

General
- Transplacental transmission
- Non-ocular (COMB)
  - Cardiac
  - Otologic
    - Sensorineural deafness
  - Mental
    - Encephalitis
  - Blood
    - Anemia
    - Thrombocytopenia
  - Hepatitis

Ocular
- Nuclear cataract, glaucoma
- Microphthalmos
- Retinitis
- Salt 'n' pepper retinopathy

Cytomegalovirus

General
- Congenital infections in 1% of infants
- Transplacental OR through mother secretions to newborn
- PCR on body secretions
- Non-ocular
  - Intrauterine growth retardation
  - Microcephaly, hydrocephalus, intracranial calcification
  - Hepatosplenomegaly, thrombocytopenia

Ocular
- Retinochoroiditis
  - Bilateral focal
  - Diffuse retinal necrosis
- Optic nerve anomalies, microphthalmos
- Uveitis, cataract

Management
- Antivirals
  - Ganciclovir/Valganciclovir /Foscarnet

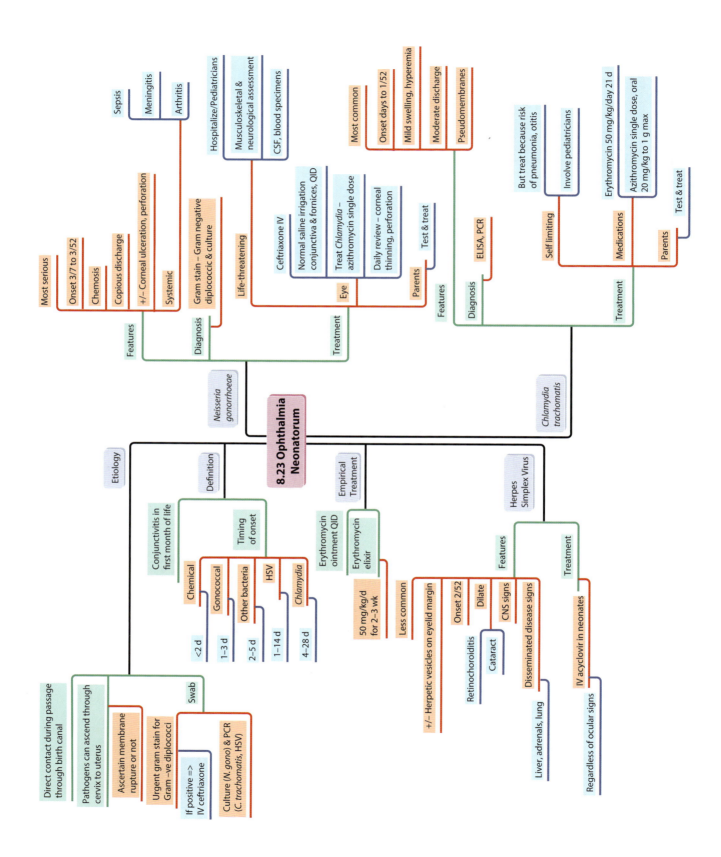

8.23 Ophthalmia Neonatorum

Etiology

Definition
- Conjunctivitis in first month of life

Timing of onset
- Chemical — <2 d
- Gonococcal — 1–3 d
- Other bacteria — 2–5 d
- HSV — 1–14 d
- Chlamydia — 4–28 d

- Direct contact during passage through birth canal
- Pathogens can ascend through cervix to uterus

Swab
- Ascertain membrane rupture or not
- Urgent gram stain for Gram –ve diplococci
- If positive => IV ceftriaxone
- Culture (N. gono) & PCR (C. trachomatis, HSV)

Neisseria gonorrhoeae

Features
- Most serious
- Onset 3/7 to 3/52
- Chemosis
- Copious discharge
- +/– Corneal ulceration, perforation
- Systemic
  - Sepsis
  - Meningitis
  - Arthritis

Diagnosis
- Gram stain – Gram negative diplococci & culture
- Life-threatening
  - Hospitalize/Pediatricians
  - Musculoskeletal & neurological assessment
  - CSF, blood specimens

Treatment
- Eye
  - Ceftriaxone IV
  - Normal saline irrigation conjunctiva & fornices, QID
  - Treat *Chlamydia* – azithromycin single dose
  - Daily review – corneal thinning, perforation
- Parents
  - Test & treat

Chlamydia trachomatis

Features
- Most common
- Onset days to 1/52
- Mild swelling, hyperemia
- Moderate discharge
- Pseudomembranes

Diagnosis
- ELISA, PCR

Treatment
- Self limiting
  - But treat because risk of pneumonia, otitis
  - Involve pediatricians
- Medications
  - Erythromycin 50 mg/kg/day 21 d
  - Azithromycin single dose, oral 20 mg/kg to 1 g max
- Parents
  - Test & treat

Empirical Treatment
- Erythromycin ointment QID
- Erythromycin elixir
  - 50 mg/kg/d for 2–3 wk

Herpes Simplex Virus

Features
- Less common
- +/– Herpetic vesicles on eyelid margin
- Onset 2/52
- Dilate
  - Retinochoroiditis
  - Cataract
- CNS signs
- Disseminated disease signs
  - Liver, adrenals, lung

Treatment
- IV acyclovir in neonates
- Regardless of ocular signs

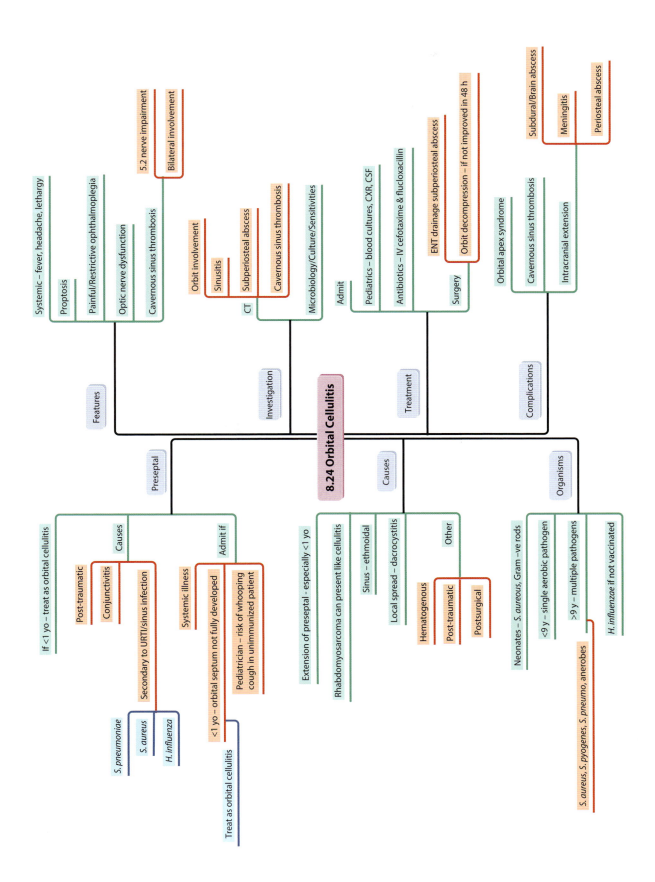

8.24 Orbital Cellulitis

Features
- Systemic – fever, headache, lethargy
- Proptosis
- Painful/Restrictive ophthalmoplegia
- Optic nerve dysfunction
- Cavernous sinus thrombosis
  - 5.2 nerve impairment
  - Bilateral involvement

Investigation
- CT
  - Orbit involvement
  - Sinusitis
  - Subperiosteal abscess
  - Cavernous sinus thrombosis
- Microbiology/Culture/Sensitivities

Treatment
- Admit
- Pediatrics – blood cultures, CXR, CSF
- Antibiotics – IV cefotaxime & flucloxacillin
- Surgery
  - ENT drainage subperiosteal abscess
  - Orbit decompression – if not improved in 48 h

Complications
- Orbital apex syndrome
- Cavernous sinus thrombosis
- Intracranial extension
  - Subdural/Brain abscess
  - Meningitis
  - Periosteal abscess

Preseptal
- If <1 yo – treat as orbital cellulitis
- Causes
  - Post-traumatic
  - Conjunctivitis
  - Secondary to URTI/sinus infection
    - S. pneumoniae
    - S. aureus
    - H. influenza
- Admit if
  - Systemic illness
  - <1 yo – orbital septum not fully developed
    - Treat as orbital cellulitis
  - Pediatrician – risk of whooping cough in unimmunized patient

Causes
- Extension of preseptal - especially <1 yo
- Rhabdomyosarcoma can present like cellulitis
- Sinus – ethmoidal
- Local spread – dacrocystitis
- Other
  - Hematogenous
  - Post-traumatic
  - Postsurgical

Organisms
- Neonates – S. aureous, Gram –ve rods
- <9 y – single aerobic pathogen
- >9 y – multiple pathogens
  - S. aureus, S. pyogenes, S. pneumo, anerobes
- H. influenzae if not vaccinated

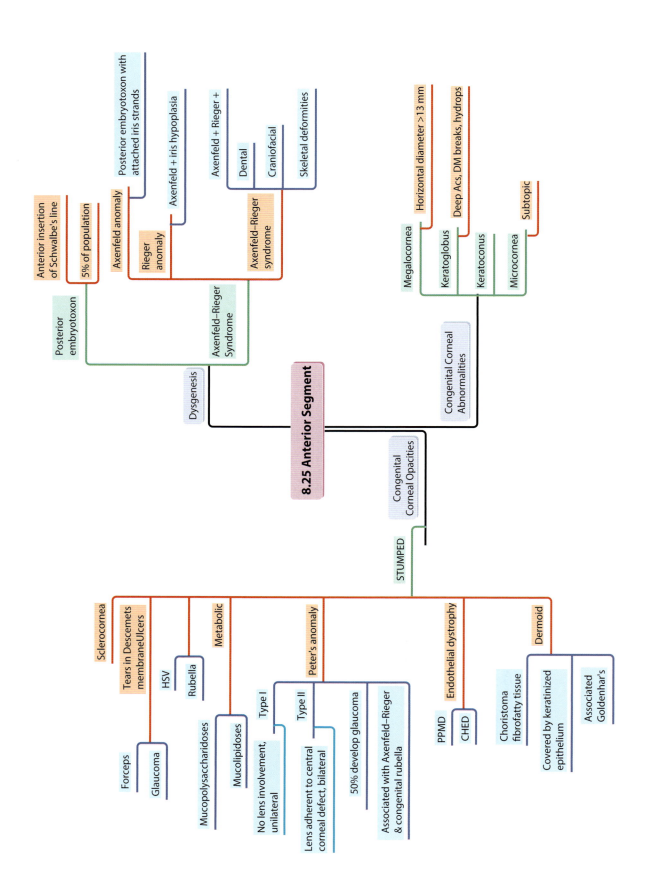

8.25 Anterior Segment

Dysgenesis

Posterior embryotoxon
- Anterior insertion of Schwalbe's line
- 5% of population

Axenfeld–Rieger Syndrome

Axenfeld anomaly
- Posterior embryotoxon with attached iris strands

Rieger anomaly
- Axenfeld + iris hypoplasia

Axenfeld–Rieger syndrome
- Axenfeld + Rieger +
  - Dental
  - Craniofacial
  - Skeletal deformities

Congenital Corneal Abnormalities

Megalocornea
- Horizontal diameter >13 mm

Keratoglobus
- Deep Acs, DM breaks, hydrops

Keratoconus

Microcornea
- Subtopic

Congenital Corneal Opacities

STUMPED

Sclerocornea
- Forceps
- Glaucoma

Tears in Descemets membrane Ulcers
- HSV
- Rubella

Metabolic
- Mucopolysaccharidoses
- Mucolipidoses

Peter's anomaly
- Type I
  - No lens involvement, unilateral
- Type II
  - Lens adherent to central corneal defect, bilateral
- 50% develop glaucoma
- Associated with Axenfeld–Rieger & congenital rubella

Endothelial dystrophy
- PPMD
- CHED

Dermoid
- Choristoma fibrofatty tissue
- Covered by keratinized epithelium
- Associated Goldenhar's

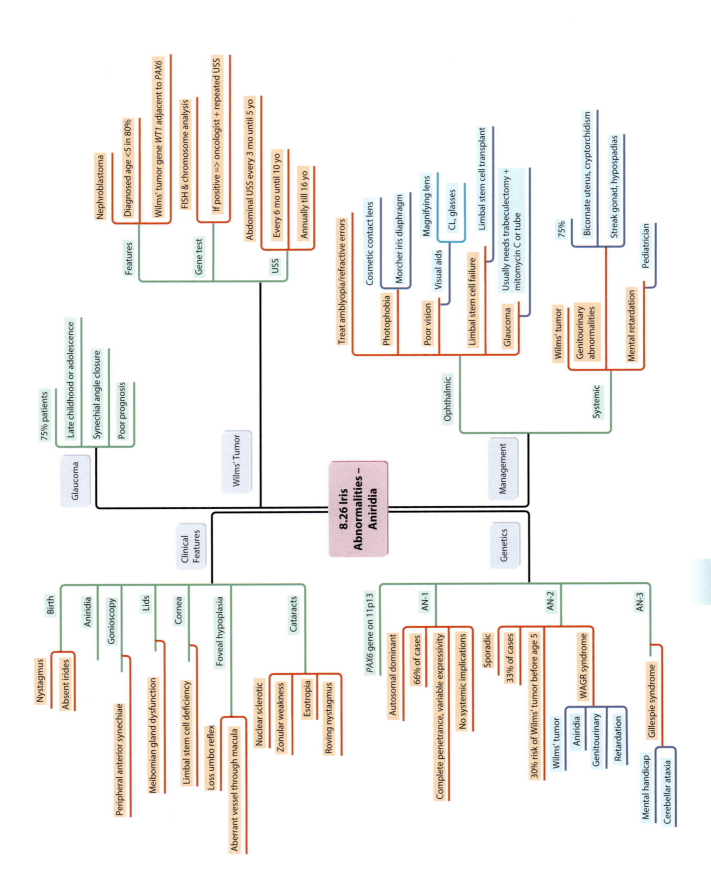

8.26 Iris Abnormalities – Aniridia

Glaucoma
- 75% patients
- Late childhood or adolescence
- Synechial angle closure
- Poor prognosis

Wilms' Tumor
- **Features**
  - Nephroblastoma
  - Diagnosed age <5 in 80%
  - Wilms' tumor gene *WT1* adjacent to *PAX6*
- **Gene test**
  - FISH & chromosome analysis
  - If positive => oncologist + repeated USS
- **USS**
  - Abdominal USS every 3 mo until 5 yo
  - Every 6 mo until 10 yo
  - Annually till 16 yo

Clinical Features
- **Birth**
  - Nystagmus
  - Absent irides
- **Aniridia**
- **Gonioscopy**
  - Peripheral anterior synechiae
- **Lids**
  - Meibomian gland dysfunction
- **Cornea**
  - Limbal stem cell deficiency
  - Loss umbo reflex
- **Foveal hypoplasia**
  - Aberrant vessel through macula
- **Cataracts**
  - Nuclear sclerotic
  - Zonular weakness
  - Esotropia
  - Roving nystagmus

Management
- **Ophthalmic**
  - Treat amblyopia/refractive errors
  - Photophobia
    - Cosmetic contact lens
    - Morcher iris diaphragm
  - Poor vision
    - Visual aids
      - Magnifying lens
      - CL, glasses
  - Limbal stem cell failure
    - Limbal stem cell transplant
  - Glaucoma
    - Usually needs trabeculectomy + mitomycin C or tube
- **Systemic**
  - Wilms' tumor — 75%
  - Genitourinary abnormalities
    - Bicornate uterus, cryptorchidism
    - Streak gonad, hypospadias
  - Mental retardation
    - Pediatrician

Genetics
- *PAX6* gene on 11p13
- **AN-1**
  - Autosomal dominant
  - 66% of cases
  - Complete penetrance, variable expressivity
  - No systemic implications
- **AN-2**
  - Sporadic
  - 33% of cases
  - 30% risk of Wilms' tumor before age 5
  - WAGR syndrome
    - Wilms' tumor
    - Aniridia
    - Genitourinary
    - Retardation
- **AN-3**
  - Gillespie syndrome
    - Mental handicap
    - Cerebellar ataxia

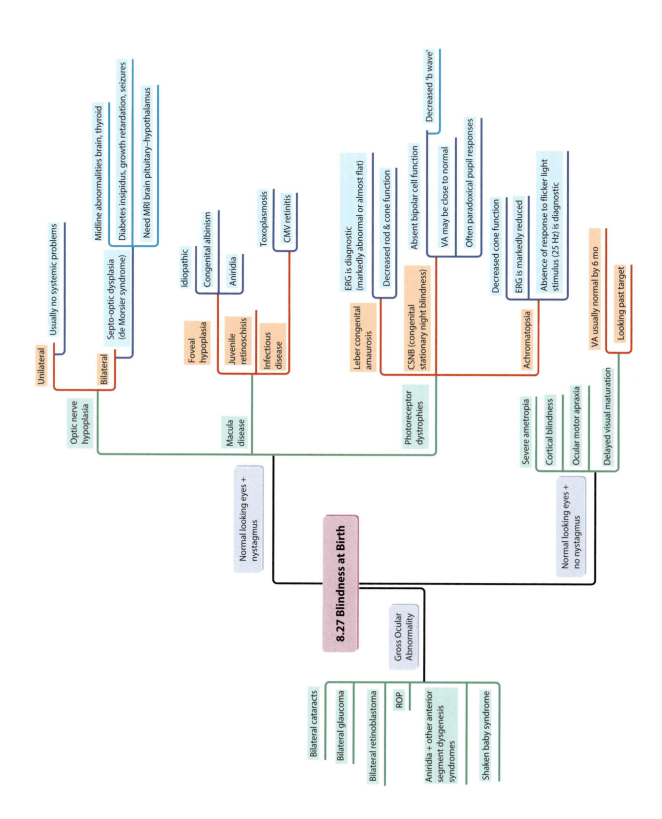

8.27 Blindness at Birth

Normal looking eyes + nystagmus

- Optic nerve hypoplasia
  - Unilateral
    - Usually no systemic problems
  - Bilateral
    - Septo-optic dysplasia (de Morsier syndrome)
      - Midline abnormalities brain, thyroid
      - Diabetes insipidus, growth retardation, seizures
      - Need MRI brain pituitary–hypothalamus
- Macula disease
  - Foveal hypoplasia
    - Idiopathic
    - Congenital albinism
    - Aniridia
  - Juvenile retinoschisis
  - Infectious disease
    - Toxoplasmosis
    - CMV retinitis
- Photoreceptor dystrophies
  - Leber congenital amaurosis
    - ERG is diagnostic (markedly abnormal or almost flat)
    - Decreased rod & cone function
  - CSNB (congenital stationary night blindness)
    - Absent bipolar cell function
      - Decreased 'b wave'
    - VA may be close to normal
    - Often paradoxical pupil responses
  - Achromatopsia
    - Decreased cone function
    - ERG is markedly reduced
    - Absence of response to flicker light stimulus (25 Hz) is diagnostic

Normal looking eyes + no nystagmus

- Severe ametropia
- Cortical blindness
- Ocular motor apraxia
- Delayed visual maturation
  - VA usually normal by 6 mo
  - Looking past target

Gross Ocular Abnormality

- Bilateral cataracts
- Bilateral glaucoma
- Bilateral retinoblastoma
- ROP
- Aniridia + other anterior segment dysgenesis syndromes
- Shaken baby syndrome

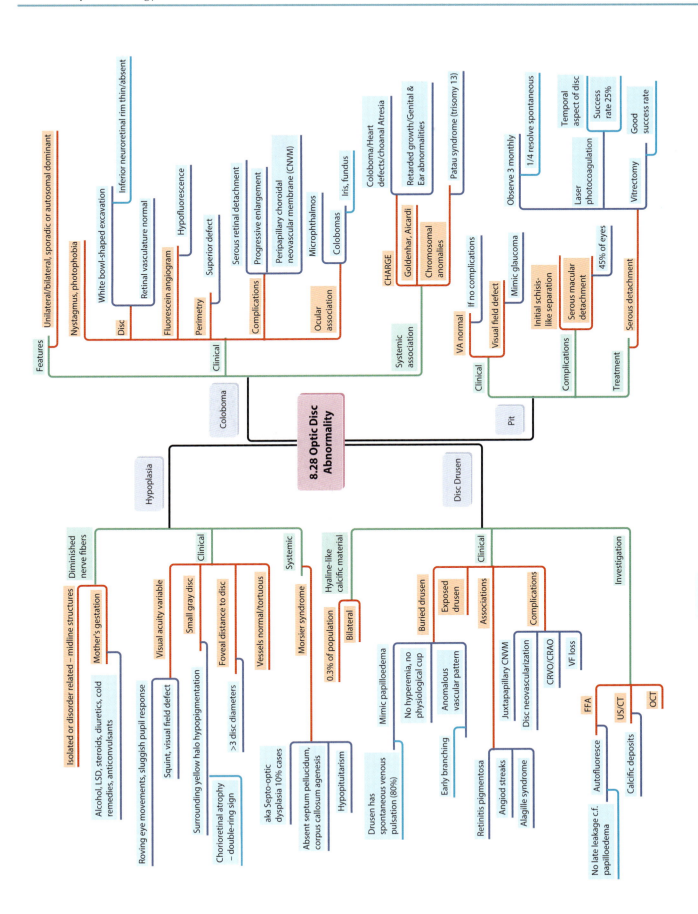

8.28 Optic Disc Abnormality

Coloboma

Features
- Unilateral/bilateral, sporadic or autosomal dominant
- Nystagmus, photophobia

Clinical
- Disc
  - White bowl-shaped excavation
  - Inferior neuroretinal rim thin/absent
  - Retinal vasculature normal
- Fluorescein angiogram
  - Hypofluorescence
- Perimetry
  - Superior defect
- Complications
  - Serous retinal detachment
  - Progressive enlargement
  - Peripapillary choroidal neovascular membrane (CNVM)
- Ocular association
  - Microphthalmos
  - Colobomas
    - Iris, fundus

Systemic association
- CHARGE
  - Coloboma/Heart defects/Genital & Ear abnormalities
  - Retarded growth/Genital & Ear abnormalities
  - Choanal Atresia
- Goldenhar, Aicardi
- Chromosomal anomalies
  - Patau syndrome (trisomy 13)

Pit

Clinical
- VA normal
  - If no complications
- Visual field defect
  - Mimic glaucoma

Complications
- Serous macular detachment
  - Initial schisis-like separation
  - 45% of eyes
- Serous detachment

Treatment
- Observe 3 monthly
  - 1/4 resolve spontaneous
- Laser photocoagulation
  - Temporal aspect of disc
  - Success rate 25%
- Vitrectomy
  - Good success rate

Hypoplasia

Clinical
- Diminished nerve fibers
  - Isolated or disorder related – midline structures
  - Mother's gestation
    - Alcohol, LSD, steroids, diuretics, cold remedies, anticonvulsants
- Roving eye movements, sluggish pupil response
- Visual acuity variable
  - Squint, visual field defect
- Small gray disc
  - Surrounding yellow halo hypopigmentation
  - Foveal distance to disc
    - Chorioretinal atrophy – double-ring sign
  - >3 disc diameters
- Vessels normal/tortuous

Systemic
- Morsier syndrome
  - aka Septo-optic dysplasia 10% cases
  - Absent septum pellucidum, corpus callosum agenesis
  - Hypopituitarism

Disc Drusen

- Hyaline-like calcific material
- 0.3% of population
- Bilateral

Clinical
- Buried drusen
  - Mimic papilloedema
- Exposed drusen
  - No hyperemia, no physiological cup
  - Anomalous vascular pattern
    - Early branching
  - Drusen has spontaneous venous pulsation (80%)
- Associations
  - Juxtapapillary CNVM
  - Retinitis pigmentosa
  - Angioid streaks
  - Alagille syndrome
- Complications
  - Disc neovascularization
  - CRVO/CRAO
  - VF loss

Investigation
- FFA
  - Autofluoresce
  - No late leakage c.f. papilloedema
- US/CT
  - Calcific deposits
- OCT

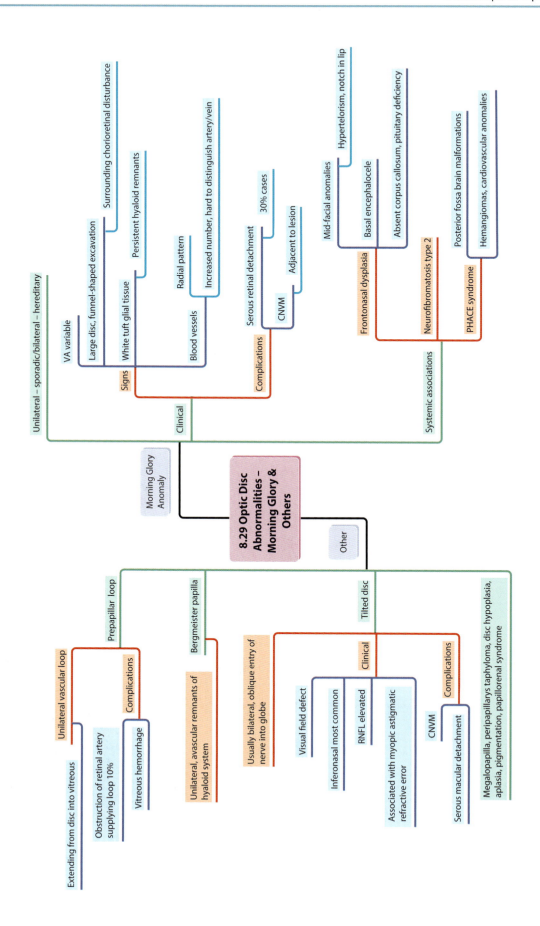

8.29 Optic Disc Abnormalities – Morning Glory & Others

Morning Glory Anomaly

- Clinical
  - Unilateral – sporadic/bilateral – hereditary
  - Signs
    - VA variable
    - Large disc, funnel-shaped excavation
      - Surrounding chorioretinal disturbance
    - White tuft glial tissue
      - Persistent hyaloid remnants
    - Blood vessels
      - Radial pattern
      - Increased number, hard to distinguish artery/vein
  - Complications
    - Serous retinal detachment
      - 30% cases
    - CNVM
      - Adjacent to lesion
  - Systemic associations
    - Frontonasal dysplasia
      - Mid-facial anomalies
        - Hypertelorism, notch in lip
      - Basal encephalocele
        - Absent corpus callosum, pituitary deficiency
    - Neurofibromatosis type 2
    - PHACE syndrome
      - Posterior fossa brain malformations
      - Hemangiomas, cardiovascular anomalies

Other

- Prepapillar loop
  - Unilateral vascular loop
    - Extending from disc into vitreous
    - Obstruction of retinal artery supplying loop 10%
  - Complications
    - Vitreous hemorrhage
- Bergmeister papilla
  - Unilateral, avascular remnants of hyaloid system
- Tilted disc
  - Usually bilateral, oblique entry of nerve into globe
  - Clinical
    - Visual field defect
    - Inferonasal most common
    - RNFL elevated
    - Associated with myopic astigmatic refractive error
  - Complications
    - CNVM
    - Serous macular detachment
    - Megalopapilla, peripapillarys taphyloma, disc hypoplasia, aplasia, pigmentation, papillorenal syndrome

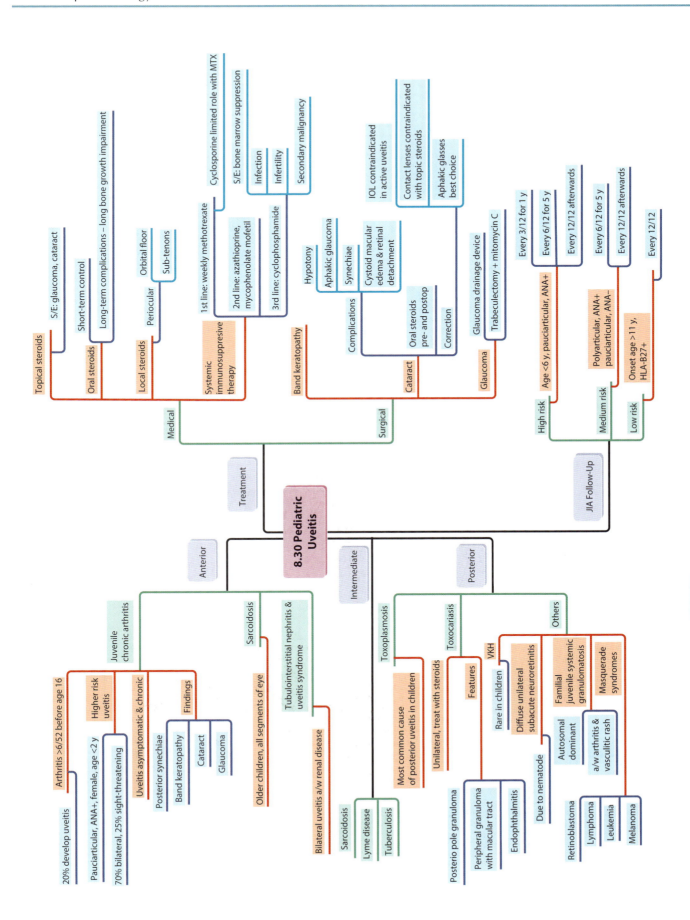

8.30 Pediatric Uveitis

Treatment

Medical

- Topical steroids
  - S/E: glaucoma, cataract
  - Short-term control
  - Long-term complications – long bone growth impairment
- Oral steroids
- Local steroids
  - Periocular
    - Orbital floor
    - Sub-tenons
- Systemic immunosuppressive therapy
  - 1st line: weekly methotrexate
    - Cyclosporine limited role with MTX
  - 2nd line: azathioprine, mycophenolate mofetil
    - S/E: bone marrow suppression
  - 3rd line: cyclophosphamide
    - Infection
    - Infertility
    - Secondary malignancy

Surgical

- Band keratopathy
- Cataract
  - Complications
    - Hypotony
    - Aphakic glaucoma
    - Synechiae
    - Cystoid macular edema & retinal detachment
  - Oral steroids pre- and postop
  - Correction
    - IOL contraindicated in active uveitis
    - Contact lenses contraindicated with topic steroids
    - Aphakic glasses best choice
- Glaucoma
  - Glaucoma drainage device
  - Trabeculectomy + mitomycin C

JIA Follow-Up

- High risk
  - Age <6 y, pauciarticular, ANA+
    - Every 3/12 for 1 y
    - Every 6/12 for 5 y
    - Every 12/12 afterwards
- Medium risk
  - Polyarticular, ANA+ pauciarticular, ANA−
    - Every 6/12 for 5 y
    - Every 12/12 afterwards
- Low risk
  - Onset age >11 y, HLA-B27+
    - Every 12/12

Anterior

- Juvenile chronic arthritis
  - Arthritis >6/52 before age 16
    - 20% develop uveitis
  - Higher risk uveitis
    - Pauciarticular, ANA+, female, age <2 y
    - 70% bilateral, 25% sight-threatening
  - Uveitis asymptomatic & chronic
  - Findings
    - Posterior synechiae
    - Band keratopathy
    - Cataract
    - Glaucoma
- Sarcoidosis
  - Older children, all segments of eye
- Tubulointerstitial nephritis & uveitis syndrome
  - Bilateral uveitis a/w renal disease
  - Sarcoidosis
  - Lyme disease
  - Tuberculosis

Intermediate

Posterior

- Toxoplasmosis
  - Most common cause of posterior uveitis in children
  - Posterio pole granuloma
  - Peripheral granuloma with macular tract
- Toxocariasis
  - Unilateral, treat with steroids
  - Due to nematode
  - Endophthalmitis
- VKH
  - Rare in children
  - Features
- Diffuse unilateral subacute neuroretinitis
  - Autosomal dominant
- Familial juvenile systemic granulomatosis
  - a/w arthritis & vasculitic rash
- Masquerade syndromes
  - Retinoblastoma
  - Lymphoma
  - Leukemia
  - Melanoma
- Others

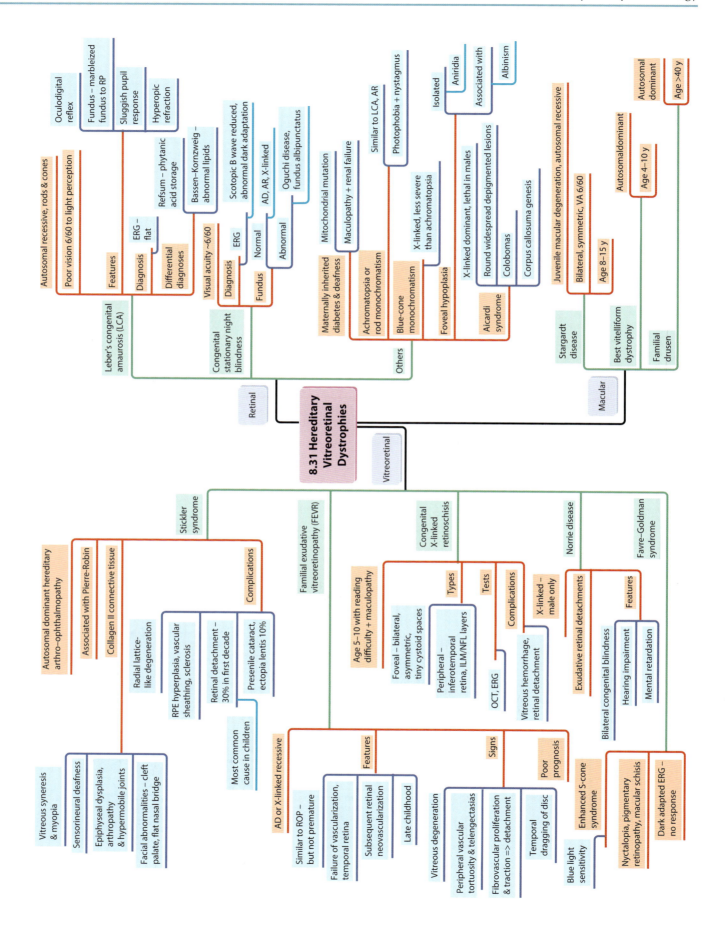

8.31 Hereditary Vitreoretinal Dystrophies

Retinal

Leber's congenital amaurosis (LCA)
- Autosomal recessive, rods & cones
- Poor vision 6/60 to light perception
- Features
  - Oculodigital reflex
  - Fundus – marbleized fundus to RP
  - Sluggish pupil response
  - Hyperopic refraction
- Diagnosis
  - ERG – flat
- Differential diagnoses

Congenital stationary night blindness
- Visual acuity ~6/60
- Diagnosis
  - ERG
    - Normal
    - Abnormal
- Fundus
  - Refsum – phytanic acid storage
  - Bassen–Kornzweig – abnormal lipids
  - Scotopic B wave reduced, abnormal dark adaptation
  - AD, AR, X-linked
  - Oguchi disease, fundus albipunctatus

Others
- Maternally inherited diabetes & deafness
  - Mitochondrial mutation
  - Maculopathy + renal failure
  - Similar to LCA, AR
- Achromatopsia or rod monochromatism
  - Photophobia + nystagmus
- Blue-cone monochromatism
  - X-linked, less severe than achromatopsia
- Foveal hypoplasia
  - Isolated
  - Associated with
    - Aniridia
    - Albinism
- Aicardi syndrome
  - X-linked dominant, lethal in males
  - Round widespread depigmented lesions
  - Colobomas
  - Corpus callosuma genesis

Macular

Stargardt disease
- Juvenile macular degeneration, autosomal recessive
- Bilateral, symmetric, VA 6/60
- Age 8–15 y

Best vitelliform dystrophy
- Autosomal dominant
- Age 4–10 y

Familial drusen
- Autosomal dominant
- Age >40 y

Vitreoretinal

Stickler syndrome
- Autosomal dominant hereditary arthro–ophthalmopathy
- Associated with Pierre-Robin
- Collagen II connective tissue
  - Vitreous syneresis & myopia
  - Sensorineural deafness
  - Epiphyseal dysplasia, arthropathy & hypermobile joints
  - Facial abnormalities – cleft palate, flat nasal bridge
- Radial lattice-like degeneration
  - RPE hyperplasia, vascular sheathing, sclerosis
- Complications
  - Retinal detachment – 30% in first decade
  - Presenile cataract, ectopia lentis 10%

Familial exudative vitreoretinopathy (FEVR)
- Most common cause in children
- AD or X-linked recessive
  - Similar to ROP – but not premature
- Features
  - Failure of vascularization, temporal retina
  - Subsequent retinal neovascularization
  - Late childhood
- Signs
  - Vitreous degeneration
  - Peripheral vascular tortuosity & telengectasias
  - Fibrovascular proliferation & traction => detachment
- Poor prognosis
  - Temporal dragging of disc

Congenital X-linked retinoschisis
- Age 5–10 with reading difficulty + maculopathy
- Types
  - Foveal – bilateral, asymmetric, tiny cystoid spaces
  - Peripheral – inferotemporal retina, ILM/NFL layers
- Tests
  - OCT, ERG
- Complications
  - Vitreous hemorrhage, retinal detachment
  - X-linked – male only

Norrie disease
- Exudative retinal detachments
- Features
  - Bilateral congenital blindness
  - Hearing impairment
  - Mental retardation

Favre–Goldman syndrome
- Enhanced S-cone syndrome
  - Blue light sensitivity
- Nyctalopia, pigmentary retinopathy, macular schisis
- Dark adapted ERG – no response

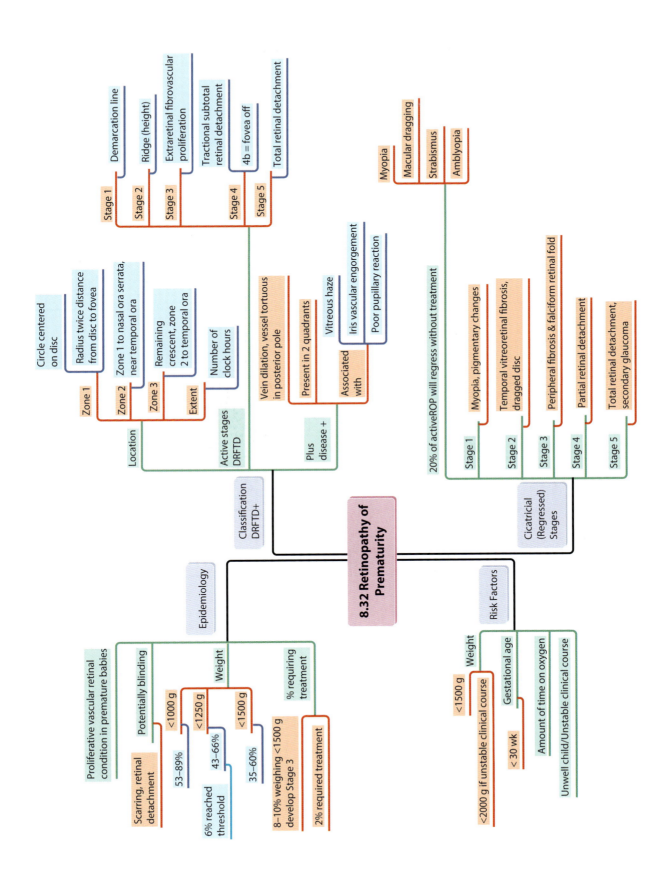

8.32 Retinopathy of Prematurity

Classification DRFTD+

Location
- Zone 1 — Circle centered on disc / Radius twice distance from disc to fovea
- Zone 2 — Zone 1 to nasal ora serrata, near temporal ora
- Zone 3 — Remaining crescent, zone 2 to temporal ora
- Extent — Number of clock hours

Active stages DRFTD
- Stage 1 — Demarcation line
- Stage 2 — Ridge (height)
- Stage 3 — Extraretinal fibrovascular proliferation
- Stage 4 — Tractional subtotal retinal detachment / 4b = fovea off
- Stage 5 — Total retinal detachment

Plus disease +
- Vein dilation, vessel tortuous in posterior pole
- Present in 2 quadrants
- Associated with
  - Vitreous haze
  - Iris vascular engorgement
  - Poor pupillary reaction

Cicatricial (Regressed) Stages
- 20% of activeROP will regress without treatment
- Stage 1 — Myopia, pigmentary changes
- Stage 2 — Temporal vitreoretinal fibrosis, dragged disc
- Stage 3 — Peripheral fibrosis & falciform retinal fold
- Stage 4 — Partial retinal detachment
- Stage 5 — Total retinal detachment, secondary glaucoma
  - Myopia
  - Macular dragging
  - Strabismus
  - Amblyopia

Epidemiology
- Proliferative vascular retinal condition in premature babies
- Potentially blinding — Scarring, retinal detachment
- Weight
  - <1000 g — 53–89%
  - <1250 g — 43–66% / 6% reached threshold
  - <1500 g — 35–60%
- % requiring treatment
  - 8–10% weighing <1500 g develop Stage 3
  - 2% required treatment

Risk Factors
- Weight
  - <1500 g
  - <2000 g if unstable clinical course
- Gestational age
  - < 30 wk
- Amount of time on oxygen
- Unwell child/Unstable clinical course

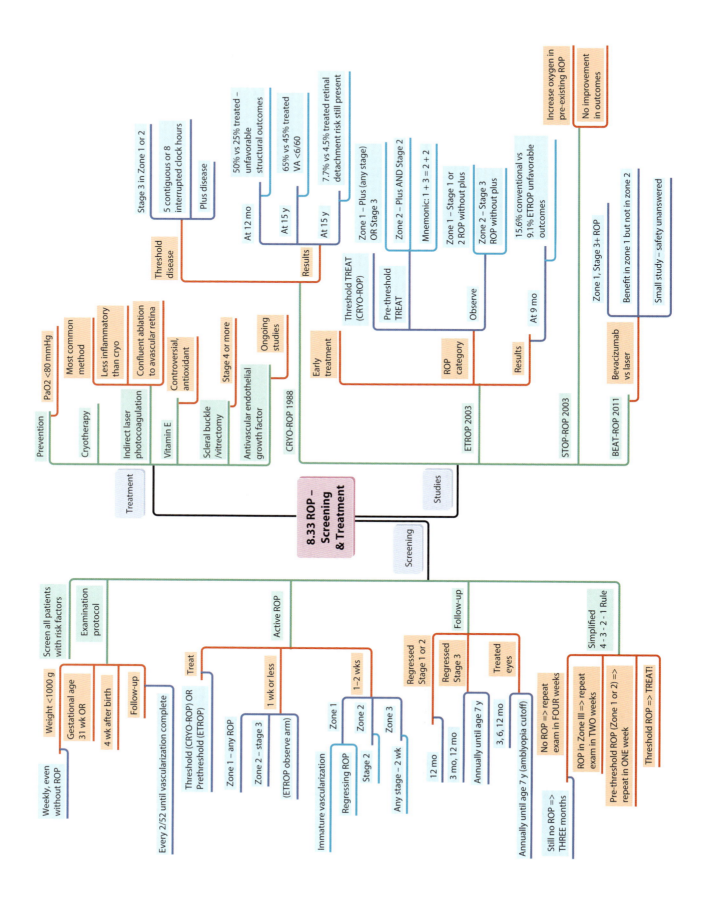

8.33 ROP – Screening & Treatment

Treatment

- Prevention
  - PaO2 <80 mmHg
- Cryotherapy
  - Most common method
  - Less inflammatory than cryo
- Indirect laser photocoagulation
  - Confluent ablation to avascular retina
- Vitamin E
  - Controversial, antioxidant
- Scleral buckle/vitrectomy
  - Stage 4 or more
- Antivascular endothelial growth factor
  - Ongoing studies

Studies

- CRYO-ROP 1988
  - Threshold disease
    - Stage 3 in Zone 1 or 2
    - 5 contiguous or 8 interrupted clock hours
    - Plus disease
  - Results
    - At 12 mo — 50% vs 25% treated – unfavorable structural outcomes
    - At 15 y — 65% vs 45% treated VA <6/60
    - At 15 y — 7.7% vs 4.5% treated retinal detachment risk still present

- ETROP 2003
  - Early treatment
    - Threshold TREAT (CRYO-ROP)
      - Zone 1 – Plus (any stage) OR Stage 3
      - Zone 2 – Plus AND Stage 2
      - Mnemonic: 1 + 3 = 2 + 2
    - Pre-threshold TREAT
    - Observe
      - Zone 1 – Stage 1 or 2 ROP without plus
      - Zone 2 – Stage 3 ROP without plus
  - ROP category
  - Results
    - At 9 mo — 15.6% conventional vs 9.1% ETROP unfavorable outcomes

- STOP-ROP 2003
  - Increase oxygen in pre-existing ROP
  - No improvement in outcomes

- BEAT-ROP 2011
  - Bevacizumab vs laser
    - Zone 1, Stage 3+ ROP
    - Benefit in zone 1 but not in zone 2
    - Small study – safety unanswered

Screening

- Screen all patients with risk factors
  - Weight <1000 g
  - Gestational age 31 wk OR
  - 4 wk after birth
  - Follow-up
- Examination protocol
  - Weekly, even without ROP
  - Every 2/52 until vascularization complete
- Active ROP
  - Treat
    - Threshold (CRYO-ROP) OR Prethreshold (ETROP)
      - Zone 1 – any ROP
      - Zone 2 – stage 3
      - (ETROP observe arm)
    - 1 wk or less
  - 1–2 wks
    - Immature vascularization
    - Regressing ROP
      - Stage 2
      - Any stage – 2 wk
    - Zone 1
    - Zone 2
    - Zone 3
- Follow-up
  - Regressed Stage 1 or 2
    - 12 mo
  - Regressed Stage 3
    - 3 mo, 12 mo
  - Treated eyes
    - Annually until age 7 y
    - 3, 6, 12 mo
  - Annually until age 7 y (amblyopia cutoff)
- Simplified 4 - 3 - 2 - 1 Rule
  - Still no ROP => THREE months
  - No ROP => repeat exam in FOUR weeks
  - ROP in Zone III => repeat exam in TWO weeks
  - Pre-threshold ROP (Zone 1 or 2) => repeat in ONE week
  - Threshold ROP => TREAT!

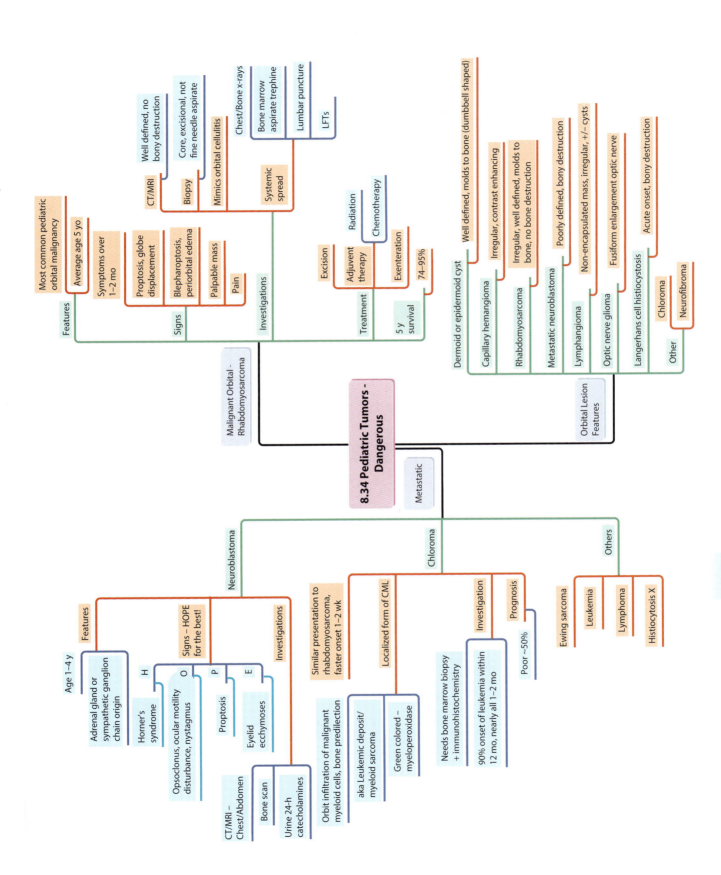

8.34 Pediatric Tumors - Dangerous

Malignant Orbital - Rhabdomyosarcoma

Features
- Most common pediatric orbital malignancy
- Average age 5 yo
- Symptoms over 1–2 mo

Signs
- Proptosis, globe displacement
- Blepharoptosis, periorbital edema
- Palpable mass
- Pain

Investigations
- CT/MRI
  - Well defined, no bony destruction
- Biopsy
  - Core, excisional, not fine needle aspirate
- Mimics orbital cellulitis
- Systemic spread
  - Chest/Bone x-rays
  - Bone marrow aspirate trephine
  - Lumbar puncture
  - LFTs

Treatment
- Excision
- Adjuvent therapy
  - Radiation
  - Chemotherapy
- Exenteration

5 y survival
- 74–95%

Orbital Lesion Features
- Dermoid or epidermoid cyst — Well defined, molds to bone (dumbbell shaped)
- Capillary hemangioma — Irregular, contrast enhancing
- Rhabdomyosarcoma — Irregular, well defined, molds to bone, no bone destruction
- Metastatic neuroblastoma — Poorly defined, bony destruction
- Lymphangioma — Non-encapsulated mass, irregular, +/− cysts
- Optic nerve glioma — Fusiform enlargement optic nerve
- Langerhans cell histiocytosis — Acute onset, bony destruction
- Other
  - Chloroma
  - Neurofibroma

Metastatic

Neuroblastoma

Features
- Age 1–4 y
- Adrenal gland or sympathetic ganglion chain origin

Signs – HOPE for the best!
- H — Horner's syndrome
- O — Opsoclonus, ocular motility disturbance, nystagmus
- P — Proptosis
- E — Eyelid ecchymoses

Investigations
- CT/MRI – Chest/Abdomen
- Bone scan
- Urine 24-h catecholamines

Chloroma
- Similar presentation to rhabdomyosarcoma, faster onset 1–2 wk
- Localized form of CML
  - Orbit infiltration of malignant myeloid cells, bone predilection
  - aka Leukemic deposit/ myeloid sarcoma
  - Green colored – myeloperoxidase
- Investigation
  - Needs bone marrow biopsy + immunohistochemistry
  - 90% onset of leukemia within 12 mo, nearly all 1–2 mo
- Prognosis
  - Poor ~50%

Others
- Ewing sarcoma
- Leukemia
- Lymphoma
- Histiocytosis X

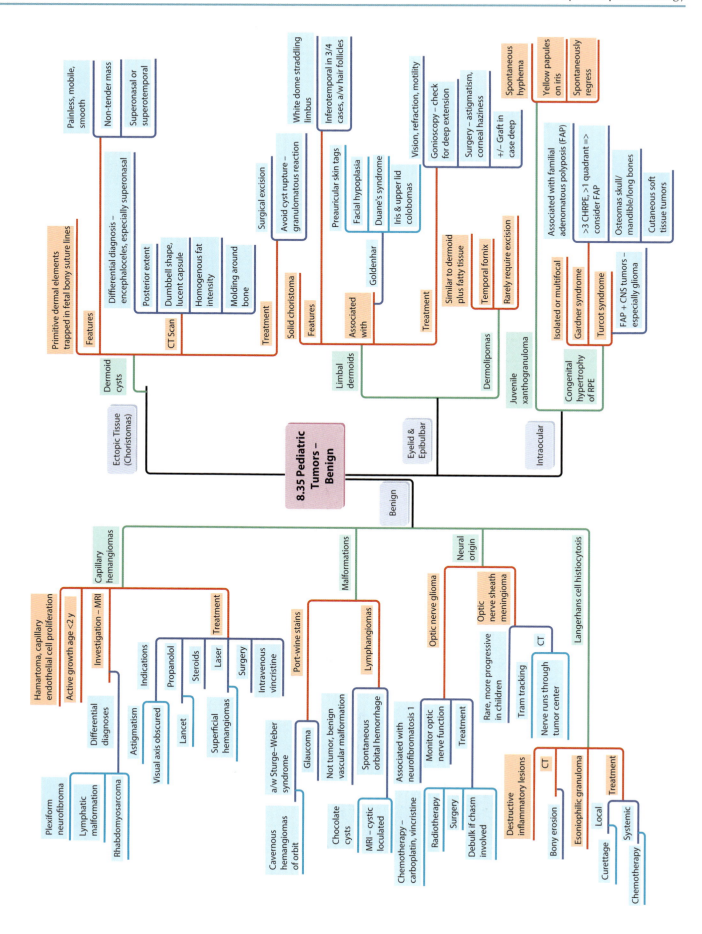

8.35 Pediatric Tumors – Benign

Ectopic Tissue (Choristomas)

Dermoid cysts
- Primitive dermal elements trapped in fetal bony suture lines
- Features
  - Painless, mobile, smooth
  - Non-tender mass
  - Superonasal or superotemporal
- Differential diagnosis – encephaloceles, especially superonasal
  - Posterior extent
- CT Scan
  - Dumbbell shape, lucent capsule
  - Homogenous fat intensity
  - Molding around bone
- Treatment
  - Surgical excision
  - Avoid cyst rupture – granulomatous reaction

Eyelid & Epibulbar

Limbal dermoids
- Solid choristoma
- Features
  - White dome straddling limbus
  - Inferotemporal in 3/4 cases, a/w hair follicles
- Associated with
  - Preauricular skin tags
  - Goldenhar
  - Facial hypoplasia
  - Duane's syndrome
  - Iris & upper lid colobomas
- Treatment
  - Vision, refraction, motility
  - Gonioscopy – check for deep extension
  - Surgery – astigmatism, corneal haziness
  - +/- Graft in case deep

Dermolipomas
- Similar to dermoid plus fatty tissue
- Temporal fornix
- Rarely require excision

Intraocular

Juvenile xanthogranuloma
- Spontaneous hyphema
- Yellow papules on iris
- Spontaneously regress

Congenital hypertrophy of RPE
- Isolated or multifocal
- Associated with familial adenomatous polyposis (FAP)
  - >3 CHRPE, >1 quadrant => consider FAP
- Gardner syndrome
  - Osteomas skull/ mandible/long bones
  - Cutaneous soft tissue tumors
- Turcot syndrome
  - FAP + CNS tumors – especially glioma

Benign

Capillary hemangiomas
- Hamartoma, capillary endothelial cell proliferation
- Active growth age <2 y
- Investigation – MRI
- Differential diagnoses
  - Plexiform neurofibroma
  - Lymphatic malformation
  - Rhabdomyosarcoma
- Indications
  - Astigmatism
  - Visual axis obscured
- Treatment
  - Propanolol
  - Steroids
    - Lancet
  - Laser
    - Superficial hemangiomas
  - Surgery
  - Intravenous vincristine

Malformations

Port-wine stains
- a/w Sturge–Weber syndrome
- Glaucoma

Cavernous hemangiomas of orbit

Lymphangiomas
- Not tumor, benign vascular malformation
- Spontaneous orbital hemorrhage
  - Chocolate cysts
  - MRI – cystic loculated
  - Chemotherapy – carboplatin, vincristine

Neural origin

Optic nerve glioma
- Associated with neurofibromatosis 1
- Monitor optic nerve function
- Treatment
  - Radiotherapy
  - Surgery
  - Debulk if chasm involved

Optic nerve sheath meningioma
- Rare, more progressive in children
- Tram tracking
- CT
  - Nerve runs through tumor center

Langerhans cell histiocytosis
- Destructive inflammatory lesions
- CT
  - Bony erosion
- Esoniophilic granuloma
- Treatment
  - Local
    - Curettage
  - Systemic
    - Chemotherapy

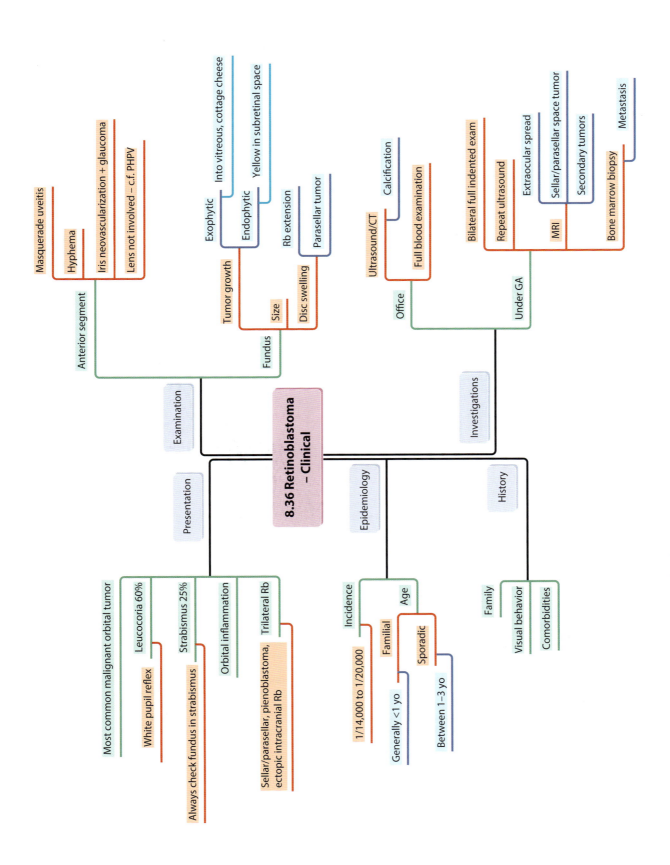

8.36 Retinoblastoma – Clinical

Examination
- Anterior segment
  - Masquerade uveitis
  - Hyphema
  - Iris neovascularization + glaucoma
  - Lens not involved – c.f. PHPV
- Fundus
  - Tumor growth
    - Exophytic
      - Into vitreous, cottage cheese
    - Endophytic
      - Yellow in subretinal space
  - Size
  - Disc swelling
  - Rb extension
    - Parasellar tumor

Investigations
- Office
  - Ultrasound/CT
    - Calcification
  - Full blood examination
- Under GA
  - Bilateral full indented exam
  - Repeat ultrasound
    - Extraocular spread
  - MRI
    - Sellar/parasellar space tumor
    - Secondary tumors
  - Bone marrow biopsy
    - Metastasis

Presentation
- Most common malignant orbital tumor
- Leucocoria 60%
  - White pupil reflex
- Strabismus 25%
  - Always check fundus in strabismus
- Orbital inflammation
- Trilateral Rb
  - Sellar/parasellar, pienoblastoma, ectopic intracranial Rb

Epidemiology
- Incidence
  - 1/14,000 to 1/20,000
  - Familial
  - Sporadic
- Age
  - Generally <1 yo
  - Between 1–3 yo

History
- Family
- Visual behavior
- Comorbidities

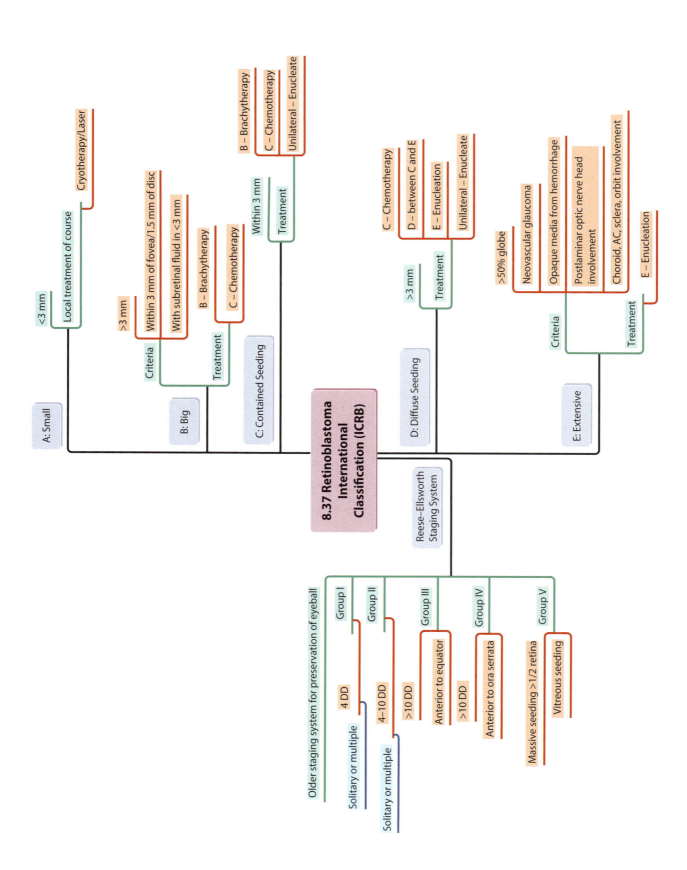

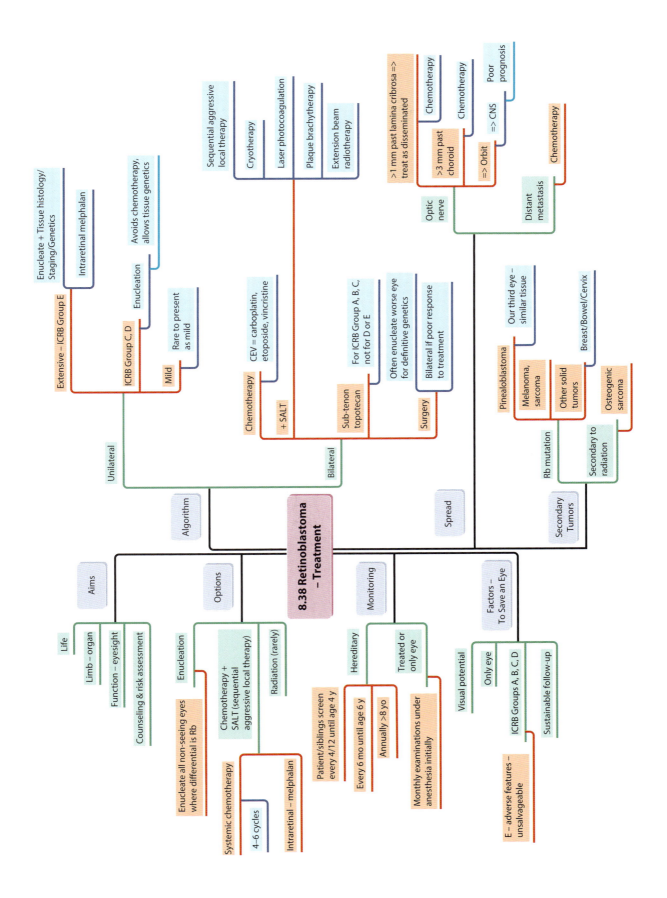

8.38 Retinoblastoma – Treatment

Algorithm

Unilateral
- ICRB Group C, D
  - Extensive – ICRB Group E
    - Enucleate + Tissue histology/Staging/Genetics
    - Intraretinal melphalan
    - Avoids chemotherapy, allows tissue genetics
  - Enucleation
- Mild
  - Rare to present as mild

Bilateral
- Chemotherapy
  - CEV = carboplatin, etoposide, vincristine
- + SALT
  - Sequential aggressive local therapy
    - Cryotherapy
    - Laser photocoagulation
    - Plaque brachytherapy
    - Extension beam radiotherapy
- Sub-tenon topotecan
  - For ICRB Group A, B, C, not for D or E
- Surgery
  - Often enucleate worse eye for definitive genetics
  - Bilateral if poor response to treatment

Spread

Optic nerve
- >1 mm past lamina cribrosa => treat as disseminated
- >3 mm past choroid => Chemotherapy
- => Orbit => Chemotherapy
  - => CNS
    - Poor prognosis

Distant metastasis
- Chemotherapy

Secondary Tumors

Rb mutation
- Pinealoblastoma
  - Our third eye – similar tissue
- Melanoma, sarcoma
- Other solid tumors
  - Breast/Bowel/Cervix

Secondary to radiation
- Osteogenic sarcoma

Aims
- Life
  - Limb – organ
- Function – eyesight
- Counseling & risk assessment

Options
- Enucleation
  - Enucleate all non-seeing eyes where differential is Rb
  - Systemic chemotherapy
    - 4–6 cycles
    - Intraretinal – melphalan
- Chemotherapy + SALT (sequential aggressive local therapy)
- Radiation (rarely)

Monitoring
- Hereditary
  - Patient/siblings screen every 4/12 until age 4 y
  - Every 6 mo until age 6 y
  - Annually >8 yo
- Treated or only eye
  - Monthly examinations under anesthesia initially

Factors – To Save an Eye
- Visual potential
- Only eye
- ICRB Groups A, B, C, D
  - E – adverse features – unsalvageable
- Sustainable follow-up

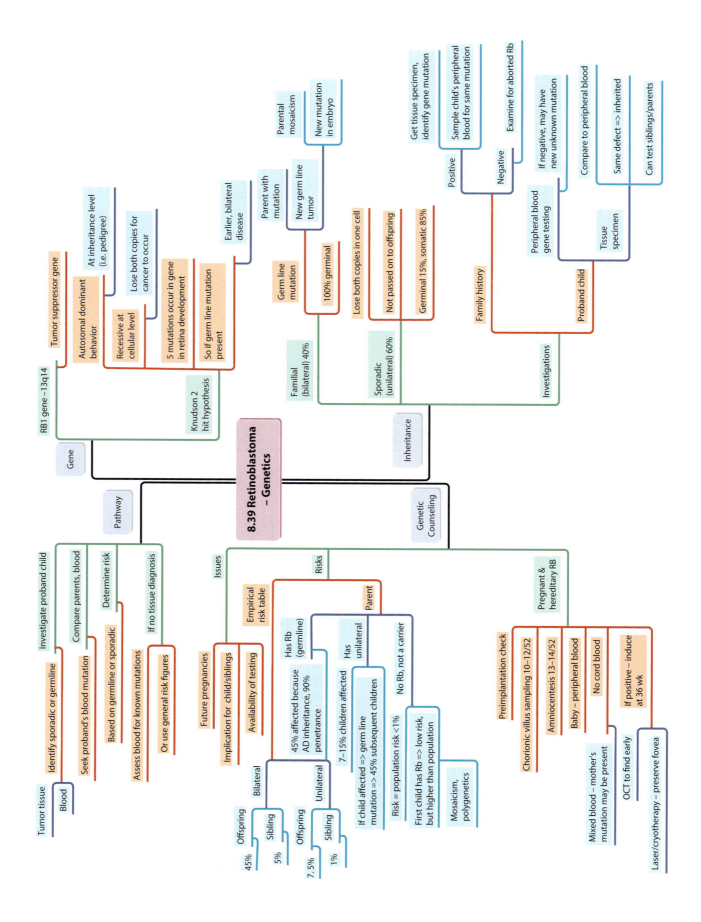

8.39 Retinoblastoma – Genetics

Gene

RB1 gene –13q14

- Tumor suppressor gene
  - Autosomal dominant behavior
    - At inheritance level (i.e. pedigree)
    - Recessive at cellular level
      - Lose both copies for cancer to occur
- Knudson 2 hit hypothesis
  - 5 mutations occur in gene in retina development
  - So if germ line mutation present
    - Earlier, bilateral disease

Pathway

- Germ line mutation
  - 100% germinal
    - Parent with mutation
      - New germ line tumor
    - Parental mosaicism
      - New mutation in embryo
  - Lose both copies in one cell
    - Not passed on to offspring
    - Germinal 15%, somatic 85%

Inheritance

- Familial (bilateral) 40%
- Sporadic (unilateral) 60%

Investigations

- Family history
- Proband child
  - Peripheral blood gene testing
    - Positive
      - Get tissue specimen, identify gene mutation
      - Sample child's peripheral blood for same mutation
    - Negative
      - Examine for aborted Rb
      - If negative, may have new unknown mutation
  - Tissue specimen
    - Compare to peripheral blood
    - Same defect => inherited
    - Can test siblings/parents

Genetic Counseling

Issues

- Investigate proband child
  - Tumor tissue
  - Blood
    - Identify sporadic or germline
    - Seek proband's blood mutation
  - Compare parents, blood
  - Determine risk
    - Based on germline or sporadic
    - Assess blood for known mutations
  - If no tissue diagnosis
    - Or use general risk figures

Risks

- Empirical risk table
  - Future pregnancies
  - Implication for child/siblings
  - Availability of testing
- Has Rb (germline)
  - Bilateral
    - Offspring 45%
    - Sibling 5%
  - Unilateral
    - Offspring 7.5%
    - Sibling 1%
  - 45% affected because AD inheritance, 90% penetrance
  - 7–15% children affected
- Parent
  - Has unilateral
    - If child affected => germ line mutation => 45% subsequent children
    - Risk = population risk <1%
  - No Rb, not a carrier
    - First child has Rb => low risk, but higher than population
    - Mosaicism, polygenetics

- Pregnant & hereditary RB
  - Preimplantation check
  - Chorionic villus sampling 10–12/52
  - Amniocentesis 13–14/52
  - Baby – peripheral blood
    - Mixed blood – mother's mutation may be present
  - No cord blood
  - If positive – induce at 36 wk
    - OCT to find early
    - Laser/cryotherapy – preserve fovea

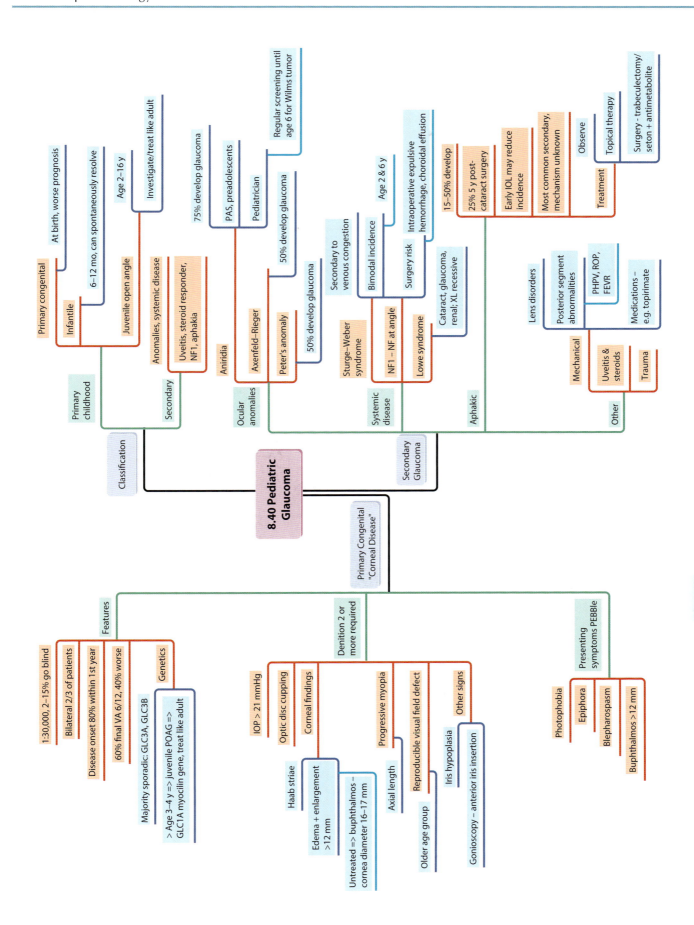

8.40 Pediatric Glaucoma

Classification

Primary childhood
- Primary congenital
  - At birth, worse prognosis
  - Infantile
    - 6–12 mo, can spontaneously resolve
  - Juvenile open angle
    - Age 2–16 y
    - Investigate/treat like adult
- Secondary
  - Anomalies, systemic disease
  - Uveitis, steroid responder, NF1, aphakia

Ocular anomalies
- Aniridia
  - 75% develop glaucoma
  - PAS, preadolescents
  - Pediatrician
  - Regular screening until age 6 for Wilms tumor
- Axenfeld–Rieger
  - 50% develop glaucoma
- Peter's anomaly
  - 50% develop glaucoma

Systemic disease
- Sturge–Weber syndrome
  - Secondary to venous congestion
  - Bimodal incidence
  - Age 2 & 6 y
- NF1 – NF at angle
- Lowe syndrome
  - Cataract, glaucoma, renal; XL recessive
  - Surgery risk
  - Intraoperative expulsive hemorrhage, choroidal effusion

Aphakic
- 15–50% develop
- 25% 5 y post-cataract surgery
- Early IOL may reduce incidence
- Most common secondary, mechanism unknown
- Treatment
  - Observe
  - Topical therapy
  - Surgery - trabeculectomy/seton + antimetabolite

Other
- Lens disorders
- Posterior segment abnormalities
  - PHPV, ROP, FEVR
- Medications – e.g. topirimate
- Mechanical
- Uveitis & steroids
- Trauma

Secondary Glaucoma

Primary Congenital "Corneal Disease"

Features
- 1:30,000, 2–15% go blind
- Bilateral 2/3 of patients
- Disease onset 80% within 1st year
- 60% final VA 6/12, 40% worse
- Genetics
  - Majority sporadic: GLC3A, GLC3B
  - > Age 3–4 y => juvenile POAG => GLC1A myocilin gene, treat like adult

Definition 2 or more required
- IOP > 21 mmHg
- Optic disc cupping
- Corneal findings
  - Haab striae
  - Edema + enlargement >12 mm
  - Untreated => buphthalmos – cornea diameter 16–17 mm
  - Axial length
- Progressive myopia
- Reproducible visual field defect
  - Older age group
- Other signs
  - Iris hypoplasia
  - Gonioscopy – anterior iris insertion

Presenting symptoms PEBBle
- Photophobia
- Epiphora
- Blepharospasm
- Buphthalmos >12 mm

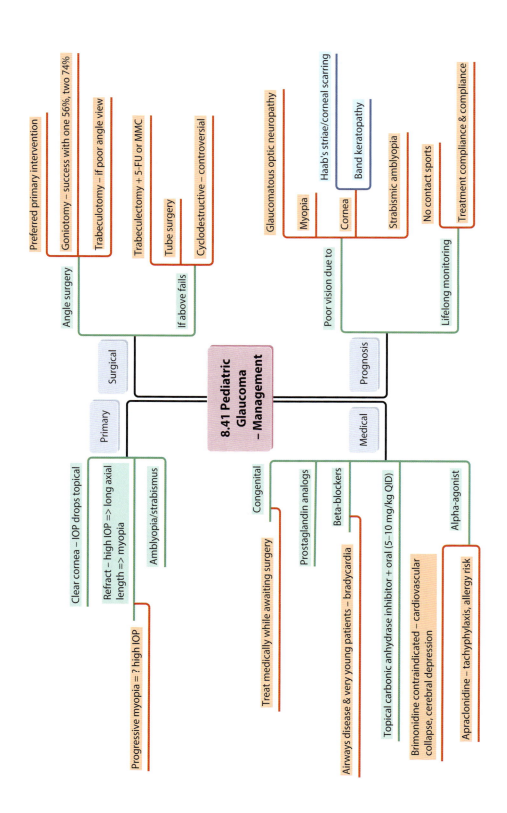

8.41 Pediatric Glaucoma – Management

Primary

Surgical

Angle surgery
- Preferred primary intervention
- Goniotomy – success with one 56%, two 74%
- Trabeculotomy – if poor angle view

If above fails
- Trabeculectomy + 5-FU or MMC
- Tube surgery
- Cyclodestructive – controversial

Clear cornea – IOP drops topical

Refract – high IOP => long axial length => myopia
- Progressive myopia = ? high IOP

Amblyopia/strabismus

Medical

Congenital – Treat medically while awaiting surgery

Prostaglandin analogs

Beta-blockers – Airways disease & very young patients – bradycardia

Topical carbonic anhydrase inhibitor + oral (5–10 mg/kg QID)
- Brimonidine contraindicated – cardiovascular collapse, cerebral depression

Alpha-agonist – Apraclonidine – tachyphylaxis, allergy risk

Prognosis

Poor vision due to
- Glaucomatous optic neuropathy
- Myopia
- Cornea
  - Haab's striae/corneal scarring
  - Band keratopathy
- Strabismic amblyopia

Lifelong monitoring
- No contact sports
- Treatment compliance & compliance

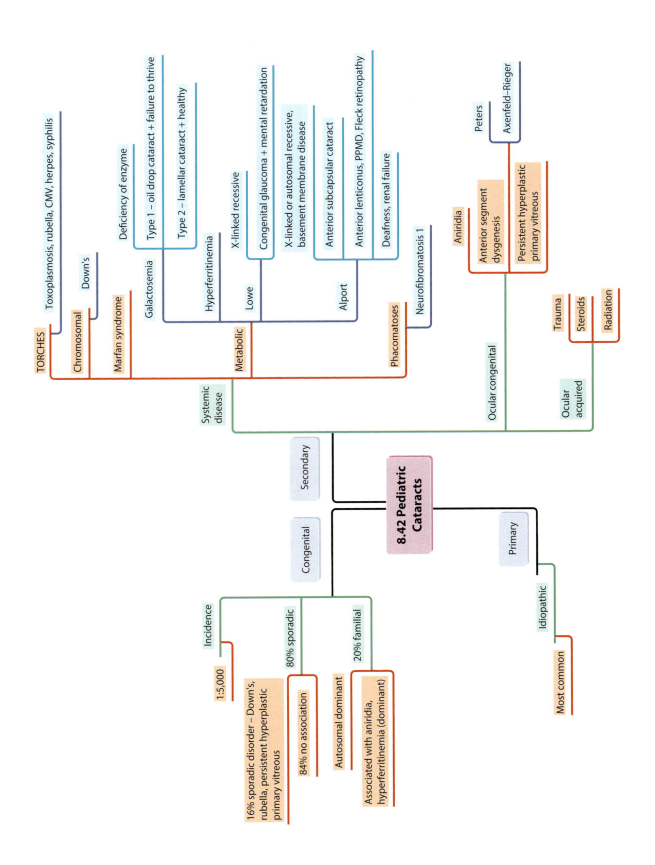

8.42 Pediatric Cataracts

Secondary

Congenital

Primary

Systemic disease

Ocular congenital

Ocular acquired

TORCHES — Toxoplasmosis, rubella, CMV, herpes, syphilis

Chromosomal — Down's

Marfan syndrome

Metabolic
- Galactosemia
  - Deficiency of enzyme
  - Type 1 – oil drop cataract + failure to thrive
  - Type 2 – lamellar cataract + healthy
- Hyperferritinemia
- Lowe
  - X-linked recessive
  - Congenital glaucoma + mental retardation
- Alport — X-linked or autosomal recessive, basement membrane disease
  - Anterior subcapsular cataract
  - Anterior lenticonus, PPMD, Fleck retinopathy
  - Deafness, renal failure

Phacomatoses — Neurofibromatosis 1

Aniridia

Anterior segment dysgenesis
- Peters
- Axenfeld–Rieger

Persistent hyperplastic primary vitreous

Trauma

Steroids

Radiation

Idiopathic — Most common

Incidence — 1:5,000

80% sporadic
- 16% sporadic disorder – Down's, rubella, persistent hyperplastic primary vitreous
- 84% no association

20% familial
- Autosomal dominant
- Associated with aniridia, hyperferritinemia (dominant)

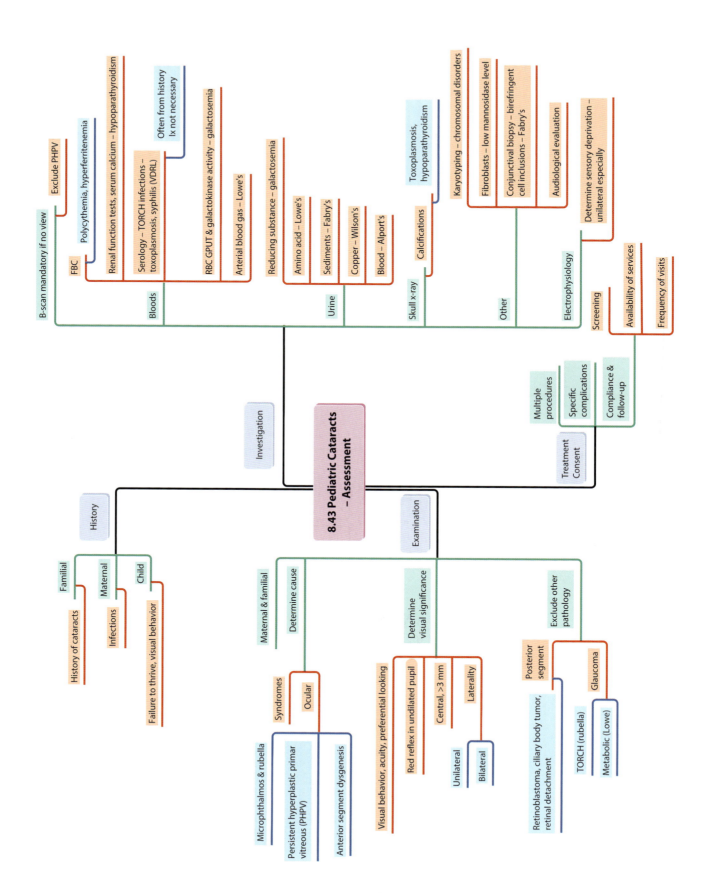

8.43 Pediatric Cataracts – Assessment

Investigation

Bloods
- B-scan mandatory if no view
  - Exclude PHPV
- FBC
  - Polycythemia, hyperferritenemia
- Renal function tests, serum calcium – hypoparathyroidism
- Serology – TORCH infections – toxoplasmosis, syphilis (VDRL)
  - Often from history Ix not necessary
- RBC GPUT & galactokinase activity – galactosemia
- Arterial blood gas – Lowe's

Urine
- Reducing substance – galactosemia
- Amino acid – Lowe's
- Sediments – Fabry's
- Copper – Wilson's
- Blood – Alport's

Skull x-ray
- Calcifications
  - Toxoplasmosis, hypoparathyroidism

Other
- Karyotyping – chromosomal disorders
- Fibroblasts – low mannosidase level
- Conjunctival biopsy – birefringent cell inclusions – Fabry's
- Audiological evaluation
- Determine sensory deprivation – unilateral especially

Electrophysiology

Screening
- Availability of services
- Frequency of visits

Treatment Consent
- Multiple procedures
- Specific complications
- Compliance & follow-up

History

Familial
- History of cataracts

Maternal
- Infections

Child
- Failure to thrive, visual behavior

Examination

Maternal & familial

Determine cause
- Syndromes
- Ocular
  - Microphthalmos & rubella
  - Persistent hyperplastic primar vitreous (PHPV)
  - Anterior segment dysgenesis

Determine visual significance
- Visual behavior, acuity, preferential looking
- Red reflex in undilated pupil
  - Central, >3 mm
  - Laterality
    - Unilateral
    - Bilateral

Exclude other pathology
- Posterior segment
  - Retinoblastoma, ciliary body tumor, retinal detachment
- Glaucoma
  - TORCH (rubella)
  - Metabolic (Lowe)

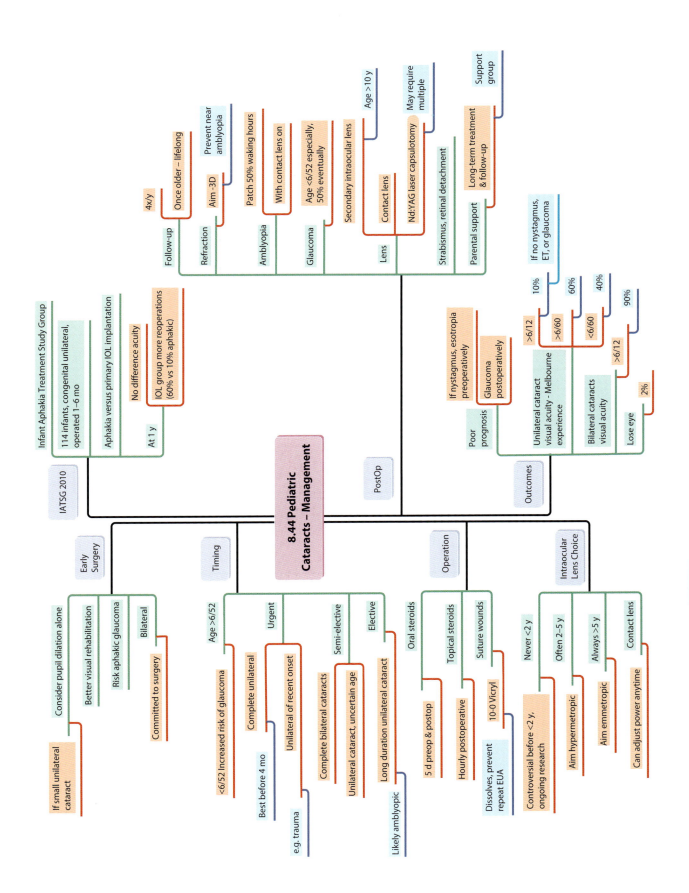

8.44 Pediatric Cataracts – Management

IATSG 2010
- Infant Aphakia Treatment Study Group
  - 114 infants, congenital unilateral, operated 1–6 mo
  - Aphakia versus primary IOL implantation
    - At 1 y
      - No difference acuity
      - IOL group more reoperations (60% vs 10% aphakic)

Early Surgery
- Consider pupil dilation alone
  - If small unilateral cataract
- Better visual rehabilitation
- Risk aphakic glaucoma
- Bilateral
  - Committed to surgery

Timing
- Age >6/52
  - <6/52 Increased risk of glaucoma
- Urgent
  - Best before 4 mo
    - e.g. trauma
  - Complete unilateral
  - Unilateral of recent onset
- Semi-elective
  - Complete bilateral cataracts
  - Unilateral cataract, uncertain age
- Elective
  - Long duration unilateral cataract
    - Likely amblyopic

Operation
- Oral steroids
  - 5 d preop & postop
- Topical steroids
  - Hourly postoperative
- Suture wounds
  - 10-0 Vicryl
    - Dissolves, prevent repeat EUA

Intraocular Lens Choice
- Never <2 y
  - Controversial before <2 y, ongoing research
- Often 2–5 y
  - Aim hypermetropic
- Always >5 y
  - Aim emmetropic
- Contact lens
  - Can adjust power anytime

PostOp
- Follow-up
  - 4x/y
  - Once older – lifelong
- Refraction
  - Prevent near amblyopia
  - Aim –3D
- Amblyopia
  - Patch 50% waking hours
  - With contact lens on
- Glaucoma
  - Age <6/52 especially, 50% eventually
- Lens
  - Secondary intraocular lens
    - Age >10 y
  - Contact lens
  - Nd:YAG laser capsulotomy
    - May require multiple
- Strabismus, retinal detachment
- Parental support
  - Long-term treatment & follow-up
    - Support group

Outcomes
- Poor prognosis
  - If nystagmus, esotropia preoperatively
  - Glaucoma postoperatively
- Unilateral cataract visual acuity - Melbourne experience
  - >6/12
    - If no nystagmus, ET, or glaucoma
    - 10%
  - >6/60
    - 60%
  - <6/60
    - 40%
- Bilateral cataracts visual acuity
  - >6/12
    - 90%
  - Lose eye
    - 2%

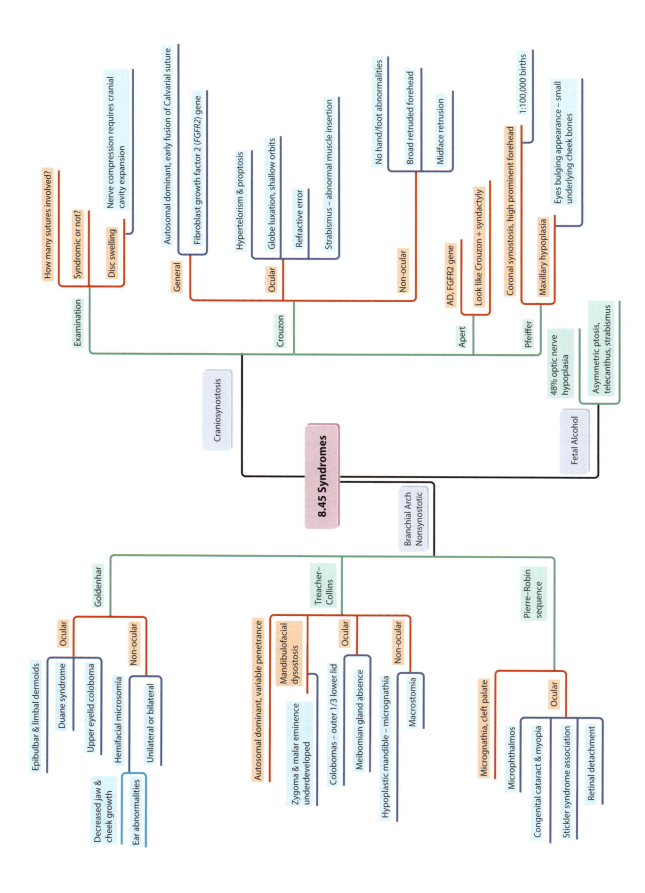

8.45 Syndromes

Craniosynostosis

Examination
- How many sutures involved?
- Syndromic or not?
- Disc swelling
  - Nerve compression requires cranial cavity expansion

Crouzon
- General
  - Autosomal dominant, early fusion of Calvarial suture
  - Fibroblast growth factor 2 (*FGFR2*) gene
- Ocular
  - Hypertelorism & proptosis
  - Globe luxation, shallow orbits
  - Refractive error
  - Strabismus – abnormal muscle insertion
- Non-ocular

Apert
- AD, FGFR2 gene
- Look like Crouzon + syndactyly
- No hand/foot abnormalities
  - Broad retruded forehead
  - Midface retrusion

Pfeiffer
- Coronal synostosis, high prominent forehead
  - 1:100,000 births
- Maxillary hypoplasia
  - Eyes bulging appearance – small underlying cheek bones

Fetal Alcohol
- 48% optic nerve hypoplasia
- Asymmetric ptosis, telecanthus, strabismus

Branchial Arch Nonsynostotic

Goldenhar
- Ocular
  - Epibulbar & limbal dermoids
  - Duane syndrome
  - Upper eyelid coloboma
- Non-ocular
  - Hemifacial microsomia
  - Unilateral or bilateral
  - Decreased jaw & cheek growth
  - Ear abnormalities

Treacher–Collins
- Mandibulofacial dysostosis
  - Autosomal dominant, variable penetrance
  - Zygoma & malar eminence underdeveloped
- Ocular
  - Colobomas – outer 1/3 lower lid
  - Meibomian gland absence
- Non-ocular
  - Hypoplastic mandible – micrognathia
  - Macrostomia

Pierre–Robin sequence
- Micrognathia, cleft palate
- Ocular
  - Microphthalmos
  - Congenital cataract & myopia
  - Stickler syndrome association
  - Retinal detachment

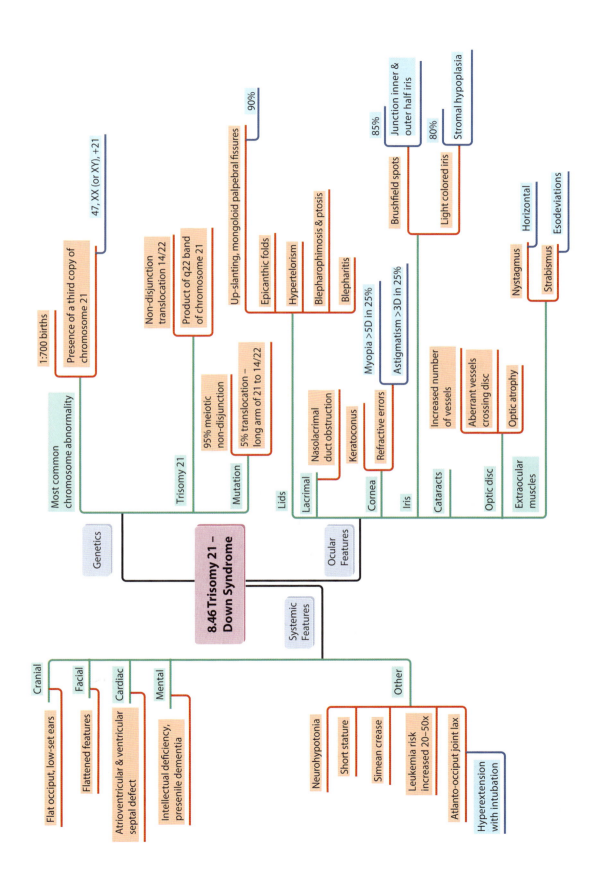

8.46 Trisomy 21 – Down Syndrome

Genetics
- Most common chromosome abnormality
  - 1:700 births
  - Presence of a third copy of chromosome 21
    - 47, XX (or XY), +21
- Trisomy 21
  - Non-disjunction translocation 14/22
  - Product of q22 band of chromosome 21
- Mutation
  - 95% meiotic non-disjunction
  - 5% translocation – long arm of 21 to 14/22

Ocular Features
- Lids
  - Up-slanting, mongoloid palpebral fissures — 90%
  - Epicanthic folds
  - Hypertelorism
  - Blepharophimosis & ptosis
  - Blepharitis
- Lacrimal
  - Nasolacrimal duct obstruction
- Cornea
  - Keratoconus
  - Refractive errors
    - Myopia >5D in 25%
    - Astigmatism >3D in 25%
- Iris
  - Brushfield spots — 85%
    - Junction inner & outer half iris
  - Light colored iris — 80%
    - Stromal hypoplasia
- Cataracts
  - Increased number of vessels
- Optic disc
  - Aberrant vessels crossing disc
  - Optic atrophy
- Extraocular muscles
  - Nystagmus
    - Horizontal
  - Strabismus
    - Esodeviations

Systemic Features
- Cranial
  - Flat occiput, low-set ears
- Facial
  - Flattened features
- Cardiac
  - Atrioventricular & ventricular septal defect
- Mental
  - Intellectual deficiency, presenile dementia
- Other
  - Neurohypotonia
  - Short stature
  - Simean crease
  - Leukemia risk increased 20–50x
  - Atlanto-occiput joint lax
    - Hyperextension with intubation

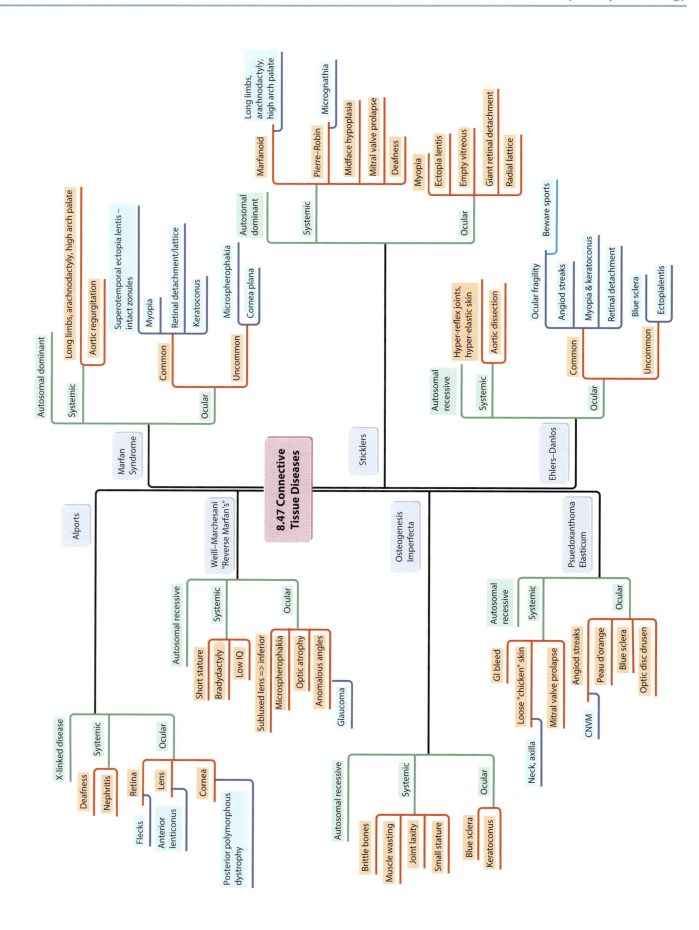

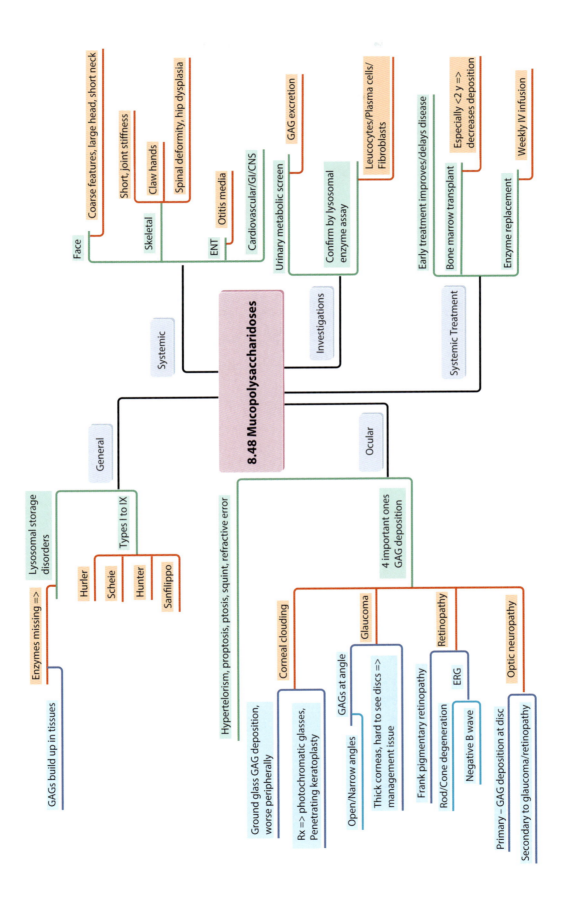

8.48 Mucopolysaccharidoses

Systemic

Face
- Coarse features, large head, short neck

Skeletal
- Short, joint stiffness
- Claw hands
- Spinal deformity, hip dysplasia

ENT
- Otitis media

Cardiovascular/GI/CNS

Investigations
- Urinary metabolic screen
  - GAG excretion
- Confirm by lysosomal enzyme assay
  - Leucocytes/Plasma cells/Fibroblasts

Systemic Treatment
- Early treatment improves/delays disease
- Bone marrow transplant
  - Especially <2 y => decreases deposition
- Enzyme replacement
  - Weekly IV infusion

General
- Lysosomal storage disorders
  - Enzymes missing =>
    - GAGs build up in tissues
- Types I to IX
  - Hurler
  - Scheie
  - Hunter
  - Sanfilippo

Ocular
- Hypertelorism, proptosis, ptosis, squint, refractive error
- 4 important ones GAG deposition
  - Corneal clouding
    - Ground glass GAG deposition, worse peripherally
    - Rx => photochromatic glasses, Penetrating keratoplasty
  - Glaucoma
    - GAGs at angle
      - Open/Narrow angles
    - Thick corneas, hard to see discs => management issue
  - Retinopathy
    - Frank pigmentary retinopathy
    - Rod/Cone degeneration
    - ERG
      - Negative B wave
  - Optic neuropathy
    - Primary – GAG deposition at disc
    - Secondary to glaucoma/retinopathy

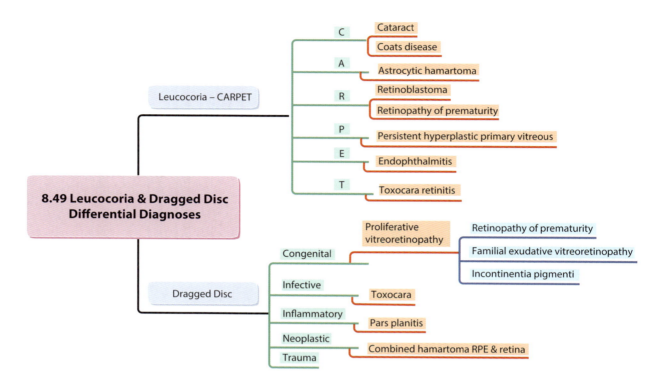

8.49 Leucocoria & Dragged Disc Differential Diagnoses

Leucocoria – CARPET

- C — Cataract
- C — Coats disease
- A — Astrocytic hamartoma
- R — Retinoblastoma
- R — Retinopathy of prematurity
- P — Persistent hyperplastic primary vitreous
- E — Endophthalmitis
- T — Toxocara retinitis

Dragged Disc

- Congenital — Proliferative vitreoretinopathy — Retinopathy of prematurity, Familial exudative vitreoretinopathy, Incontinentia pigmenti
- Infective — Toxocara
- Inflammatory — Pars planitis
- Neoplastic — Combined hamartoma RPE & retina
- Trauma

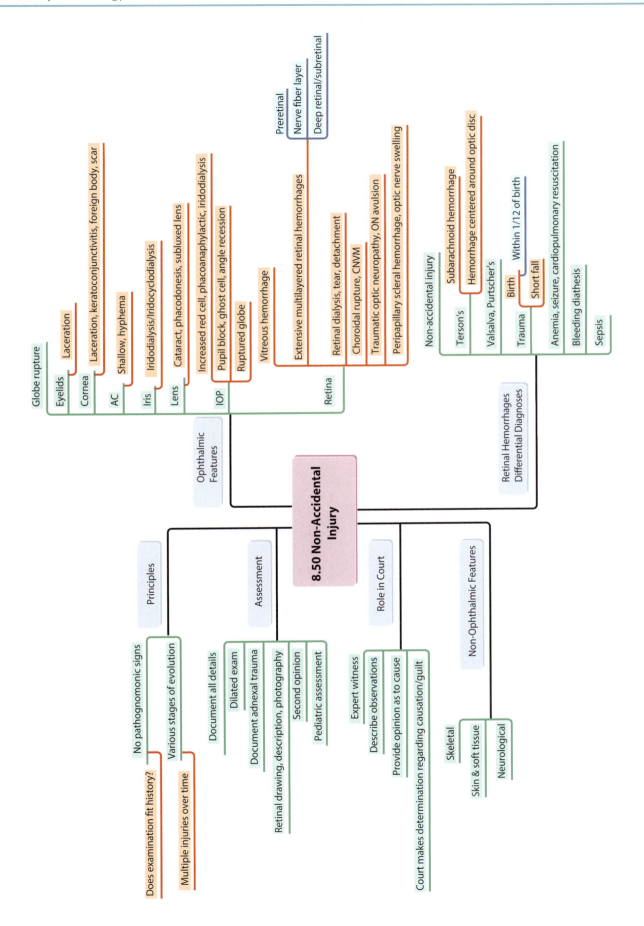

8.50 Non-Accidental Injury

Ophthalmic Features

Globe rupture

Eyelids — Laceration

Cornea — Laceration, keratoconjunctivitis, foreign body, scar

AC — Shallow, hyphema

Iris — Iridodialysis/Iridocyclodialysis

Lens — Cataract, phacodonesis, subluxed lens

IOP — Increased red cell, phacoanaphylactic, iridodialysis
— Pupil block, ghost cell, angle recession
— Ruptured globe

Retina — Vitreous hemorrhage
— Extensive multilayered retinal hemorrhages
— Retinal dialysis, tear, detachment
— Choroidal rupture, CNVM
— Traumatic optic neuropathy, ON avulsion
— Peripapillary scleral hemorrhage, optic nerve swelling

Preretinal
Nerve fiber layer
Deep retinal/subretinal

Retinal Hemorrhages Differential Diagnoses

Non-accidental injury
Terson's — Subarachnoid hemorrhage
Valsalva, Purtscher's — Hemorrhage centered around optic disc
Trauma — Birth — Within 1/12 of birth
— Short fall
Anemia, seizure, cardiopulmonary resuscitation
Bleeding diathesis
Sepsis

Principles

No pathognomonic signs
Various stages of evolution — Does examination fit history?
— Multiple injuries over time

Assessment

Document all details
Dilated exam
Document adnexal trauma
Retinal drawing, description, photography
Second opinion
Pediatric assessment

Role in Court

Expert witness
Describe observations
Provide opinion as to cause
Court makes determination regarding causation/guilt

Non-Ophthalmic Features

Skeletal
Skin & soft tissue
Neurological

9 Retina and Vitreous

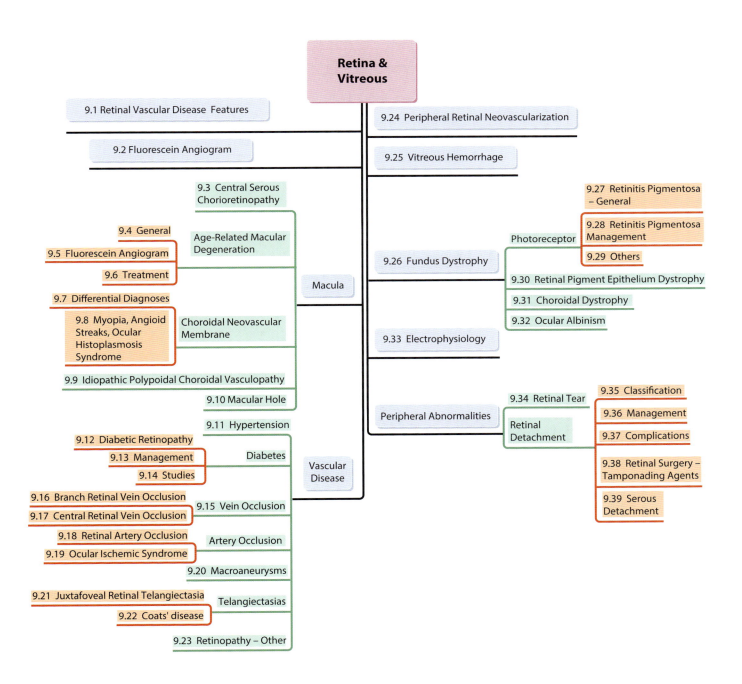

Retina & Vitreous

9.1 Retinal Vascular Disease Features

9.2 Fluorescein Angiogram

Macula

9.3 Central Serous Chorioretinopathy

Age-Related Macular Degeneration
- 9.4 General
- 9.5 Fluorescein Angiogram
- 9.6 Treatment
- 9.7 Differential Diagnoses
- 9.8 Myopia, Angioid Streaks, Ocular Histoplasmosis Syndrome

Choroidal Neovascular Membrane

9.9 Idiopathic Polypoidal Choroidal Vasculopathy

9.10 Macular Hole

Vascular Disease

Diabetes
- 9.11 Hypertension
- 9.12 Diabetic Retinopathy
- 9.13 Management
- 9.14 Studies

Vein Occlusion
- 9.16 Branch Retinal Vein Occlusion
- 9.17 Central Retinal Vein Occlusion
- 9.15 Vein Occlusion

Artery Occlusion
- 9.18 Retinal Artery Occlusion
- 9.19 Ocular Ischemic Syndrome

9.20 Macroaneurysms

Telangiectasias
- 9.21 Juxtafoveal Retinal Telangiectasia
- 9.22 Coats' disease

9.23 Retinopathy – Other

9.24 Peripheral Retinal Neovascularization

9.25 Vitreous Hemorrhage

9.26 Fundus Dystrophy

Photoreceptor
- 9.27 Retinitis Pigmentosa – General
- 9.28 Retinitis Pigmentosa Management
- 9.29 Others

9.30 Retinal Pigment Epithelium Dystrophy

9.31 Choroidal Dystrophy

9.32 Ocular Albinism

9.33 Electrophysiology

Peripheral Abnormalities

9.34 Retinal Tear

Retinal Detachment
- 9.35 Classification
- 9.36 Management
- 9.37 Complications
- 9.38 Retinal Surgery – Tamponading Agents
- 9.39 Serous Detachment

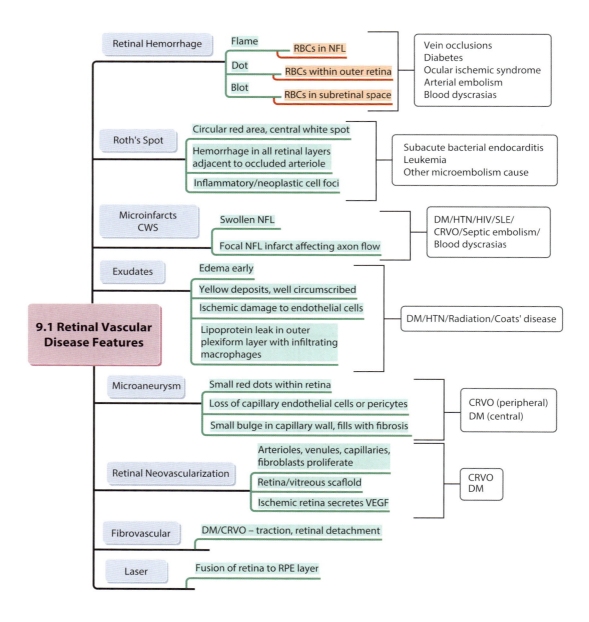

Retinal Hemorrhage
- Flame — RBCs in NFL
- Dot — RBCs within outer retina
- Blot — RBCs in subretinal space

Vein occlusions
Diabetes
Ocular ischemic syndrome
Arterial embolism
Blood dyscrasias

Roth's Spot
- Circular red area, central white spot
- Hemorrhage in all retinal layers adjacent to occluded arteriole
- Inflammatory/neoplastic cell foci

Subacute bacterial endocarditis
Leukemia
Other microembolism cause

Microinfarcts CWS
- Swollen NFL
- Focal NFL infarct affecting axon flow

DM/HTN/HIV/SLE/CRVO/Septic embolism/Blood dyscrasias

Exudates
- Edema early
- Yellow deposits, well circumscribed
- Ischemic damage to endothelial cells
- Lipoprotein leak in outer plexiform layer with infiltrating macrophages

DM/HTN/Radiation/Coats' disease

9.1 Retinal Vascular Disease Features

Microaneurysm
- Small red dots within retina
- Loss of capillary endothelial cells or pericytes
- Small bulge in capillary wall, fills with fibrosis

CRVO (peripheral)
DM (central)

Retinal Neovascularization
- Arterioles, venules, capillaries, fibroblasts proliferate
- Retina/vitreous scaflold
- Ischemic retina secretes VEGF

CRVO
DM

Fibrovascular
- DM/CRVO – traction, retinal detachment

Laser
- Fusion of retina to RPE layer

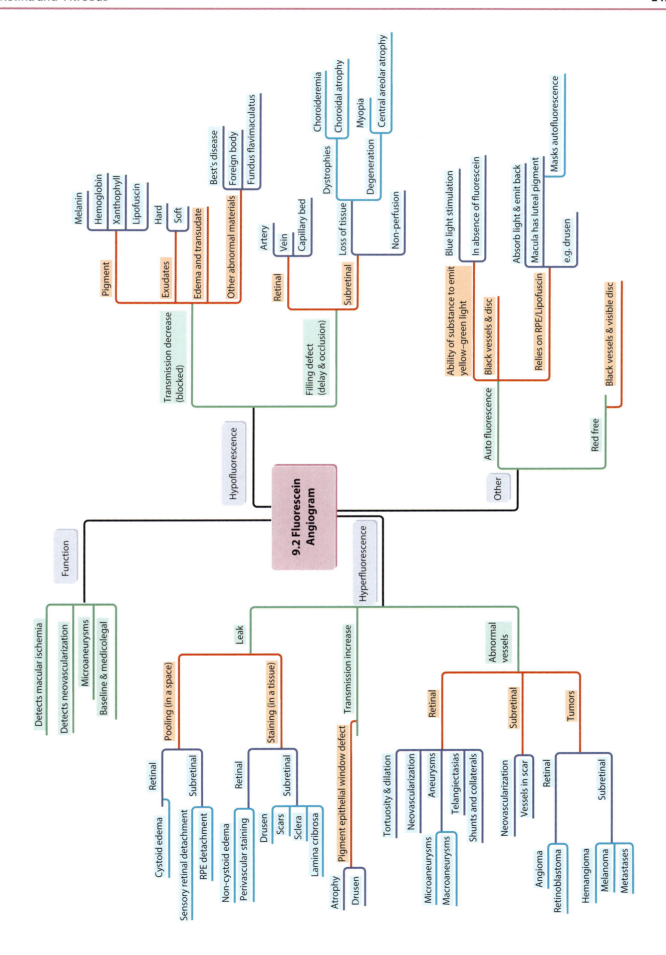

9.2 Fluorescein Angiogram

Hypofluorescence

Transmission decrease (blocked)
- Pigment
  - Melanin
  - Hemoglobin
  - Xanthophyll
  - Lipofuscin
- Exudates
  - Hard
  - Soft
- Edema and transudate
- Other abnormal materials
  - Best's disease
  - Foreign body
  - Fundus flavimaculatus

Filling defect (delay & occlusion)
- Retinal
  - Artery
  - Vein
  - Capillary bed
- Subretinal
  - Loss of tissue
    - Dystrophies
      - Choroideremia
      - Choroidal atrophy
    - Degeneration
      - Myopia
      - Central areolar atrophy
  - Non-perfusion

Other

Auto fluorescence
- Ability of substance to emit yellow–green light
  - Blue light stimulation
  - In absence of fluorescein
- Black vessels & disc
- Relies on RPE/Lipofuscin
  - Absorb light & emit back
  - Macula has luteal pigment
    - Masks autofluorescence
  - e.g. drusen

Red free
- Black vessels & visible disc

Function
- Detects macular ischemia
- Detects neovascularization
- Microaneurysms
- Baseline & medicolegal

Hyperfluorescence

Leak
- Pooling (in a space)
  - Retinal
    - Cystoid edema
  - Subretinal
    - Sensory retinal detachment
    - RPE detachment
- Staining (in a tissue)
  - Retinal
    - Non-cystoid edema
    - Perivascular staining
  - Subretinal
    - Drusen
    - Scars
    - Sclera
    - Lamina cribrosa

Transmission increase
- Pigment epithelial window defect
  - Atrophy
  - Drusen

Abnormal vessels
- Retinal
  - Tortuosity & dilation
  - Neovascularization
  - Aneurysms
    - Microaneurysms
    - Macroaneurysms
  - Telangiectasias
  - Shunts and collaterals
- Subretinal
  - Neovascularization
  - Vessels in scar
- Tumors
  - Retinal
    - Angioma
    - Retinoblastoma
  - Subretinal
    - Hemangioma
    - Melanoma
    - Metastases

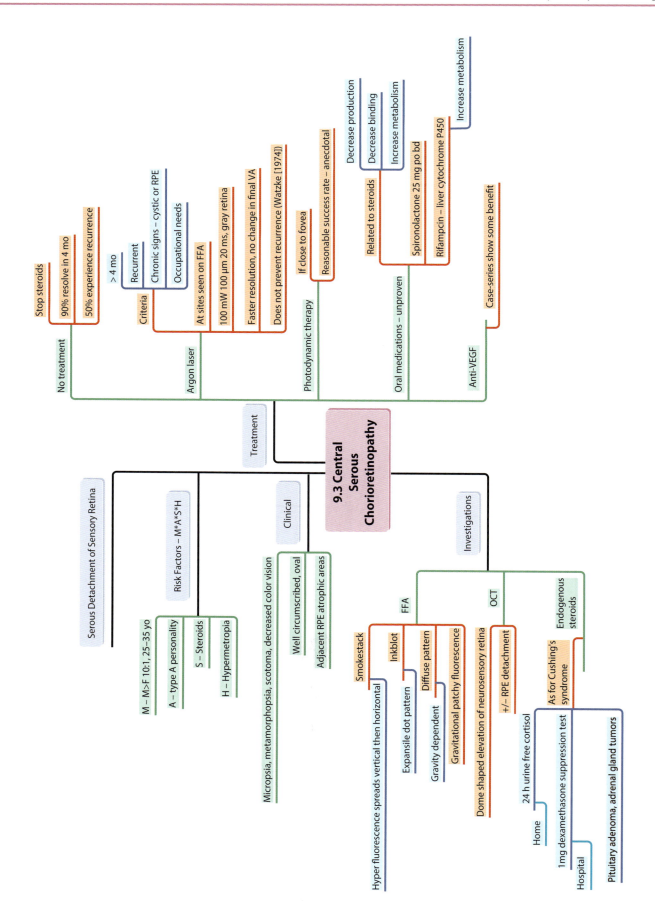

9.3 Central Serous Chorioretinopathy

Treatment

No treatment
- Stop steroids
- 90% resolve in 4 mo
- 50% experience recurrence

Argon laser
- Criteria
  - > 4 mo
  - Recurrent
  - Chronic signs – cystic or RPE
  - Occupational needs
- At sites seen on FFA
- 100 mW 100 μm 20 ms, gray retina
- Faster resolution, no change in final VA
- Does not prevent recurrence (Watzke [1974])

Photodynamic therapy
- If close to fovea
- Reasonable success rate – anecdotal

Oral medications – unproven
- Related to steroids
  - Decrease production
  - Decrease binding
  - Increase metabolism
- Spironolactone 25 mg po bd
- Rifampcin – liver cytochrome P450
  - Increase metabolism

Anti-VEGF
- Case-series show some benefit

Clinical

Serous Detachment of Sensory Retina

Risk Factors – M*A*S*H
- M – M>F 10:1, 25–35 yo
- A – type A personality
- S – Steroids
- H – Hypermetropia

Micropsia, metamorphopsia, scotoma, decreased color vision

- Well circumscribed, oval
- Adjacent RPE atrophic areas

Investigations

FFA
- Smokestack
  - Hyper fluorescence spreads vertical then horizontal
- Inkblot
  - Expansile dot pattern
- Diffuse pattern
  - Gravity dependent
  - Gravitational patchy fluorescence

OCT
- Dome shaped elevation of neurosensory retina
- +/– RPE detachment

Endogenous steroids
- As for Cushing's syndrome
  - 24 h urine free cortisol
    - Home
  - 1mg dexamethasone suppression test
    - Hospital
  - Pituitary adenoma, adrenal gland tumors

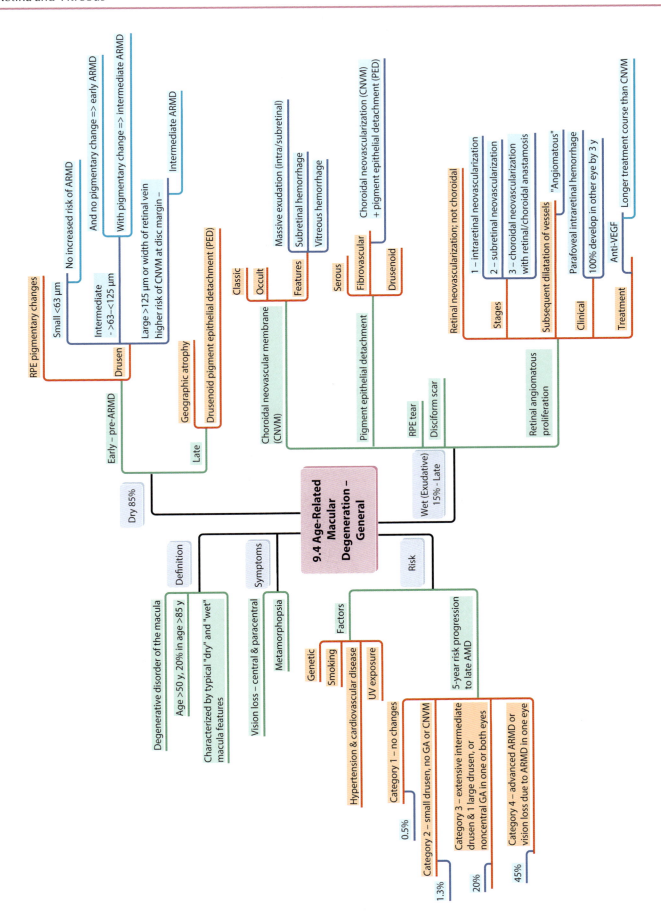

9.4 Age-Related Macular Degeneration – General

Definition
- Degenerative disorder of the macula
- Age >50 y, 20% in age >85 y
- Characterized by typical "dry" and "wet" macula features

Symptoms
- Vision loss – central & paracentral
- Metamorphopsia

Risk
- Factors
  - Genetic
  - Smoking
  - Hypertension & cardiovascular disease
  - UV exposure
- 5-year risk progression to late AMD
  - Category 1 – no changes — 0.5%
  - Category 2 – small drusen, no GA or CNVM — 1.3%
  - Category 3 – extensive intermediate drusen & 1 large drusen, or noncentral GA in one or both eyes — 20%
  - Category 4 – advanced ARMD or vision loss due to ARMD in one eye — 45%

Dry 85%
- Early – pre-ARMD
  - RPE pigmentary changes
  - Drusen
    - Small <63 μm — No increased risk of ARMD
    - Intermediate – >63–<125 μm
      - And no pigmentary change => early ARMD
      - With pigmentary change => intermediate ARMD
    - Large >125 μm or width of retinal vein higher risk of CNVM at disc margin – Intermediate ARMD
- Late
  - Geographic atrophy
  - Drusenoid pigment epithelial detachment (PED)

Wet (Exudative) 15% – Late
- Choroidal neovascular membrane (CNVM)
  - Classic
  - Occult
  - Features
    - Massive exudation (intra/subretinal)
    - Subretinal hemorrhage
    - Vitreous hemorrhage
- Pigment epithelial detachment
  - Serous
  - Fibrovascular
  - Drusenoid — Choroidal neovascularization (CNVM) + pigment epithelial detachment (PED)
- RPE tear
- Disciform scar
- Retinal angiomatous proliferation
  - Retinal neovascularization; not choroidal
  - Stages
    - 1 – intraretinal neovascularization
    - 2 – subretinal neovascularization
    - 3 – choroidal neovascularization with retinal/choroidal anastomosis
  - Subsequent dilatation of vessels — "Angiomatous"
  - Clinical
    - Parafoveal intraretinal hemorrhage
    - 100% develop in other eye by 3 y
  - Treatment
    - Anti-VEGF
    - Longer treatment course than CNVM

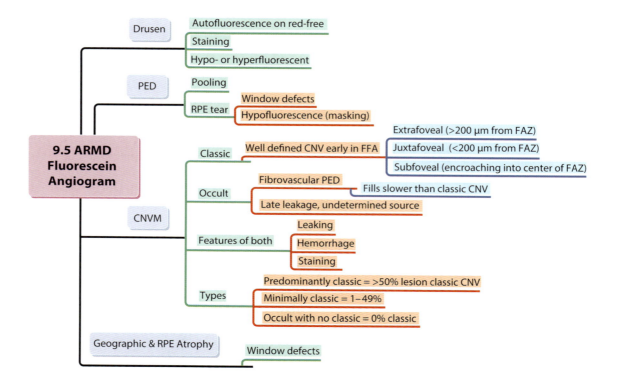

9.5 ARMD Fluorescein Angiogram

Drusen
- Autofluorescence on red-free
- Staining
- Hypo- or hyperfluorescent

PED
- Pooling
- RPE tear
  - Window defects
  - Hypofluorescence (masking)

CNVM
- Classic — Well defined CNV early in FFA
  - Extrafoveal (>200 μm from FAZ)
  - Juxtafoveal (<200 μm from FAZ)
  - Subfoveal (encroaching into center of FAZ)
- Occult
  - Fibrovascular PED — Fills slower than classic CNV
  - Late leakage, undetermined source
- Features of both
  - Leaking
  - Hemorrhage
  - Staining
- Types
  - Predominantly classic = >50% lesion classic CNV
  - Minimally classic = 1–49%
  - Occult with no classic = 0% classic

Geographic & RPE Atrophy
- Window defects

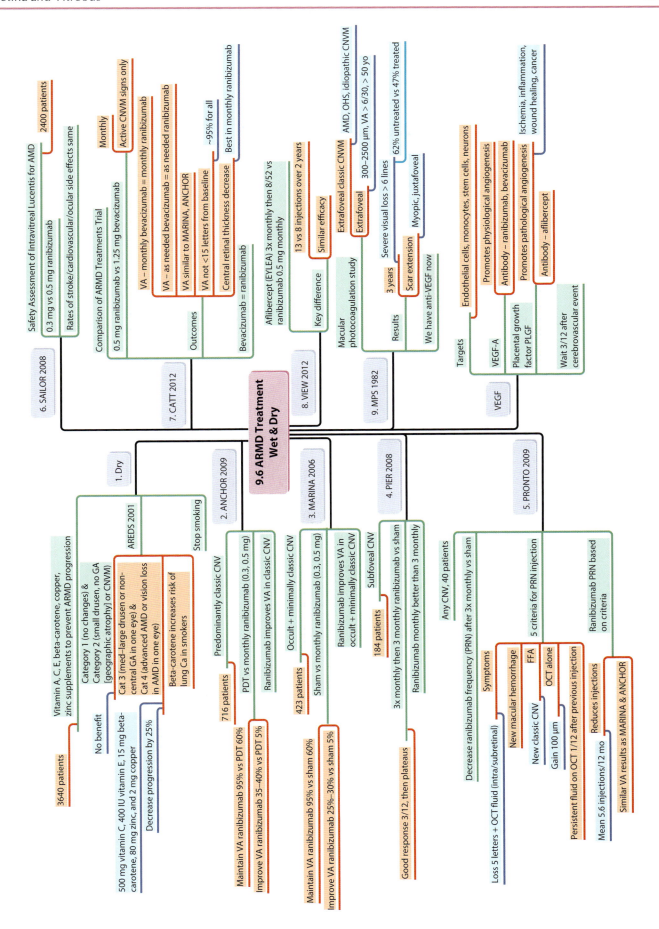

9.6 ARMD Treatment Wet & Dry

1. Dry

AREDS 2001

- Vitamin A, C, E, beta-carotene, copper, zinc supplements to prevent ARMD progression
  - 3640 patients
  - Category 1 (no changes) & Category 2 (small drusen, no GA [geographic atrophy] or CNVM)
    - No benefit
    - 500 mg vitamin C, 400 IU vitamin E, 15 mg beta-carotene, 80 mg zinc, and 2 mg copper
  - Cat 3 (med–large drusen or non-central GA in one eye) & Cat 4 (advanced AMD or vision loss in AMD in one eye)
    - Decrease progression by 25%
    - Beta-carotene increases risk of lung Ca in smokers
- Stop smoking

2. ANCHOR 2009

- Predominantly classic CNV
  - 716 patients
  - PDT vs monthly ranibizumab (0.3, 0.5 mg)
    - Maintain VA ranibizumab 95% vs PDT 60%
    - Improve VA ranibizumab 35–40% vs PDT 5%
  - Ranibizumab improves VA in classic CNV

3. MARINA 2006

- Occult + minimally classic CNV
  - 423 patients
  - Sham vs monthly ranibizumab (0.3, 0.5 mg)
    - Maintain VA ranibizumab 95% vs sham 60%
    - Improve VA ranibizumab 25%–30% vs sham 5%
  - Ranibizumab improves VA in occult + minimally classic CNV

4. PIER 2008

- Subfoveal CNV
  - 184 patients
  - 3x monthly then 3 monthly ranibizumab vs sham
    - Good response 3/12, then plateaus
  - Ranibizumab monthly better than 3 monthly

5. PRONTO 2009

- Any CNV, 40 patients
  - Decrease ranibizumab frequency (PRN) after 3x monthly vs sham
    - Loss 5 letters + OCT fluid (intra/subretinal)
  - 5 criteria for PRN injection
    - Symptoms
    - New macular hemorrhage
    - New classic CNV
    - FFA
    - OCT alone
    - Gain 100 µm
    - Persistent fluid on OCT 1/12 after previous injection
  - Ranibizumab PRN based on criteria
    - Reduces injections
    - Mean 5.6 injections/12 mo
    - Similar VA results as MARINA & ANCHOR

6. SAILOR 2008

- Safety Assessment of Intravitreal Lucentis for AMD
  - 2400 patients
  - 0.3 mg vs 0.5 mg ranibizumab
  - Rates of stroke/cardiovascular/ocular side effects same

7. CATT 2012

- Comparison of ARMD Treatments Trial
  - 0.5 mg ranibizumab vs 1.25 mg bevacizumab
    - Monthly
    - Active CNVM signs only
  - Outcomes
    - VA – monthly bevacizumab = monthly ranibizumab
    - VA – as needed bevacizumab = as needed ranibizumab
    - VA similar to MARINA, ANCHOR
    - VA not <15 letters from baseline
    - ~95% for all
    - Central retinal thickness decrease
    - Best in monthly ranibizumab
  - Bevacizumab = ranibizumab

8. VIEW 2012

- Aflibercept (EYLEA) 3x monthly then 8/52 vs ranibizumab 0.5 mg monthly
  - 13 vs 8 injections over 2 years
  - Similar efficacy
  - Key difference
    - Extrafoveal classic CNVM
    - Extrafoveal

9. MPS 1982

- Macular photocoagulation study
  - AMD, OHS, idiopathic CNVM
  - 300–2500 µm, VA > 6/30, > 50 yo
  - Severe visual loss > 6 lines
    - 62% untreated vs 47% treated
    - Myopic, juxtafoveal
  - Results
    - 3 years
      - Scar extension
    - We have anti-VEGF now

VEGF

- Targets
  - Endothelial cells, monocytes, stem cells, neurons
- VEGF-A
  - Promotes physiological angiogenesis
  - Antibody – ranibizumab, bevacizumab
- Placental growth factor PLGF
  - Promotes pathological angiogenesis
  - Antibody – aflibercept
  - Ischemia, inflammation, wound healing, cancer
- Wait 3/12 after cerebrovascular event

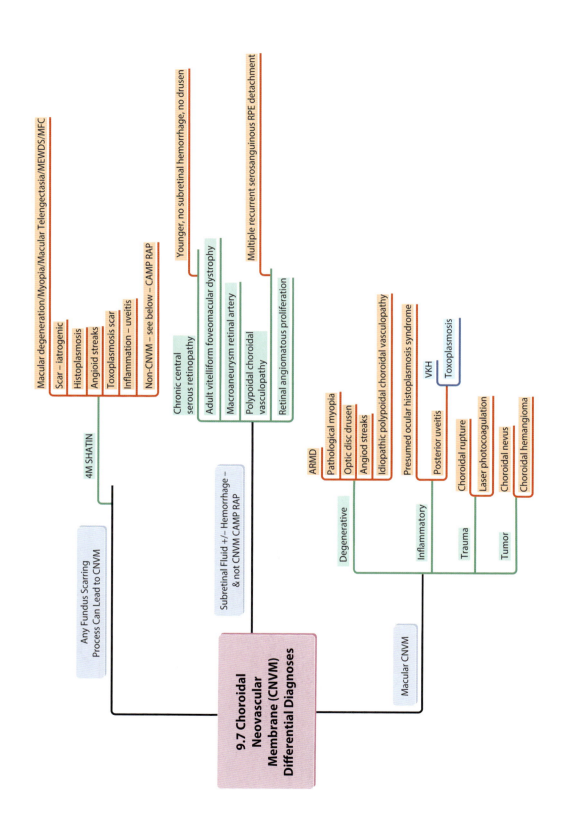

9.7 Choroidal Neovascular Membrane (CNVM) Differential Diagnoses

Any Fundus Scarring Process Can Lead to CNVM

4M SHATIN

Macular degeneration/Myopia/Macular Telengectasia/MEWDS/MFC
Scar – iatrogenic
Histoplasmosis
Angioid streaks
Toxoplasmosis scar
Inflammation – uveitis
Non-CNVM – see below – CAMP RAP

Subretinal Fluid +/– Hemorrhage – & not CNVM CAMP RAP

Chronic central serous retinopathy
Adult vitelliform foveomacular dystrophy — Younger, no subretinal hemorrhage, no drusen
Macroaneurysm retinal artery
Polypoidal choroidal vasculopathy — Multiple recurrent serosanguinous RPE detachment
Retinal angiomatous proliferation

Macular CNVM

Degenerative
ARMD
Pathological myopia
Optic disc drusen
Angioid streaks
Idiopathic polypoidal choroidal vasculopathy

Inflammatory
Presumed ocular histoplasmosis syndrome
VKH
Toxoplasmosis
Posterior uveitis

Trauma
Choroidal rupture
Laser photocoagulation

Tumor
Choroidal nevus
Choroidal hemangioma

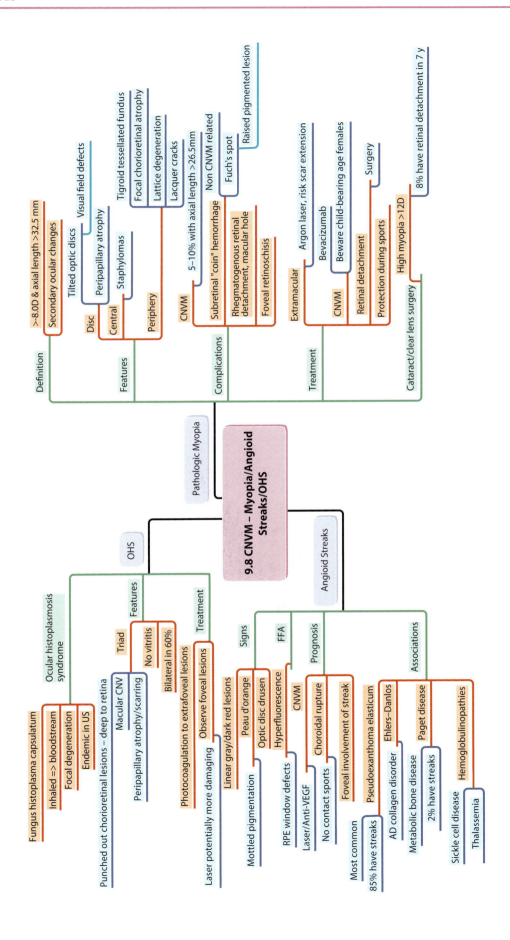

9.8 CNVM – Myopia/Angioid Streaks/OHS

Pathologic Myopia

Definition
- >8.0D & axial length >32.5 mm

Features
- Secondary ocular changes
- Disc
  - Tilted optic discs
  - Visual field defects
  - Peripapillary atrophy
- Central
  - Staphylomas
  - Tigroid tessellated fundus
  - Focal chorioretinal atrophy
  - Lattice degeneration
  - Lacquer cracks
- Periphery

Complications
- CNVM
  - 5–10% with axial length >26.5mm
  - Non CNVM related
  - Fuch's spot
  - Raised pigmented lesion
- Subretinal "coin" hemorrhage
- Rhegmatogenous retinal detachment, macular hole
- Foveal retinoschisis

Treatment
- Extramacular
  - Argon laser, risk scar extension
- CNVM
  - Bevacizumab
- Retinal detachment
  - Beware child-bearing age females
- Protection during sports
  - Surgery
- High myopia >12D
- Cataract/clear lens surgery
  - 8% have retinal detachment in 7 y

OHS

Ocular histoplasmosis syndrome
- Fungus histoplasma capsulatum
- Inhaled => bloodstream
- Focal degeneration
- Endemic in US
- Punched out chorioretinal lesions – deep to retina

Features
- Triad
  - Macular CNV
  - Peripapillary atrophy/scarring
  - No vitritis
  - Bilateral in 60%

Treatment
- Photocoagulation to extrafoveal lesions
- Observe foveal lesions
- Laser potentially more damaging

Angioid Streaks

Signs
- Linear gray/dark red lesions
- Peau d'orange
- Mottled pigmentation
- Optic disc drusen

FFA
- Hyperfluorescence
- RPE window defects

Prognosis
- CNVM
  - Laser/Anti-VEGF
  - No contact sports
- Choroidal rupture
- Foveal involvement of streak

Associations
- Pseudoexanthoma elasticum
  - Most common
  - 85% have streaks
  - AD collagen disorder
- Ehlers–Danlos
- Metabolic bone disease
- Paget disease
  - 2% have streaks
- Hemoglobulinopathies
  - Sickle cell disease
  - Thalassemia

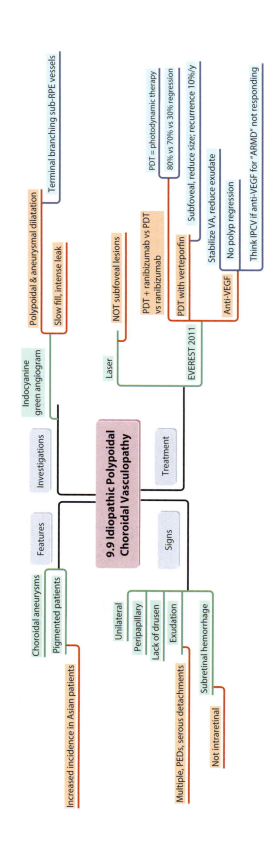

9.9 Idiopathic Polypoidal Choroidal Vasculopathy

Features
- Choroidal aneurysms
- Pigmented patients
  - Increased incidence in Asian patients

Investigations
- Indocyanine green angiogram
  - Polypoidal & aneurysmal dilatation
    - Terminal branching sub-RPE vessels
  - Slow fill, intense leak

Signs
- Unilateral
- Peripapillary
- Lack of drusen
- Exudation
  - Multiple, PEDs, serous detachments
- Subretinal hemorrhage
  - Not intraretinal

Treatment
- Laser
  - NOT subfoveal lesions
- EVEREST 2011
  - PDT + ranibizumab vs PDT vs ranibizumab
  - PDT with verteporfin
    - PDT = photodynamic therapy
    - 80% vs 70% vs 30% regression
    - Subfoveal, reduce size; recurrence 10%/y
    - Stabilize VA, reduce exudate
  - Anti-VEGF
    - No polyp regression
    - Think IPCV if anti-VEGF for "ARMD" not responding

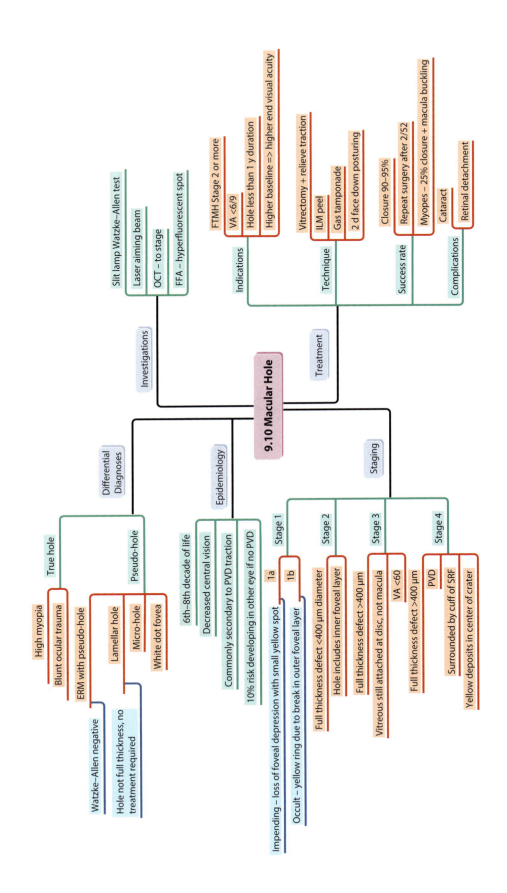

9.10 Macular Hole

Investigations
- Slit lamp Watzke–Allen test
- Laser aiming beam
- OCT – to stage
- FFA – hyperfluorescent spot

Treatment
- Indications
  - FTMH Stage 2 or more
  - VA <6/9
  - Hole less than 1 y duration
  - Higher baseline => higher end visual acuity
- Technique
  - Vitrectomy + relieve traction
  - ILM peel
  - Gas tamponade
  - 2 d face down posturing
- Success rate
  - Closure 90–95%
  - Repeat surgery after 2/52
  - Myopes – 25% closure + macula buckling
- Complications
  - Cataract
  - Retinal detachment

Differential Diagnoses
- True hole
  - High myopia
  - Blunt ocular trauma
  - ERM with pseudo-hole
- Pseudo-hole
  - Lamellar hole
  - Micro-hole
  - White dot fovea
    - Watzke–Allen negative
    - Hole not full thickness, no treatment required

Epidemiology
- 6th–8th decade of life
- Decreased central vision
- Commonly secondary to PVD traction
- 10% risk developing in other eye if no PVD

Staging
- Stage 1
  - 1a
  - 1b
    - Impending – loss of foveal depression with small yellow spot
    - Occult – yellow ring due to break in outer foveal layer
- Stage 2
  - Full thickness defect <400 μm diameter
  - Hole includes inner foveal layer
- Stage 3
  - Full thickness defect >400 μm
  - Vitreous still attached at disc, not macula
  - VA <60
- Stage 4
  - Full thickness defect >400 μm
  - PVD
  - Surrounded by cuff of SRF
  - Yellow deposits in center of crater

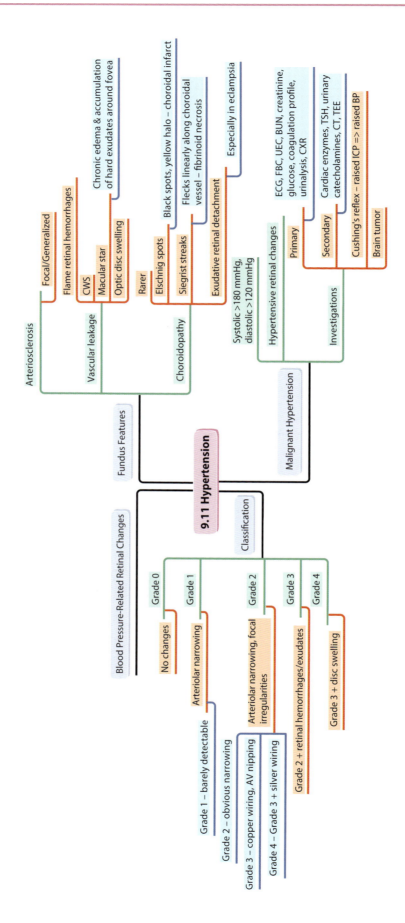

9.11 Hypertension

Fundus Features

Arteriosclerosis

Vascular leakage
- Focal/Generalized
- Flame retinal hemorrhages
- CWS
- Macular star
- Optic disc swelling
  - Chronic edema & accumulation of hard exudates around fovea

Choroidopathy
- Rarer
- Elschnig spots
  - Black spots, yellow halo – choroidal infarct
- Siegrist streaks
  - Flecks linearly along choroidal vessel – fibrinoid necrosis
- Exudative retinal detachment
  - Especially in eclampsia

Malignant Hypertension
- Systolic >180 mmHg, diastolic >120 mmHg
- Hypertensive retinal changes
- Investigations
  - Primary
    - ECG, FBC, UEC, BUN, creatinine, glucose, coagulation profile, urinalysis, CXR
  - Secondary
    - Cardiac enzymes, TSH, urinary catecholamines, CT, TEE
    - Cushing's reflex – raised ICP => raised BP
    - Brain tumor

Classification

Blood Pressure-Related Retinal Changes
- Grade 0
  - No changes
- Grade 1
  - Arteriolar narrowing
    - Grade 1 – barely detectable
    - Grade 2 – obvious narrowing
    - Grade 3 – copper wiring, AV nipping
    - Grade 4 – Grade 3 + silver wiring
- Grade 2
  - Arteriolar narrowing, focal irregularities
- Grade 3
  - Grade 2 + retinal hemorrhages/exudates
- Grade 4
  - Grade 3 + disc swelling

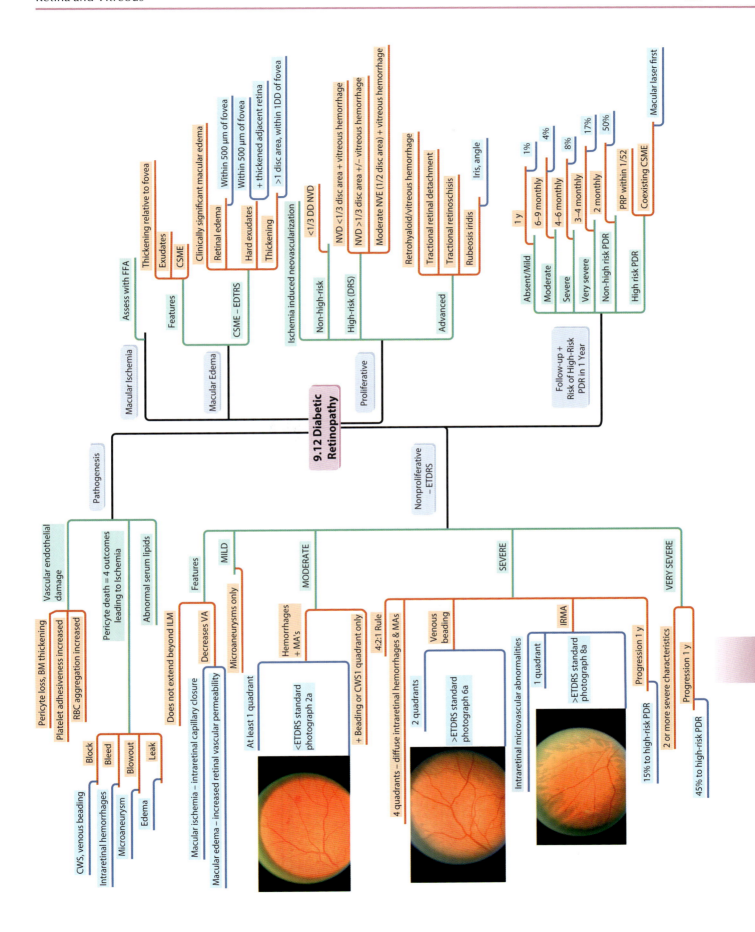

9.12 Diabetic Retinopathy

Macular Ischemia
- Assess with FFA
  - Thickening relative to fovea
  - Exudates
  - CSME

Macular Edema
- Features
  - Retinal edema — Clinically significant macular edema
  - Hard exudates — Within 500 μm of fovea
    - Within 500 μm of fovea
    - + thickened adjacent retina
  - Thickening — >1 disc area, within 1DD of fovea
- CSME – EDTRS

Proliferative
- Ischemia induced neovascularization
  - Non-high-risk — <1/3 DD NVD
  - High-risk (DRS)
    - NVD <1/3 disc area + vitreous hemorrhage
    - NVD >1/3 disc area +/− vitreous hemorrhage
    - Moderate NVE (1/2 disc area) + vitreous hemorrhage
  - Advanced
    - Retrohyaloid/vitreous hemorrhage
    - Tractional retinal detachment
    - Tractional retinoschisis
    - Rubeosis iridis
    - Iris, angle

Follow-up + Risk of High-Risk PDR in 1 Year
- Absent/Mild — 1 y — 1%
- Moderate — 6–9 monthly — 4%
- Severe — 4–6 monthly — 8%
- Very severe — 3–4 monthly — 17%
- Non-high risk PDR — 2 monthly — 50%
- High risk PDR — PRP within 1/52
  - Coexisting CSME — Macular laser first

Pathogenesis
- Vascular endothelial damage
  - Pericyte loss, BM thickening
  - Platelet adhesiveness increased
  - RBC aggregation increased
- Pericyte death = 4 outcomes leading to Ischemia
  - Block — CWS, venous beading
  - Bleed — Intraretinal hemorrhages
  - Blowout — Microaneurysm
  - Leak — Edema
- Abnormal serum lipids

Nonproliferative – ETDRS
- Features
  - Does not extend beyond ILM
  - Decreases VA
    - Macular ischemia – intraretinal capillary closure
    - Macular edema – increased retinal vascular permeability
- MILD
  - Microaneurysms only
- MODERATE
  - Hemorrhages + MA's
    - At least 1 quadrant — <ETDRS standard photograph 2a
    - + Beading or CWS1 quadrant only
  - 4:2:1 Rule
- SEVERE
  - Hemorrhages and MAs — 4 quadrants – diffuse intraretinal
  - Venous beading — 2 quadrants — >ETDRS standard photograph 6a
  - IRMA — Intraretinal microvascular abnormalities — 1 quadrant — >ETDRS standard photograph 8a
  - Progression 1 y — 15% to high-risk PDR
- VERY SEVERE
  - 2 or more severe characteristics
  - Progression 1 y — 45% to high-risk PDR

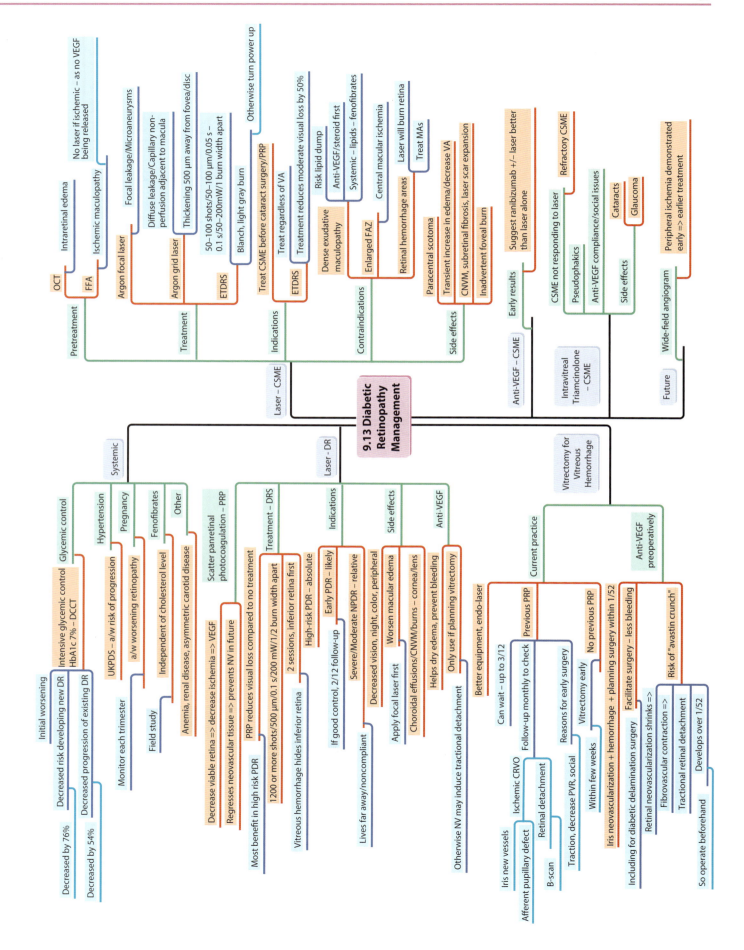

9.13 Diabetic Retinopathy Management

Laser – CSME

Pretreatment
- OCT — Intraretinal edema
- FFA
  - Ischemic maculopathy — No laser if ischemic — as no VEGF being released

Treatment
- Argon focal laser
  - Focal leakage/Microaneurysms
  - Diffuse leakage/Capillary non-perfusion adjacent to macula
- Argon grid laser — Thickening 500 μm away from fovea/disc
- ETDRS
  - 50–100 shots/50–100 μm/0.05 s – 0.1 s/50–200mW/1 burn width apart
  - Blanch, light gray burn
  - Otherwise turn power up

Indications
- ETDRS
  - Treat CSME before cataract surgery/PRP
  - Treat regardless of VA
  - Treatment reduces moderate visual loss by 50%

Contraindications
- Dense exudative maculopathy — Risk lipid dump
  - Anti-VEGF/steroid first
  - Systemic – lipids – fenofibrates
- Enlarged FAZ — Central macular ischemia
- Retinal hemorrhage areas — Treat MAs
- Paracentral scotoma — Laser will burn retina

Side effects
- Transient increase in edema/decrease VA
- CNVM, subretinal fibrosis, laser scar expansion
- Inadvertent foveal burn

Anti-VEGF – CSME
- Early results — Suggest ranibizumab +/– laser better than laser alone
- CSME not responding to laser — Refractory CSME
- Pseudophakics
- Anti-VEGF compliance/social issues
- Side effects
  - Cataracts
  - Glaucoma

Intravitreal Triamcinolone – CSME

Future
- Wide-field angiogram — Peripheral ischemia demonstrated early => earlier treatment

Systemic
- Glycemic control
  - Intensive glycemic control
    - Initial worsening
    - Decreased risk developing new DR — Decreased by 76%
    - Decreased progression of existing DR — Decreased by 54%
  - HbA1c 7% – DCCT
- Hypertension
  - UKPDS – a/w risk of progression
  - a/w worsening retinopathy
- Pregnancy
  - Monitor each trimester
- Fenofibrates
  - Field study
  - Independent of cholesterol level
- Other
  - Anemia, renal disease, asymmetric carotid disease

Laser – DR

Treatment – DRS
Scatter panretinal photocoagulation – PRP
- Decrease viable retina => decrease ischemia => VEGF
- Regresses neovascular tissue => prevents NV in future
- PRP reduces visual loss compared to no treatment
  - Most benefit in high risk PDR
- 1200 or more shots/500 μm/0.1 s/200 mW/1/2 burn width apart
- 2 sessions, inferior retina first
  - Vitreous hemorrhage hides inferior retina

Indications
- Early PDR – likely
- High-risk PDR – absolute
- Severe/Moderate NPDR – relative
  - If good control, 2/12 follow-up
  - Lives far away/noncompliant

Side effects
- Decreased vision, night, color, peripheral
- Worsen macular edema — Apply focal laser first
- Choroidal effusions/CNVM/burns – cornea/lens
- Helps dry edema, prevent bleeding

Anti-VEGF
- Only use if planning vitrectomy
  - Otherwise NV may induce tractional detachment

Vitrectomy for Vitreous Hemorrhage

Current practice
- Better equipment, endo-laser
- Previous PRP
  - Can wait – up to 3/12
  - Follow-up monthly to check
    - Ischemic CRVO
      - Iris new vessels
      - Afferent pupillary defect
    - Retinal detachment — B-scan
- No previous PRP
  - Reasons for early surgery
    - Vitrectomy early — Within few weeks
    - Iris neovascularization + hemorrhage + planning surgery within 1/52
    - Traction, decrease PVR, social
    - Facilitate surgery – less bleeding

Anti-VEGF preoperatively
- Including for diabetic delamination surgery
- Retinal neovascularization shrinks =>
  - Fibrovascular contraction =>
  - Tractional retinal detachment
- Risk of "avastin crunch"
  - Develops over 1/52
  - So operate beforehand

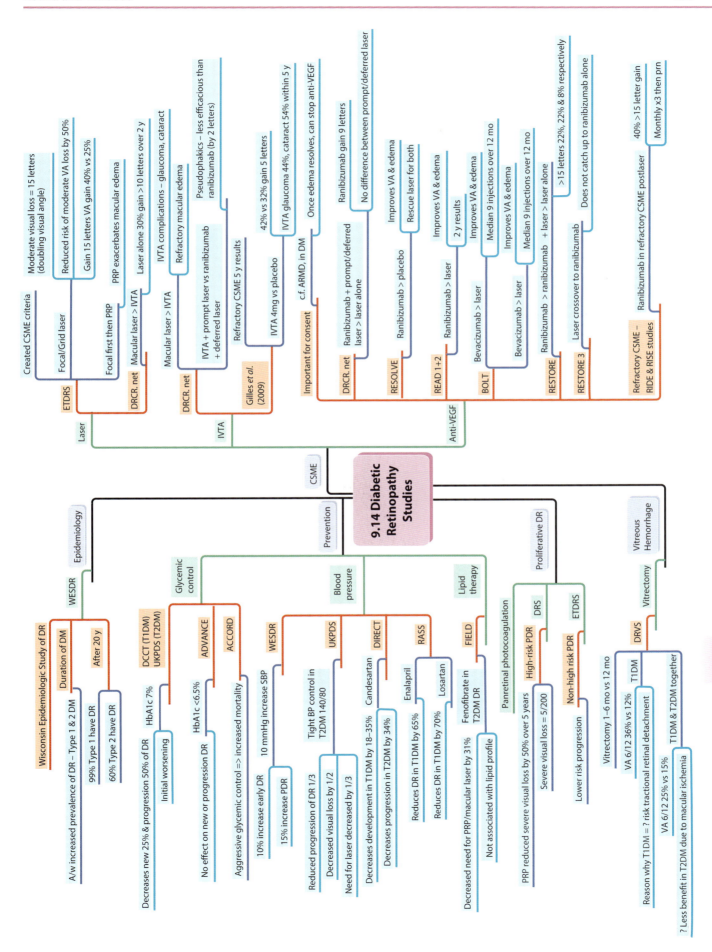

9.14 Diabetic Retinopathy Studies

CSME

Laser

ETDRS
- Created CSME criteria
  - Moderate visual loss = 15 letters (doubling visual angle)
- Focal/Grid laser
  - Reduced risk of moderate VA loss by 50%
  - Gain 15 letters VA gain 40% vs 25%
- Focal first then PRP
  - PRP exacerbates macular edema

DRCR. net
- Macular laser > IVTA
  - Laser alone 30% gain >10 letters over 2 y
  - IVTA complications – glaucoma, cataract

DRCR. net
- Macular laser > IVTA
  - Refractory macular edema

IVTA

Gilles et al. (2009)
- IVTA + prompt laser vs ranibizumab + deferred laser
  - Pseudophakics – less efficacious than ranibizumab (by 2 letters)
- Refractory CSME 5 y results
  - 42% vs 32% gain 5 letters
  - IVTA glaucoma 44%, cataract 54% within 5 y
- IVTA 4mg vs placebo
  - Once edema resolves, can stop anti-VEGF

Anti-VEGF

Important for consent
- c.f. ARMD, in DM

DRCR. net
- Ranibizumab + prompt/deferred laser > laser alone
  - Ranibizumab gain 9 letters
  - No difference between prompt/deferred laser

RESOLVE
- Ranibizumab > placebo
  - Improves VA & edema
  - Rescue laser for both

READ 1+2
- Ranibizumab > laser
  - Improves VA & edema
  - 2 y results
  - Improves VA & edema

BOLT
- Bevacizumab > laser
  - Median 9 injections over 12 mo
- Bevacizumab > laser
  - Improves VA & edema
  - Median 9 injections over 12 mo

RESTORE
- Ranibizumab > ranibizumab + laser > laser alone
  - >15 letters 22%, 22% & 8% respectively

RESTORE 3
- Laser crossover to ranibizumab
  - Does not catch up to ranibizumab alone

Refractory CSME – RIDE & RISE studies
- Ranibizumab in refractory CSME postlaser
  - 40% >15 letter gain
  - Monthly x3 then prn

Epidemiology

WESDR

Wisconsin Epidemiologic Study of DR
- A/w increased prevalence of DR – Type 1 & 2 DM
- Duration of DM
  - 99% Type 1 have DR
  - After 20 y
    - 60% Type 2 have DR

Prevention

Glycemic control

DCCT (T1DM) UKPDS (T2DM)
- HbA1c < 7%
  - Decreases new 25% & progression 50% of DR
  - Initial worsening

ADVANCE
- HbA1c < 6.5%
  - No effect on new or progression DR

ACCORD
- Aggressive glycemic control => increased mortality

Blood pressure

WESDR
- 10 mmHg increase SBP
  - 10% increase early DR
  - 15% increase PDR

UKPDS
- Tight BP control in T2DM 140/80
  - Reduced progression of DR 1/3
  - Decreased visual loss by 1/2
  - Need for laser decreased by 1/3

DIRECT
- Candesartan
  - Decreases development in T1DM by 18–35%
  - Decreases progression in T2DM by 34%

RASS
- Enalapril
  - Reduces DR in T1DM by 65%
- Losartan
  - Reduces DR in T1DM by 70%

Lipid therapy

FIELD
- Fenofibrate in T2DM DR
  - Decreased need for PRP/macular laser by 31%
  - Not associated with lipid profile

Proliferative DR

- Panretinal photocoagulation

DRS
- High-risk PDR
  - PRP reduced severe visual loss by 50% over 5 years
  - Severe visual loss = 5/200

ETDRS
- Non-high risk PDR
  - Lower risk progression

Vitreous Hemorrhage

Vitrectomy

DRVS
- T1DM
  - Vitrectomy 1–6 mo vs 12 mo
  - VA 6/12 36% vs 12%
  - Reason why T1DM = ? risk tractional retinal detachment
- T1DM & T2DM together
  - VA 6/12 25% vs 15%
  - ? Less benefit in T2DM due to macular ischemia

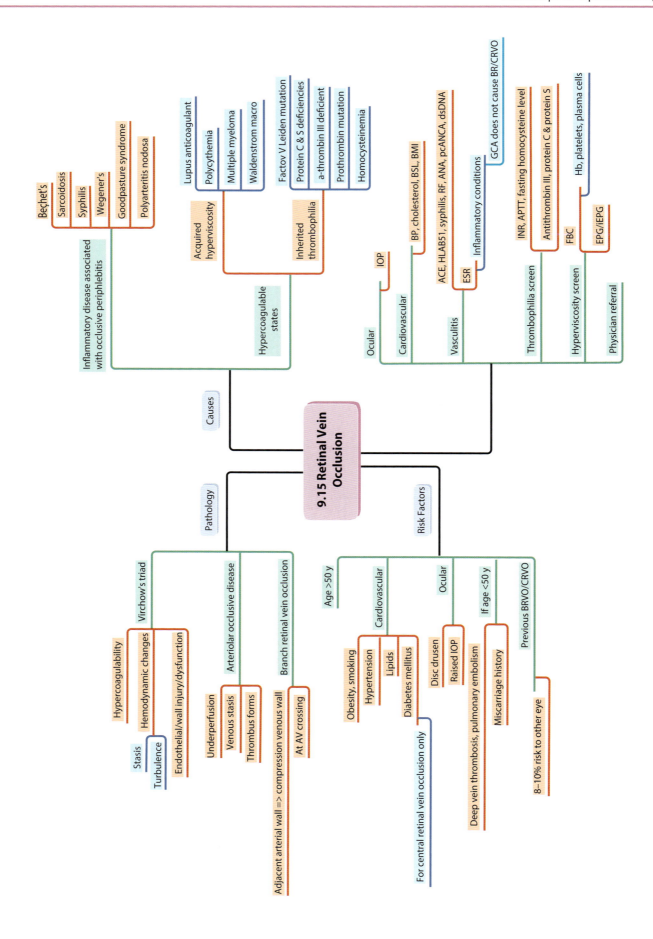

9.15 Retinal Vein Occlusion

Causes

Inflammatory disease associated with occlusive periphlebitis
- Bechet's
- Sarcoidosis
- Syphilis
- Wegener's
- Goodpasture syndrome
- Polyarteritis nodosa

Hypercoagulable states
- Acquired hyperviscosity
  - Lupus anticoagulant
  - Polycythemia
  - Multiple myeloma
  - Waldenstrom macro
- Inherited thrombophilia
  - Factov V Leiden mutation
  - Protein C & S deficiencies
  - a-thrombin III deficient
  - Prothrombin mutation
  - Homocysteinemia

Ocular
- IOP

Cardiovascular
- BP, cholesterol, BSL, BMI

Vasculitis
- ACE, HLAB51, syphilis, RF, ANA, pcANCA, dsDNA
- ESR
- Inflammatory conditions
- GCA does not cause BR/CRVO

Thrombophilia screen
- INR, APTT, fasting homocysteine level
- Antithrombin III, protein C & protein S

Hyperviscosity screen
- FBC
  - Hb, platelets, plasma cells
- EPG/iEPG

Physician referral

Pathology

Virchow's triad
- Hypercoagulability
- Hemodynamic changes
  - Stasis
  - Turbulence
- Endothelial/wall injury/dysfunction

Arteriolar occlusive disease
- Underperfusion
- Venous stasis
- Thrombus forms

Branch retinal vein occlusion
- At AV crossing
- Adjacent arterial wall => compression venous wall

Risk Factors

Age >50 y

Cardiovascular
- Obesity, smoking
- Hypertension
- Lipids
- Diabetes mellitus

Ocular
- Disc drusen
- Raised IOP
  - For central retinal vein occlusion only

If age <50 y
- Deep vein thrombosis, pulmonary embolism
- Miscarriage history

Previous BRVO/CRVO
- 8–10% risk to other eye

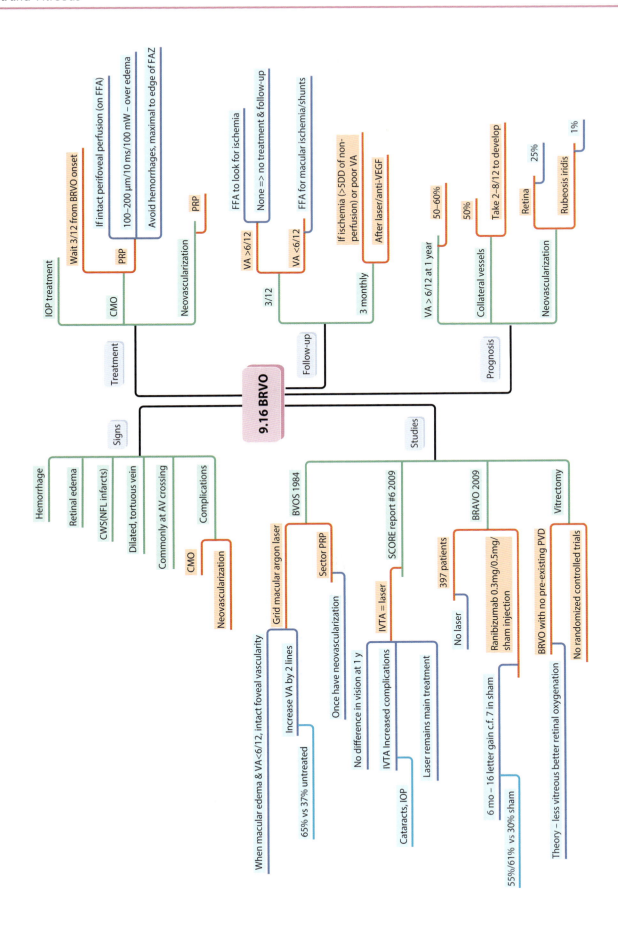

9.16 BRVO

Treatment

IOP treatment

CMO
- Wait 3/12 from BRVO onset
- PRP
  - If intact perifoveal perfusion (on FFA)
  - 100–200 μm/10 ms/100 mW – over edema
  - Avoid hemorrhages, maximal to edge of FAZ

Neovascularization
- PRP

Follow-up

3/12
- VA >6/12
  - FFA to look for ischemia
  - None => no treatment & follow-up
- VA <6/12
  - FFA for macular ischemia/shunts

3 monthly
- If ischemia (>5DD of non-perfusion) or poor VA
- After laser/anti-VEGF

Prognosis

- VA > 6/12 at 1 year — 50–60%
- Collateral vessels — 50%
- Neovascularization — Take 2–8/12 to develop
  - Retina — 25%
  - Rubeosis iridis — 1%

Signs

- Hemorrhage
- Retinal edema
- CWS(NFL infarcts)
- Dilated, tortuous vein
- Commonly at AV crossing
- Complications
  - CMO
  - Neovascularization

Studies

BVOS 1984
- Grid macular argon laser
  - When macular edema & VA<6/12, intact foveal vascularity
  - Increase VA by 2 lines
    - 65% vs 37% untreated
- Sector PRP
  - Once have neovascularization

SCORE report #6 2009
- IVTA = laser
  - No difference in vision at 1 y
  - IVTA Increased complications
    - Cataracts, IOP
  - Laser remains main treatment

BRAVO 2009
- 397 patients
  - No laser
- Ranibizumab 0.3mg/0.5mg/sham injection
  - 6 mo – 16 letter gain c.f. 7 in sham
  - 55%/61% vs 30% sham

Vitrectomy
- BRVO with no pre-existing PVD
  - Theory – less vitreous better retinal oxygenation
- No randomized controlled trials

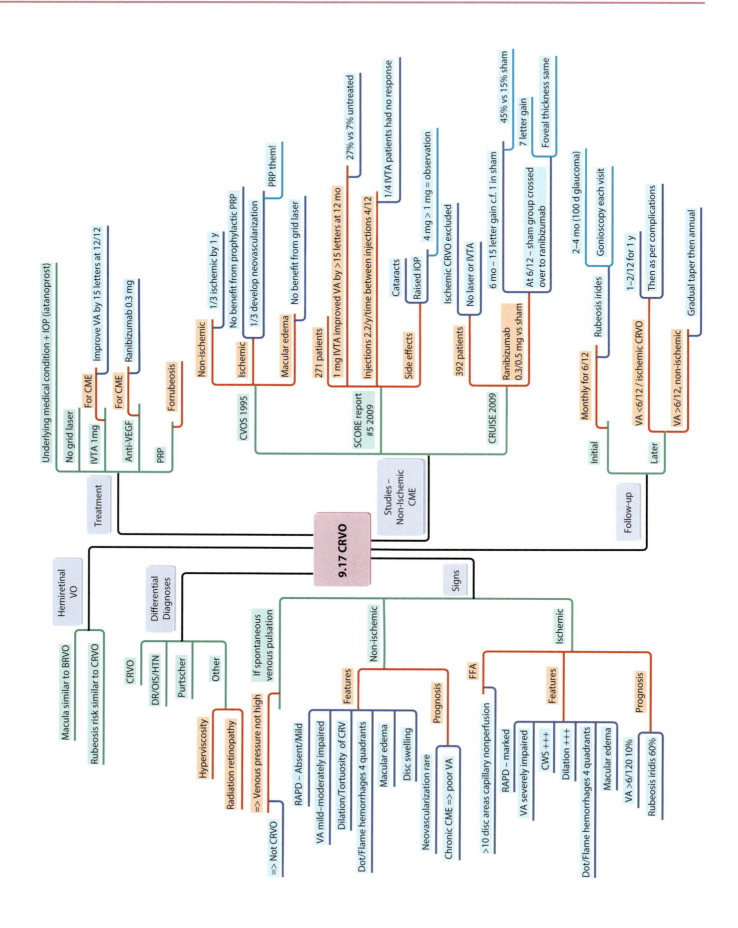

9.17 CRVO

Treatment

Non-ischemic CME
- No grid laser
- IVTA 1mg — For CME
- Anti-VEGF — For CME
  - Improve VA by 15 letters at 12/12
  - Ranibizumab 0.3 mg
- PRP — Forrubeosis
- Underlying medical condition + IOP (latanoprost)

Studies – Non-Ischemic CME

CVOS 1995
- Non-ischemic — 1/3 ischemic by 1 y
- Ischemic
  - No benefit from prophylactic PRP
  - 1/3 develop neovascularization — PRP them!
- Macular edema — No benefit from grid laser

SCORE report #5 2009
- 271 patients
- 1 mg IVTA improved VA by >15 letters at 12 mo — 27% vs 7% untreated
- Injections 2.2/y/time between injections 4/12 — 1/4 IVTA patients had no response
- Side effects
  - Cataracts
  - Raised IOP — 4 mg > 1 mg = observation

CRUISE 2009
- Ischemic CRVO excluded
- 392 patients
- No laser or IVTA
- Ranibizumab 0.3/0.5 mg vs sham
  - 6 mo – 15 letter gain c.f. 1 in sham — 45% vs 15% sham
  - At 6/12 – sham group crossed over to ranibizumab — 7 letter gain
  - Foveal thickness same

Follow-up

Initial
- Monthly for 6/12 — Rubeosis irides — 2–4 mo (100 d glaucoma) — Gonioscopy each visit

Later
- VA <6/12 / ischemic CRVO — 1–2/12 for 1 y — Then as per complications
- VA >6/12, non-ischemic — Gradual taper then annual

Hemiretinal VO
- Macula similar to BRVO
- Rubeosis risk similar to CRVO

Differential Diagnoses
- CRVO
- DR/OIS/HTN
- Purtscher
- Other
  - Hyperviscosity
  - Radiation retinopathy — => Venous pressure not high => Not CRVO

Signs
- If spontaneous venous pulsation => Not CRVO

Non-ischemic
- Features
  - RAPD – Absent/Mild
  - VA mild–moderately impaired
  - Dilation/Tortuosity of CRV
  - Dot/Flame hemorrhages 4 quadrants
  - Macular edema
  - Disc swelling
- Prognosis
  - Neovascularization rare
  - Chronic CME => poor VA

Ischemic
- FFA — >10 disc areas capillary nonperfusion
- Features
  - RAPD – marked
  - VA severely impaired
  - CWS +++
  - Dilation +++
  - Dot/Flame hemorrhages 4 quadrants
  - Macular edema
- Prognosis
  - VA >6/120 10%
  - Rubeosis iridis 60%

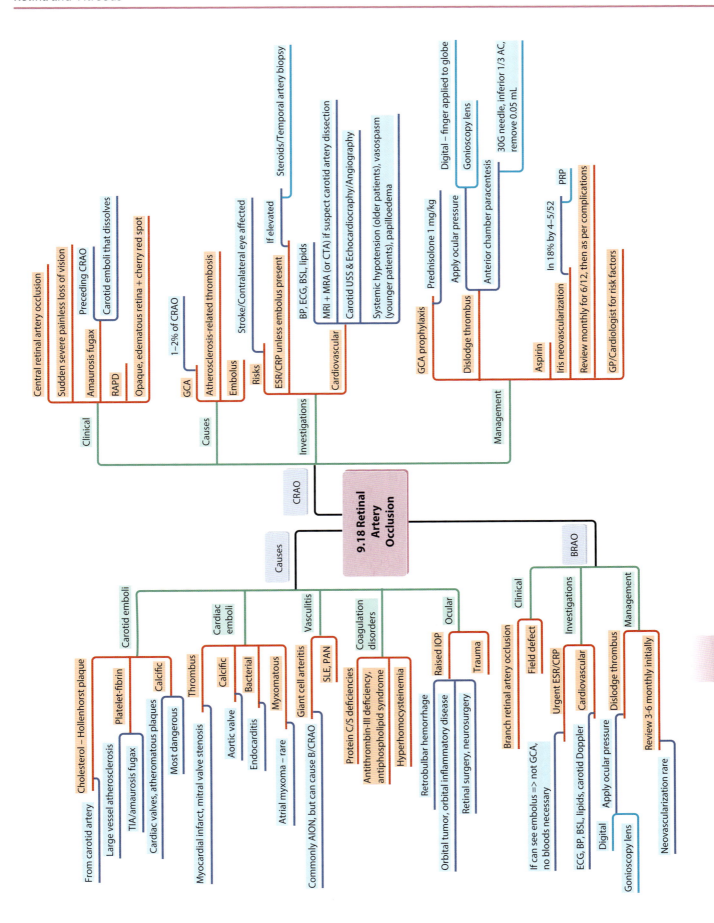

9.18 Retinal Artery Occlusion

CRAO

Clinical — Central retinal artery occlusion
- Sudden severe painless loss of vision
- Amaurosis fugax — Preceding CRAO
- RAPD
- Opaque, edematous retina + cherry red spot
- Carotid emboli that dissolves

Causes
- GCA — 1–2% of CRAO
- Atherosclerosis-related thrombosis
- Embolus

Investigations
- Risks — Stroke/Contralateral eye affected
- ESR/CRP unless embolus present — If elevated — Steroids/Temporal artery biopsy
- Cardiovascular
  - BP, ECG, BSL, lipids
  - MRI + MRA (or CTA) if suspect carotid artery dissection
  - Carotid USS & Echocardiography/Angiography
  - Systemic hypotension (older patients), vasospasm (younger patients), papilloedema

Management
- GCA prophylaxis — Prednisolone 1 mg/kg
- Dislodge thrombus
  - Apply ocular pressure
    - Digital – finger applied to globe
    - Gonioscopy lens
  - Anterior chamber paracentesis — 30G needle, inferior 1/3 AC, remove 0.05 mL
- Aspirin
- Iris neovascularization — In 18% by 4–5/52 — PRP
- Review monthly for 6/12, then as per complications
- GP/Cardiologist for risk factors

Causes

Carotid emboli
- Cholesterol – Hollenhorst plaque
  - From carotid artery
  - Large vessel atherosclerosis
  - TIA/amaurosis fugax
- Platelet-fibrin
- Calcific — Cardiac valves, atheromatous plaques

Cardiac emboli
- Thrombus
  - Most dangerous
  - Myocardial infarct, mitral valve stenosis
- Calcific — Aortic valve
- Bacterial — Endocarditis
- Myxomatous — Atrial myxoma – rare

Vasculitis
- Giant cell arteritis — Commonly AION, but can cause B/CRAO
- SLE, PAN

Coagulation disorders
- Protein C/S deficiencies
- Antithrombin-III deficiency, antiphospholipid syndrome
- Hyperhomocysteinemia

Ocular
- Raised IOP — Retrobulbar hemorrhage
- Trauma
  - Orbital tumor, orbital inflammatory disease
  - Retinal surgery, neurosurgery

BRAO

Clinical
- Branch retinal artery occlusion
- Field defect

Investigations
- Urgent ESR/CRP — If can see embolus => not GCA, no bloods necessary
- Cardiovascular — ECG, BP, BSL, lipids, carotid Doppler

Management
- Dislodge thrombus
  - Apply ocular pressure
    - Digital
    - Gonioscopy lens
- Review 3-6 monthly initially
- Neovascularization rare

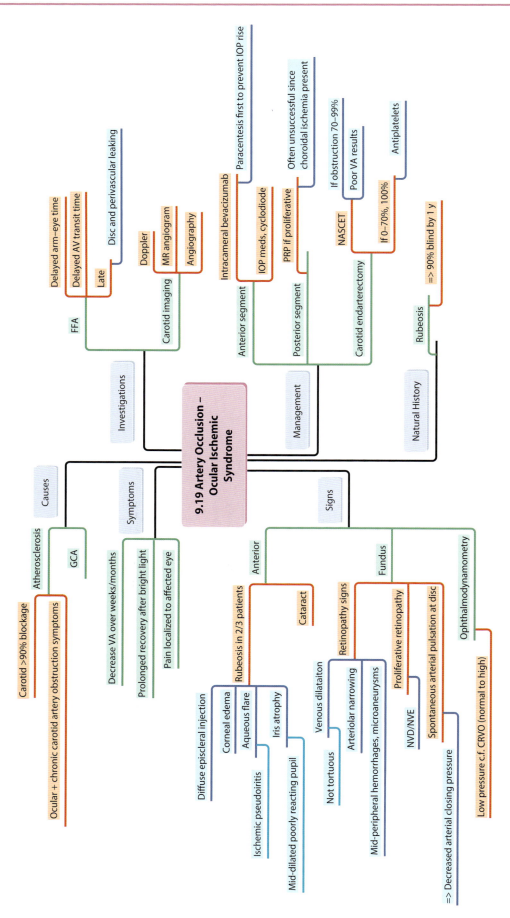

9.19 Artery Occlusion – Ocular Ischemic Syndrome

Investigations

FFA
- Delayed arm–eye time
- Delayed AV transit time
- Late
  - Disc and perivascular leaking

Carotid imaging
- Doppler
- MR angiogram
- Angiography

Management

Anterior segment
- Intracameral bevacizumab
  - Paracentesis first to prevent IOP rise
- IOP meds, cyclodiode

Posterior segment
- PRP if proliferative
  - Often unsuccessful since choroidal ischemia present

Carotid endarterectomy
- NASCET
  - If obstruction 70–99%
  - Poor VA results
- If 0–70%, 100%

Rubeosis
- Antiplatelets

Natural History
- => 90% blind by 1 y

Causes
- Atherosclerosis
  - Carotid >90% blockage
- GCA
  - Ocular + chronic carotid artery obstruction symptoms

Symptoms
- Decrease VA over weeks/months
- Prolonged recovery after bright light
- Pain localized to affected eye

Signs

Anterior
- Diffuse episcleral injection
- Corneal edema
- Aqueous flare
  - Ischemic pseudoiritis
- Iris atrophy
  - Mid-dilated poorly reacting pupil
- Rubeosis in 2/3 patients
- Cataract

Fundus
- Retinopathy signs
  - Venous dilataiton
    - Not tortuous
  - Arteriolar narrowing
  - Mid-peripheral hemorrhages, microaneurysms
- Proliferative retinopathy
  - NVD/NVE
- Spontaneous arterial pulsation at disc
  - Decreased arterial closing pressure

Ophthalmodynamometry
- Low pressure c.f. CRVO (normal to high)

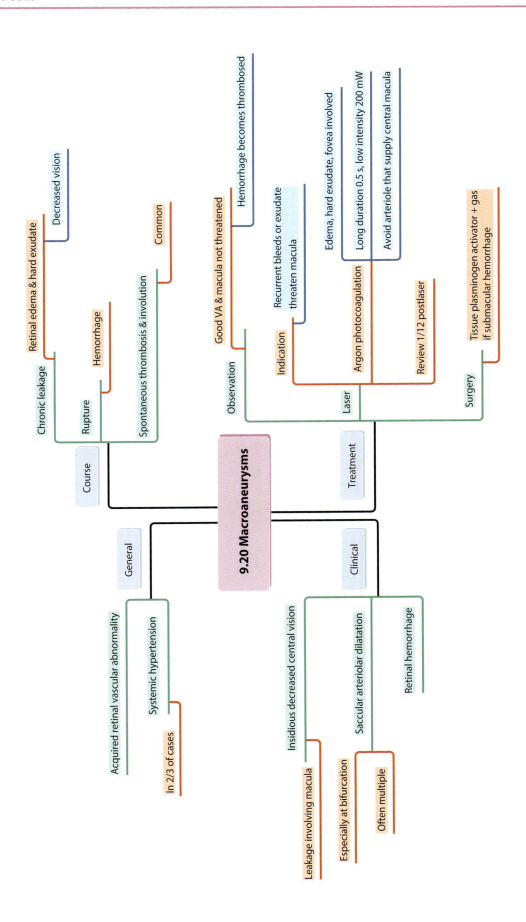

9.20 Macroaneurysms

General
- Acquired retinal vascular abnormality
- Systemic hypertension
  - In 2/3 of cases

Clinical
- Insidious decreased central vision
  - Leakage involving macula
- Saccular arteriolar dilatation
  - Especially at bifurcation
  - Often multiple
- Retinal hemorrhage

Course
- Chronic leakage
  - Retinal edema & hard exudate
    - Decreased vision
- Rupture
  - Hemorrhage
- Spontaneous thrombosis & involution
  - Common

Treatment
- Observation
  - Good VA & macula not threatened
    - Hemorrhage becomes thrombosed
- Laser
  - Indication
    - Recurrent bleeds or exudate threaten macula
  - Argon photocoagulation
    - Edema, hard exudate, fovea involved
    - Long duration 0.5 s, low intensity 200 mW
    - Avoid arteriole that supply central macula
  - Review 1/12 postlaser
- Surgery
  - Tissue plasminogen activator + gas if submacular hemorrhage

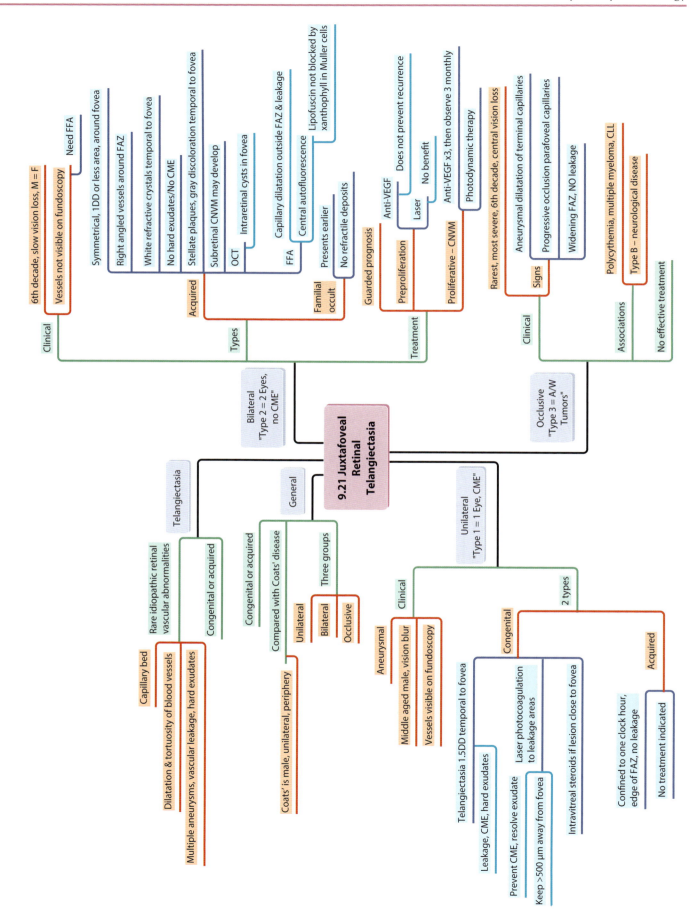

9.21 Juxtafoveal Retinal Telangiectasia

General
- Congenital or acquired
- Compared with Coats' disease
  - Coats' is male, unilateral, periphery
- Three groups
  - Unilateral
  - Bilateral
  - Occlusive

Telangiectasia
- Rare idiopathic retinal vascular abnormalities
- Congenital or acquired
  - Capillary bed
  - Dilatation & tortuosity of blood vessels
  - Multiple aneurysms, vascular leakage, hard exudates

Unilateral "Type 1 = 1 Eye, CME"
- Clinical
  - Aneurysmal
  - Middle aged male, vision blur
  - Vessels visible on fundoscopy
- 2 types
  - Congenital
    - Telangiectasia 1.5DD temporal to fovea
    - Leakage, CME, hard exudates
    - Laser photocoagulation to leakage areas
      - Prevent CME, resolve exudate
      - Keep >500 μm away from fovea
    - Intravitreal steroids if lesion close to fovea
  - Acquired
    - Confined to one clock hour, edge of FAZ, no leakage
    - No treatment indicated

Bilateral "Type 2 = 2 Eyes, no CME"
- Clinical
  - 6th decade, slow vision loss, M = F
  - Vessels not visible on fundoscopy
    - Need FFA
- Types
  - Acquired
    - Symmetrical, 1DD or less area, around fovea
    - Right angled vessels around FAZ
    - White refractive crystals temporal to fovea
    - No hard exudates/No CME
    - Stellate plaques, gray discoloration temporal to fovea
    - Subretinal CNVM may develop
    - OCT
      - Intraretinal cysts in fovea
    - FFA
      - Capillary dilatation outside FAZ & leakage
      - Central autofluorescence
        - Lipofuscin not blocked by xanthophyll in Muller cells
  - Familial occult
    - Presents earlier
    - No refractile deposits
- Treatment
  - Guarded prognosis
  - Preproliferation
    - Anti-VEGF
      - Does not prevent recurrence
    - Laser
      - No benefit
  - Proliferative – CNVM
    - Anti-VEGF x3, then observe 3 monthly
    - Photodynamic therapy

Occlusive "Type 3 = A/W Tumors"
- Clinical
  - Rarest, most severe, 6th decade, central vision loss
  - Signs
    - Aneurysmal dilatation of terminal capillaries
    - Progressive occlusion parafoveal capillaries
    - Widening FAZ, NO leakage
- Associations
  - Polycythemia, multiple myeloma, CLL
  - Type B – neurological disease
- No effective treatment

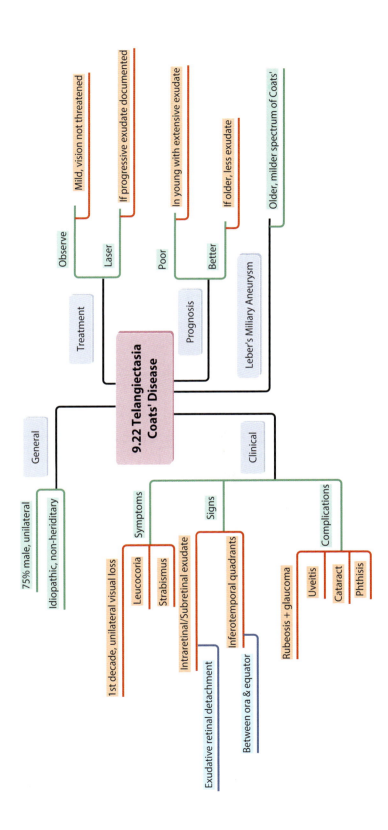

9.22 Telangiectasia Coats' Disease

General
- 75% male, unilateral
- Idiopathic, non-heriditary

Treatment
- Observe
  - Mild, vision not threatened
- Laser
  - If progressive exudate documented

Prognosis
- Poor
  - In young with extensive exudate
- Better
  - If older, less exudate
- Older, milder spectrum of Coats'

Leber's Miliary Aneurysm

Clinical
- Symptoms
  - 1st decade, unilateral visual loss
  - Leucocoria
  - Strabismus
- Signs
  - Intraretinal/Subretinal exudate
  - Inferotemporal quadrants
    - Exudative retinal detachment
    - Between ora & equator
- Complications
  - Rubeosis + glaucoma
  - Uveitis
  - Cataract
  - Phthisis

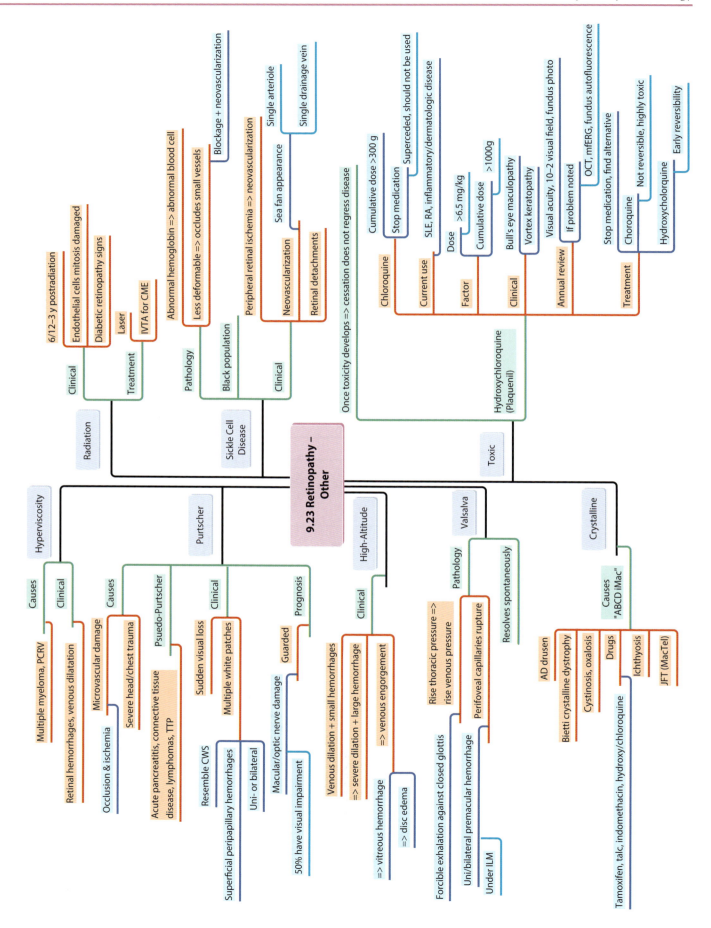

9.23 Retinopathy – Other

Radiation

Clinical
- 6/12–3 y postradiation
- Endothelial cells mitosis damaged
- Diabetic retinopathy signs

Treatment
- Laser
- IVTA for CME

Sickle Cell Disease

Pathology
- Abnormal hemoglobin => abnormal blood cell
- Less deformable => occludes small vessels
- Blockage + neovascularization

Black population

Clinical
- Peripheral retinal ischemia => neovascularization
- Neovascularization
  - Sea fan appearance
  - Single arteriole
  - Single drainage vein
- Retinal detachments

Toxic

Once toxicity develops => cessation does not regress disease

Hydroxychloroquine (Plaquenil)

Chloroquine
- Cumulative dose >300 g
- Stop medication
- Superceded, should not be used

Current use
- SLE, RA, inflammatory/dermatologic disease

Factor
- Dose => >6.5 mg/kg
- Cumulative dose => >1000g

Clinical
- Bull's eye maculopathy
- Vortex keratopathy

Annual review
- Visual acuity, 10–2 visual field, fundus photo
- If problem noted
- OCT, mfERG, fundus autofluorescence

Treatment
- Stop medication, find alternative
- Choroquine — Not reversible, highly toxic
- Hydroxychlorquine — Early reversibility

Hyperviscosity

Causes
- Multiple myeloma, PCRV

Clinical
- Retinal hemorrhages, venous dilatation
- Occlusion & ischemia

Purtscher

Causes
- Microvascular damage
- Severe head/chest trauma
- Psuedo-Purtscher
  - Acute pancreatitis, connective tissue disease, lymphomas, TTP

Clinical
- Sudden visual loss
- Multiple white patches
  - Resemble CWS
  - Superficial peripapillary hemorrhages
  - Uni- or bilateral
  - Macular/optic nerve damage

Prognosis
- Guarded
- 50% have visual impairment

High-Altitude

Clinical
- Venous dilation + small hemorrhages
- => severe dilation + large hemorrhage
- => venous engorgement
  - => vitreous hemorrhage
  - => disc edema

Valsalva

Pathology
- Rise thoracic pressure => rise venous pressure
- Perifoveal capillaries rupture
  - Forcible exhalation against closed glottis
  - Uni/bilateral premacular hemorrhage
  - Under ILM

Resolves spontaneously

Crystalline

Causes
"ABCD iMac"
- AD drusen
- Bietti crystalline dystrophy
- Cystinosis, oxalosis
- Drugs
  - Tamoxifen, talc, indomethacin, hydroxy/chloroquine
- Ichthyosis
- JFT (MacTel)

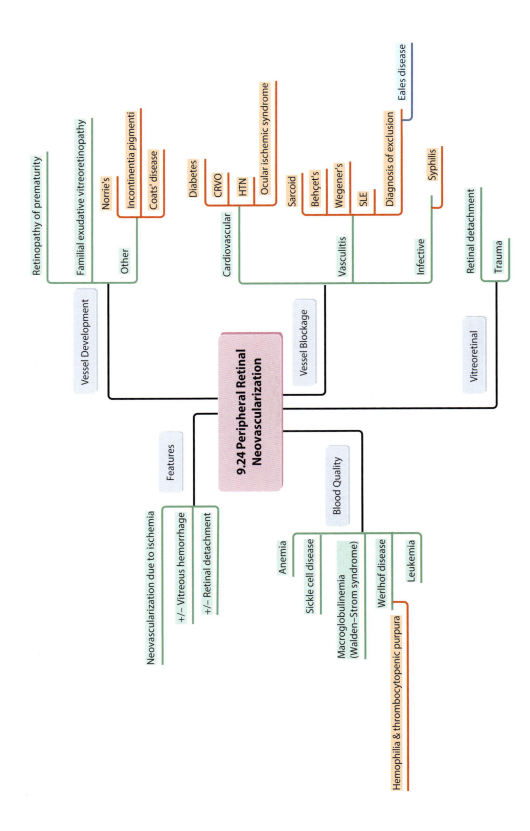

9.24 Peripheral Retinal Neovascularization

Features
- Neovascularization due to ischemia
  - +/– Vitreous hemorrhage
  - +/– Retinal detachment

Vessel Development
- Retinopathy of prematurity
- Familial exudative vitreoretinopathy
- Other
  - Norrie's
  - Incontinentia pigmenti
  - Coats' disease

Vessel Blockage
- Cardiovascular
  - Diabetes
  - CRVO
  - HTN
  - Ocular ischemic syndrome
- Vasculitis
  - Sarcoid
  - Behçet's
  - Wegener's
  - SLE
  - Diagnosis of exclusion
    - Eales disease
- Infective
  - Syphilis

Blood Quality
- Anemia
- Sickle cell disease
- Macroglobulinemia (Walden–Strom syndrome)
- Werlhof disease
- Leukemia
- Hemophilia & thrombocytopenic purpura

Vitreoretinal
- Retinal detachment
- Trauma

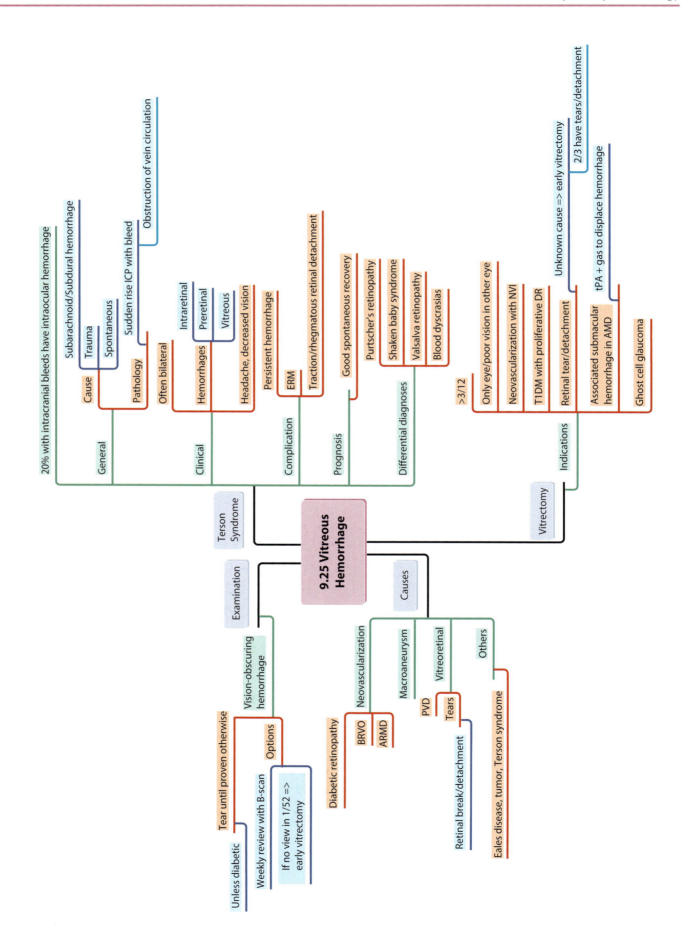

9.25 Vitreous Hemorrhage

Terson Syndrome

General
- 20% with intracranial bleeds have intraocular hemorrhage
- Cause
  - Subarachnoid/Subdural hemorrhage
  - Trauma
  - Spontaneous
- Pathology
  - Sudden rise ICP with bleed
  - Obstruction of vein circulation

Clinical
- Often bilateral
- Hemorrhages
  - Intraretinal
  - Preretinal
  - Vitreous
- Headache, decreased vision

Complication
- Persistent hemorrhage
- ERM
- Traction/rhegmatous retinal detachment

Prognosis
- Good spontaneous recovery

Differential diagnoses
- Purtscher's retinopathy
- Shaken baby syndrome
- Valsalva retinopathy
- Blood dyscrasias

Vitrectomy

Indications
- >3/12
- Only eye/poor vision in other eye
- Neovascularization with NVI
- T1DM with proliferative DR
- Retinal tear/detachment
  - Unknown cause => early vitrectomy
  - 2/3 have tears/detachment
- Associated submacular hemorrhage in AMD
  - tPA + gas to displace hemorrhage
- Ghost cell glaucoma

Examination

Vision-obscuring hemorrhage
- Tear until proven otherwise
  - Unless diabetic
- Options
  - Weekly review with B-scan
  - If no view in 1/52 => early vitrectomy

Causes

- Neovascularization
  - Diabetic retinopathy
  - BRVO
  - ARMD
- Macroaneurysm
- Vitreoretinal
  - PVD
  - Tears
  - Retinal break/detachment
- Others
  - Eales disease, tumor, Terson syndrome

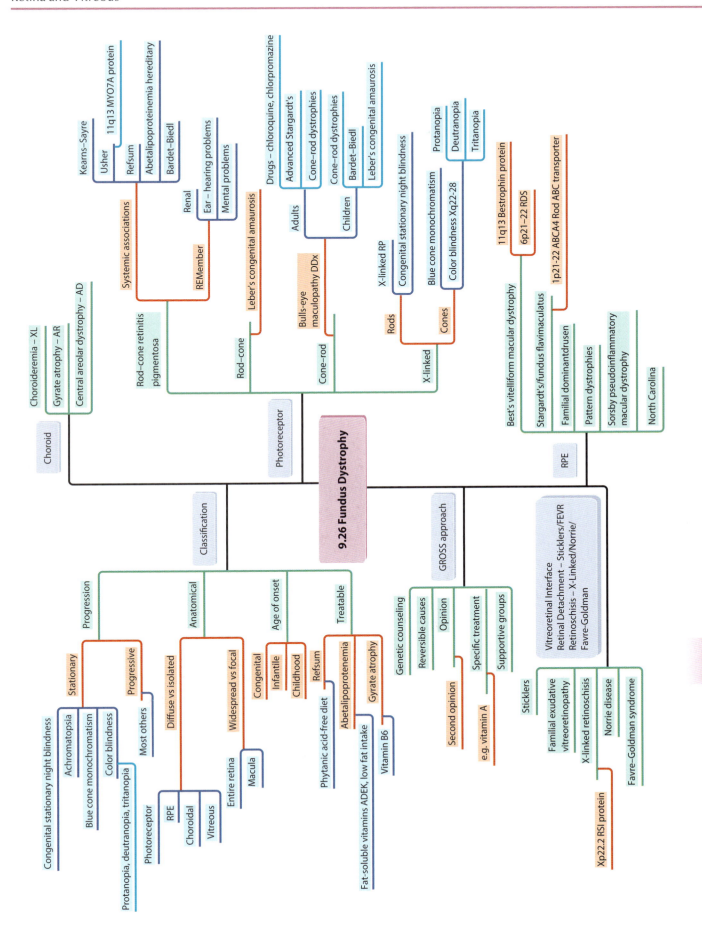

9.26 Fundus Dystrophy

Choroid
- Choroideremia – XL
- Gyrate atrophy – AR
- Central areolar dystrophy – AD

Photoreceptor

Rod–cone retinitis pigmentosa
- Rod–cone
  - Systemic associations
    - Kearns–Sayre
    - Usher — 11q13 MYO7A protein
    - Refsum
    - Abetalipoproteinemia hereditary
    - Bardet–Biedl
  - REMember
    - Renal
    - Ear – hearing problems
    - Mental problems
- Leber's congenital amaurosis

Cone–rod
- Bulls-eye maculopathy DDx
  - Adults
    - Drugs – chloroquine, chlorpromazine
    - Advanced Stargardt's
    - Cone–rod dystrophies
  - Children
    - Cone–rod dystrophies
    - Bardet–Biedl
    - Leber's congenital amaurosis

X-linked
- Rods
  - X-linked RP
  - Congenital stationary night blindness
- Cones
  - Blue cone monochromatism
  - Color blindness Xq22-28
    - Protanopia
    - Deutranopia
    - Tritanopia

RPE
- Best's vitelliform macular dystrophy — 11q13 Bestrophin protein
- Stargardt's/fundus flavimaculatus — 6p21–22 RDS
- Familial dominantdrusen — 1p21-22 ABCA4 Rod ABC transporter
- Pattern dystrophies
- Sorsby pseudoinflammatory macular dystrophy
- North Carolina

Classification

Progression
- Stationary
  - Congenital stationary night blindness
  - Achromatopsia
  - Blue cone monochromatism
  - Color blindness
    - Protanopia, deutranopia, tritanopia
- Progressive
  - Most others

Anatomical
- Diffuse vs isolated
  - Photoreceptor
  - RPE
  - Choroidal
  - Vitreous
- Widespread vs focal
  - Entire retina
  - Macula

Age of onset
- Congenital
- Infantile
- Childhood

Treatable
- Refsum — Phytanic acid-free diet
- Abetalipoproteinemia — Fat-soluble vitamins ADEK, low fat intake
- Gyrate atrophy — Vitamin B6

GROSS approach
- Genetic counseling
- Reversible causes
- Opinion
  - Second opinion
- Specific treatment
  - e.g. vitamin A
- Supportive groups

Vitreoretinal Interface
Retinal Detachment – Sticklers/FEVR
Retinoschisis – X-Linked/Norrie/
Favre-Goldman
- Sticklers
- Familial exudative vitreoretinopathy
- X-linked retinoschisis — Xp22.2 RS1 protein
- Norrie disease
- Favre–Goldman syndrome

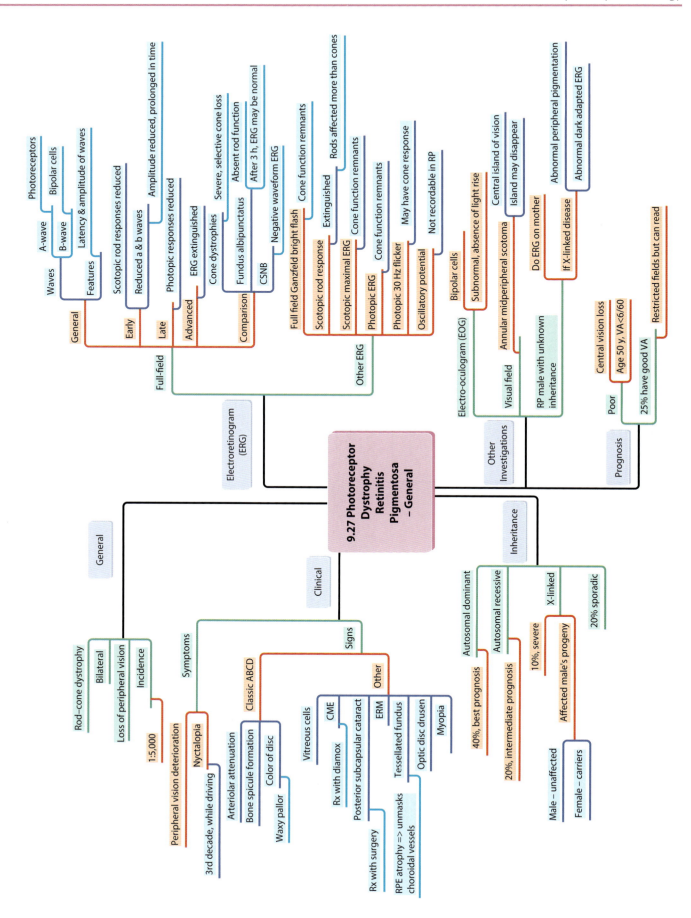

9.27 Photoreceptor Dystrophy Retinitis Pigmentosa – General

Electroretinogram (ERG)

Full-field

General
- Waves
  - A-wave
  - B-wave
- Features
  - Photoreceptors
  - Bipolar cells
  - Latency & amplitude of waves

Early
- Scotopic rod responses reduced
- Reduced a & b waves
  - Amplitude reduced, prolonged in time

Late
- Photopic responses reduced

Advanced
- ERG extinguished

Comparison
- Cone dystrophies
  - Severe, selective cone loss
- Fundus albipunctatus
  - Absent rod function
  - After 3 h, ERG may be normal
- CSNB
  - Negative waveform ERG

Other ERG
- Full field Ganzfeld bright flash
  - Cone function remnants
- Scotopic rod response
  - Extinguished
  - Rods affected more than cones
- Scotopic maximal ERG
  - Cone function remnants
- Photopic ERG
  - Cone function remnants
- Photopic 30 Hz flicker
  - May have cone response
- Oscillatory potential
  - Not recordable in RP

Other Investigations

Electro-oculogram (EOG)
- Bipolar cells
- Subnormal, absence of light rise

Visual field
- Annular midperipheral scotoma
- Central island of vision
- Island may disappear

RP male with unknown inheritance
- Do ERG on mother
- If X-linked disease
  - Abnormal peripheral pigmentation
  - Abnormal dark adapted ERG

Prognosis

Poor
- Central vision loss
- Age 50 y, VA <6/60

- 25% have good VA
- Restricted fields but can read

General

Rod–cone dystrophy
Bilateral
Loss of peripheral vision
Incidence
- 1:5,000

Clinical

Symptoms
- Peripheral vision deterioration
- Nyctalopia
  - 3rd decade, while driving

Signs
Classic ABCD
- Arteriolar attenuation
- Bone spicule formation
- Color of disc
  - Waxy pallor

Other
- Vitreous cells
- CME
  - Rx with diamox
- Posterior subcapsular cataract
  - Rx with surgery
- ERM
- Tessellated fundus
  - RPE atrophy => unmasks choroidal vessels
- Optic disc drusen
- Myopia

Inheritance
- Autosomal dominant
  - 40%, best prognosis
- Autosomal recessive
  - 20%, intermediate prognosis
- X-linked
  - 10%, severe
  - Affected male's progeny
    - Male – unaffected
    - Female – carriers
- 20% sporadic

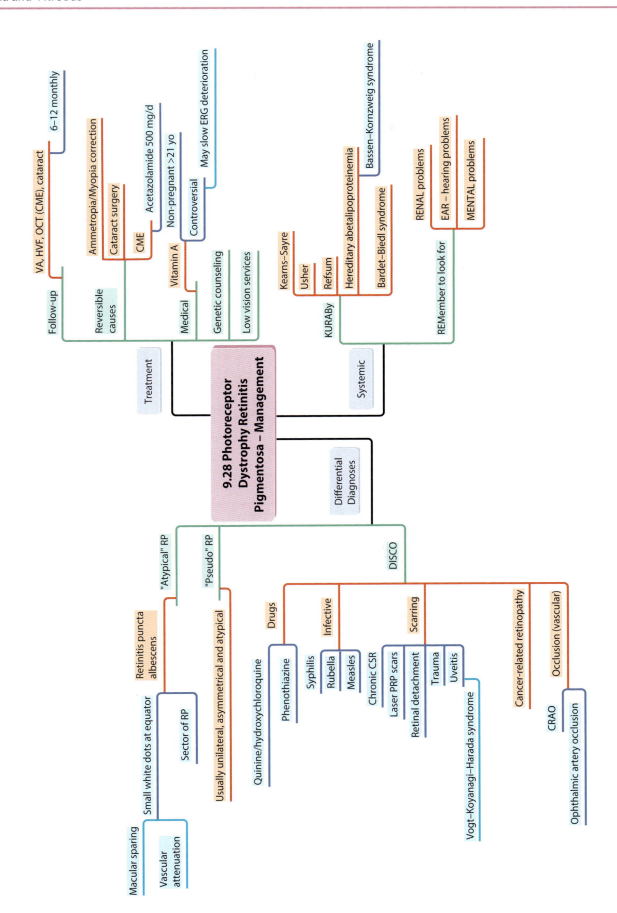

9.28 Photoreceptor Dystrophy Retinitis Pigmentosa – Management

Treatment

Follow-up
- VA, HVF, OCT (CME), cataract
- 6–12 monthly

Reversible causes
- Ammetropia/Myopia correction
- Cataract surgery
  - CME
- Acetazolamide 500 mg/d
  - Non-pregnant >21 yo
  - Controversial

Medical
- Vitamin A
  - May slow ERG deterioration
- Genetic counseling
- Low vision services

Systemic

KURABy
- Kearns–Sayre
- Usher
- Refsum
- Hereditary abetalipoproteinemia
- Bardet–Biedl syndrome
- Bassen–Kornzweig syndrome

REMember to look for
- RENAL problems
- EAR – hearing problems
- MENTAL problems

Differential Diagnoses

"Atypical" RP
- Retinitis puncta albescens
- Small white dots at equator
- Sector of RP
  - Macular sparing
  - Vascular attenuation

"Pseudo" RP
- Usually unilateral, asymmetrical and atypical

DISCO
- Drugs
  - Quinine/hydroxychloroquine
  - Phenothiazine
- Infective
  - Syphilis
  - Rubella
  - Measles
- Scarring
  - Chronic CSR
  - Laser PRP scars
  - Retinal detachment
  - Trauma
  - Uveitis
  - Vogt–Koyanagi–Harada syndrome
- Cancer-related retinopathy
- Occlusion (vascular)
  - CRAO
  - Ophthalmic artery occlusion

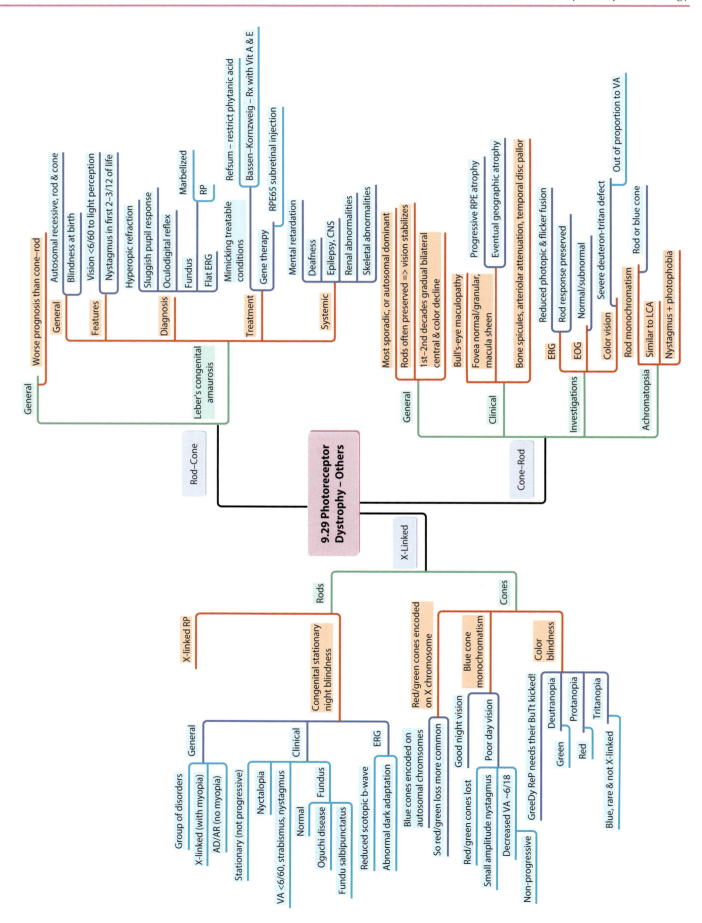

9.29 Photoreceptor Dystrophy – Others

Rod–Cone

General
- Worse prognosis than cone–rod

Leber's congenital amaurosis
- General
  - Autosomal recessive, rod & cone
  - Blindness at birth
- Features
  - Vision <6/60 to light perception
  - Nystagmus in first 2–3/12 of life
  - Hyperopic refraction
  - Sluggish pupil response
  - Oculodigital reflex
- Diagnosis
  - Fundus
    - Marbelized
    - RP
  - Flat ERG
  - Mimicking treatable conditions
- Treatment
  - Gene therapy
    - Refsum – restrict phytanic acid
    - Bassen–Kornzweig – Rx with Vit A & E
    - RPE65 subretinal injection
- Systemic
  - Mental retardation
  - Deafness
  - Epilepsy, CNS
  - Renal abnormalities
  - Skeletal abnormalities

Cone–Rod

General
- Most sporadic, or autosomal dominant
- Rods often preserved => vision stabilizes
- 1st–2nd decades gradual bilateral central & color decline

Clinical
- Bull's-eye maculopathy
- Fovea normal/granular, macula sheen
- Bone spicules, arteriolar attenuation, temporal disc pallor
  - Progressive RPE atrophy
  - Eventual geographic atrophy

Investigations
- ERG
  - Reduced photopic & flicker fusion
  - Rod response preserved
- EOG
  - Normal/subnormal
- Color vision
  - Severe deuteron-tritan defect

Achromatopsia
- Rod monochromatism
  - Rod or blue cone
- Similar to LCA
- Nystagmus + photophobia
- Out of proportion to VA

X-Linked

Rods
- X-linked RP
- Congenital stationary night blindness
  - General
    - Group of disorders
    - X-linked (with myopia)
    - AD/AR (no myopia)
    - Stationary (not progressive)
  - Clinical
    - Nyctalopia
    - VA <6/60, strabismus, nystagmus
    - Fundus
      - Normal
      - Oguchi disease
      - Fundu salbipunctatus
  - ERG
    - Reduced scotopic b-wave
    - Abnormal dark adaptation

Cones
- Red/green cones encoded on X chromosome
  - Blue cones encoded on autosomal chromsomes
  - So red/green loss more common
- Blue cone monochromatism
  - Good night vision
  - Poor day vision
  - Red/green cones lost
  - Small amplitude nystagmus
  - Decreased VA ~6/18
  - Non-progressive
- Color blindness
  - GreeDy ReP needs their BuTt kicked!
  - Deutranopia
    - Green
  - Protanopia
    - Red
  - Tritanopia
    - Blue, rare & not X-linked

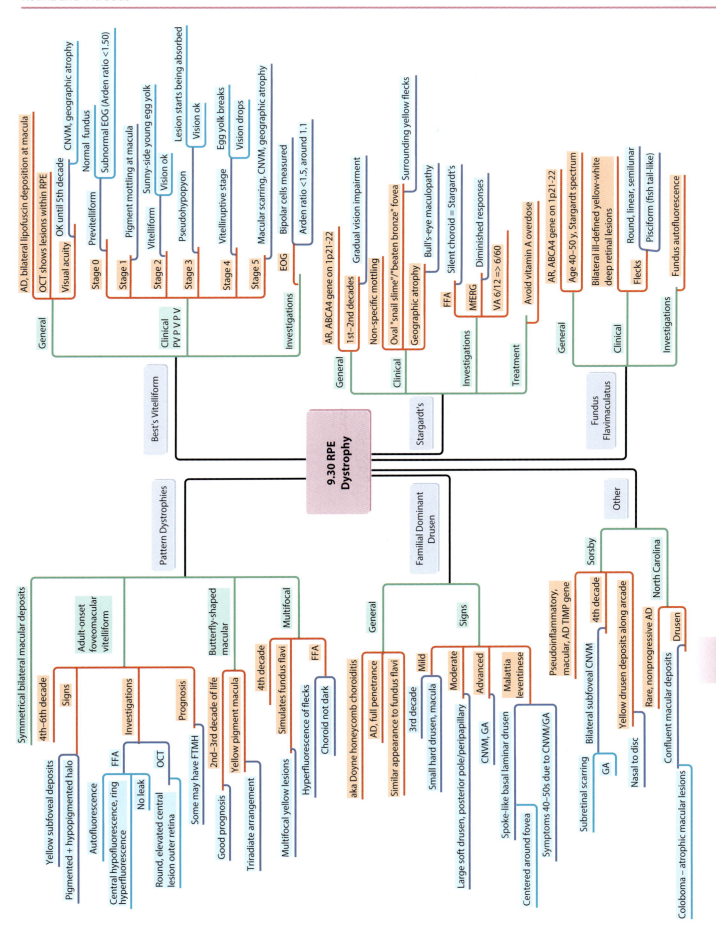

9.30 RPE Dystrophy

Best's Vitelliform

General
- AD, bilateral lipofuscin deposition at macula
- OCT shows lesions within RPE
- Visual acuity
  - OK until 5th decade
  - CNVM, geographic atrophy

Clinical (PV PV PV PV)
- Stage 0 – Previtelliform
  - Normal fundus
  - Subnormal EOG (Arden ratio <1.50)
- Stage 1 – Pigment mottling at macula
- Stage 2 – Vitelliform
  - Sunny-side young egg yolk
  - Vision ok
- Stage 3 – Pseudohypopyon
  - Lesion starts being absorbed
  - Vision ok
- Stage 4 – Vitelliruptive stage
  - Egg yolk breaks
  - Vision drops
- Stage 5 – Macular scarring, CNVM, geographic atrophy

Investigations
- EOG
  - Bipolar cells measured
  - Arden ratio <1.5, around 1.1

Stargardt's

General
- AR, ABCA4 gene on 1p21-22
- 1st–2nd decades
- Gradual vision impairment
- Non-specific mottling

Clinical
- Oval "snail slime"/"beaten bronze" fovea
- Geographic atrophy
- Bull's-eye maculopathy
- Surrounding yellow flecks

Investigations
- FFA – Silent choroid = Stargardt's
- mfERG – Diminished responses
- VA 6/12 => 6/60

Treatment
- Avoid vitamin A overdose

Fundus Flavimaculatus

General
- AR, ABCA4 gene on 1p21-22
- Age 40–50 y, Stargardt spectrum

Clinical
- Bilateral ill-defined yellow-white deep retinal lesions
- Flecks
  - Round, linear, semilunar
  - Pisciform (fish tail-like)

Investigations
- Fundus autofluorescence

Pattern Dystrophies

Adult-onset foveomacular vitelliform
- Symmetrical bilateral macular deposits
- 4th–6th decade
- Signs
  - Yellow subfoveal deposits
  - Pigmented + hypopigmented halo
- Investigations
  - Autofluorescence
  - FFA
    - Central hypofluorescence, ring hyperfluorescence
    - No leak
  - OCT
    - Round, elevated central lesion outer retina
- Prognosis
  - Some may have FTMH
  - Good prognosis

Butterfly-shaped macular
- 2nd–3rd decade of life
- Yellow pigment macula
- Triradiate arrangement

Multifocal
- 4th decade
- Simulates fundus flavi
- FFA
  - Hyperfluorescence of flecks
  - Choroid not dark
- Multifocal yellow lesions

Familial Dominant Drusen

General
- aka Doyne honeycomb choroiditis
- AD, full penetrance
- Similar appearance to fundus flavi
- 3rd decade

Signs
- Mild
  - Small hard drusen, macula
- Moderate
  - CNVM, GA
- Advanced
  - Large soft drusen, posterior pole/peripapillary
- Malattia leventinese
  - Spoke-like basal laminar drusen
  - Centered around fovea
  - Symptoms 40–50s due to CNVM/GA

Other

Sorsby
- Pseudoinflammatory, macular, AD TIMP gene
- 4th decade
- Bilateral subfoveal CNVM
  - Subretinal scarring
  - GA

North Carolina
- Rare, nonprogressive AD
- Yellow drusen deposits along arcade
  - Nasal to disc
- Drusen
  - Confluent macular deposits
  - Coloboma – atrophic macular lesions

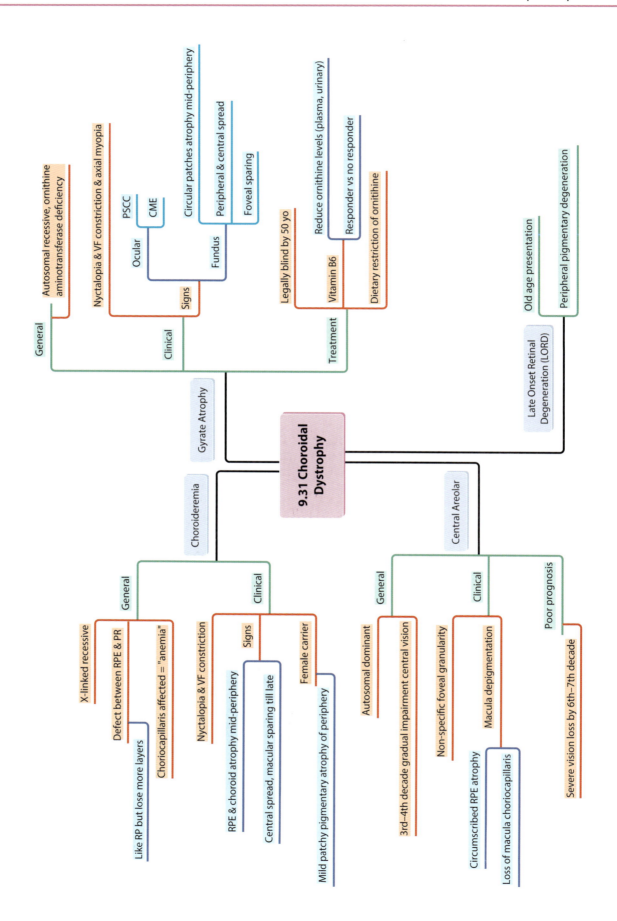

9.31 Choroidal Dystrophy

Gyrate Atrophy

General
- Autosomal recessive, ornithine aminotransferase deficiency

Clinical
- Nyctalopia & VF constriction & axial myopia
- Signs
  - Ocular
    - PSCC
    - CME
  - Fundus
    - Circular patches atrophy mid-periphery
    - Peripheral & central spread
    - Foveal sparing

Treatment
- Legally blind by 50 yo
- Vitamin B6
  - Reduce ornithine levels (plasma, urinary)
  - Responder vs no responder
- Dietary restriction of ornithine

Late Onset Retinal Degeneration (LORD)
- Old age presentation
- Peripheral pigmentary degeneration

Choroideremia

General
- X-linked recessive
- Defect between RPE & PR
  - Like RP but lose more layers
- Choriocapillaris affected = "anemia"

Clinical
- Nyctalopia & VF constriction
- Signs
  - RPE & choroid atrophy mid-periphery
  - Central spread, macular sparing till late
- Female carrier
  - Mild patchy pigmentary atrophy of periphery

Central Areolar

General
- Autosomal dominant
- 3rd–4th decade gradual impairment central vision

Clinical
- Non-specific foveal granularity
- Macula depigmentation
  - Circumscribed RPE atrophy
  - Loss of macula choriocapillaris

Poor prognosis
- Severe vision loss by 6th–7th decade

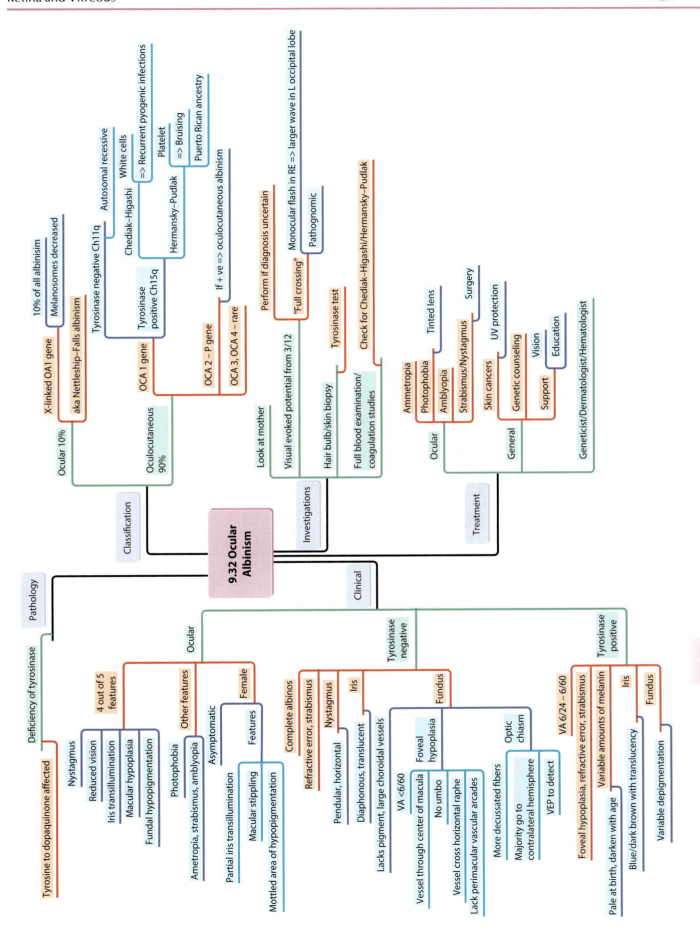

9.32 Ocular Albinism

Classification

Ocular 10%
- X-linked OA1 gene
- aka Nettleship–Falls albinism
  - 10% of all albinisim
  - Melanosomes decreased

Oculocutaneous 90%
- OCA 1 gene
  - Tyrosinase negative Ch11q
  - Tyrosinase positive Ch15q
    - Chediak–Higashi
      - Autosomal recessive
      - White cells
        - => Recurrent pyogenic infections
    - Hermansky–Pudlak
      - Platelet
        - => Bruising
      - Puerto Rican ancestry
- OCA 2 – P gene
- OCA 3, OCA 4 – rare
  - If + ve => oculocutaneous albinism

Investigations
- Look at mother
- Visual evoked potential from 3/12
  - Perform if diagnosis uncertain
  - "Full crossing"
  - Monocular flash in RE => larger wave in L occipital lobe
  - Pathognomic
- Hair bulb/skin biopsy
  - Tyrosinase test
- Full blood examination/ coagulation studies
  - Check for Chediak–Higashi/Hermansky–Pudlak

Treatment
- Ocular
  - Ammetropia
  - Photophobia
    - Tinted lens
  - Amblyopia
  - Strabismus/Nystagmus
    - Surgery
  - UV protection
- General
  - Skin cancers
  - Genetic counseling
    - Vision
    - Support
    - Education
- Geneticist/Dermatologist/Hematologist

Pathology
- Deficiency of tyrosinase
  - Tyrosine to dopaquinone affected

Clinical

Ocular
- 4 out of 5 features
  - Nystagmus
  - Reduced vision
  - Iris transillumination
  - Macular hypoplasia
  - Fundal hypopigmentation
- Other features
  - Photophobia
  - Ametropia, strabismus, amblyopia
- Female
  - Asymptomatic
  - Features
    - Partial iris transillumination
    - Macular stippling
    - Mottled area of hypopigmentation

Tyrosinase negative
- Complete albinos
  - Refractive error, strabismus
  - Nystagmus
    - Pendular, horizontal
- Iris
  - Diaphonous, translucent
  - Lacks pigment, large choroidal vessels
- Fundus
  - Foveal hypoplasia
    - VA <6/60
    - Vessel through center of macula
    - No umbo
    - Vessel cross horizontal raphe
    - Lack perimacular vascular arcades
  - Optic chiasm
    - More decussated fibers
    - Majority go to contralateral hemisphere
    - VEP to detect

Tyrosinase positive
- VA 6/24 – 6/60
  - Foveal hypoplasia, refractive error, strabismus
  - Variable amounts of melanin
- Iris
  - Pale at birth, darken with age
  - Blue/dark brown with translucency
- Fundus
  - Variable depigmentation

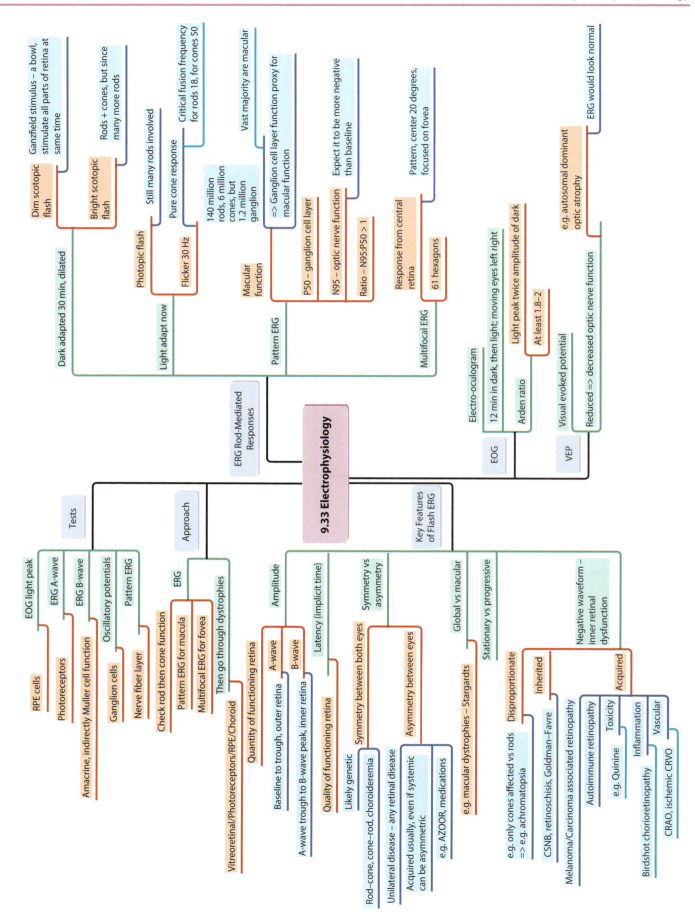

9.33 Electrophysiology

Tests
- EOG light peak — RPE cells
- ERG A-wave — Photoreceptors
- ERG B-wave — Amacrine, indirectly Muller cell function
- Oscillatory potentials
- Ganglion cells
- Pattern ERG — Nerve fiber layer

Approach
- Check rod then cone function
- Pattern ERG for macula
- Multifocal ERG for fovea
- Then go through dystrophies
  - Vitreoretinal/Photoreceptors/RPE/Choroid
- ERG
  - Quantity of functioning retina
    - Amplitude
      - A-wave — Baseline to trough, outer retina
      - B-wave — A-wave trough to B-wave peak, inner retina
    - Latency (implicit time) — Quality of functioning retina
      - Likely genetic — Rod–cone, cone–rod, choroideremia
      - Acquired usually, even if systemic can be asymmetric — Unilateral disease – any retinal disease
      - e.g. AZOOR, medications

Key Features of Flash ERG
- Symmetry vs asymmetry
  - Symmetry between both eyes
  - Asymmetry between eyes
- Global vs macular
  - e.g. macular dystrophies – Stargardts
- Stationary vs progressive
- Disproportionate
  - e.g. only cones affected vs rods => e.g. achromatopsia
- Inherited
  - CSNB, retinoschisis, Goldman–Favre
- Negative waveform – inner retinal dysfunction
  - Melanoma/Carcinoma associated retinopathy
  - Autoimmune retinopathy
  - Acquired
    - Toxicity — e.g. Quinine
    - Inflammation — Birdshot chorioretinopathy
    - Vascular — CRAO, ischemic CRVO

ERG Rod-Mediated Responses
- Dark adapted 30 min, dilated
  - Dim scotopic flash — Ganzfield stimulus – a bowl, stimulate all parts of retina at same time
  - Bright scotopic flash — Rods + cones, but since many more rods — Still many rods involved
- Light adapt now
  - Photopic flash — Pure cone response
  - Flicker 30 Hz — Critical fusion frequency for rods 18, for cones 50
- Macular function — Vast majority are macular
  - 140 million rods, 6 million cones, but 1.2 million ganglion
- Pattern ERG
  - P50 – ganglion cell layer => Ganglion cell layer function proxy for macular function
  - N95 – optic nerve function — Expect it to be more negative than baseline
  - Ratio – N95:P50 > 1
- Multifocal ERG
  - Response from central retina — Pattern, center 20 degrees, focused on fovea
  - 61 hexagons

EOG
- Electro-oculogram — 12 min in dark, then light; moving eyes left right
- Arden ratio — Light peak twice amplitude of dark
  - At least 1.8–2

VEP
- Visual evoked potential
- Reduced => decreased optic nerve function
  - e.g. autosomal dominant optic atrophy — ERG would look normal

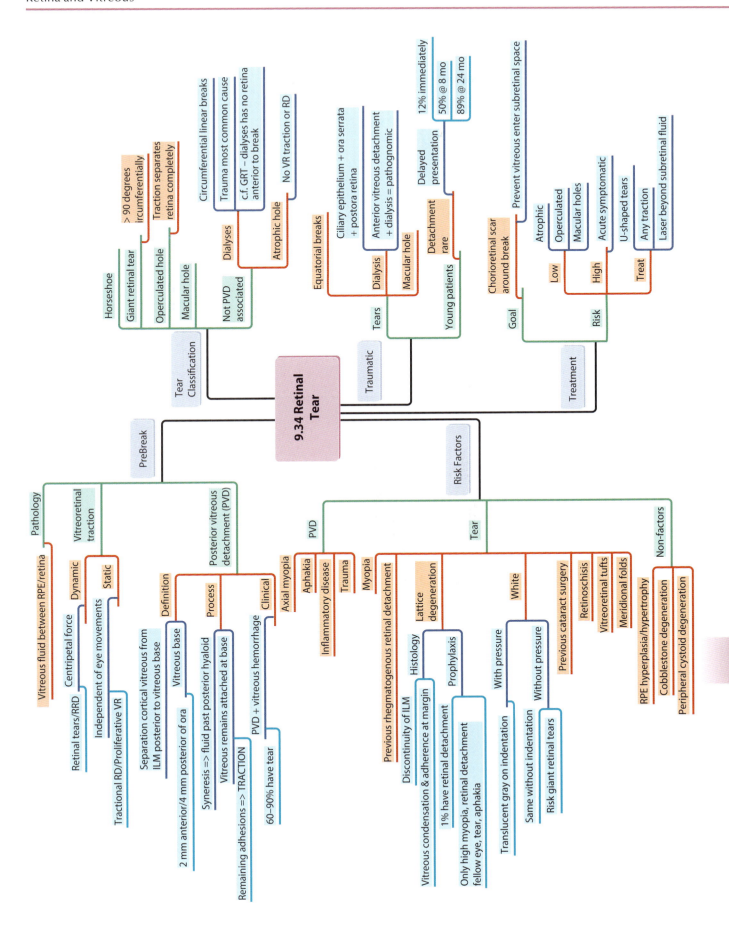

9.34 Retinal Tear

Tear Classification
- Horseshoe
  - > 90 degrees circumferentially
  - Traction separates retina completely
- Giant retinal tear
- Operculated hole
- Macular hole
- Not PVD associated
  - Dialyses
    - Circumferential linear breaks
    - Trauma most common cause
    - c.f. GRT – dialyses has no retina anterior to break
  - Atrophic hole
    - No VR traction or RD

Traumatic
- Tears
  - Equatorial breaks
  - Dialysis
    - Ciliary epithelium + ora serrata + postora retina
    - Anterior vitreous detachment + dialysis = pathognomic
  - Macular hole
    - Delayed presentation
      - 12% immediately
      - 50% @ 8 mo
      - 89% @ 24 mo
  - Detachment rare
- Young patients

Treatment
- Goal
  - Chorioretinal scar around break
  - Prevent vitreous enter subretinal space
- Risk
  - Low
    - Atrophic
    - Operculated
    - Macular holes
  - High
    - Acute symptomatic
    - U-shaped tears
    - Any traction
  - Treat
    - Laser beyond subretinal fluid

PreBreak
- Pathology
  - Vitreoretinal traction
    - Vitreous fluid between RPE/retina
    - Centripetal force
      - Retinal tears/RRD
    - Dynamic
      - Independent of eye movements
    - Static
      - Tractional RD/Proliferative VR
  - Posterior vitreous detachment (PVD)
    - Definition
      - Separation cortical vitreous from ILM posterior to vitreous base
    - Vitreous base
      - 2 mm anterior/4 mm posterior of ora
    - Process
      - Syneresis => fluid past posterior hyaloid
      - Vitreous remains attached at base
    - Remaining adhesions => TRACTION
    - Clinical
      - PVD + vitreous hemorrhage
      - 60–90% have tear

Risk Factors
- PVD
  - Axial myopia
  - Aphakia
  - Inflammatory disease
  - Trauma
  - Myopia
- Tear
  - Previous rhegmatogenous retinal detachment
  - Lattice degeneration
    - Histology
      - Discontinuity of ILM
      - Vitreous condensation & adherence at margin
    - Prophylaxis
      - 1% have retinal detachment
      - Only high myopia, retinal detachment fellow eye, tear, aphakia
  - White
    - With pressure
      - Translucent gray on indentation
    - Without pressure
      - Same without indentation
      - Risk giant retinal tears
  - Previous cataract surgery
  - Retinoschisis
  - Vitreoretinal tufts
  - Meridional folds
- Non-factors
  - RPE hyperplasia/hypertrophy
  - Cobblestone degeneration
  - Peripheral cystoid degeneration

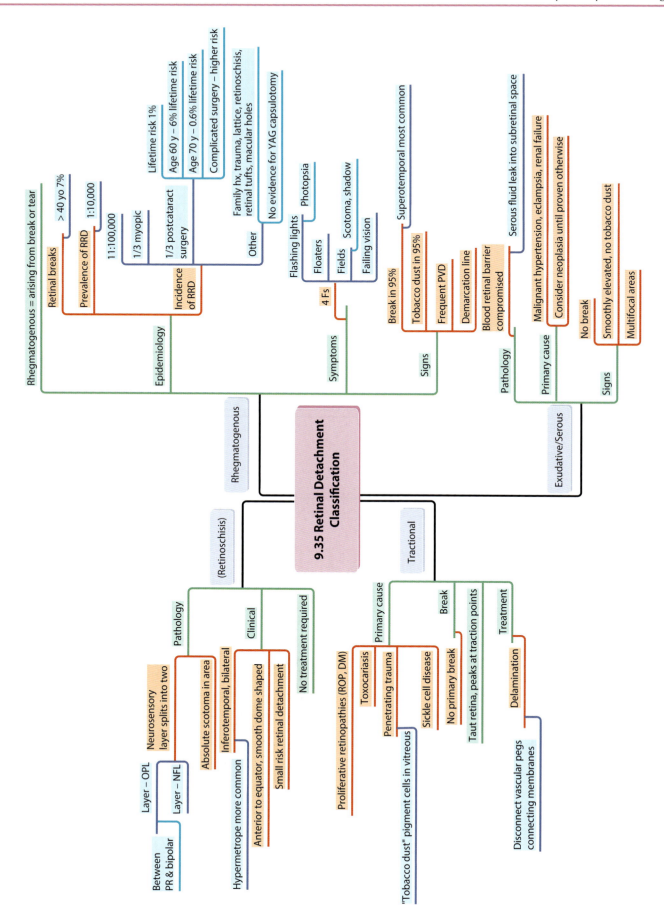

9.35 Retinal Detachment Classification

Rhegmatogenous

Rhegmatogenous = arising from break or tear

Epidemiology

Incidence of RRD
- Prevalence of RRD
  - Retinal breaks — > 40 yo 7%
  - 1:10,000
  - 1:100,000
- 1/3 myopic
- 1/3 postcataract surgery
  - Lifetime risk 1%
  - Age 60 y – 6% lifetime risk
  - Age 70 y – 0.6% lifetime risk
  - Complicated surgery – higher risk
- Other
  - Family hx, trauma, lattice, retinoschisis, retinal tufts, macular holes
  - No evidence for YAG capsulotomy

Symptoms
- 4 Fs
  - Flashing lights — Photopsia
  - Floaters
  - Fields — Scotoma, shadow
  - Failing vision

Signs
- Superotemporal most common
- Break in 95%
- Tobacco dust in 95%
- Frequent PVD
- Demarcation line
- Blood retinal barrier compromised

Exudative/Serous

Pathology
- Serous fluid leak into subretinal space

Primary cause
- Malignant hypertension, eclampsia, renal failure
- Consider neoplasia until proven otherwise

Signs
- No break
- Smoothly elevated, no tobacco dust
- Multifocal areas

(Retinoschisis)

Pathology
- Neurosensory layer splits into two
  - Layer – OPL — Between PR & bipolar
  - Layer – NFL
- Hypermetrope more common
- Anterior to equator, smooth dome shaped

Clinical
- Absolute scotoma in area
- Inferotemporal, bilateral
- Small risk retinal detachment
- No treatment required

Tractional

Primary cause
- Proliferative retinopathies (ROP, DM)
- Toxocariasis
- Penetrating trauma — "Tobacco dust" pigment cells in vitreous
- Sickle cell disease

Break
- No primary break
- Taut retina, peaks at traction points

Treatment
- Delamination — Disconnect vascular pegs connecting membranes

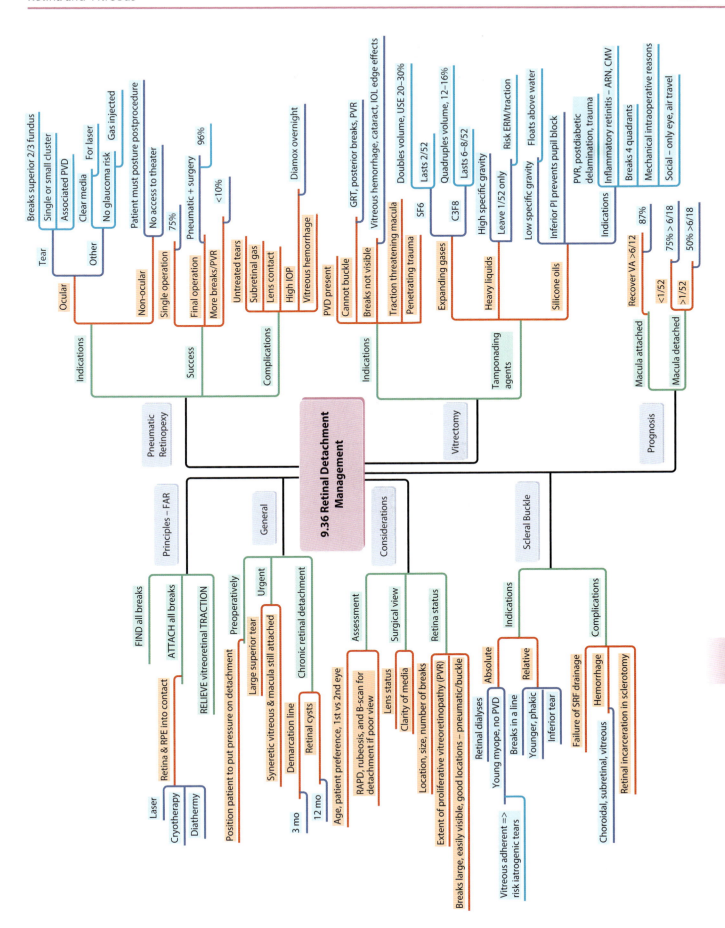

9.36 Retinal Detachment Management

Pneumatic Retinopexy

Indications
- Tear
  - Breaks superior 2/3 fundus
  - Single or small cluster
  - Associated PVD
- Other
  - Clear media
    - For laser
  - No glaucoma risk
    - Gas injected

Non-ocular
- Patient must posture postprocedure
- No access to theater

Success
- Single operation — 75%
- Final operation — 96%
  - Pneumatic + surgery
  - <10%
- More breaks/PVR

Complications
- Untreated tears
- Subretinal gas
- Lens contact
- High IOP
  - Diamox overnight
- Vitreous hemorrhage

Vitrectomy

Indications
- PVD present
- Cannot buckle
  - GRT, posterior breaks, PVR
- Breaks not visible
  - Vitreous hemorrhage, cataract, IOL edge effects
- Traction threatening macula
- Penetrating trauma

Tamponading agents
- Expanding gases
  - SF6
    - Doubles volume, USE 20–30%
    - Lasts 2/52
  - C3F8
    - Quadruples volume, 12–16%
    - Lasts 6–8/52
- Heavy liquids
  - High specific gravity
    - Leave 1/52 only
  - Low specific gravity
    - Risk ERM/traction
    - Floats above water
- Silicone oils
  - Inferior PI prevents pupil block
  - Indications
    - PVR, postdiabetic delamination, trauma
    - Inflammatory retinitis – ARN, CMV
    - Breaks 4 quadrants
    - Mechanical intraoperative reasons
    - Social – only eye, air travel

Prognosis

Macula attached
- Recover VA >6/12 — 87%

Macula detached
- <1/52 — 75% > 6/18
- >1/52 — 50% >6/18

Principles – FAR
- FIND all breaks
- ATTACH all breaks
  - Retina & RPE into contact
    - Laser
    - Cryotherapy
    - Diathermy
  - Position patient to put pressure on detachment
- RELIEVE vitreoretinal TRACTION

General

Preoperatively
- Urgent
  - Large superior tear
  - Syneretic vitreous & macula still attached
- Chronic retinal detachment
  - Demarcation line
    - 3 mo
    - 12 mo
  - Retinal cysts

Considerations

Assessment
- Age, patient preference, 1st vs 2nd eye
- RAPD, rubeosis, and B-scan for detachment if poor view

Surgical view
- Lens status
- Clarity of media

Retina status
- Location, size, number of breaks
- Extent of proliferative vitreoretinopathy (PVR)
- Breaks large, easily visible, good locations – pneumatic/buckle
- Vitreous adherent => risk iatrogenic tears

Scleral Buckle

Indications
- Absolute
  - Retinal dialyses
  - Young myope, no PVD
  - Breaks in a line
- Relative
  - Younger, phakic
  - Inferior tear

Complications
- Failure of SRF drainage
  - Hemorrhage
    - Choroidal, subretinal, vitreous
  - Retinal incarceration in sclerotomy

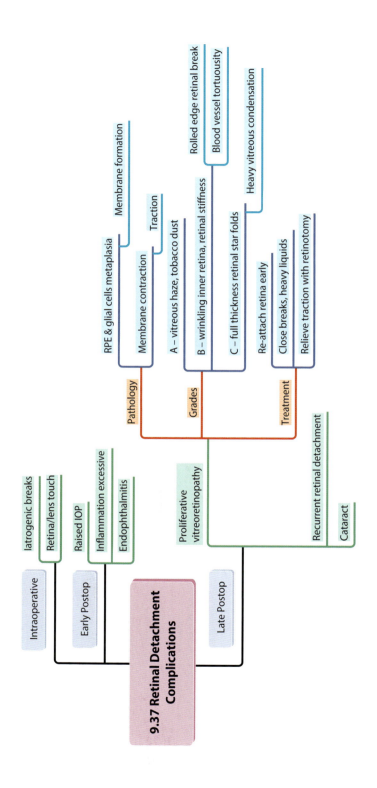

9.37 Retinal Detachment Complications

Intraoperative
- Iatrogenic breaks
- Retina/lens touch

Early Postop
- Raised IOP
- Inflammation excessive
- Endophthalmitis

Late Postop
- Proliferative vitreoretinopathy
- Recurrent retinal detachment
- Cataract

Proliferative vitreoretinopathy

Pathology
- RPE & glial cells metaplasia
  - Membrane formation
- Membrane contraction
  - Traction

Grades
- A – vitreous haze, tobacco dust
- B – wrinkling inner retina, retinal stiffness
  - Rolled edge retinal break
  - Blood vessel tortuousity
- C – full thickness retinal star folds
  - Heavy vitreous condensation

Treatment
- Re-attach retina early
- Close breaks, heavy liquids
- Relieve traction with retinotomy

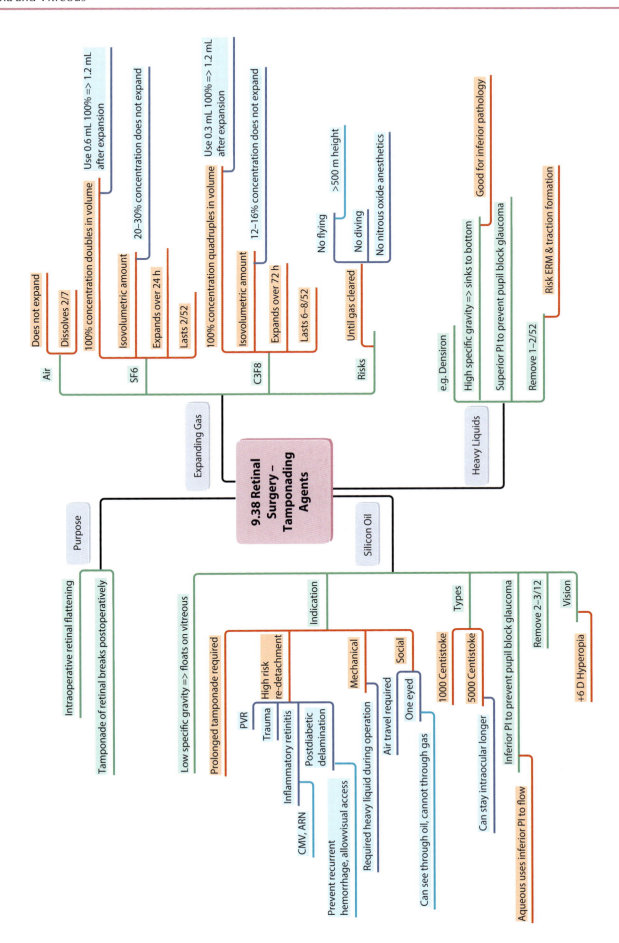

9.38 Retinal Surgery – Tamponading Agents

Expanding Gas

- Air
  - Does not expand
  - Dissolves 2/7
- SF6
  - 100% concentration doubles in volume
    - Use 0.6 mL 100% => 1.2 mL after expansion
  - 20–30% concentration does not expand
  - Isovolumetric amount
  - Expands over 24 h
  - Lasts 2/52
- C3F8
  - 100% concentration quadruples in volume
    - Use 0.3 mL 100% => 1.2 mL after expansion
  - 12–16% concentration does not expand
  - Isovolumetric amount
  - Expands over 72 h
  - Lasts 6–8/52
- Risks
  - Until gas cleared
  - No flying
    - >500 m height
  - No diving
  - No nitrous oxide anesthetics

Heavy Liquids
- e.g. Densiron
- High specific gravity => sinks to bottom
- Superior PI to prevent pupil block glaucoma
  - Good for inferior pathology
- Remove 1–2/52
  - Risk ERM & traction formation

Purpose
- Intraoperative retinal flattening
- Tamponade of retinal breaks postoperatively

Silicon Oil
- Low specific gravity => floats on vitreous
- Prolonged tamponade required
- Indication
  - High risk re-detachment
    - PVR
    - Trauma
    - Inflammatory retinitis
      - CMV, ARN
    - Postdiabetic delamination
      - Prevent recurrent hemorrhage, allow visual access
  - Mechanical
    - Required heavy liquid during operation
    - Air travel required
    - One eyed
      - Can see through oil, cannot through gas
  - Social
- Types
  - 1000 Centistoke
  - 5000 Centistoke
    - Can stay intraocular longer
- Inferior PI to prevent pupil block glaucoma
  - Aqueous uses inferior PI to flow
- Remove 2–3/12
- Vision
  - +6 D Hyperopia

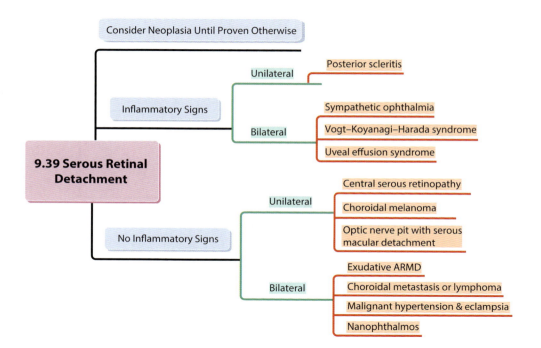

9.39 Serous Retinal Detachment

- Consider Neoplasia Until Proven Otherwise
- Inflammatory Signs
  - Unilateral
    - Posterior scleritis
  - Bilateral
    - Sympathetic ophthalmia
    - Vogt–Koyanagi–Harada syndrome
    - Uveal effusion syndrome
- No Inflammatory Signs
  - Unilateral
    - Central serous retinopathy
    - Choroidal melanoma
    - Optic nerve pit with serous macular detachment
  - Bilateral
    - Exudative ARMD
    - Choroidal metastasis or lymphoma
    - Malignant hypertension & eclampsia
    - Nanophthalmos

10 Trauma

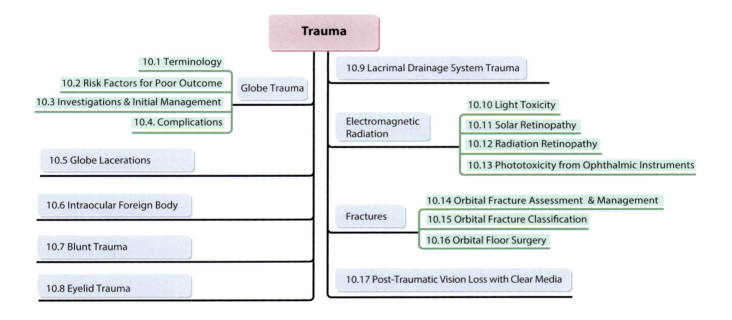

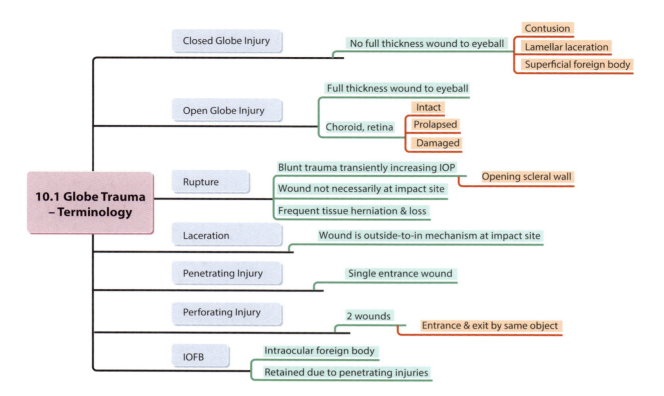

Closed Globe Injury — No full thickness wound to eyeball
- Contusion
- Lamellar laceration
- Superficial foreign body

Open Globe Injury
- Full thickness wound to eyeball
- Choroid, retina
  - Intact
  - Prolapsed
  - Damaged

10.1 Globe Trauma – Terminology

Rupture
- Blunt trauma transiently increasing IOP — Opening scleral wall
- Wound not necessarily at impact site
- Frequent tissue herniation & loss

Laceration — Wound is outside-to-in mechanism at impact site

Penetrating Injury — Single entrance wound

Perforating Injury
- 2 wounds — Entrance & exit by same object

IOFB
- Intraocular foreign body
- Retained due to penetrating injuries

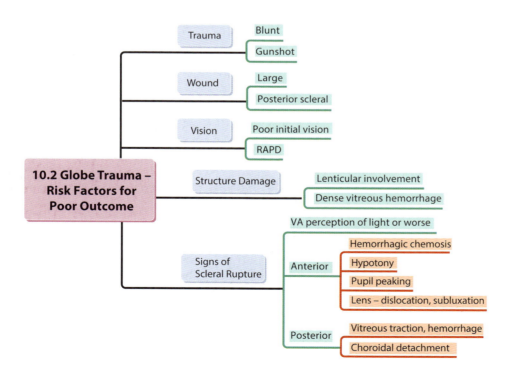

Trauma
- Blunt
- Gunshot

Wound
- Large
- Posterior scleral

Vision
- Poor initial vision
- RAPD

10.2 Globe Trauma – Risk Factors for Poor Outcome

Structure Damage
- Lenticular involvement
- Dense vitreous hemorrhage

Signs of Scleral Rupture
- VA perception of light or worse
- Anterior
  - Hemorrhagic chemosis
  - Hypotony
  - Pupil peaking
  - Lens – dislocation, subluxation
- Posterior
  - Vitreous traction, hemorrhage
  - Choroidal detachment

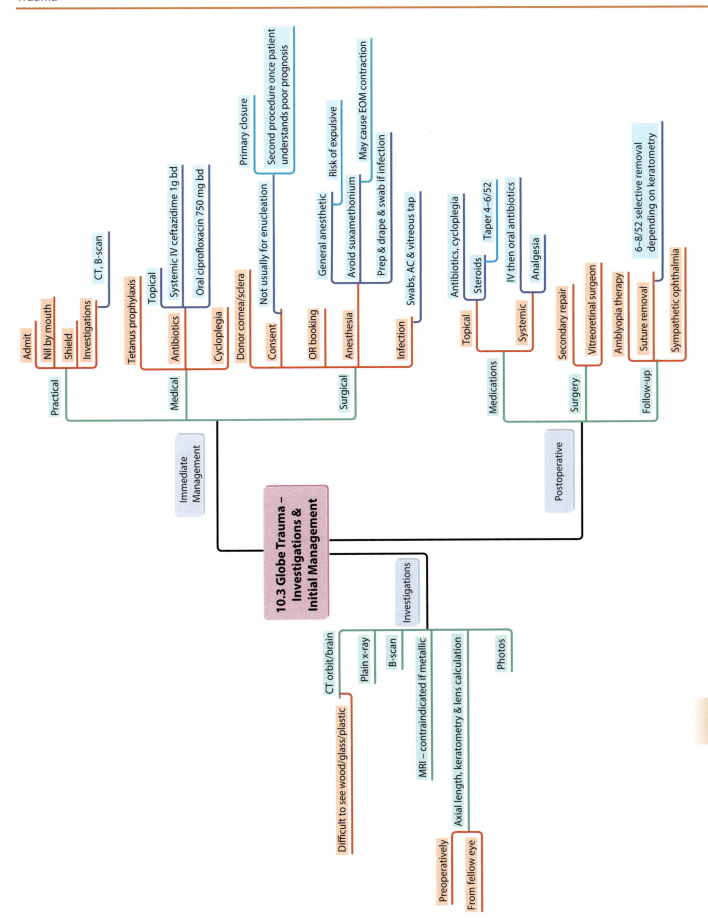

10.3 Globe Trauma – Investigations & Initial Management

Immediate Management

Practical
- Admit
- Nil by mouth
- Shield
- Investigations
  - CT, B-scan

Medical
- Tetanus prophylaxis
- Antibiotics
  - Topical
  - Systemic IV ceftazidime 1g bd
  - Oral ciprofloxacin 750 mg bd
- Cycloplegia

Surgical
- Donor cornea/sclera
- Consent
  - Primary closure
  - Second procedure once patient understands poor prognosis
  - Not usually for enucleation
- OR booking
- Anesthesia
  - General anesthetic
  - Risk of expulsive
  - Avoid suxamethonium
  - May cause EOM contraction
  - Prep & drape & swab if infection
- Infection
  - Swabs, AC & vitreous tap

Postoperative

Medications
- Topical
  - Antibiotics, cycloplegia
  - Steroids
    - Taper 4–6/52
- Systemic
  - IV then oral antibiotics
  - Analgesia

Surgery
- Secondary repair
- Vitreoretinal surgeon

Follow-up
- Amblyopia therapy
- Suture removal
  - 6–8/52 selective removal depending on keratometry
- Sympathetic ophthalmia

Investigations

- CT orbit/brain
  - Difficult to see wood/glass/plastic
- Plain x-ray
- B-scan
- MRI – contraindicated if metallic
- Axial length, keratometry & lens calculation
  - Preoperatively
  - From fellow eye
- Photos

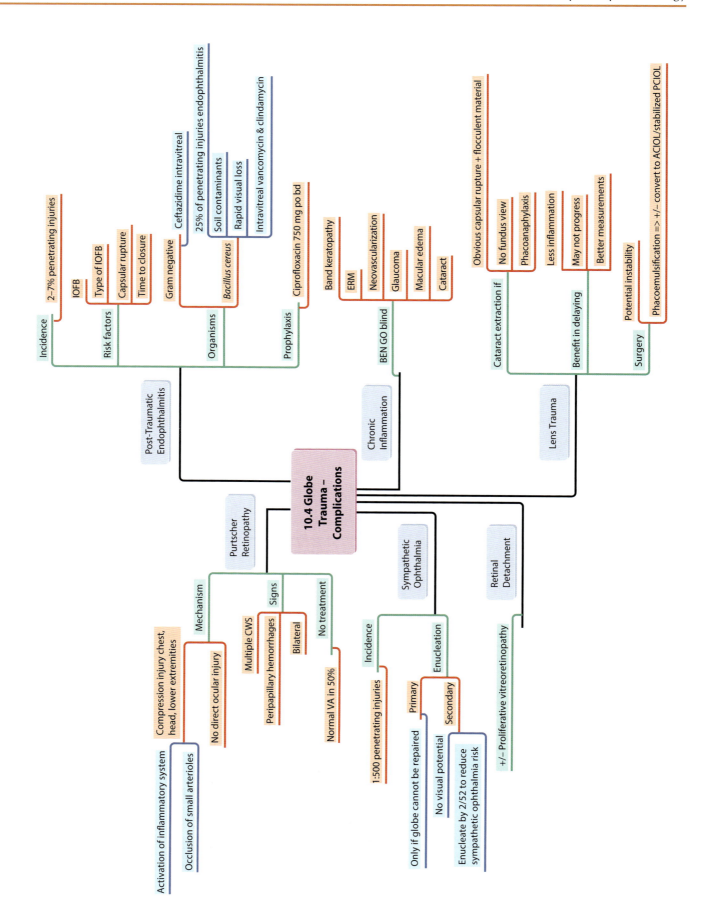

10.4 Globe Trauma – Complications

Post-Traumatic Endophthalmitis

- Incidence
  - 2–7% penetrating injuries
- Risk factors
  - IOFB
  - Type of IOFB
  - Capsular rupture
  - Time to closure
- Organisms
  - Gram negative
  - *Bacillus cereus*
    - Ceftazidime intravitreal
    - 25% of penetrating injuries endophthalmitis
    - Soil contaminants
    - Rapid visual loss
    - Intravitreal vancomycin & clindamycin
- Prophylaxis
  - Ciprofloxacin 750 mg po bd

Chronic Inflammation

- BEN GO blind
  - Band keratopathy
  - ERM
  - Neovascularization
  - Glaucoma
  - Macular edema
  - Cataract

Lens Trauma

- Cataract extraction if
  - Obvious capsular rupture + flocculent material
  - No fundus view
  - Phacoanaphylaxis
- Benefit in delaying
  - Less inflammation
  - May not progress
  - Better measurements
- Surgery
  - Potential instability
  - Phacoemulsification => +/– convert to ACIOL/stabilized PCIOL

Purtscher Retinopathy

- Mechanism
  - Compression injury chest, head, lower extremities
  - No direct ocular injury
  - Activation of inflammatory system
  - Occlusion of small arterioles
- Signs
  - Multiple CWS
  - Peripapillary hemorrhages
  - Bilateral
- No treatment
  - Normal VA in 50%

Sympathetic Ophthalmia

- Incidence
  - 1:500 penetrating injuries
- Enucleation
  - Primary
    - Only if globe cannot be repaired
    - No visual potential
  - Secondary
    - Enucleate by 2/52 to reduce sympathetic ophthalmia risk

Retinal Detachment

- +/– Proliferative vitreoretinopathy

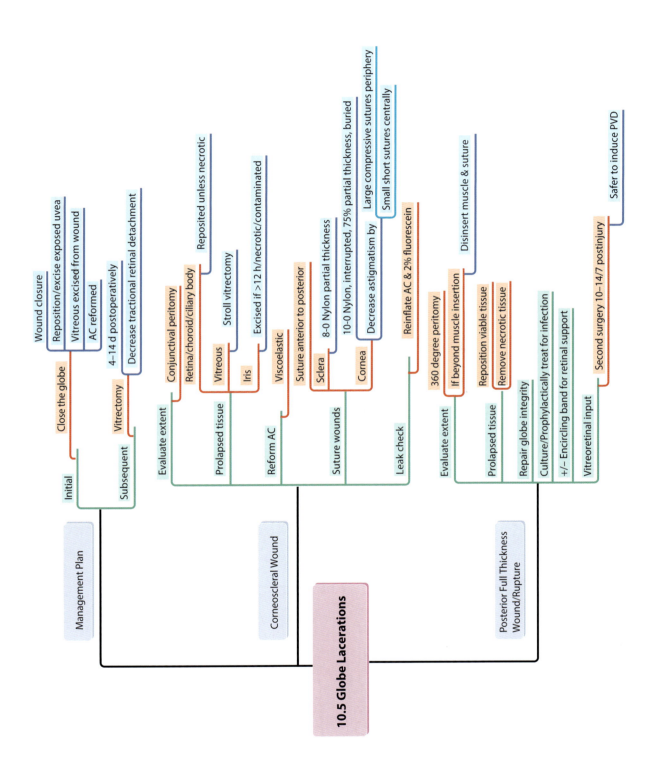

10.5 Globe Lacerations

Management Plan
- Initial
- Subsequent

Initial
- Close the globe
  - Wound closure
    - Reposition/excise exposed uvea
    - Vitreous excised from wound
    - AC reformed

Subsequent
- Vitrectomy
  - 4–14 d postoperatively
  - Decrease tractional retinal detachment

Corneoscleral Wound
- Evaluate extent
  - Conjunctival peritomy
  - Retina/choroid/ciliary body
    - Reposited unless necrotic
- Prolapsed tissue
  - Vitreous
    - Stroll vitrectomy
  - Iris
    - Excised if >12 h/necrotic/contaminated
- Reform AC
  - Viscoelastic
- Suture wounds
  - Suture anterior to posterior
  - Sclera
    - 8-0 Nylon partial thickness
  - Cornea
    - 10-0 Nylon, interrupted, 75% partial thickness, buried
    - Decrease astigmatism by
      - Large compressive sutures periphery
      - Small short sutures centrally
- Leak check
  - Reinflate AC & 2% fluorescein

Posterior Full Thickness Wound/Rupture
- Evaluate extent
  - 360 degree peritomy
  - If beyond muscle insertion
    - Disinsert muscle & suture
- Prolapsed tissue
  - Reposition viable tissue
  - Remove necrotic tissue
- Repair globe integrity
- Culture/Prophylactically treat for infection
- +/– Encircling band for retinal support
- Vitreoretinal input
  - Second surgery 10–14/7 postinjury
    - Safer to induce PVD

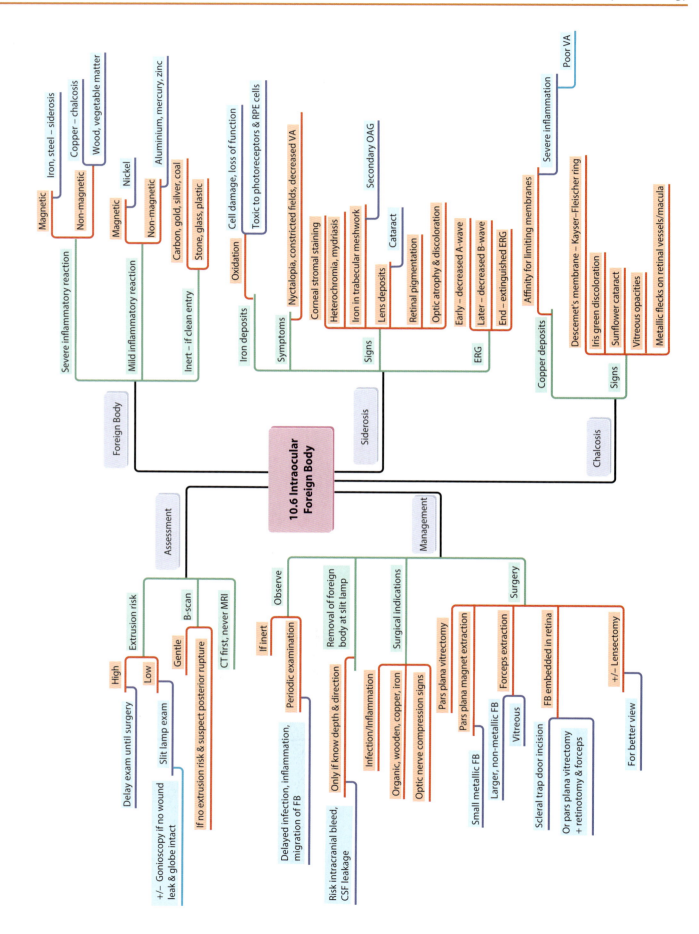

10.6 Intraocular Foreign Body

Foreign Body
- Severe inflammatory reaction
  - Magnetic
    - Iron, steel – siderosis
  - Non-magnetic
    - Copper – chalcosis
    - Wood, vegetable matter
- Mild inflammatory reaction
  - Magnetic
    - Nickel
  - Non-magnetic
    - Aluminium, mercury, zinc
    - Carbon, gold, silver, coal
- Inert – if clean entry
  - Stone, glass, plastic

Siderosis
- Iron deposits
  - Oxidation
    - Cell damage, loss of function
    - Toxic to photoreceptors & RPE cells
- Symptoms
  - Nyctalopia, constricted fields, decreased VA
- Signs
  - Corneal stromal staining
  - Heterochromia, mydriasis
  - Iron in trabecular meshwork
    - Secondary OAG
  - Lens deposits
    - Cataract
  - Retinal pigmentation
  - Optic atrophy & discoloration
- ERG
  - Early – decreased A-wave
  - Later – decreased B-wave
  - End – extinguished ERG

Chalcosis
- Copper deposits
  - Affinity for limiting membranes
  - Severe inflammation
    - Poor VA
- Signs
  - Descemet's membrane – Kayser–Fleischer ring
  - Iris green discoloration
  - Sunflower cataract
  - Vitreous opacities
  - Metallic flecks on retinal vessels/macula

Assessment
- Extrusion risk
  - High
    - Delay exam until surgery
      - +/– Gonioscopy if no wound leak & globe intact
  - Low
    - Slit lamp exam
    - If no extrusion risk & suspect posterior rupture
- B-scan
  - Gentle
- CT first, never MRI

Management
- Observe
  - If inert
    - Periodic examination
- Removal of foreign body at slit lamp
  - Only if know depth & direction
    - Delayed infection, inflammation, migration of FB
    - Risk intracranial bleed, CSF leakage
- Surgical indications
  - Infection/Inflammation
  - Organic, wooden, copper, iron
  - Optic nerve compression signs
- Surgery
  - Pars plana vitrectomy
    - Small metallic FB
  - Pars plana magnet extraction
    - Larger, non-metallic FB
  - Forceps extraction
    - Vitreous
    - FB embedded in retina
      - Scleral trap door incision
      - Or pars plana vitrectomy + retinotomy & forceps
  - +/– Lensectomy
    - For better view

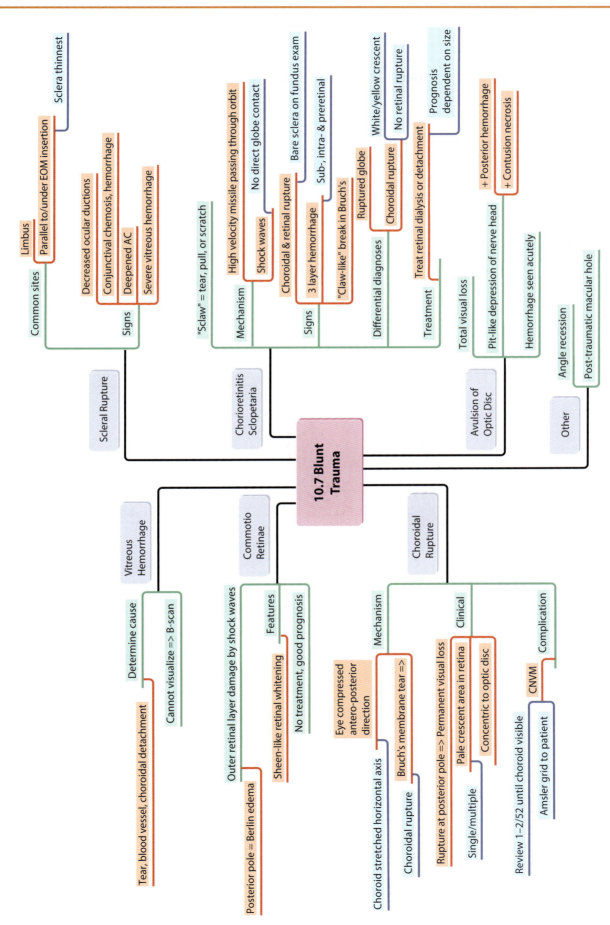

10.7 Blunt Trauma

Scleral Rupture
- Common sites
  - Limbus
  - Parallel to/under EOM insertion
    - Sclera thinnest
- Signs
  - Decreased ocular ductions
  - Conjunctival chemosis, hemorrhage
  - Deepened AC
  - Severe vitreous hemorrhage

Chorioretinitis Sclopetaria
- "Sclaw" = tear, pull, or scratch
- Mechanism
  - High velocity missile passing through orbit
  - No direct globe contact
  - Shock waves
- Signs
  - Choroidal & retinal rupture
    - Bare sclera on fundus exam
  - 3 layer hemorrhage
    - Sub-, intra- & preretinal
  - "Claw-like" break in Bruch's
    - Ruptured globe
- Differential diagnoses
  - Choroidal rupture
    - White/yellow crescent
    - No retinal rupture
  - Treat retinal dialysis or detachment
- Treatment
  - Prognosis dependent on size

Avulsion of Optic Disc
- Total visual loss
- Pit-like depression of nerve head
  - + Posterior hemorrhage
  - + Contusion necrosis
- Hemorrhage seen acutely

Other
- Angle recession
- Post-traumatic macular hole

Vitreous Hemorrhage
- Determine cause
  - Tear, blood vessel, choroidal detachment
- Cannot visualize => B-scan

Commotio Retinae
- Outer retinal layer damage by shock waves
  - Posterior pole = Berlin edema
- Features
  - Sheen-like retinal whitening
  - No treatment, good prognosis

Choroidal Rupture
- Mechanism
  - Eye compressed antero-posterior direction
    - Bruch's membrane tear =>
  - Choroid stretched horizontal axis
  - Choroidal rupture
  - Rupture at posterior pole => Permanent visual loss
- Clinical
  - Pale crescent area in retina
  - Concentric to optic disc
  - Single/multiple
  - Review 1–2/52 until choroid visible
- Complication
  - CNVM
  - Amsler grid to patient

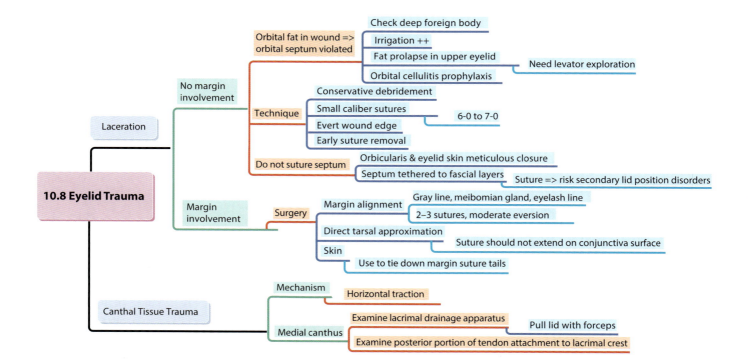

10.8 Eyelid Trauma

Laceration
- No margin involvement
  - Orbital fat in wound => orbital septum violated
    - Check deep foreign body
    - Irrigation ++
    - Fat prolapse in upper eyelid — Need levator exploration
    - Orbital cellulitis prophylaxis
  - Technique
    - Conservative debridement
    - Small caliber sutures — 6-0 to 7-0
    - Evert wound edge
    - Early suture removal
  - Do not suture septum
    - Orbicularis & eyelid skin meticulous closure
    - Septum tethered to fascial layers — Suture => risk secondary lid position disorders
- Margin involvement
  - Surgery
    - Margin alignment — Gray line, meibomian gland, eyelash line
    - 2–3 sutures, moderate eversion
    - Direct tarsal approximation — Suture should not extend on conjunctiva surface
    - Skin
    - Use to tie down margin suture tails

Canthal Tissue Trauma
- Mechanism
  - Horizontal traction
- Medial canthus
  - Examine lacrimal drainage apparatus — Pull lid with forceps
  - Examine posterior portion of tendon attachment to lacrimal crest

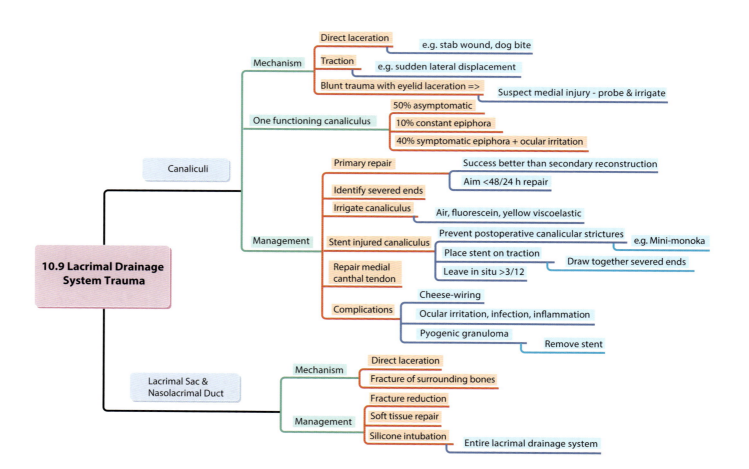

10.9 Lacrimal Drainage System Trauma

Canaliculi
- Mechanism
  - Direct laceration — e.g. stab wound, dog bite
  - Traction — e.g. sudden lateral displacement
  - Blunt trauma with eyelid laceration => — Suspect medial injury - probe & irrigate
- One functioning canaliculus
  - 50% asymptomatic
  - 10% constant epiphora
  - 40% symptomatic epiphora + ocular irritation
- Management
  - Primary repair — Success better than secondary reconstruction
    - Aim <48/24 h repair
  - Identify severed ends
  - Irrigate canaliculus — Air, fluorescein, yellow viscoelastic
  - Stent injured canaliculus
    - Prevent postoperative canalicular strictures — e.g. Mini-monoka
    - Place stent on traction — Draw together severed ends
    - Leave in situ >3/12
  - Repair medial canthal tendon
  - Complications
    - Cheese-wiring
    - Ocular irritation, infection, inflammation
    - Pyogenic granuloma — Remove stent

Lacrimal Sac & Nasolacrimal Duct
- Mechanism
  - Direct laceration
  - Fracture of surrounding bones
- Management
  - Fracture reduction
  - Soft tissue repair
  - Silicone intubation — Entire lacrimal drainage system

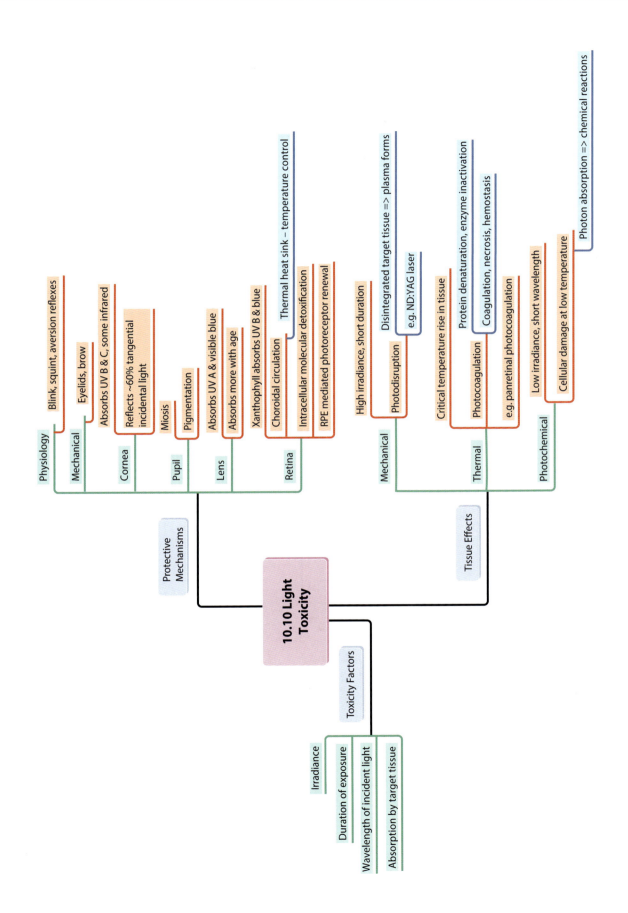

10.10 Light Toxicity

Protective Mechanisms

Physiology
- Blink, squint, aversion reflexes

Mechanical
- Eyelids, brow

Cornea
- Absorbs UV B & C, some infrared
- Reflects ~60% tangential incidental light

Pupil
- Miosis
- Pigmentation

Lens
- Absorbs UV A & visible blue
- Absorbs more with age
- Xanthophyll absorbs UV B & blue

Retina
- Choroidal circulation — Thermal heat sink – temperature control
- Intracellular molecular detoxification
- RPE mediated photoreceptor renewal

Tissue Effects

Mechanical
- High irradiance, short duration
- Photodisruption — Disintegrated target tissue => plasma forms
  - e.g. ND:YAG laser

Thermal
- Critical temperature rise in tissue
- Photocoagulation — Protein denaturation, enzyme inactivation
  - Coagulation, necrosis, hemostasis
  - e.g. panretinal photocoagulation

Photochemical
- Low irradiance, short wavelength
- Cellular damage at low temperature — Photon absorption => chemical reactions

Toxicity Factors
- Irradiance
- Duration of exposure
- Wavelength of incident light
- Absorption by target tissue

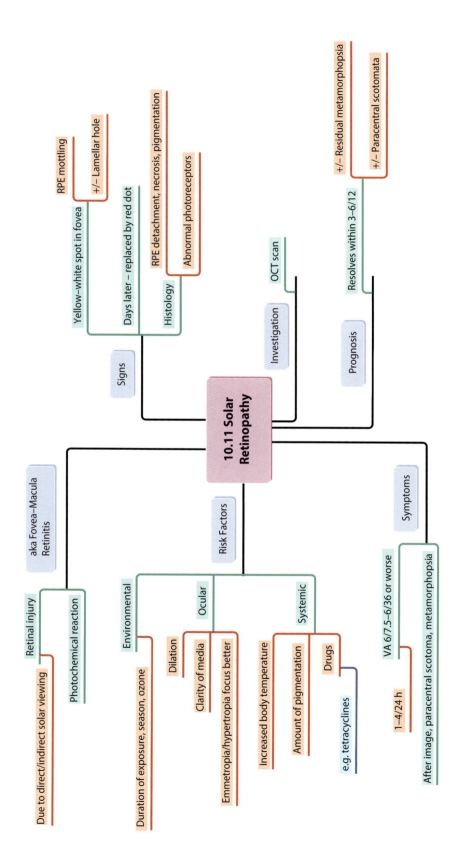

10.11 Solar Retinopathy

aka Fovea–Macula Retinitis

Signs
- Yellow–white spot in fovea
  - RPE mottling
  - +/– Lamellar hole
- Days later – replaced by red dot
- Histology
  - RPE detachment, necrosis, pigmentation
  - Abnormal photoreceptors

Investigation
- OCT scan

Prognosis
- Resolves within 3–6/12
  - +/– Residual metamorphopsia
  - +/– Paracentral scotomata

Risk Factors
- Retinal injury
- Photochemical reaction
- Environmental
  - Due to direct/indirect solar viewing
  - Duration of exposure, season, ozone
- Ocular
  - Dilation
  - Clarity of media
  - Emmetropia/hypertropia focus better
- Systemic
  - Increased body temperature
  - Amount of pigmentation
  - Drugs
    - e.g. tetracyclines

Symptoms
- VA 6/7.5–6/36 or worse
  - 1–4/24 h
- After image, paracentral scotoma, metamorphopsia

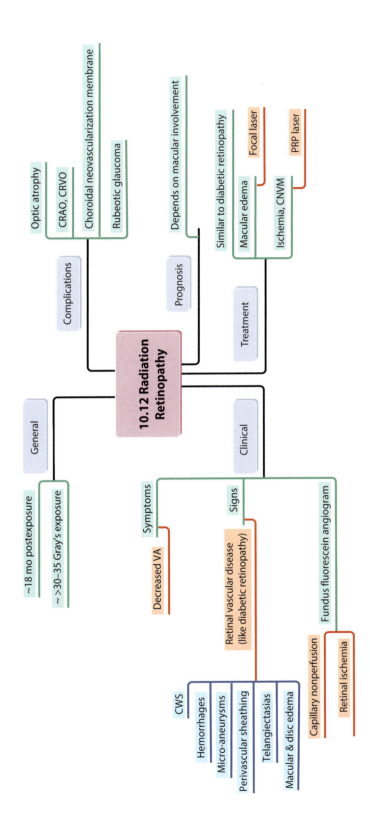

10.12 Radiation Retinopathy

General
- ~18 mo postexposure
- ~ >30–35 Gray's exposure

Complications
- Optic atrophy
- CRAO, CRVO
- Choroidal neovascularization membrane
- Rubeotic glaucoma

Prognosis
- Depends on macular involvement

Treatment
- Similar to diabetic retinopathy
- Macular edema → Focal laser
- Ischemia, CNVM → PRP laser

Clinical
- Symptoms
  - Decreased VA
- Signs
  - Retinal vascular disease (like diabetic retinopathy)
    - CWS
    - Hemorrhages
    - Micro-aneurysms
    - Perivascular sheathing
    - Telangiectasias
    - Macular & disc edema
  - Fundus fluorescein angiogram
    - Capillary nonperfusion
    - Retinal ischemia

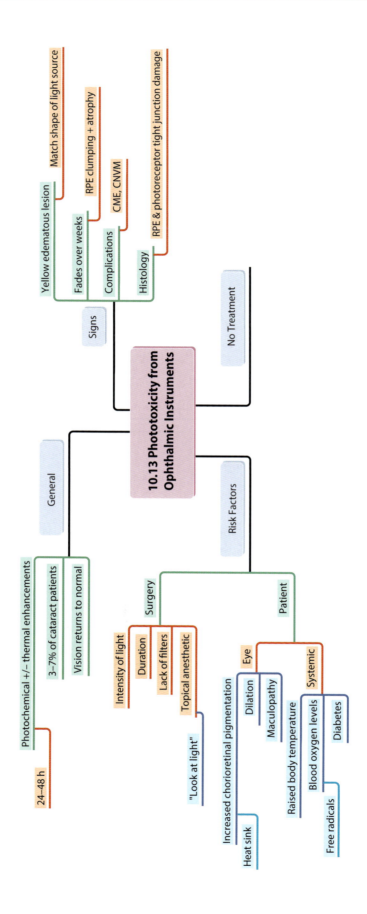

10.13 Phototoxicity from Ophthalmic Instruments

Signs
- Yellow edematous lesion — Match shape of light source
- Fades over weeks
- Complications
  - RPE clumping + atrophy
  - CME, CNVM
- Histology — RPE & photoreceptor tight junction damage

No Treatment

General
- Photochemical +/- thermal enhancements — 24–48 h
- 3–7% of cataract patients
- Vision returns to normal

Risk Factors
- Surgery
  - Intensity of light
  - Duration
  - Lack of filters
  - Topical anesthetic — "Look at light"
- Patient
  - Eye
    - Increased chorioretinal pigmentation — Heat sink
    - Dilation
    - Maculopathy
  - Systemic
    - Raised body temperature
    - Blood oxygen levels — Free radicals
    - Diabetes

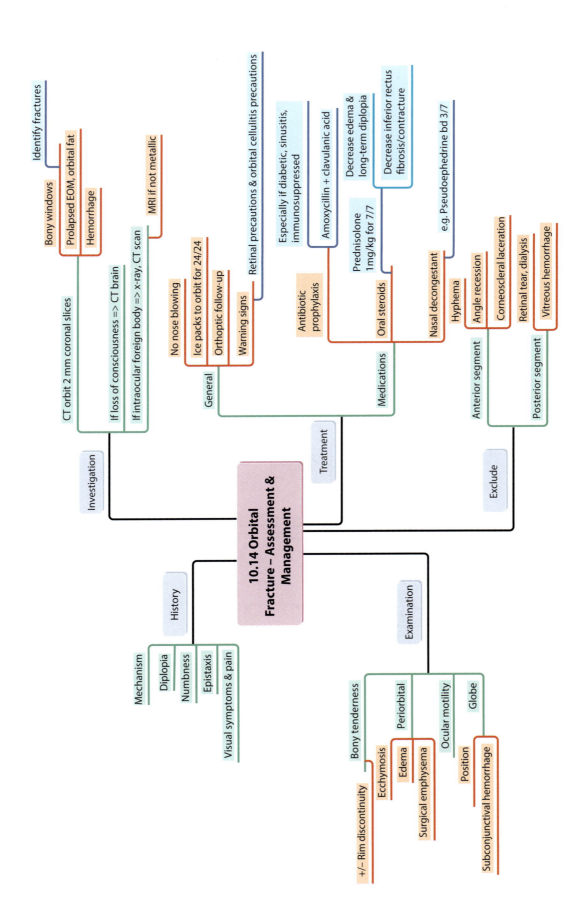

10.14 Orbital Fracture – Assessment & Management

History
- Mechanism
- Diplopia
- Numbness
- Epistaxis
- Visual symptoms & pain

Examination
- Bony tenderness
  - +/- Rim discontinuity
- Periorbital
  - Ecchymosis
  - Edema
  - Surgical emphysema
- Ocular motility
- Globe
  - Position
  - Subconjunctival hemorrhage

Investigation
- CT orbit 2 mm coronal slices
  - Bony windows — Identify fractures
  - Prolapsed EOM, orbital fat
  - Hemorrhage
- If loss of consciousness => CT brain
- If intraocular foreign body => x-ray, CT scan
  - MRI if not metallic

Treatment
- General
  - No nose blowing
  - Ice packs to orbit for 24/24
  - Orthoptic follow-up
  - Warning signs — Retinal precautions & orbital cellulitis precautions
- Medications
  - Antibiotic prophylaxis
    - Especially if diabetic, sinusitis, immunosuppressed
    - Amoxycillin + clavulanic acid
  - Oral steroids
    - Prednisolone 1mg/kg for 7/7
      - Decrease edema & long-term diplopia
      - Decrease inferior rectus fibrosis/contracture
  - Nasal decongestant
    - e.g. Pseudoephedrine bd 3/7

Exclude
- Anterior segment
  - Hyphema
  - Angle recession
  - Corneoscleral laceration
- Posterior segment
  - Retinal tear, dialysis
  - Vitreous hemorrhage

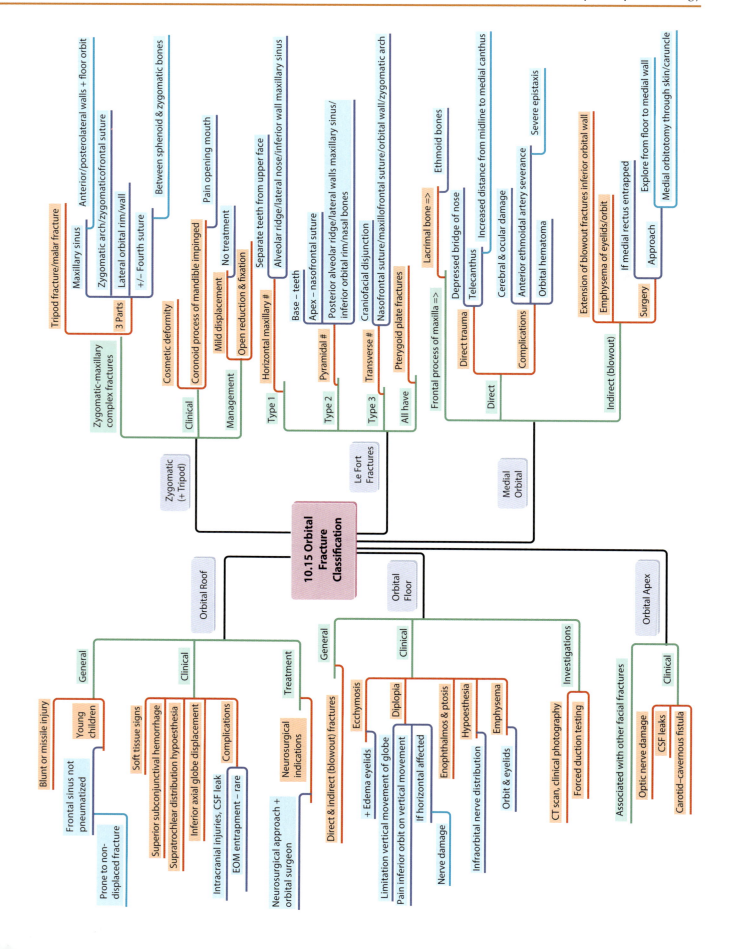

10.15 Orbital Fracture Classification

Zygomatic (+ Tripod)

Zygomatic-maxillary complex fractures
- Tripod fracture/malar fracture
  - Maxillary sinus — Anterior/posterolateral walls + floor orbit
  - Zygomatic arch/zygomaticofrontal suture
  - Lateral orbital rim/wall
  - +/− Fourth suture
  - Between sphenoid & zygomatic bones
- 3 Parts

Clinical
- Cosmetic deformity
- Coronoid process of mandible impinged — Pain opening mouth

Management
- Mild displacement — No treatment
- Open reduction & fixation

Le Fort Fractures

Type 1
- Horizontal maxillary # — Separate teeth from upper face
- Alveolar ridge/lateral nose/inferior wall maxillary sinus
- Base – teeth

Type 2
- Pyramidal # — Apex – nasofrontal suture
- Posterior alveolar ridge/lateral walls maxillary sinus/inferior orbital rim/nasal bones

Type 3
- Transverse # — Craniofacial disjunction
- Nasofrontal suture/maxillofrontal suture/orbital wall/zygomatic arch

All have
- Pterygoid plate fractures

Medial Orbital

Direct
- Frontal process of maxilla =>
- Lacrimal bone =>
  - Ethmoid bones
- Direct trauma
  - Depressed bridge of nose
  - Telecanthus — Increased distance from midline to medial canthus
- Complications
  - Cerebral & ocular damage
  - Anterior ethmoidal artery severance — Severe epistaxis
  - Orbital hematoma

Indirect (blowout)
- Extension of blowout fractures inferior orbital wall
- Emphysema of eyelids/orbit
- If medial rectus entrapped
- Surgery
  - Approach — Explore from floor to medial wall
  - Medial orbitotomy through skin/caruncle

Orbital Roof

General
- Blunt or missile injury
- Young children
- Frontal sinus not pneumatized — Prone to non-displaced fracture

Clinical
- Soft tissue signs
- Superior subconjunctival hemorrhage
- Supratrochlear distribution hypoesthesia
- Inferior axial globe displacement
- Complications
  - Intracranial injuries, CSF leak
  - EOM entrapment – rare

Treatment
- Neurosurgical indications — Neurosurgical approach + orbital surgeon

Orbital Floor

General
- Direct & indirect (blowout) fractures

Clinical
- Ecchymosis — + Edema eyelids
- Diplopia
  - Limitation vertical movement of globe
  - Pain inferior orbit on vertical movement
  - If horizontal affected — Nerve damage
- Enophthalmos & ptosis
- Hypoesthesia — Infraorbital nerve distribution
- Emphysema — Orbit & eyelids

Investigations
- CT scan, clinical photography
- Forced duction testing

Orbital Apex

- Associated with other facial fractures

Clinical
- Optic nerve damage
- CSF leaks
- Carotid–cavernous fistula

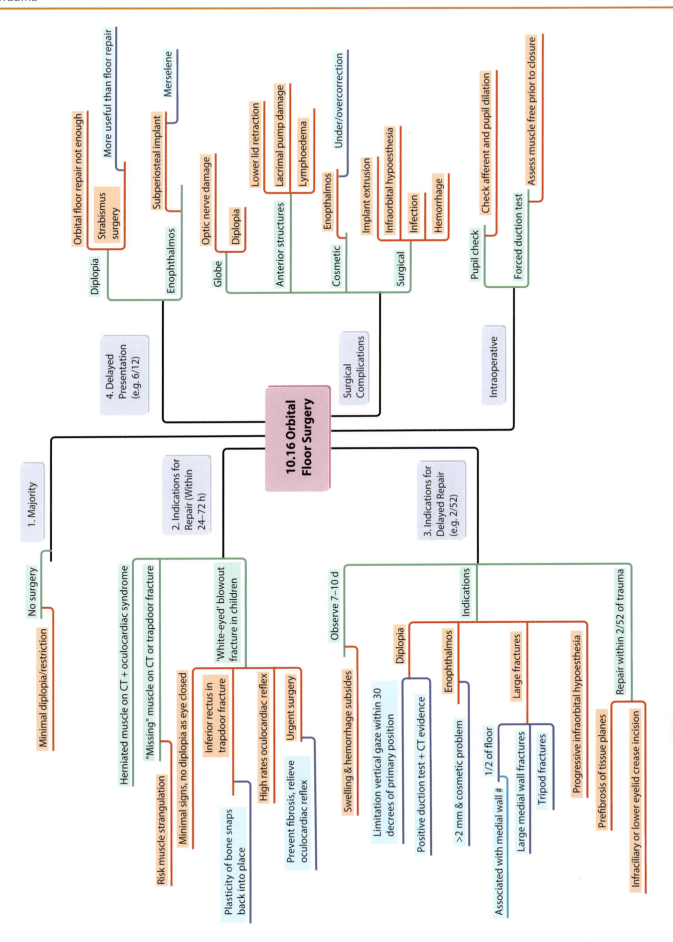

10.16 Orbital Floor Surgery

1. Majority
- No surgery
  - Minimal diplopia/restriction

2. Indications for Repair (Within 24–72 h)
- Herniated muscle on CT + oculocardiac syndrome
  - Risk muscle strangulation
- "Missing" muscle on CT or trapdoor fracture
  - Minimal signs, no diplopia as eye closed
    - Plasticity of bone snaps back into place
- 'White-eyed' blowout fracture in children
  - Inferior rectus in trapdoor fracture
  - High rates oculocardiac reflex
  - Urgent surgery
    - Prevent fibrosis, relieve oculocardiac reflex

3. Indications for Delayed Repair (e.g. 2/52)
- Observe 7–10 d
  - Swelling & hemorrhage subsides
- Indications
  - Diplopia
    - Limitation vertical gaze within 30 decrees of primary position
    - Positive duction test + CT evidence
  - Enophthalmos
    - >2 mm & cosmetic problem
  - Large fractures
    - 1/2 of floor
    - Associated with medial wall #
    - Large medial wall fractures
    - Tripod fractures
  - Progressive infraorbital hypoesthesia
    - Prefibrosis of tissue planes
  - Repair within 2/52 of trauma
    - Infraciliary or lower eyelid crease incision

4. Delayed Presentation (e.g. 6/12)
- Diplopia
  - Orbital floor repair not enough
  - Strabismus surgery
    - More useful than floor repair
- Enophthalmos
  - Subperiosteal implant
    - Merselene

Surgical Complications
- Globe
  - Optic nerve damage
  - Diplopia
- Anterior structures
  - Lower lid retraction
  - Lacrimal pump damage
  - Lymphoedema
- Cosmetic
  - Enophthalmos
  - Under/overcorrection
- Surgical
  - Implant extrusion
  - Infraorbital hypoesthesia
  - Infection
  - Hemorrhage

Intraoperative
- Pupil check
  - Check afferent and pupil dilation
- Forced duction test
  - Assess muscle free prior to closure

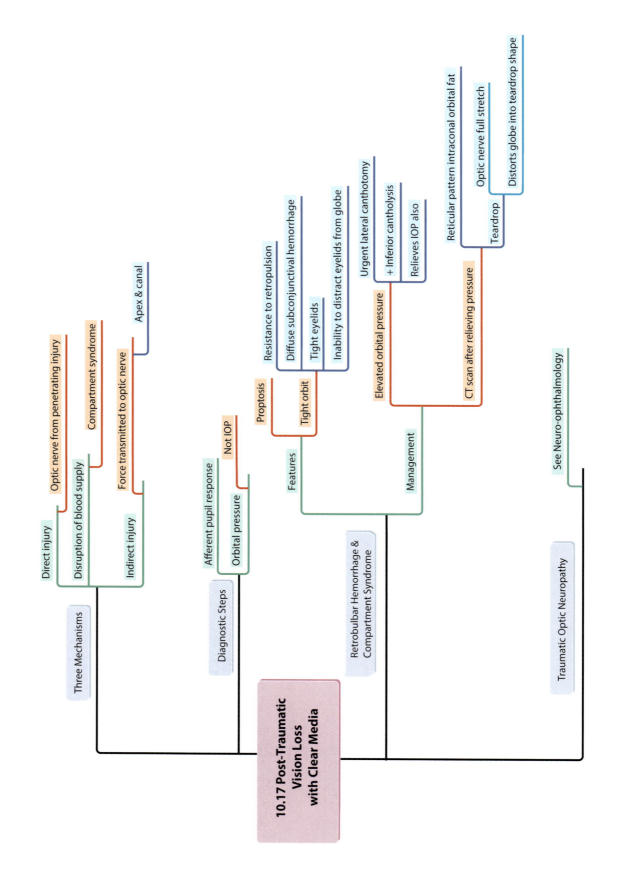

10.17 Post-Traumatic Vision Loss with Clear Media

- Three Mechanisms
  - Direct injury
    - Optic nerve from penetrating injury
  - Disruption of blood supply
    - Compartment syndrome
  - Indirect injury
    - Force transmitted to optic nerve
      - Apex & canal
- Diagnostic Steps
  - Afferent pupil response
  - Orbital pressure
    - Not IOP
- Retrobulbar Hemorrhage & Compartment Syndrome
  - Features
    - Proptosis
    - Tight orbit
      - Resistance to retropulsion
      - Diffuse subconjunctival hemorrhage
      - Tight eyelids
      - Inability to distract eyelids from globe
  - Management
    - Elevated orbital pressure
      - Urgent lateral canthotomy
      - + Inferior cantholysis
      - Relieves IOP also
    - CT scan after relieving pressure
      - Reticular pattern intraconal orbital fat
      - Teardrop
        - Optic nerve full stretch
        - Distorts globe into teardrop shape
- Traumatic Optic Neuropathy
  - See Neuro-ophthalmology

11 Uveitis and Inflammatory Eye Disease

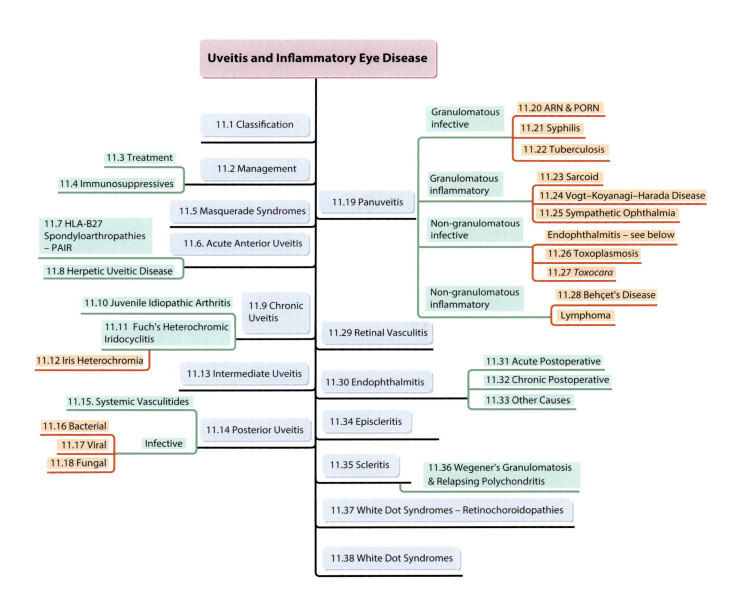

Uveitis and Inflammatory Eye Disease

11.1 Classification

11.3 Treatment

11.2 Management

11.4 Immunosuppressives

11.5 Masquerade Syndromes

11.7 HLA-B27 Spondyloarthropathies – PAIR

11.6. Acute Anterior Uveitis

11.8 Herpetic Uveitic Disease

11.10 Juvenile Idiopathic Arthritis

11.9 Chronic Uveitis

11.11 Fuch's Heterochromic Iridocyclitis

11.12 Iris Heterochromia

11.13 Intermediate Uveitis

11.15. Systemic Vasculitides

11.16 Bacterial

11.14 Posterior Uveitis

11.17 Viral

Infective

11.18 Fungal

11.19 Panuveitis

Granulomatous infective

11.20 ARN & PORN

11.21 Syphilis

11.22 Tuberculosis

Granulomatous inflammatory

11.23 Sarcoid

11.24 Vogt–Koyanagi–Harada Disease

11.25 Sympathetic Ophthalmia

Non-granulomatous infective

Endophthalmitis – see below

11.26 Toxoplasmosis

11.27 *Toxocara*

Non-granulomatous inflammatory

11.28 Behçet's Disease

Lymphoma

11.29 Retinal Vasculitis

11.30 Endophthalmitis

11.31 Acute Postoperative

11.32 Chronic Postoperative

11.33 Other Causes

11.34 Episcleritis

11.35 Scleritis

11.36 Wegener's Granulomatosis & Relapsing Polychondritis

11.37 White Dot Syndromes – Retinochoroidopathies

11.38 White Dot Syndromes

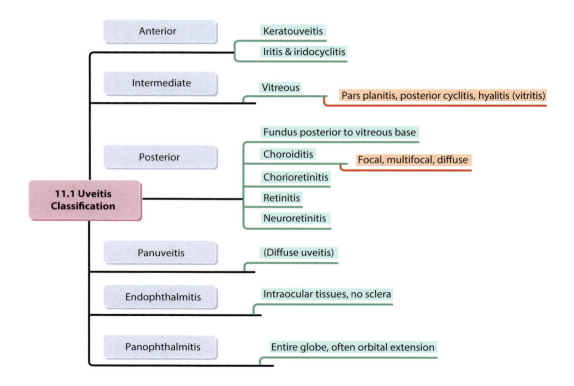

Anterior
- Keratouveitis
- Iritis & iridocyclitis

Intermediate
- Vitreous
  - Pars planitis, posterior cyclitis, hyalitis (vitritis)

Posterior
- Fundus posterior to vitreous base
- Choroiditis
  - Focal, multifocal, diffuse
- Chorioretinitis
- Retinitis
- Neuroretinitis

11.1 Uveitis Classification

Panuveitis
- (Diffuse uveitis)

Endophthalmitis
- Intraocular tissues, no sclera

Panophthalmitis
- Entire globe, often orbital extension

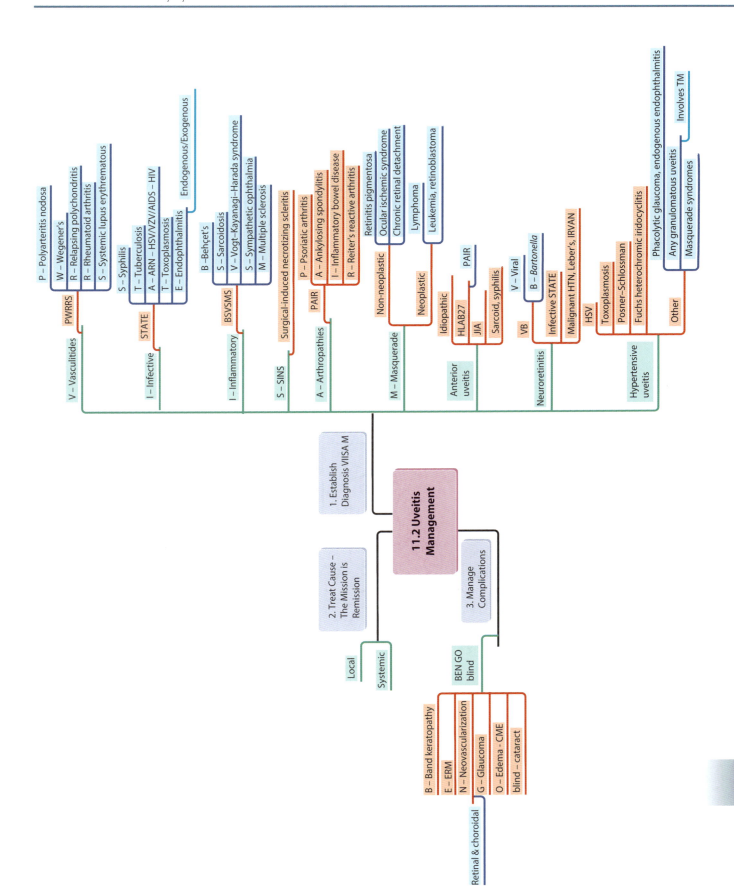

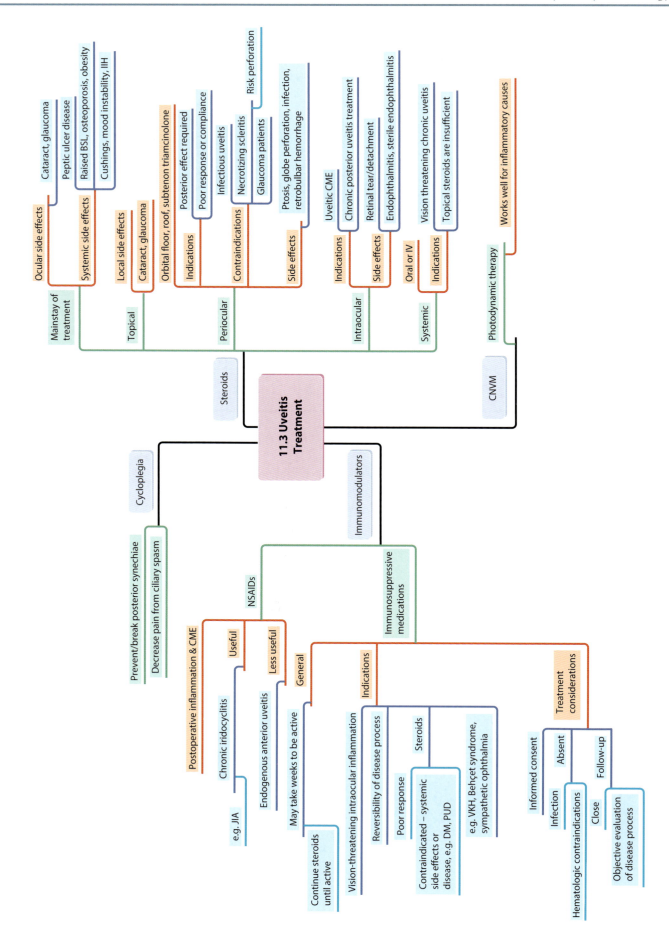

11.3 Uveitis Treatment

Steroids

Mainstay of treatment
- Ocular side effects
  - Cataract, glaucoma
- Systemic side effects
  - Peptic ulcer disease
  - Raised BSL, osteoporosis, obesity
  - Cushings, mood instability, IIH

Topical
- Local side effects
  - Cataract, glaucoma

Periocular
- Orbital floor, roof, subtenon triamcinolone
- Indications
  - Posterior effect required
  - Poor response or compliance
- Contraindications
  - Infectious uveitis
  - Necrotizing scleritis
  - Glaucoma patients
- Side effects
  - Ptosis, globe perforation, infection, retrobulbar hemorrhage
  - Risk perforation

Intraocular
- Indications
  - Uveitic CME
  - Chronic posterior uveitis treatment
- Side effects
  - Retinal tear/detachment
  - Endophthalmitis, sterile endophthalmitis

Systemic
- Oral or IV
- Indications
  - Vision threatening chronic uveitis
  - Topical steroids are insufficient

Photodynamic therapy
- Works well for inflammatory causes

CNVM

Cycloplegia
- Prevent/break posterior synechiae
- Decrease pain from ciliary spasm

NSAIDs
- Postoperative inflammation & CME
  - Useful
- Chronic iridocyclitis
  - e.g. JIA
- Less useful
  - Endogenous anterior uveitis

Immunomodulators

Immunosuppressive medications
- General
  - May take weeks to be active
  - Continue steroids until active
- Indications
  - Vision-threatening intraocular inflammation
  - Reversibility of disease process
  - Poor response
    - Steroids
      - Contraindicated – systemic side effects or disease, e.g. DM, PUD
  - e.g. VKH, Behçet syndrome, sympathetic ophthalmia
- Treatment considerations
  - Informed consent
  - Absent
    - Infection
    - Hematologic contraindications
  - Close
    - Follow-up
    - Objective evaluation of disease process

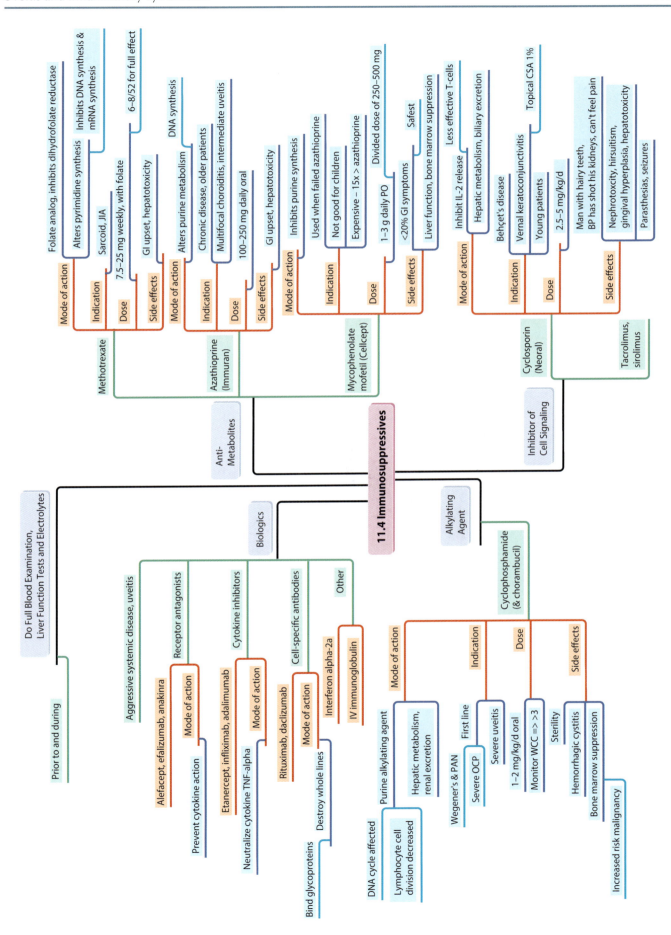

11.4 Immunosuppressives

Anti-Metabolites

Methotrexate
- Mode of action
  - Folate analog, inhibits dihydrofolate reductase
  - Alters pyrimidine synthesis
  - Inhibits DNA synthesis & mRNA synthesis
  - 6–8/52 for full effect
- Indication
  - Sarcoid, JIA
- Dose
  - 7.5–25 mg weekly, with folate
- Side effects
  - GI upset, hepatotoxicity

Azathioprine (Immuran)
- Mode of action
  - DNA synthesis
  - Alters purine metabolism
- Indication
  - Chronic disease, older patients
  - Multifocal choroiditis, intermediate uveitis
- Dose
  - 100–250 mg daily oral
- Side effects
  - GI upset, hepatotoxicity

Mycophenolate mofetil (Cellcept)
- Mode of action
  - Inhibits purine synthesis
- Indication
  - Used when failed azathioprine
  - Not good for children
  - Expensive – 15x > azathioprine
- Dose
  - Divided dose of 250–500 mg
  - 1–3 g daily PO
- Side effects
  - <20% GI symptoms
  - Safest
  - Liver function, bone marrow suppression

Inhibitor of Cell Signaling

Cyclosporin (Neoral)
- Mode of action
  - Less effective T-cells
  - Inhibit IL-2 release
  - Hepatic metabolism, biliary excretion
- Indication
  - Behçet's disease
  - Vernal keratoconjunctivitis
  - Young patients
  - Topical CSA 1%
- Dose
  - 2.5–5 mg/kg/d
- Side effects
  - Man with hairy teeth, BP has shot his kidneys, can't feel pain
  - Nephrotoxcity, hirsuitism, gingival hyperplasia, hepatotoxicity
  - Parasthesias, seizures

Tacrolimus, sirolimus

Do Full Blood Examination, Liver Function Tests and Electrolytes
- Prior to and during

Biologics
- Aggressive systemic disease, uveitis
- Receptor antagonists
  - Alefacept, efalizumab, anakinra
  - Mode of action
    - Prevent cytokine action
- Cytokine inhibitors
  - Etanercept, infliximab, adalimumab
  - Mode of action
    - Neutralize cytokine TNF-alpha
- Cell-specific antibodies
  - Rituximab, daclizumab
  - Mode of action
    - Destroy whole lines
    - Bind glycoproteins
- Other
  - Interferon alpha-2a
  - IV immunoglobulin

Alkylating Agent

Cyclophosphamide (& chorambucil)
- Mode of action
  - Purine alkylating agent
  - DNA cycle affected
  - Lymphocyte cell division decreased
  - Hepatic metabolism, renal excretion
- Indication
  - First line
  - Wegener's & PAN
  - Severe OCP
  - Severe uveitis
- Dose
  - 1–2 mg/kg/d oral
  - Monitor WCC => >3
- Side effects
  - Sterility
  - Hemorrhagic cystitis
  - Bone marrow suppression
  - Increased risk malignancy

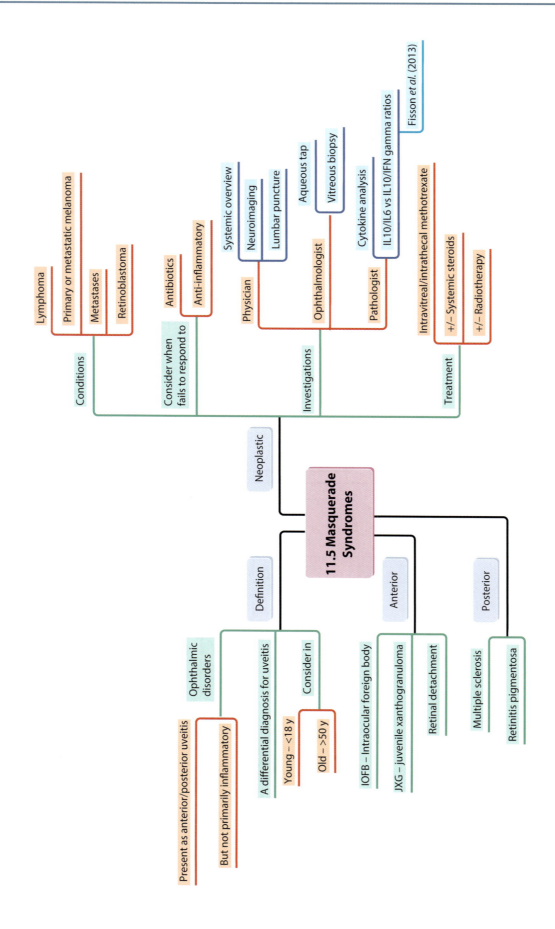

11.5 Masquerade Syndromes

Definition
- Ophthalmic disorders
  - Present as anterior/posterior uveitis
  - But not primarily inflammatory
- A differential diagnosis for uveitis
- Consider in
  - Young – <18 y
  - Old – >50 y

Neoplastic
- Conditions
  - Lymphoma
    - Primary or metastatic melanoma
  - Metastases
  - Retinoblastoma
- Consider when fails to respond to
  - Antibiotics
  - Anti-inflammatory
- Investigations
  - Physician
    - Systemic overview
    - Neuroimaging
    - Lumbar puncture
  - Ophthalmologist
    - Aqueous tap
    - Vitreous biopsy
  - Pathologist
    - Cytokine analysis
    - IL10/IL6 vs IL10/IFN gamma ratios
      - Fisson *et al.* (2013)
- Treatment
  - Intravitreal/intrathecal methotrexate
  - +/– Systemic steroids
  - +/– Radiotherapy

Anterior
- IOFB – Intraocular foreign body
- JXG – juvenile xanthogranuloma
- Retinal detachment

Posterior
- Multiple sclerosis
- Retinitis pigmentosa

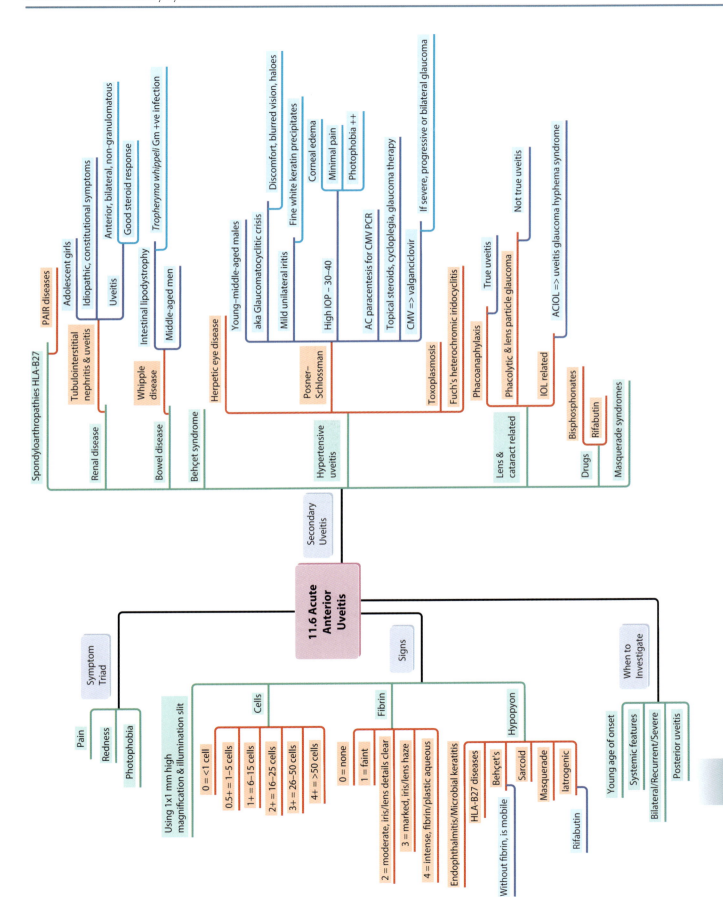

11.6 Acute Anterior Uveitis

Symptom Triad
- Pain
- Redness
- Photophobia

Signs

Cells
- Using 1x1 mm high magnification & illumination slit
- 0 = <1 cell
- 0.5+ = 1–5 cells
- 1+ = 6–15 cells
- 2+ = 16–25 cells
- 3+ = 26–50 cells
- 4+ = >50 cells

Fibrin
- 0 = none
- 1 = faint
- 2 = moderate, iris/lens details clear
- 3 = marked, iris/lens haze
- 4 = intense, fibrin/plastic aqueous

Hypopyon
- Endophthalmitis/Microbial keratitis
- HLA-B27 diseases
- Behçet's
- Sarcoid
- Masquerade
- Iatrogenic
  - Without fibrin, is mobile
  - Rifabutin

When to Investigate
- Young age of onset
- Systemic features
- Bilateral/Recurrent/Severe
- Posterior uveitis

Secondary Uveitis

Spondyloarthropathies HLA-B27
- PAIR diseases

Renal disease
- Tubulointerstitial nephritis & uveitis
  - Adolescent girls
  - Idiopathic, constitutional symptoms
  - Uveitis
    - Anterior, bilateral, non-granulomatous
    - Good steroid response

Bowel disease
- Whipple disease
  - Intestinal lipodystrophy
  - Middle-aged men
    - Tropheryma whippeli Gm +ve infection

Behçet syndrome

Hypertensive uveitis
- Herpetic eye disease
- Posner–Schlossman
  - Young–middle-aged males
  - aka Glaucomatocyclitic crisis
  - Mild unilateral iritis
    - Discomfort, blurred vision, haloes
    - Fine white keratin precipitates
    - Corneal edema
    - Minimal pain
    - Photophobia ++
  - High IOP – 30–40
  - AC paracentesis for CMV PCR
  - Topical steroids, cycloplegia, glaucoma therapy
  - CMV => valganciclovir
    - If severe, progressive or bilateral glaucoma
- Toxoplasmosis
- Fuch's heterochromic iridocyclitis

Lens & cataract related
- Phacoanaphylaxis
  - True uveitis
- Phacolytic & lens particle glaucoma
- IOL related
  - Not true uveitis
  - ACIOL => uveitis glaucoma hyphema syndrome

Drugs
- Bisphosphonates
- Rifabutin

Masquerade syndromes

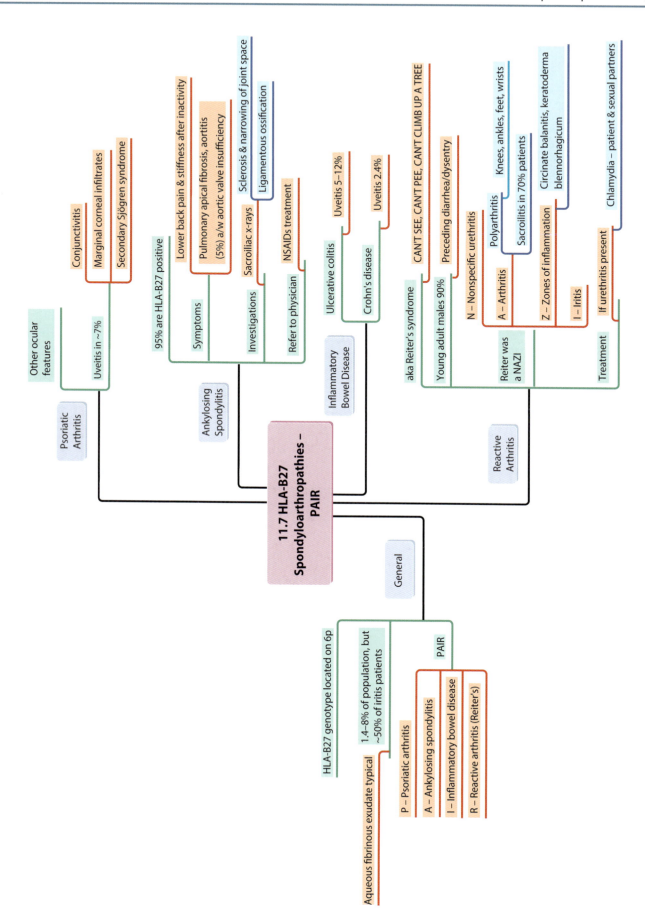

11.7 HLA-B27 Spondyloarthropathies – PAIR

Psoriatic Arthritis
- Other ocular features
  - Uveitis in ~7%
  - Conjunctivitis
  - Marginal corneal infiltrates
  - Secondary Sjögren syndrome

Ankylosing Spondylitis
- 95% are HLA-B27 positive
- Symptoms
  - Lower back pain & stiffness after inactivity
  - Pulmonary apical fibrosis, aortitis (5%) a/w aortic valve insufficiency
- Investigations
  - Sacroiliac x-rays
  - Sclerosis & narrowing of joint space
  - Ligamentous ossification
- Refer to physician
  - NSAIDs treatment

Inflammatory Bowel Disease
- Ulcerative colitis — Uveitis 5–12%
- Crohn's disease — Uveitis 2.4%

Reactive Arthritis
- aka Reiter's syndrome
  - CAN'T SEE, CAN'T PEE, CAN'T CLIMB UP A TREE
- Young adult males 90%
  - Preceding diarrhea/dysentry
- Reiter was a NAZI
  - N – Nonspecific urethritis
  - A – Arthritis
    - Polyarthritis
    - Knees, ankles, feet, wrists
    - Sacroilitis in 70% patients
  - Z – Zones of inflammation
    - Circinate balanitis, keratoderma blennorhagicum
  - I – Iritis
- Treatment
  - If urethritis present
    - Chlamydia – patient & sexual partners

General
- HLA-B27 genotype located on 6p
  - Aqueous fibrinous exudate typical
- 1.4–8% of population, but ~50% of iritis patients
- PAIR
  - P – Psoriatic arthritis
  - A – Ankylosing spondylitis
  - I – Inflammatory bowel disease
  - R – Reactive arthritis (Reiter's)

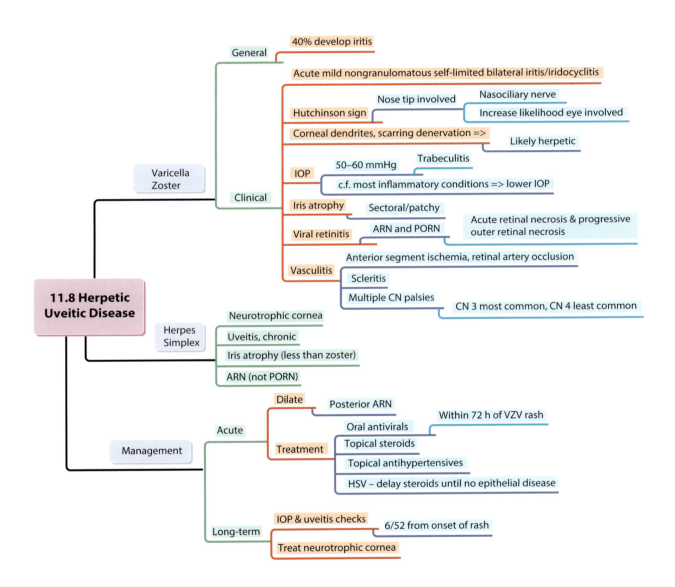

11.8 Herpetic Uveitic Disease

Varicella Zoster
- General
  - 40% develop iritis
- Clinical
  - Acute mild nongranulomatous self-limited bilateral iritis/iridocyclitis
  - Hutchinson sign — Nose tip involved — Nasociliary nerve — Increase likelihood eye involved
  - Corneal dendrites, scarring denervation => Likely herpetic
  - IOP — 50–60 mmHg — Trabeculitis — c.f. most inflammatory conditions => lower IOP
  - Iris atrophy — Sectoral/patchy
  - Viral retinitis — ARN and PORN — Acute retinal necrosis & progressive outer retinal necrosis
  - Vasculitis — Anterior segment ischemia, retinal artery occlusion
  - Scleritis
  - Multiple CN palsies — CN 3 most common, CN 4 least common

Herpes Simplex
- Neurotrophic cornea
- Uveitis, chronic
- Iris atrophy (less than zoster)
- ARN (not PORN)

Management
- Acute
  - Dilate — Posterior ARN
  - Treatment
    - Oral antivirals — Within 72 h of VZV rash
    - Topical steroids
    - Topical antihypertensives
    - HSV – delay steroids until no epithelial disease
- Long-term
  - IOP & uveitis checks — 6/52 from onset of rash
  - Treat neurotrophic cornea

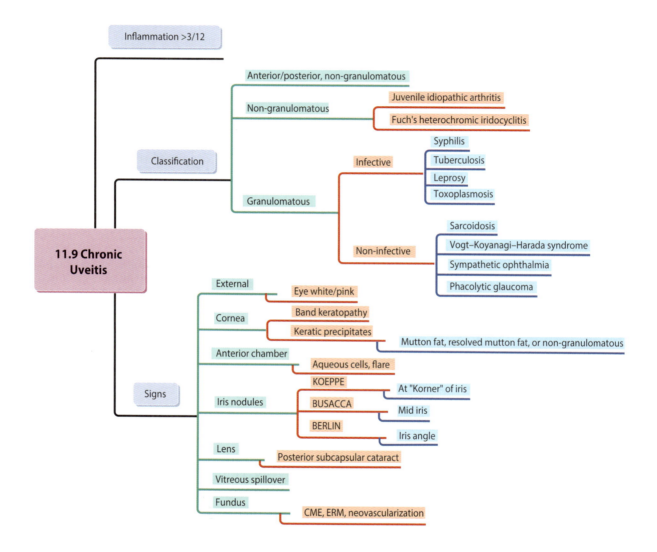

Inflammation >3/12

Classification

11.9 Chronic Uveitis

Signs

Non-granulomatous
- Anterior/posterior, non-granulomatous
- Juvenile idiopathic arthritis
- Fuch's heterochromic iridocyclitis

Granulomatous
- Infective
  - Syphilis
  - Tuberculosis
  - Leprosy
  - Toxoplasmosis
- Non-infective
  - Sarcoidosis
  - Vogt–Koyanagi–Harada syndrome
  - Sympathetic ophthalmia
  - Phacolytic glaucoma

External
- Eye white/pink

Cornea
- Band keratopathy
- Keratic precipitates
  - Mutton fat, resolved mutton fat, or non-granulomatous

Anterior chamber
- Aqueous cells, flare

Iris nodules
- KOEPPE — At "Korner" of iris
- BUSACCA — Mid iris
- BERLIN — Iris angle

Lens
- Posterior subcapsular cataract

Vitreous spillover

Fundus
- CME, ERM, neovascularization

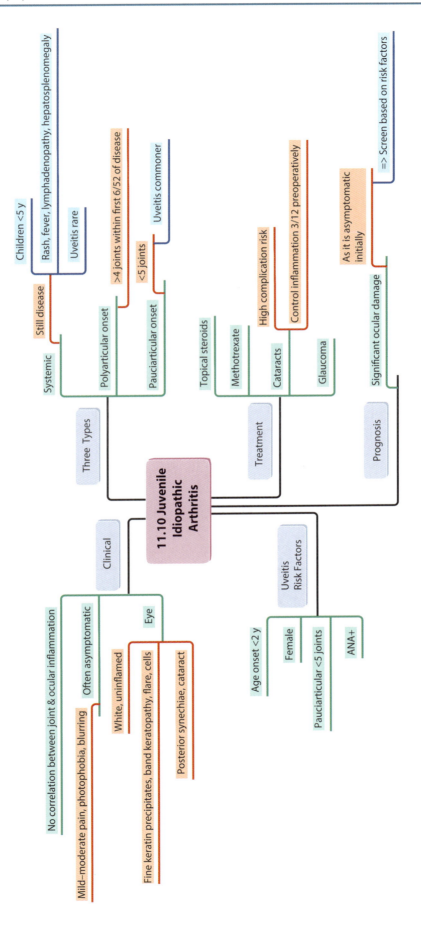

11.10 Juvenile Idiopathic Arthritis

Three Types
- Systemic
  - Still disease
    - Children <5 y
    - Rash, fever, lymphadenopathy, hepatosplenomegaly
    - Uveitis rare
- Polyarticular onset
  - >4 joints within first 6/52 of disease
- Pauciarticular onset
  - <5 joints
  - Uveitis commoner

Treatment
- Topical steroids
- Methotrexate
- Cataracts
  - High complication risk
  - Control inflammation 3/12 preoperatively
- Glaucoma

Prognosis
- Significant ocular damage
- As it is asymptomatic initially
  - => Screen based on risk factors

Clinical
- No correlation between joint & ocular inflammation
- Mild–moderate pain, photophobia, blurring
  - Often asymptomatic
- Eye
  - White, uninflamed
  - Fine keratin precipitates, band keratopathy, flare, cells
  - Posterior synechiae, cataract

Uveitis Risk Factors
- Age onset <2 y
- Female
- Pauciarticular <5 joints
- ANA+

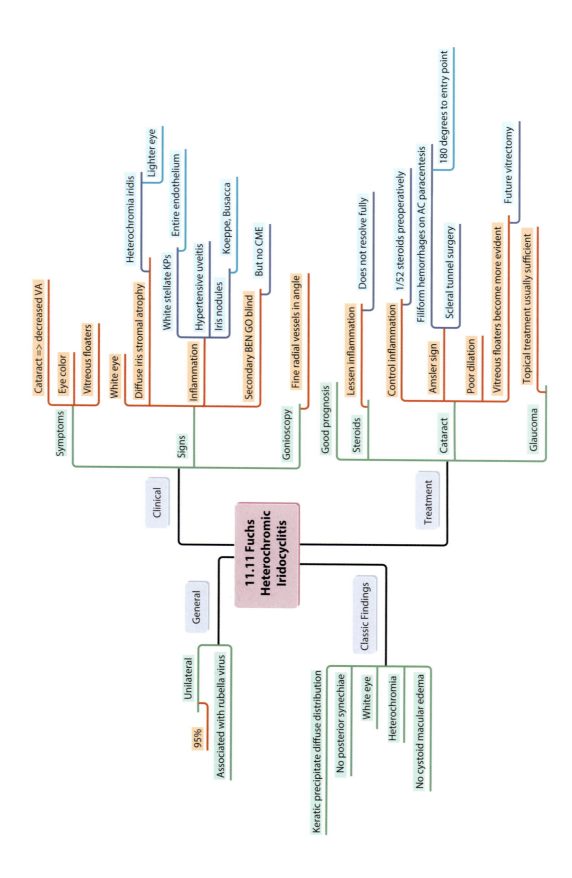

11.11 Fuchs Heterochromic Iridocyclitis

General
- Unilateral
  - 95%
  - Associated with rubella virus

Classic Findings
- Keratic precipitate diffuse distribution
- No posterior synechiae
- White eye
- Heterochromia
- No cystoid macular edema

Clinical
- Symptoms
  - Cataract => decreased VA
  - Eye color
  - Vitreous floaters
- Signs
  - White eye
  - Diffuse iris stromal atrophy
    - Heterochromia iridis
      - Lighter eye
  - White stellate KPs
    - Entire endothelium
  - Inflammation
    - Hypertensive uveitis
    - Iris nodules
      - Koeppe, Busacca
  - Secondary BEN GO blind
    - But no CME
- Gonioscopy
  - Fine radial vessels in angle

Treatment
- Good prognosis
- Steroids
  - Lessen inflammation
    - Does not resolve fully
  - Control inflammation
    - 1/52 steroids preoperatively
- Cataract
  - Amsler sign
    - Filiform hemorrhages on AC paracentesis
    - 180 degrees to entry point
  - Scleral tunnel surgery
  - Poor dilation
  - Vitreous floaters become more evident
    - Future vitrectomy
- Glaucoma
  - Topical treatment usually sufficient

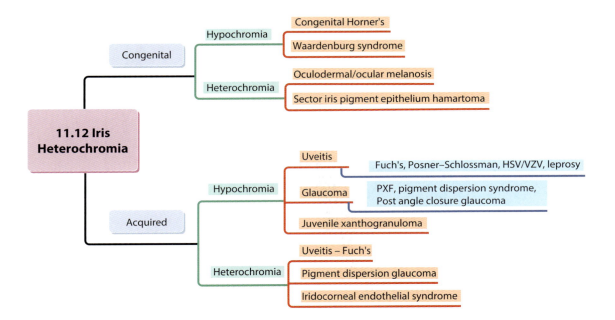

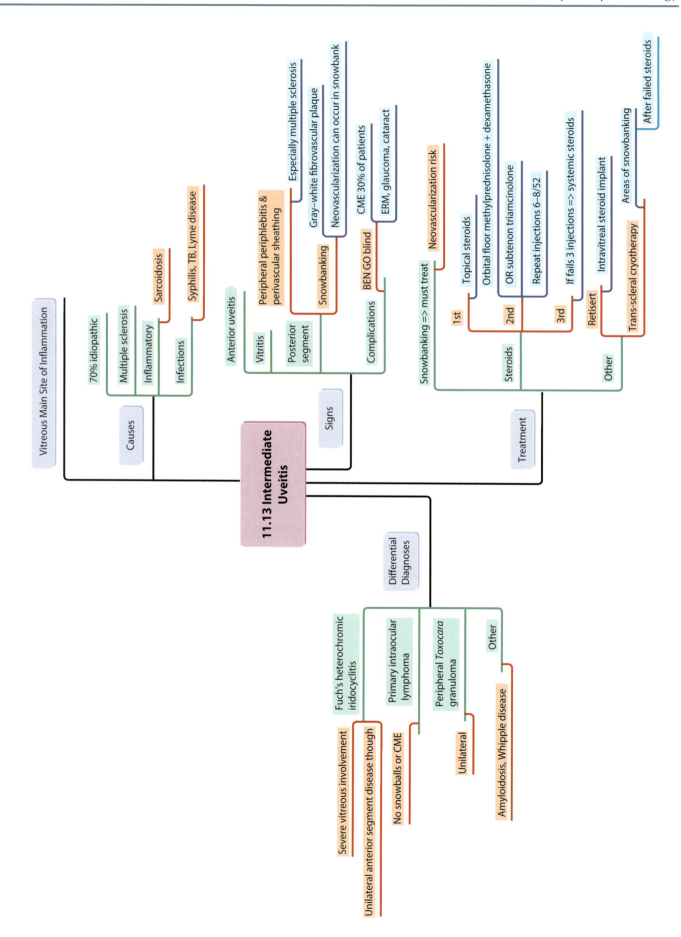

11.13 Intermediate Uveitis

Causes
- Vitreous Main Site of Inflammation
  - 70% idiopathic
  - Multiple sclerosis
  - Inflammatory
    - Sarcoidosis
  - Infections
    - Syphilis, TB, Lyme disease

Signs
- Anterior uveitis
- Vitritis
  - Peripheral periphlebitis & perivascular sheathing
- Posterior segment
  - Snowbanking
    - Especially multiple sclerosis
    - Gray–white fibrovascular plaque
    - Neovascularization can occur in snowbank
- Complications
  - BEN GO blind
    - CME 30% of patients
    - ERM, glaucoma, cataract

Treatment
- Snowbanking => must treat
  - Neovascularization risk
- Steroids
  - 1st
    - Topical steroids
  - 2nd
    - Orbital floor methylprednisolone + dexamethasone
    - OR subtenon triamcinolone
    - Repeat injections 6–8/52
  - 3rd
    - If fails 3 injections => systemic steroids
  - Retisert
    - Intravitreal steroid implant
- Other
  - Trans-scleral cryotherapy
    - Areas of snowbanking
    - After failed steroids

Differential Diagnoses
- Fuch's heterochromic iridocyclitis
  - Severe vitreous involvement
  - Unilateral anterior segment disease though
  - No snowballs or CME
- Primary intraocular lymphoma
- Peripheral *Toxocara* granuloma
  - Unilateral
- Other
  - Amyloidosis, Whipple disease

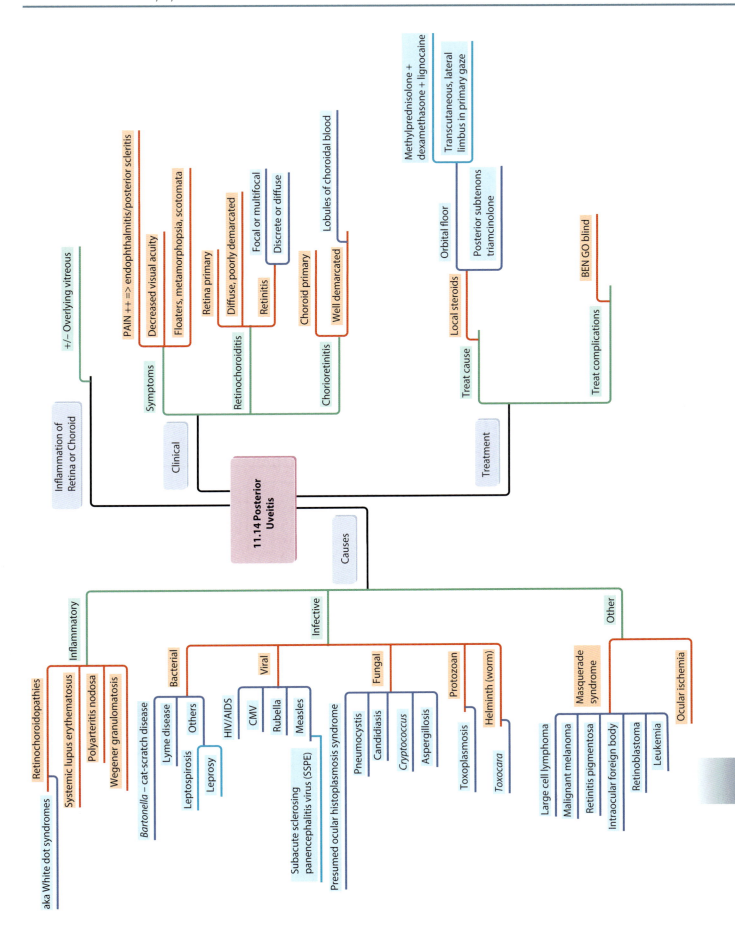

11.14 Posterior Uveitis

Inflammation of Retina or Choroid

Clinical

Symptoms
- +/− Overlying vitreous
- PAIN ++ => endophthalmitis/posterior scleritis
- Decreased visual acuity
- Floaters, metamorphopsia, scotomata

Retinochoroiditis
- Retina primary
- Diffuse, poorly demarcated
- Retinitis
  - Focal or multifocal
  - Discrete or diffuse

Chorioretinitis
- Choroid primary
- Well demarcated
- Lobules of choroidal blood

Treatment

Treat cause
- Local steroids
  - Methylprednisolone + dexamethasone + lignocaine
    - Transcutaneous, lateral limbus in primary gaze
  - Orbital floor
  - Posterior subtenons triamcinolone

Treat complications
- BEN GO blind

Causes

Inflammatory
- Retinochoroidopathies
  - aka White dot syndromes
- Systemic lupus erythematosus
- Polyarteritis nodosa
- Wegener granulomatosis

Infective
- Bacterial
  - Bartonella – cat-scratch disease
  - Lyme disease
  - Others
    - Leptospirosis
    - Leprosy
- Viral
  - HIV/AIDS
  - CMV
  - Rubella
  - Measles
    - Subacute sclerosing panencephalitis virus (SSPE)
  - Presumed ocular histoplasmosis syndrome
- Fungal
  - Pneumocystis
  - Candidiasis
  - Cryptococcus
  - Aspergillosis
- Protozoan
  - Toxoplasmosis
- Helminth (worm)
  - Toxocara

Other
- Masquerade syndrome
  - Large cell lymphoma
  - Malignant melanoma
  - Retinitis pigmentosa
  - Intraocular foreign body
  - Retinoblastoma
  - Leukemia
- Ocular ischemia

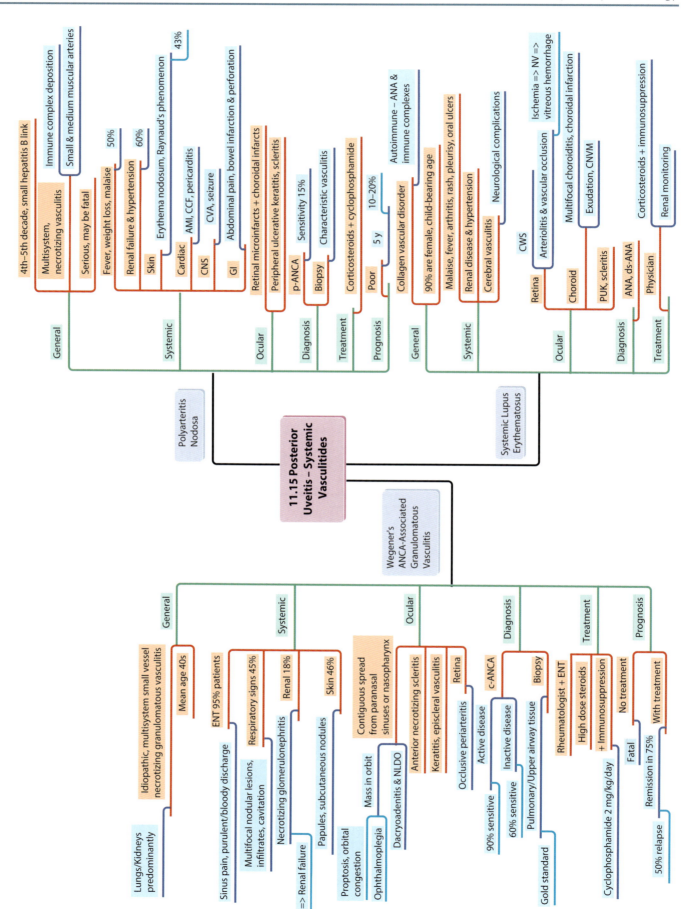

11.15 Posterior Uveitis – Systemic Vasculitides

Polyarteritis Nodosa

General
- 4th–5th decade, small hepatitis B link
- Immune complex deposition
- Small & medium muscular arteries
- Multisystem, necrotizing vasculitis
- Serious, may be fatal

Systemic
- Fever, weight loss, malaise — 50%
- Skin — Renal failure & hypertension — 60%
  - Erythema nodosum, Raynaud's phenomenon — 43%
- Cardiac — AMI, CCF, pericarditis
- CNS — CVA, seizure
- GI — Abdominal pain, bowel infarction & perforation

Ocular
- Retinal microinfarcts + choroidal infarcts
- Peripheral ulcerative keratitis, scleritis

Diagnosis
- p-ANCA — Sensitivity 15%
- Biopsy — Characteristic vasculitis

Treatment
- Corticosteroids + cyclophosphamide

Prognosis
- Poor — 5 y — 10–20%

Systemic Lupus Erythematosus

General
- Autoimmune – ANA & immune complexes
- Collagen vascular disorder
- 90% are female, child-bearing age

Systemic
- Malaise, fever, arthritis, rash, pleurisy, oral ulcers
- Renal disease & hypertension
- Cerebral vasculitis — Neurological complications

Ocular
- Retina — CWS
  - Arteriolitis & vascular occlusion
  - Ischemia => NV => vitreous hemorrhage
- Choroid — Multifocal choroiditis, choroidal infarction
  - Exudation, CNVM

Diagnosis
- PUK, scleritis
- ANA, ds-ANA

Treatment
- Physician — Corticosteroids + immunosuppression
- Renal monitoring

Wegener's ANCA-Associated Granulomatous Vasculitis

General
- Idiopathic, multisystem small vessel necrotizing granulomatous vasculitis
- Lungs/Kidneys predominantly
- Mean age 40s

Systemic
- ENT 95% patients — Sinus pain, purulent/bloody discharge
- Respiratory signs 45% — Multifocal nodular lesions, infiltrates, cavitation
- Renal 18% — Necrotizing glomerulonephritis => Renal failure
- Skin 46% — Papules, subcutaneous nodules

Ocular
- Contiguous spread from paranasal sinuses or nasopharynx
  - Proptosis, orbital congestion
  - Mass in orbit
  - Ophthalmoplegia
  - Dacryoadenitis & NLDO
- Anterior necrotizing scleritis
- Keratitis, episcleral vasculitis
- Retina — Occlusive periarteritis

Diagnosis
- c-ANCA — Active disease — 90% sensitive
  - Inactive disease — 60% sensitive
- Biopsy — Pulmonary/Upper airway tissue — Gold standard

Treatment
- Rheumatologist + ENT
- High dose steroids
- + Immunosuppression — Cyclophosphamide 2 mg/kg/day

Prognosis
- No treatment — Fatal
- With treatment — Remission in 75% — 50% relapse

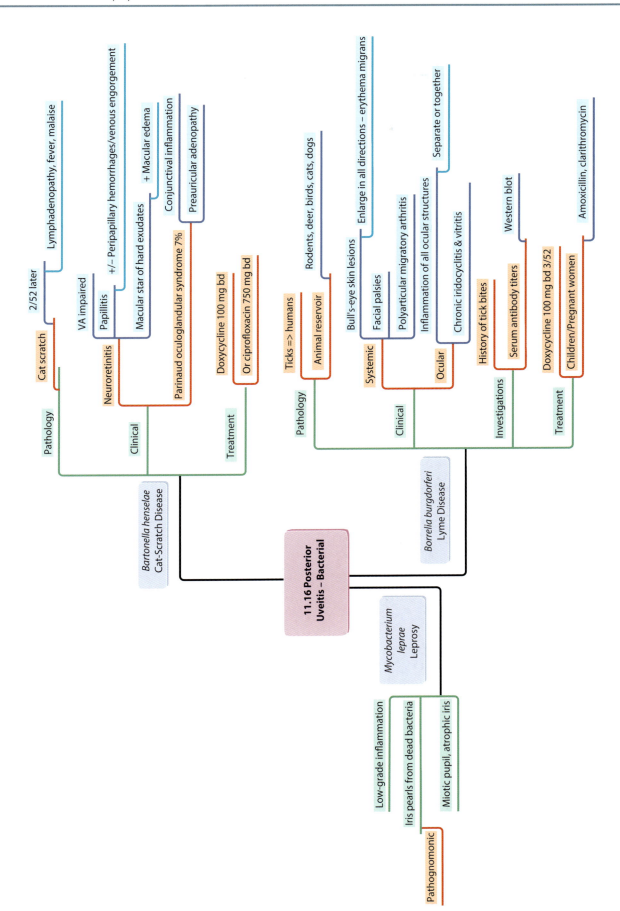

11.16 Posterior Uveitis – Bacterial

Bartonella henselae Cat-Scratch Disease

Pathology
- Cat scratch
  - 2/52 later
    - Lymphadenopathy, fever, malaise

Clinical
- VA impaired
- Papillitis
  - +/– Peripapillary hemorrhages/venous engorgement
- Neuroretinitis
- Macular star of hard exudates
  - + Macular edema
- Parinaud oculoglandular syndrome 7%
  - Conjunctival inflammation
  - Preauricular adenopathy

Treatment
- Doxycycline 100 mg bd
- Or ciprofloxacin 750 mg bd

Borrelia burgdorferi Lyme Disease

Pathology
- Ticks => humans
- Animal reservoir
  - Rodents, deer, birds, cats, dogs

Clinical
- Systemic
  - Bull's-eye skin lesions
    - Enlarge in all directions – erythema migrans
  - Facial palsies
  - Polyarticular migratory arthritis
- Ocular
  - Inflammation of all ocular structures
    - Separate or together
  - Chronic iridocyclitis & vitritis

Investigations
- History of tick bites
- Serum antibody titers
  - Western blot

Treatment
- Doxycycline 100 mg bd 3/52
- Children/Pregnant women
  - Amoxicillin, clarithromycin

Mycobacterium leprae Leprosy
- Low-grade inflammation
- Iris pearls from dead bacteria
- Miotic pupil, atrophic iris
  - Pathognomonic

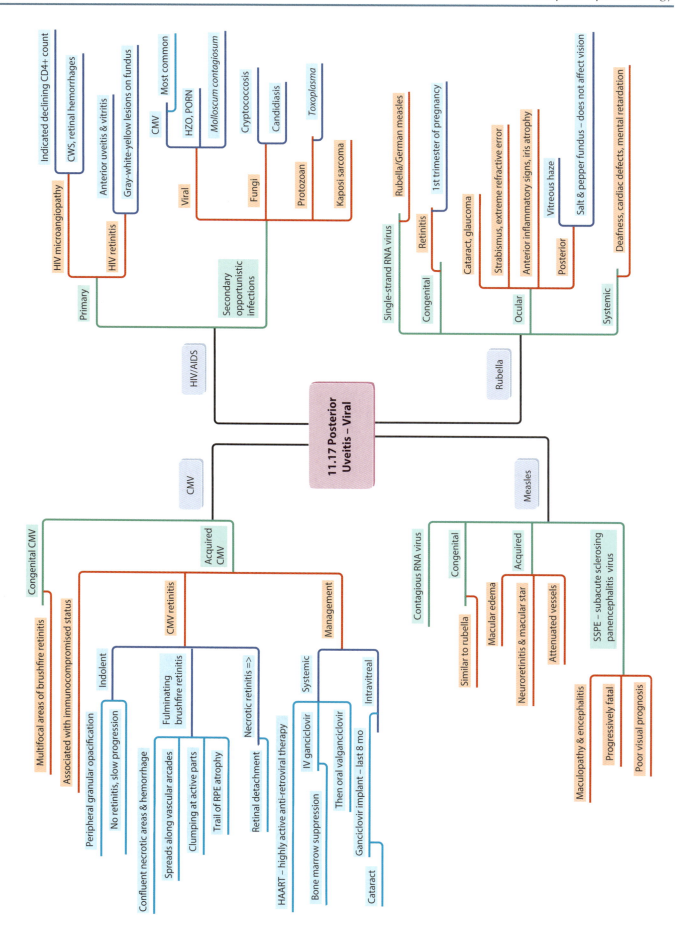

11.17 Posterior Uveitis – Viral

HIV/AIDS

Primary

HIV microangiopathy
- Indicated declining CD4+ count
- CWS, retinal hemorrhages

HIV retinitis
- Anterior uveitis & vitritis
- Gray-white-yellow lesions on fundus

Secondary opportunistic infections

Viral
- CMV — Most common
- HZO, PORN
- *Molloscum contagiosum*

Fungi
- Cryptococcosis
- Candidiasis

Protozoan
- *Toxoplasma*

Kaposi sarcoma

Rubella

Single-strand RNA virus

Congenital
- Rubella/German measles
- 1st trimester of pregnancy

Retinitis

Ocular
- Cataract, glaucoma
- Strabismus, extreme refractive error
- Anterior inflammatory signs, iris atrophy

Posterior
- Vitreous haze
- Salt & pepper fundus – does not affect vision

Systemic
- Deafness, cardiac defects, mental retardation

CMV

Congenital CMV

Acquired CMV
- Multifocal areas of brushfire retinitis
- Associated with immunocompromised status

CMV retinitis

Indolent
- Peripheral granular opacification
- No retinitis, slow progression

Fulminating brushfire retinitis
- Confluent necrotic areas & hemorrhage
- Spreads along vascular arcades
- Clumping at active parts
- Trail of RPE atrophy

Necrotic retinitis =>
- Retinal detachment

Management

Systemic
- HAART – highly active anti-retroviral therapy
- IV ganciclovir
- Bone marrow suppression
- Then oral valganciclovir

Intravitreal
- Ganciclovir implant – last 8 mo
- Cataract

Measles

Contagious RNA virus

Congenital
- Similar to rubella

Acquired
- Macular edema
- Neuroretinitis & macular star
- Attenuated vessels

SSPE – subacute sclerosing panencephalitis virus
- Maculopathy & encephalitis
- Progressively fatal
- Poor visual prognosis

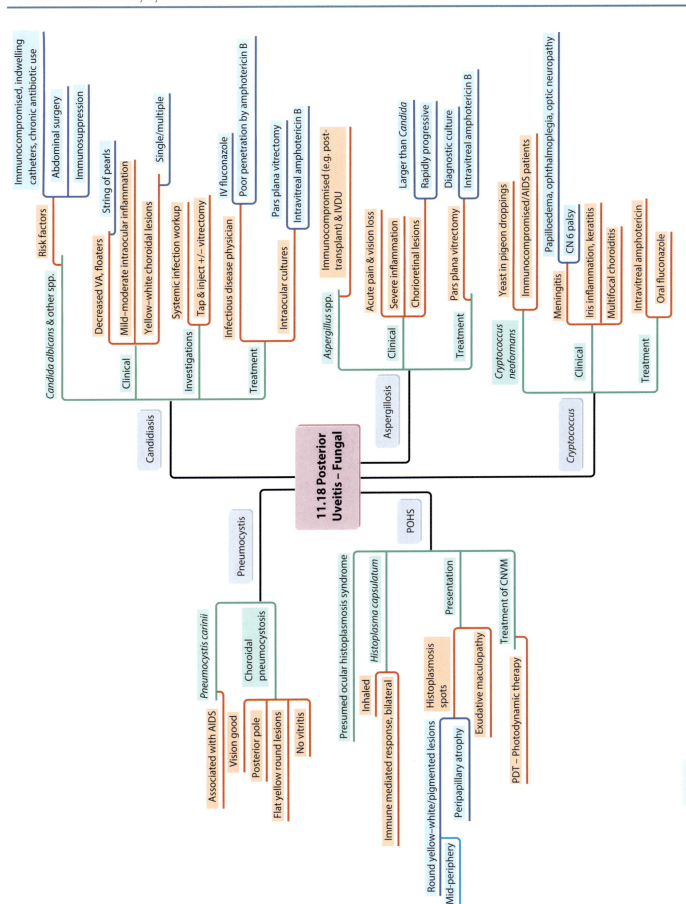

11.18 Posterior Uveitis – Fungal

Candidiasis

Candida albicans & other spp.

Risk factors
- Immunocompromised, indwelling catheters, chronic antibiotic use
- Abdominal surgery
- Immunosuppression

Clinical
- Decreased VA, floaters
- Mild–moderate intraocular inflammation
- String of pearls
- Yellow–white choroidal lesions
- Single/multiple

Investigations
- Systemic infection workup
- Tap & inject +/– vitrectomy

Treatment
- Infectious disease physician
- IV fluconazole
- Poor penetration by amphotericin B
- Intraocular cultures
- Pars plana vitrectomy
- Intravitreal amphotericin B

Aspergillosis

Aspergillus spp.
- Immunocompromised (e.g. post-transplant) & IVDU

Clinical
- Acute pain & vision loss
- Severe inflammation
- Chorioretinal lesions
- Larger than *Candida*
- Rapidly progressive

Treatment
- Pars plana vitrectomy
- Diagnostic culture
- Intravitreal amphotericin B

Cryptococcus

Cryptococcus neoformans
- Yeast in pigeon droppings
- Immunocompromised/AIDS patients

Clinical
- Meningitis
- Papilloedema, ophthalmoplegia, optic neuropathy
- CN 6 palsy
- Iris inflammation, keratitis
- Multifocal choroiditis

Treatment
- Intravitreal amphotericin
- Oral fluconazole

Pneumocystis

Pneumocystis carinii

Choroidal pneumocystosis
- Associated with AIDS
- Vision good
- Posterior pole
- Flat yellow round lesions
- No vitritis

POHS

Presumed ocular histoplasmosis syndrome

Histoplasma capsulatum
- Inhaled
- Immune mediated response, bilateral

Presentation
- Histoplasmosis spots
- Round yellow–white/pigmented lesions
- Mid-periphery
- Peripapillary atrophy
- Exudative maculopathy

Treatment of CNVM
- PDT – Photodynamic therapy

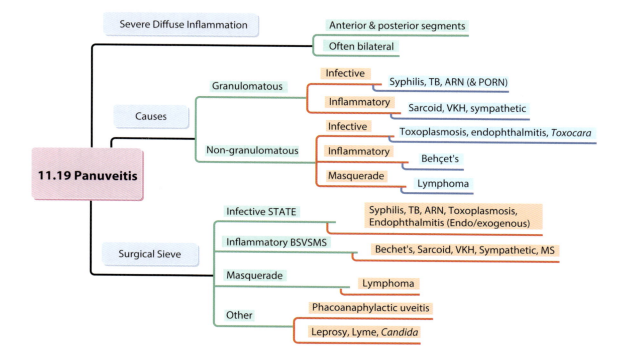

Severe Diffuse Inflammation
- Anterior & posterior segments
- Often bilateral

11.19 Panuveitis

Causes
- Granulomatous
  - Infective — Syphilis, TB, ARN (& PORN)
  - Inflammatory — Sarcoid, VKH, sympathetic
- Non-granulomatous
  - Infective — Toxoplasmosis, endophthalmitis, *Toxocara*
  - Inflammatory — Behçet's
  - Masquerade — Lymphoma

Surgical Sieve
- Infective STATE — Syphilis, TB, ARN, Toxoplasmosis, Endophthalmitis (Endo/exogenous)
- Inflammatory BSVSMS — Bechet's, Sarcoid, VKH, Sympathetic, MS
- Masquerade — Lymphoma
- Other
  - Phacoanaphylactic uveitis
  - Leprosy, Lyme, *Candida*

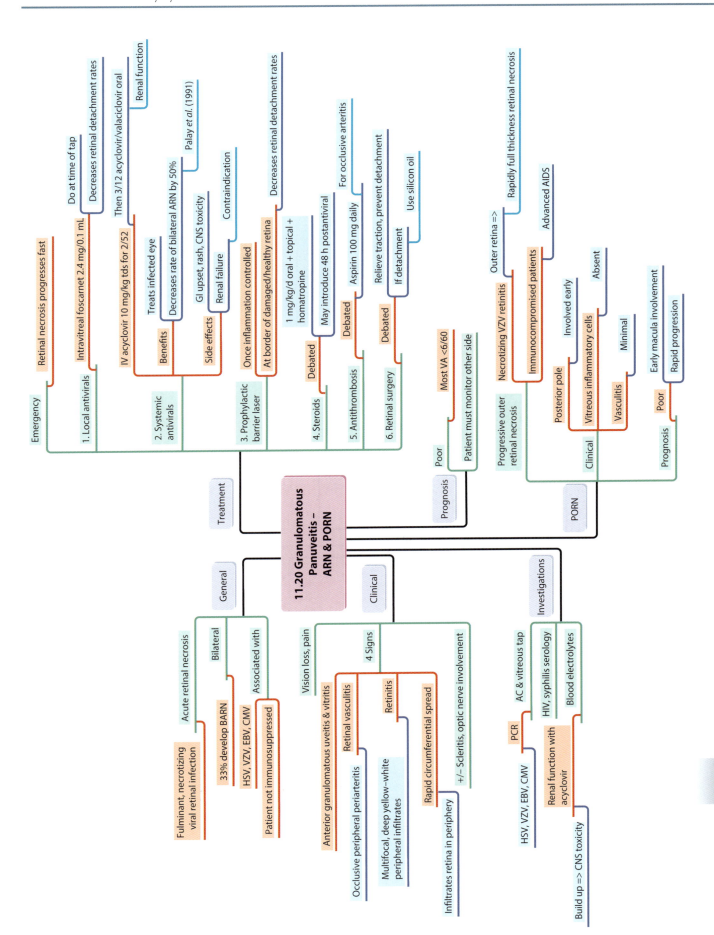

11.20 Granulomatous Panuveitis – ARN & PORN

Treatment

Emergency — Retinal necrosis progresses fast

1. Local antivirals
- Intravitreal foscarnet 2.4 mg/0.1 mL
  - Do at time of tap
  - Decreases retinal detachment rates

2. Systemic antivirals
- IV acyclovir 10 mg/kg tds for 2/52
  - Then 3/12 acyclovir/valaciclovir oral
    - Renal function
- Benefits
  - Treats infected eye
  - Decreases rate of bilateral ARN by 50%
    - Palay et al. (1991)
- Side effects
  - GI upset, rash, CNS toxicity
  - Renal failure
    - Contraindication

3. Prophylactic barrier laser
- Once inflammation controlled
- At border of damaged/healthy retina
  - Decreases retinal detachment rates

4. Steroids
- Debated
  - 1 mg/kg/d oral + topical + homatropine
- Debated
  - May introduce 48 h postantiviral
    - For occlusive arteritis
    - Aspirin 100 mg daily

5. Antithrombosis
- Debated
  - Relieve traction, prevent detachment
  - If detachment
    - Use silicon oil

6. Retinal surgery

Prognosis
- Poor — Most VA <6/60
- Patient must monitor other side

PORN

Progressive outer retinal necrosis
- Outer retina =>
  - Rapidly full thickness retinal necrosis
- Necrotizing VZV retinitis
  - Immunocompromised patients
    - Advanced AIDS

Clinical
- Posterior pole
  - Involved early
- Vitreous inflammatory cells
  - Absent
  - Minimal
- Vasculitis

Prognosis
- Poor
  - Early macula involvement
  - Rapid progression

General
- Acute retinal necrosis
- Bilateral
  - 33% develop BARN
- Associated with
  - HSV, VZV, EBV, CMV
  - Patient not immunosuppressed
- Fulminant, necrotizing viral retinal infection

Clinical
- Vision loss, pain
- 4 Signs
  - Anterior granulomatous uveitis & vitritis
  - Retinal vasculitis
    - Occlusive peripheral periarteritis
  - Retinitis
    - Multifocal, deep yellow–white peripheral infiltrates
    - Rapid circumferential spread
      - Infiltrates retina in periphery
  - +/– Scleritis, optic nerve involvement

Investigations
- AC & vitreous tap
  - PCR
    - HSV, VZV, EBV, CMV
- HIV, syphilis serology
- Blood electrolytes
  - Renal function with acyclovir
    - Build up => CNS toxicity

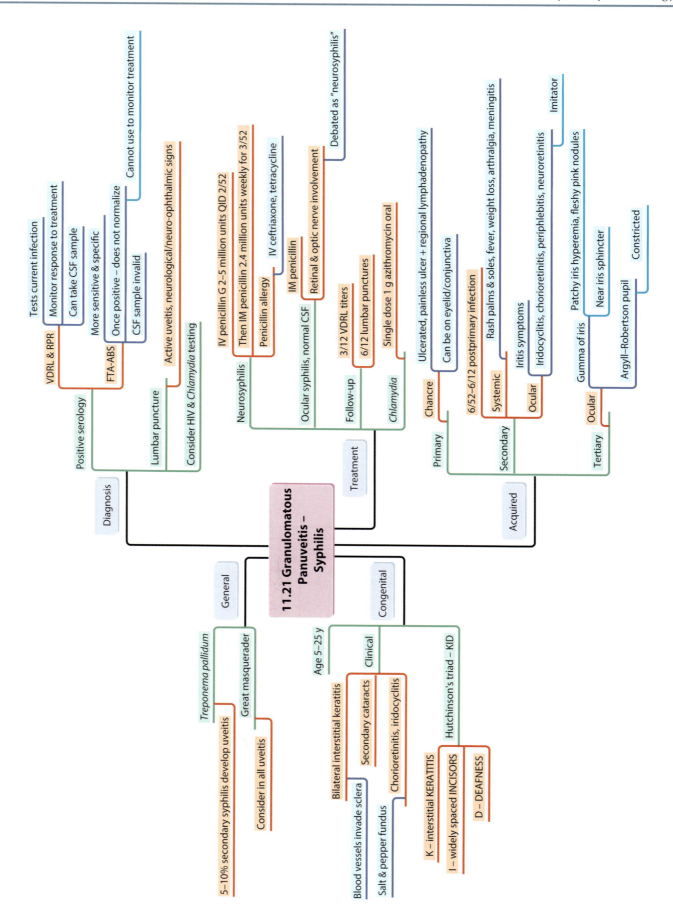

11.21 Granulomatous Panuveitis – Syphilis

General
- *Treponema pallidum*
- Great masquerader
  - 5–10% secondary syphilis develop uveitis
  - Consider in all uveitis

Diagnosis
- Positive serology
  - VDRL & RPR
    - Tests current infection
    - Monitor response to treatment
    - Can take CSF sample
    - More sensitive & specific
  - FTA-ABS
    - Once positive – does not normalize
    - CSF sample invalid
    - Cannot use to monitor treatment
- Lumbar puncture
  - Active uveitis, neurological/neuro-ophthalmic signs
- Consider HIV & *Chlamydia* testing

Treatment
- Neurosyphilis
  - IV penicillin G 2–5 million units QID 2/52
  - Then IM penicillin 2.4 million units weekly for 3/52
  - Penicillin allergy
    - IV ceftriaxone, tetracycline
  - IM penicillin
  - Retinal & optic nerve involvement
    - Debated as "neurosyphilis"
- Ocular syphilis, normal CSF
- Follow-up
  - 3/12 VDRL titers
  - 6/12 lumbar punctures
- *Chlamydia*
  - Single dose 1 g azithromycin oral

Acquired
- Primary
  - Chancre
    - Ulcerated, painless ulcer + regional lymphadenopathy
    - Can be on eyelid/conjunctiva
- Secondary
  - 6/52–6/12 postprimary infection
  - Systemic
    - Rash palms & soles, fever, weight loss, arthralgia, meningitis
  - Ocular
    - Iritis symptoms
    - Iridocyclitis, chorioretinitis, periphlebitis, neuroretinitis
    - Imitator
- Tertiary
  - Ocular
    - Gumma of iris
      - Patchy iris hyperemia, fleshy pink nodules
    - Argyll–Robertson pupil
      - Near iris sphincter
      - Constricted

Congenital
- Age 5–25 y
- Clinical
  - Bilateral interstitial keratitis
    - Blood vessels invade sclera
  - Secondary cataracts
  - Chorioretinitis, iridocyclitis
    - Salt & pepper fundus
  - Hutchinson's triad – KID
    - K – interstitial KERATITIS
    - I – widely spaced INCISORS
    - D – DEAFNESS

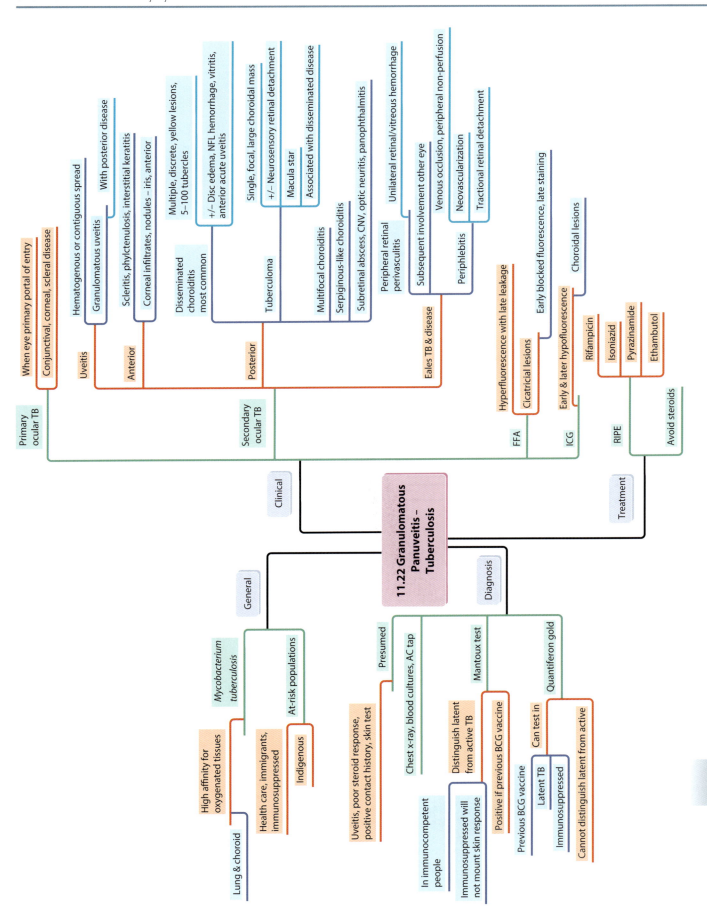

11.22 Granulomatous Panuveitis – Tuberculosis

Clinical

Primary ocular TB
- When eye primary portal of entry
  - Conjunctival, corneal, scleral disease

Secondary ocular TB
- Uveitis
  - Hematogenous or contiguous spread
  - Granulomatous uveitis
    - With posterior disease
- Anterior
  - Scleritis, phlyctenulosis, interstitial keratitis
  - Corneal infiltrates, nodules – iris, anterior
- Posterior
  - Disseminated choroiditis most common
    - Multiple, discrete, yellow lesions, 5–100 tubercles
    - +/– Disc edema, NFL hemorrhage, vitritis, anterior acute uveitis
  - Tuberculoma
    - Single, focal, large choroidal mass
    - +/– Neurosensory retinal detachment
    - Macula star
    - Associated with disseminated disease
  - Multifocal choroiditis
  - Serpiginous-like choroiditis
  - Subretinal abscess, CNV, optic neuritis, panophthalmitis
- Eales TB & disease
  - Peripheral retinal perivasculitis
  - Subsequent involvement other eye
    - Unilateral retinal/vitreous hemorrhage
    - Venous occlusion, peripheral non-perfusion
    - Neovascularization
    - Tractional retinal detachment
  - Periphlebitis

FFA
- Hyperfluorescence with late leakage
- Cicatricial lesions
  - Early blocked fluorescence, late staining

ICG
- Early & later hypofluorescence
  - Choroidal lesions

Treatment

RIPE
- Rifampicin
- Isoniazid
- Pyrazinamide
- Ethambutol

Avoid steroids

General

Mycobacterium tuberculosis
- High affnity for oxygenated tissues
  - Lung & choroid
- At-risk populations
  - Health care, immigrants, immunosuppressed
  - Indigenous

Diagnosis

Presumed
- Uveitis, poor steroid response, positive contact history, skin test
- Chest x-ray, blood cultures, AC tap

Mantoux test
- Distinguish latent from active TB
  - In immunocompetent people
  - Immunosuppressed will not mount skin response
- Positive if previous BCG vaccine
  - Previous BCG vaccine

Quantiferon gold
- Can test in
  - Latent TB
  - Immunosuppressed
- Cannot distinguish latent from active

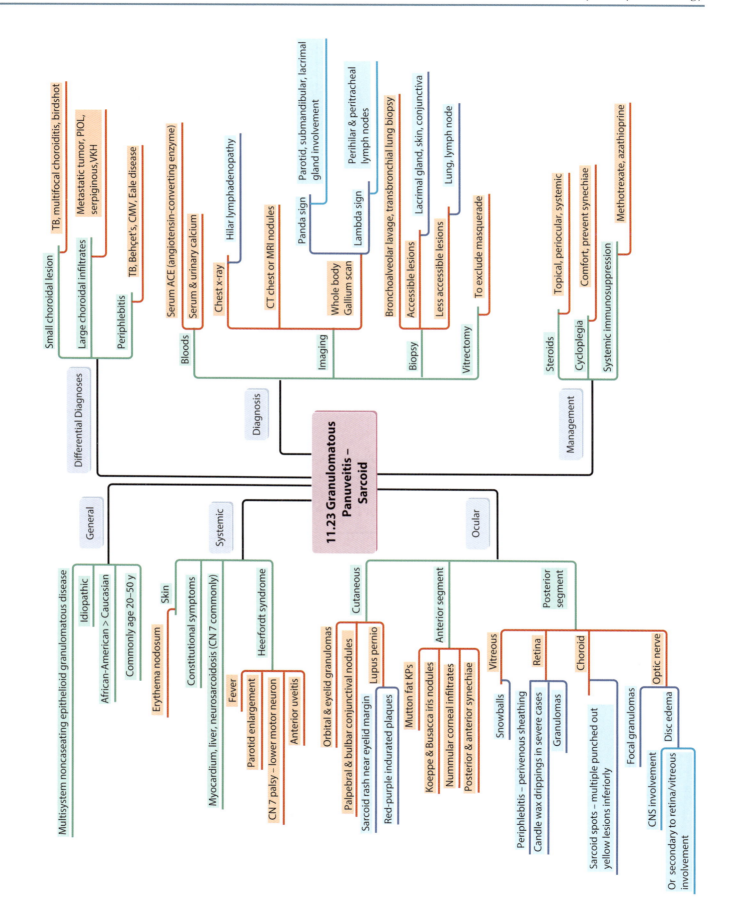

11.23 Granulomatous Panuveitis – Sarcoid

Differential Diagnoses

Small choroidal lesion
- TB, multifocal choroiditis, birdshot

Large choroidal infiltrates
- Metastatic tumor, PIOL, serpiginous, VKH

Periphlebitis
- TB, Behçet's, CMV, Eale disease

Diagnosis

Bloods
- Serum ACE (angiotensin-converting enzyme)
- Serum & urinary calcium

Imaging
- Chest x-ray
  - Hilar lymphadenopathy
- CT chest or MRI nodules
- Whole body Gallium scan
  - Panda sign
    - Parotid, submandibular, lacrimal gland involvement
  - Lambda sign
    - Perihilar & peritracheal lymph nodes

Biopsy
- Accessible lesions
  - Lacrimal gland, skin, conjunctiva
- Less accessible lesions
  - Bronchoalveolar lavage, transbronchial lung biopsy
  - Lung, lymph node

Vitrectomy
- To exclude masquerade

Management

Steroids
- Topical, periocular, systemic

Cycloplegia
- Comfort, prevent synechiae

Systemic immunosuppression
- Methotrexate, azathioprine

General
- Multisystem noncaseating epithelioid granulomatous disease
- Idiopathic
- African-American > Caucasian
- Commonly age 20–50 y

Systemic
- Skin
  - Erythema nodosum
- Constitutional symptoms
- Myocardium, liver, neurosarcoidosis (CN 7 commonly)
- Heerfordt syndrome
  - Fever
  - Parotid enlargement
  - CN 7 palsy – lower motor neuron
  - Anterior uveitis
- Cutaneous
  - Orbital & eyelid granulomas
  - Palpebral & bulbar conjunctival nodules
  - Sarcoid rash near eyelid margin
  - Lupus pernio
  - Red-purple indurated plaques

Ocular
- Anterior segment
  - Mutton fat KPs
  - Koeppe & Busacca iris nodules
  - Nummular corneal infiltrates
  - Posterior & anterior synechiae
- Posterior segment
  - Vitreous
    - Snowballs
  - Retina
    - Periphlebitis – perivenous sheathing
    - Candle wax drippings in severe cases
    - Granulomas
    - Sarcoid spots – multiple punched out yellow lesions inferiorly
  - Choroid
    - Focal granulomas
  - Optic nerve
    - CNS involvement
    - Disc edema
    - Or secondary to retina/vitreous involvement

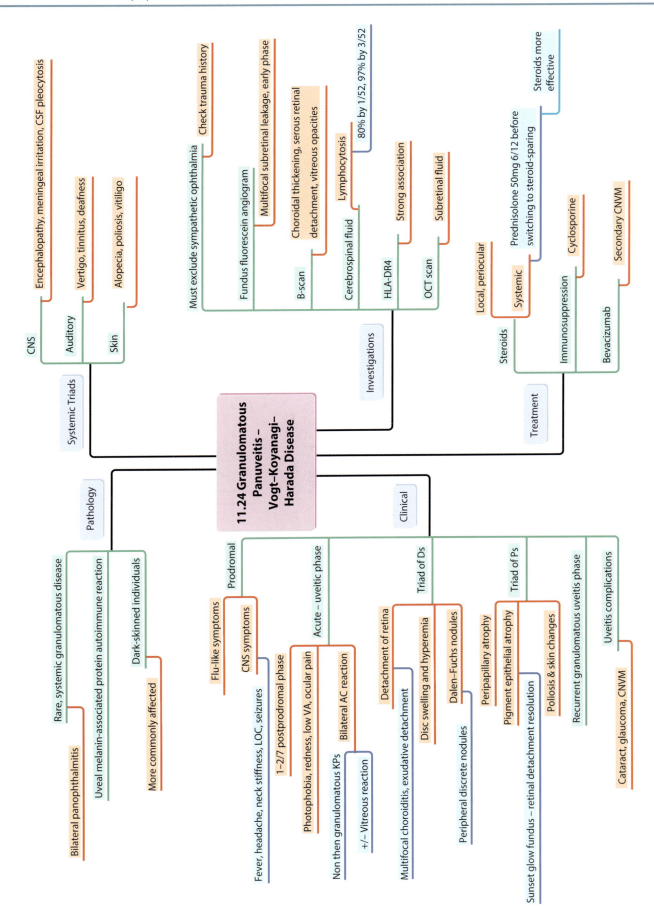

11.24 Granulomatous Panuveitis – Vogt–Koyanagi–Harada Disease

Systemic Triads

CNS
- Encephalopathy, meningeal irritation, CSF pleocytosis

Auditory
- Vertigo, tinnitus, deafness

Skin
- Alopecia, poliosis, vitiligo

Investigations
- Must exclude sympathetic ophthalmia
  - Check trauma history
- Fundus fluorescein angiogram
  - Multifocal subretinal leakage, early phase
- B-scan
  - Choroidal thickening, serous retinal detachment, vitreous opacities
- Cerebrospinal fluid
  - Lymphocytosis
  - 80% by 1/52, 97% by 3/52
- HLA-DR4
  - Strong association
- OCT scan
  - Subretinal fluid

Treatment

Steroids
- Local, periocular
- Systemic
  - Prednisolone 50mg 6/12 before switching to steroid-sparing

Immunosuppression
- Cyclosporine
  - Steroids more effective

Bevacizumab
- Secondary CNVM

Pathology
- Rare, systemic granulomatous disease
- Bilateral panophthalmitis
- Uveal melanin-associated protein autoimmune reaction
- Dark-skinned individuals
- More commonly affected

Clinical

Prodromal
- Flu-like symptoms
- CNS symptoms
  - Fever, headache, neck stiffness, LOC, seizures
  - 1–2/7 postprodromal phase

Acute – uveitic phase
- Photophobia, redness, low VA, ocular pain
- Bilateral AC reaction
- Non then granulomatous KPs
- +/– Vitreous reaction

Triad of Ds
- Detachment of retina
  - Multifocal choroiditis, exudative detachment
- Disc swelling and hyperemia
- Dalen–Fuchs nodules
  - Peripheral discrete nodules

Triad of Ps
- Peripapillary atrophy
- Pigment epithelial atrophy
  - Sunset glow fundus – retinal detachment resolution
- Poliosis & skin changes

Recurrent granulomatous uveitis phase

Uveitis complications
- Cataract, glaucoma, CNVM

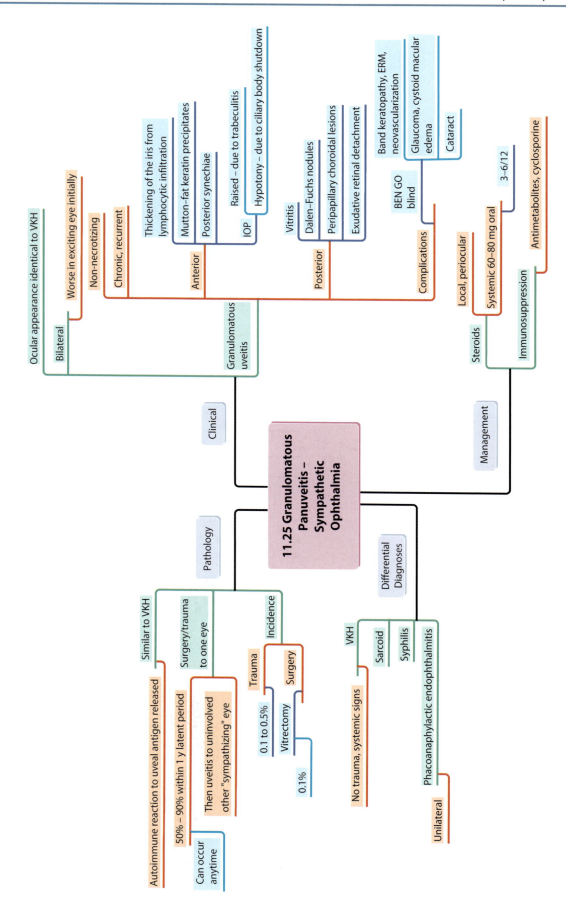

11.25 Granulomatous Panuveitis – Sympathetic Ophthalmia

Clinical

Granulomatous uveitis

Bilateral
- Ocular appearance identical to VKH

Worse in exciting eye initially

Non-necrotizing

Chronic, recurrent

Anterior
- Thickening of the iris from lymphocytic infiltration
- Mutton–fat keratin precipitates
- Posterior synechiae
- IOP
  - Raised – due to trabeculitis
  - Hypotony – due to ciliary body shutdown

Posterior
- Vitritis
- Dalen–Fuchs nodules
- Peripapillary choroidal lesions
- Exudative retinal detachment

Complications
- BEN GO blind
- Band keratopathy, ERM, neovascularization
- Glaucoma, cystoid macular edema
- Cataract

Management

Steroids
- Local, periocular
- Systemic 60–80 mg oral
  - 3–6/12

Immunosuppression
- Antimetabolites, cyclosporine

Pathology

Similar to VKH
- Autoimmune reaction to uveal antigen released
- 50% – 90% within 1 y latent period
  - Can occur anytime

Surgery/trauma to one eye
- Then uveitis to uninvolved other "sympathizing" eye

Incidence
- Trauma
  - 0.1 to 0.5%
- Surgery
  - Vitrectomy
    - 0.1%

Differential Diagnoses

VKH
- No trauma, systemic signs

Sarcoid

Syphilis

Phacoanaphylactic endophthalmitis
- Unilateral

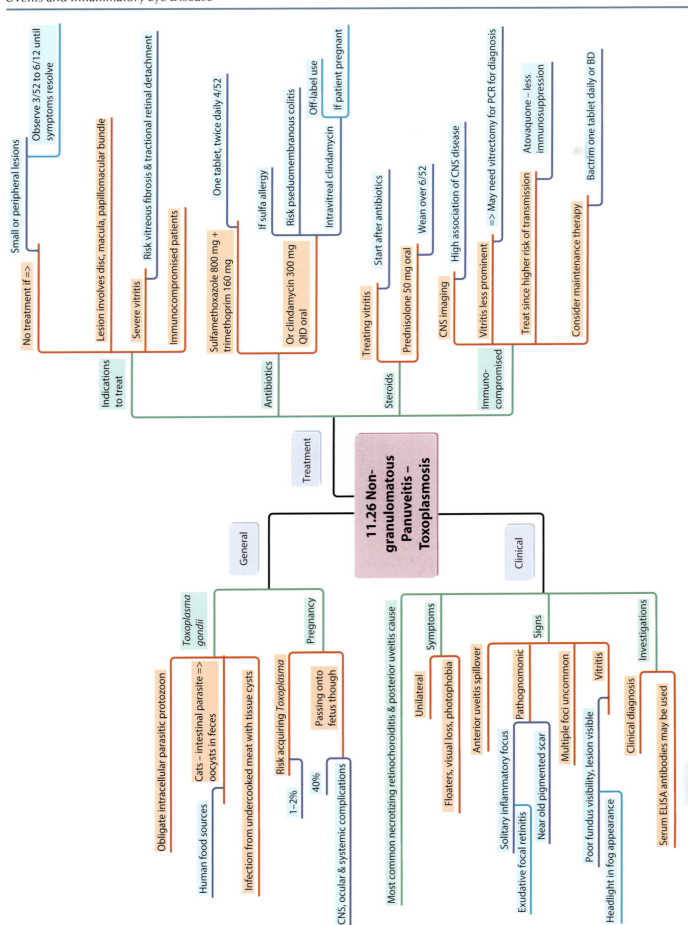

11.26 Non-granulomatous Panuveitis – Toxoplasmosis

Treatment

Indications to treat
- No treatment if =>
  - Small or peripheral lesions
  - Observe 3/52 to 6/12 until symptoms resolve
- Lesion involves disc, macula, papillomacular bundle
- Severe vitritis
  - Risk vitreous fibrosis & tractional retinal detachment
- Immunocompromised patients

Antibiotics
- Sulfamethoxazole 800 mg + trimethoprim 160 mg
  - One tablet, twice daily 4/52
- Or clindamycin 300 mg QID oral
  - If sulfa allergy
  - Risk pseuodomembranous colitis
  - Intravitreal clindamycin
    - Off-label use
    - If patient pregnant

Steroids
- Treating vitritis
  - Start after antibiotics
- Prednisolone 50 mg oral
  - Wean over 6/52

Immuno-compromised
- CNS imaging
  - High association of CNS disease
- Vitritis less prominent
  - => May need vitrectomy for PCR for diagnosis
- Treat since higher risk of transmission
  - Atovaquone – less immunosuppression
- Consider maintenance therapy
  - Bactrim one tablet daily or BD

General

Toxoplasma gondii
- Obligate intracellular parasitic protozoon
- Cats – intestinal parasite => oocysts in feces
- Human food sources
- Infection from undercooked meat with tissue cysts

Pregnancy
- Risk acquiring Toxoplasma
  - 1–2%
- Passing onto fetus though
  - 40%
- CNS, ocular & systemic complications

Clinical

- Most common necrotizing retinochoroiditis & posterior uveitis cause

Symptoms
- Unilateral
- Floaters, visual loss, photophobia

Signs
- Anterior uveitis spillover
- Pathognomonic
  - Solitary inflammatory focus
  - Exudative focal retinitis
  - Near old pigmented scar
- Multiple foci uncommon
- Vitritis
  - Poor fundus visibility, lesion visible
  - Headlight in fog appearance

Investigations
- Clinical diagnosis
- Serum ELISA antibodies may be used

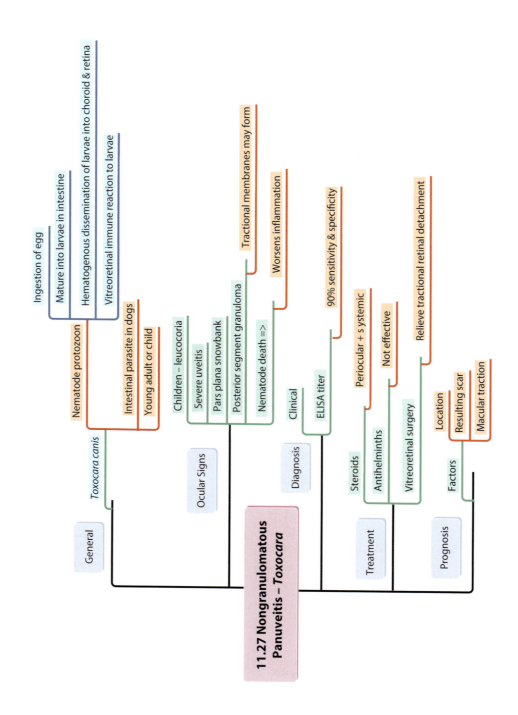

11.27 Nongranulomatous Panuveitis – Toxocara

General

Toxocara canis
- Nematode protozoon
  - Ingestion of egg
  - Mature into larvae in intestine
  - Hematogenous dissemination of larvae into choroid & retina
  - Vitreoretinal immune reaction to larvae
- Intestinal parasite in dogs
- Young adult or child

Ocular Signs
- Children – leucocoria
- Severe uveitis
- Pars plana snowbank
- Posterior segment granuloma
  - Tractional membranes may form
- Nematode death =>
  - Worsens inflammation

Diagnosis
- Clinical
- ELISA titer
  - 90% sensitivity & specificity

Treatment
- Steroids
  - Periocular + s ystemic
- Antihelminths
  - Not effective
- Vitreoretinal surgery
  - Relieve tractional retinal detachment

Prognosis
- Factors
  - Location
  - Resulting scar
  - Macular traction

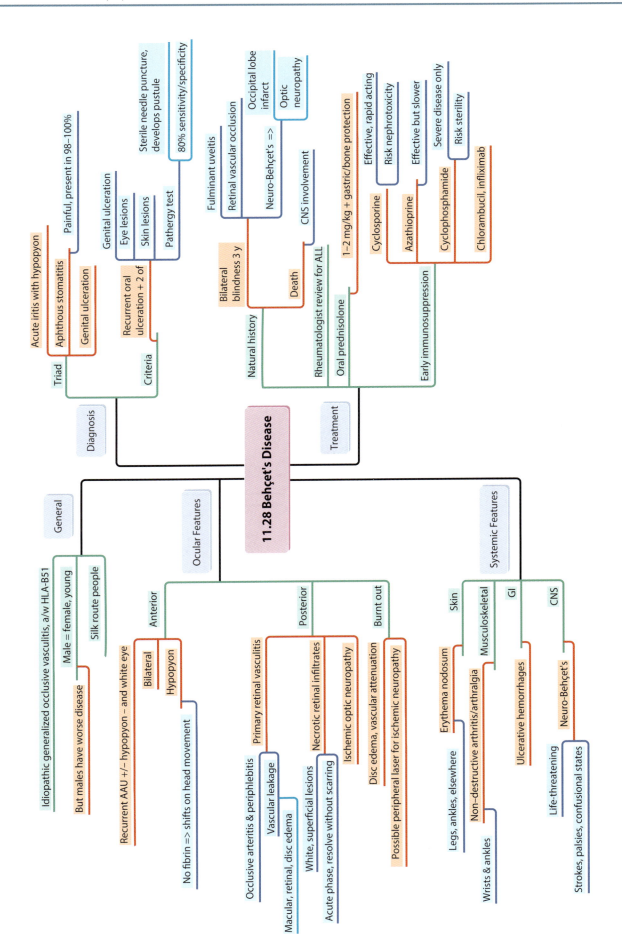

11.28 Behçet's Disease

Diagnosis

Triad
- Acute iritis with hypopyon
- Aphthous stomatitis — Painful, present in 98–100%
- Genital ulceration

Criteria
- Recurrent oral ulceration + 2 of
  - Genital ulceration
  - Eye lesions
  - Skin lesions
  - Pathergy test — Sterile needle puncture, develops pustule — 80% sensitivity/specificity

Treatment

Natural history
- Fulminant uveitis
- Retinal vascular occlusion
- Neuro-Behçet's => — Occipital lobe infarct / Optic neuropathy
- CNS involvement
- Bilateral blindness 3 y
- Death

Rheumatologist review for ALL

Oral prednisolone — 1–2 mg/kg + gastric/bone protection

Early immunosuppression
- Cyclosporine — Effective, rapid acting / Risk nephrotoxicity
- Azathioprine — Effective but slower
- Cyclophosphamide — Severe disease only / Risk sterility
- Chlorambucil, infliximab

General
- Idiopathic generalized occlusive vasculitis, a/w HLA-B51
- Male = female, young — But males have worse disease
- Silk route people

Ocular Features

Anterior
- Recurrent AAU +/- hypopyon – and white eye
  - Bilateral
  - Hypopyon — No fibrin => shifts on head movement

Posterior
- Primary retinal vasculitis
  - Occlusive arteritis & periphlebitis
  - Vascular leakage — Macular, retinal, disc edema
- Necrotic retinal infiltrates — White, superficial lesions / Acute phase, resolve without scarring
- Ischemic optic neuropathy — Disc edema, vascular attenuation / Possible peripheral laser for ischemic neuropathy

Burnt out

Systemic Features

Skin
- Erythema nodosum — Legs, ankles, elsewhere

Musculoskeletal
- Non-destructive arthritis/arthralgia — Wrists & ankles

GI
- Ulcerative hemorrhages

CNS
- Neuro-Behçet's — Life-threatening / Strokes, palsies, confusional states

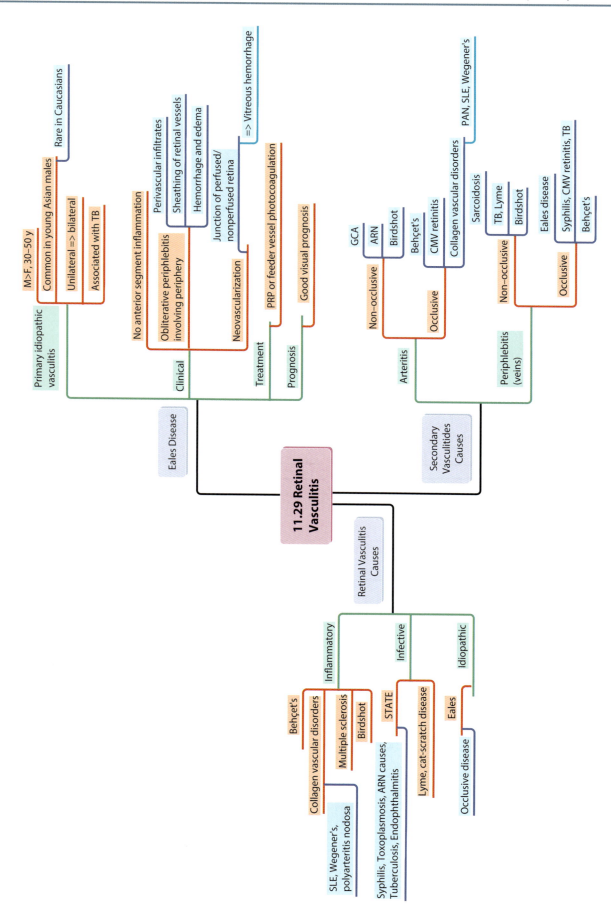

11.29 Retinal Vasculitis

Eales Disease

Primary idiopathic vasculitis
- M>F, 30–50 y
- Common in young Asian males
  - Unilateral => bilateral
  - Associated with TB
- Rare in Caucasians

Clinical
- No anterior segment inflammation
- Obliterative periphlebitis involving periphery
  - Perivascular infiltrates
  - Sheathing of retinal vessels
  - Hemorrhage and edema
- Neovascularization
  - Junction of perfused/nonperfused retina
  - => Vitreous hemorrhage

Treatment
- PRP or feeder vessel photocoagulation

Prognosis
- Good visual prognosis

Secondary Vasculitides Causes

Arteritis
- Non-occlusive
  - GCA
  - ARN
  - Birdshot
- Occlusive
  - Behçet's
  - CMV retinitis
  - Collagen vascular disorders
    - Sarcoidosis
    - PAN, SLE, Wegener's

Periphlebitis (veins)
- Non-occlusive
  - TB, Lyme
  - Birdshot
  - Sarcoidosis
- Occlusive
  - Eales disease
  - Syphilis, CMV retinitis, TB
  - Behçet's

Retinal Vasculitis Causes

Inflammatory
- Behçet's
- Collagen vascular disorders
  - SLE, Wegener's, polyarteritis nodosa
- Multiple sclerosis
- Birdshot

Infective
- STATE
  - Syphilis, Toxoplasmosis, ARN causes, Tuberculosis, Endophthalmitis
- Lyme, cat-scratch disease

Idiopathic
- Eales
- Occlusive disease

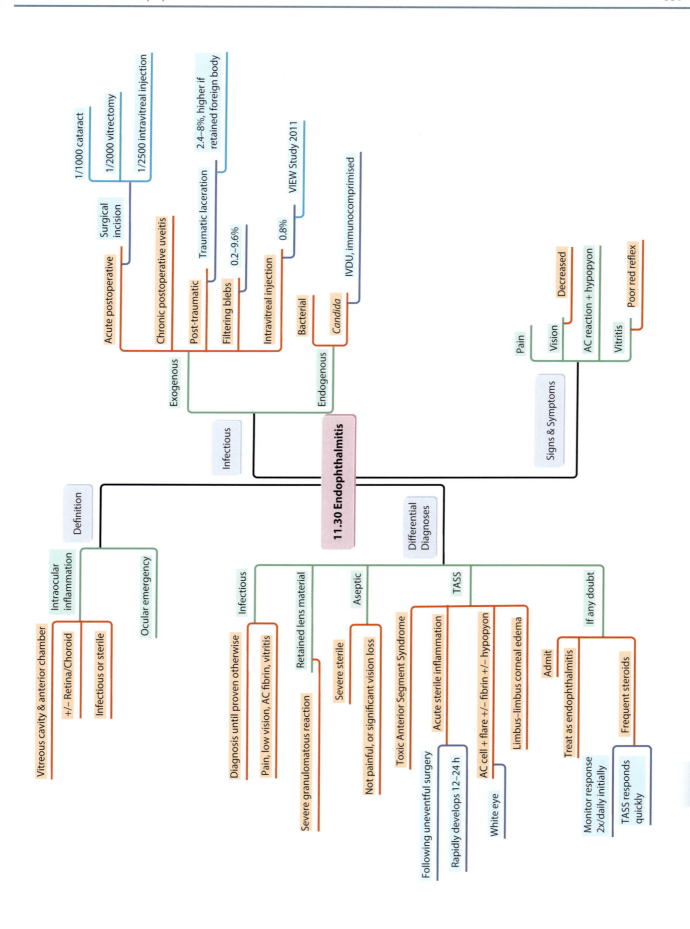

11.30 Endophthalmitis

Definition
- Intraocular inflammation
  - Vitreous cavity & anterior chamber
  - +/− Retina/Choroid
  - Infectious or sterile
- Ocular emergency

Infectious
- Exogenous
  - Acute postoperative
    - Surgical incision
      - 1/1000 cataract
      - 1/2000 vitrectomy
      - 1/2500 intravitreal injection
  - Chronic postoperative uveitis
  - Post-traumatic
    - Traumatic laceration
      - 2.4–8%, higher if retained foreign body
  - Filtering blebs
    - 0.2–9.6%
  - Intravitreal injection
    - 0.8%
      - VIEW Study 2011
- Endogenous
  - Bacterial
  - Candida
    - IVDU, immunocomprimised

Signs & Symptoms
- Pain
- Vision
  - Decreased
- AC reaction + hypopyon
- Vitritis
- Poor red reflex

Differential Diagnoses
- Infectious
  - Diagnosis until proven otherwise
  - Pain, low vision, AC fibrin, vitritis
- Retained lens material
  - Severe granulomatous reaction
- Aseptic
  - Severe sterile
  - Not painful, or significant vision loss
- TASS
  - Toxic Anterior Segment Syndrome
    - Following uneventful surgery
  - Acute sterile inflammation
    - Rapidly develops 12–24 h
  - AC cell + flare +/− fibrin +/− hypopyon
    - White eye
  - Limbus–limbus corneal edema
  - If any doubt
    - Admit
    - Treat as endophthalmitis
    - Frequent steroids
      - Monitor response 2x/daily initially
      - TASS responds quickly

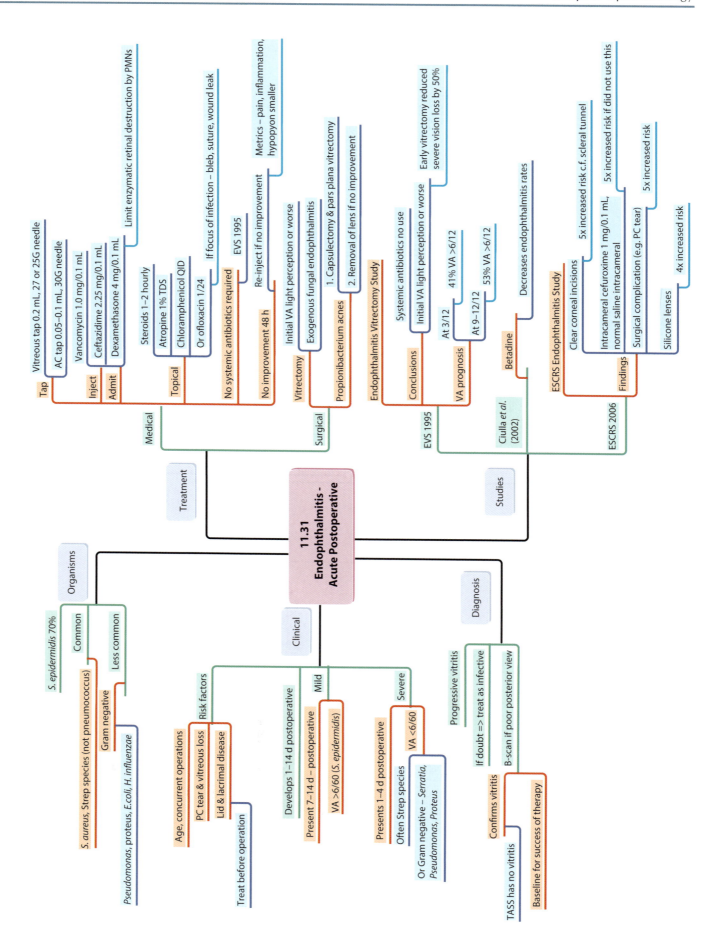

11.31 Endophthalmitis – Acute Postoperative

Treatment

Medical

- **Tap**
  - Vitreous tap 0.2 mL, 27 or 25G needle
  - AC tap 0.05–0.1 mL, 30G needle
- **Inject**
  - Vancomycin 1.0 mg/0.1 mL
  - Ceftazidime 2.25 mg/0.1 mL
  - Dexamethasone 4 mg/0.1 mL
    - Limit enzymatic retinal destruction by PMNs
- **Admit**
- **Topical**
  - Steroids 1–2 hourly
  - Atropine 1% TDS
  - Chloramphenicol QID
  - Or ofloxacin 1/24
- No systemic antibiotics required
  - If focus of infection – bleb, suture, wound leak
- No improvement 48 h
  - Re-inject if no improvement
    - EVS 1995
      - Metrics – pain, inflammation, hypopyon smaller

Surgical

- **Vitrectomy**
  - Initial VA light perception or worse
- Exogenous fungal endophthalmitis
  - 1. Capsulectomy & pars plana vitrectomy
  - 2. Removal of lens if no improvement
- Propionibacterium acnes

Studies

EVS 1995

- Endophthalmitis Vitrectomy Study
- **Conclusions**
  - Systemic antibiotics no use
  - Initial VA light perception or worse
    - Early vitrectomy reduced severe vision loss by 50%
- **VA prognosis**
  - At 3/12
    - 41% VA >6/12
  - At 9-12/12
    - 53% VA >6/12

Ciulla et al. (2002)

- Betadine
  - Decreases endophthalmitis rates

ESCRS 2006

- ESCRS Endophthalmitis Study
- **Findings**
  - Clear corneal incisions
    - 5x increased risk c.f. scleral tunnel
  - Intracameral cefuroxime 1 mg/0.1 mL, normal saline intracameral
    - 5x increased risk if did not use this
  - Surgical complication (e.g. PC tear)
    - 5x increased risk
  - Silicone lenses
    - 4x increased risk

Clinical

Organisms

- **Common**
  - S. epidermidis 70%
  - S. aureus, Strep species (not pneumococcus)
- **Less common**
  - Gram negative
    - Pseudomonas, proteus, E.coli, H. influenzae

Risk factors

- Age, concurrent operations
- PC tear & vitreous loss
- Lid & lacrimal disease
  - Treat before operation

Mild

- Develops 1–14 d postoperative
- Present 7–14 d – postoperative
- VA >6/60 (S. epidermidis)

Severe

- Presents 1–4 d postoperative
- Often Strep species
- Or Gram negative – Serratia, Pseudomonas, Proteus
- VA <6/60

Diagnosis

- Progressive vitritis
- If doubt => treat as infective
- B-scan if poor posterior view
  - Confirms vitritis
  - TASS has no vitritis
  - Baseline for success of therapy

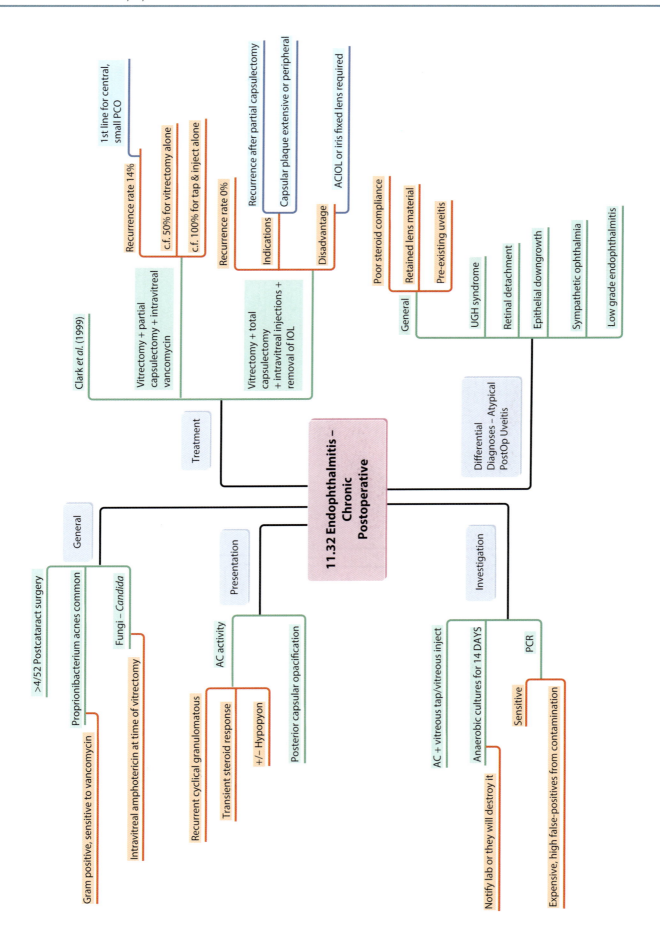

11.32 Endophthalmitis – Chronic Postoperative

Treatment

Clark et al. (1999)

Vitrectomy + partial capsulectomy + intravitreal vancomycin
- Recurrence rate 14%
  - c.f. 50% for vitrectomy alone
  - c.f. 100% for tap & inject alone
  - 1st line for central, small PCO

Vitrectomy + total capsulectomy + intravitreal injections + removal of IOL
- Recurrence rate 0%
- Indications
  - Recurrence after partial capsulectomy
  - Capsular plaque extensive or peripheral
- Disadvantage
  - ACIOL or iris fixed lens required

Differential Diagnoses – Atypical PostOp Uveitis

General
- Poor steroid compliance
- Retained lens material
- Pre-existing uveitis

- UGH syndrome
- Retinal detachment
- Epithelial downgrowth
- Sympathetic ophthalmia
- Low grade endophthalmitis

General
- >4/52 Postcataract surgery
- Proprionibacterium acnes common
  - Gram positive, sensitive to vancomycin
- Fungi – Candida
  - Intravitreal amphotericin at time of vitrectomy

Presentation
- AC activity
  - Recurrent cyclical granulomatous
  - Transient steroid response
  - +/– Hypopyon
- Posterior capsular opacification

Investigation
- AC + vitreous tap/vitreous inject
  - Anaerobic cultures for 14 DAYS
    - Notify lab or they will destroy it
  - PCR
    - Sensitive
    - Expensive, high false-positives from contamination

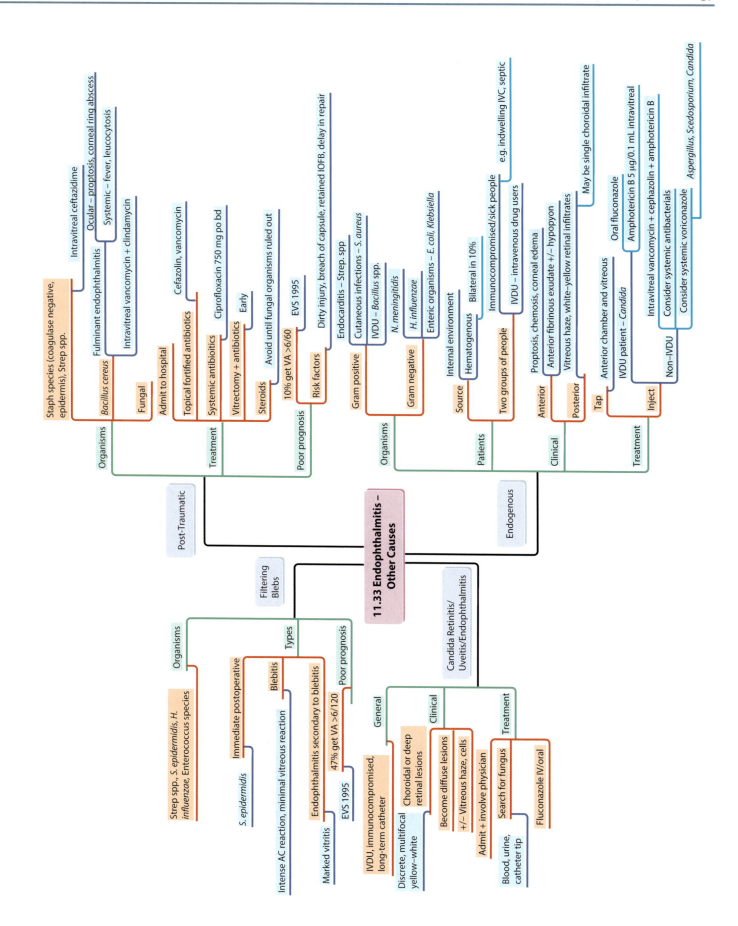

11.33 Endophthalmitis – Other Causes

Post-Traumatic

Organisms
- Staph species (coagulase negative, epidermis), Strep spp.
  - Intravitreal ceftazidime
- *Bacillus cereus*
  - Fulminant endophthalmitis
    - Ocular – proptosis, corneal ring abscess
    - Systemic – fever, leucocytosis
  - Intravitreal vancomycin + clindamycin
- Fungal

Treatment
- Admit to hospital
- Topical fortified antibiotics
  - Cefazolin, vancomycin
- Systemic antibiotics
  - Ciprofloxacin 750 mg po bd
- Vitrectomy + antibiotics
  - Early
- Steroids
  - Avoid until fungal organisms ruled out

Poor prognosis
- 10% get VA >6/60
  - EVS 1995
- Risk factors
  - Dirty injury, breach of capsule, retained IOFB, delay in repair

Endogenous

Organisms
- Gram positive
  - Endocarditis – Strep. spp
  - Cutaneous infections – *S. aureus*
  - IVDU – *Bacillus* spp.
- Gram negative
  - *N. meningitidis*
  - *H. influenzae*
  - Enteric organisms – *E. coli, Klebsiella*

Source
- Internal environment
- Hematogenous
  - Bilateral in 10%

Patients
- Two groups of people
  - Immunocompromised/sick people
    - e.g. indwelling IVC, septic
  - IVDU – intravenous drug users

Clinical
- Anterior
  - Proptosis, chemosis, corneal edema
  - Anterior fibrinous exudate +/- hypopyon
- Posterior
  - Vitreous haze, white–yellow retinal infiltrates
  - May be single choroidal infiltrate

Treatment
- Tap
  - Anterior chamber and vitreous
- Inject
  - IVDU patient – *Candida*
    - Oral fluconazole
    - Amphotericin B 5 µg/0.1 mL intravitreal
  - Non-IVDU
    - Intravitreal vancomycin + cephazolin + amphotericin B
    - Consider systemic antibacterials
    - Consider systemic voriconazole
      - *Aspergillus, Scedosporium, Candida*

Filtering Blebs

Organisms
- Strep spp., *S. epidermidis, H. influenzae,* Enterococcus species

Types
- Immediate postoperative
  - *S. epidermidis*
- Blebitis
  - Intense AC reaction, minimal vitreous reaction
  - Marked vitritis
- Endophthalmitis secondary to blebitis
  - IVDU, immunocompromised, long-term catheter

Poor prognosis
- 47% get VA >6/120
  - EVS 1995

Candida Retinitis/Uveitis/Endophthalmitis

General
- Discrete, multifocal yellow–white
  - Choroidal or deep retinal lesions

Clinical
- Become diffuse lesions
- +/- Vitreous haze, cells

Treatment
- Admit + involve physician
- Search for fungus
  - Blood, urine, catheter tip
- Fluconazole IV/oral

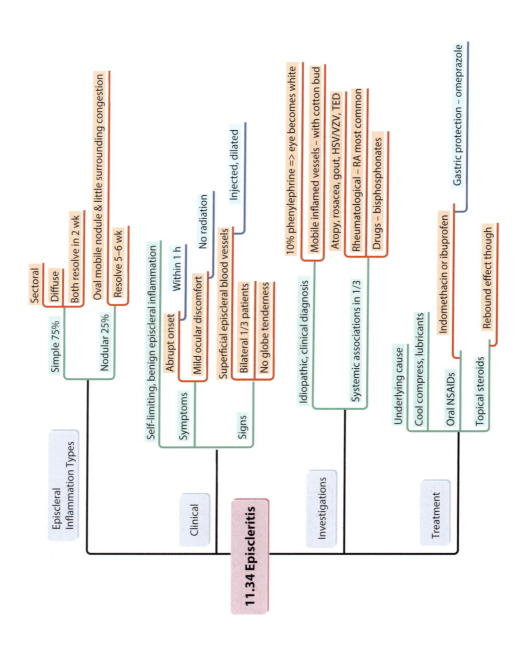

11.34 Episcleritis

Episcleral Inflammation Types
- Simple 75%
  - Sectoral
  - Diffuse
  - Both resolve in 2 wk
- Nodular 25%
  - Oval mobile nodule & little surrounding congestion
  - Resolve 5–6 wk

Clinical
- Self-limiting, benign episcleral inflammation
- Symptoms
  - Abrupt onset
  - Within 1 h
  - Mild ocular discomfort
  - No radiation
- Signs
  - Superficial episcleral blood vessels
  - Injected, dilated
  - Bilateral 1/3 patients
  - No globe tenderness

Investigations
- Idiopathic, clinical diagnosis
  - 10% phenylephrine => eye becomes white
  - Mobile inflamed vessels – with cotton bud
- Systemic associations in 1/3
  - Atopy, rosacea, gout, HSV/VZV, TED
  - Rheumatological – RA most common
  - Drugs – bisphosphonates

Treatment
- Underlying cause
- Cool compress, lubricants
- Oral NSAIDs
  - Indomethacin or ibuprofen
  - Gastric protection – omeprazole
- Topical steroids
  - Rebound effect though

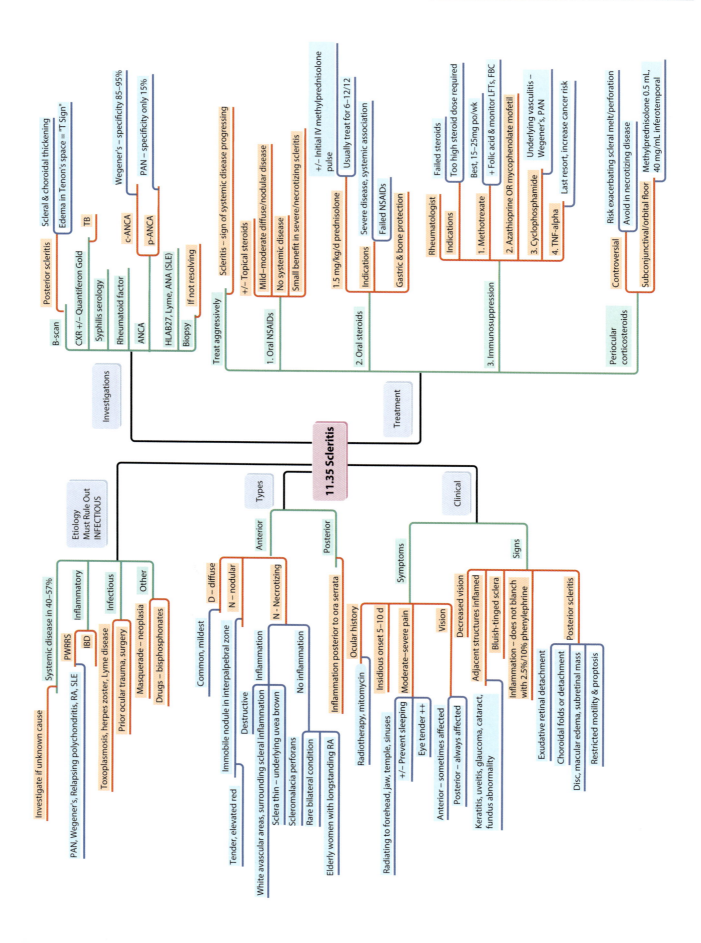

11.35 Scleritis

Investigations

- B-scan
  - Posterior scleritis
    - Scleral & choroidal thickening
    - Edema in Tenon's space = "T Sign"
- CXR +/– Quantiferon Gold
  - TB
- Syphilis serology
- Rheumatoid factor
- ANCA
  - c-ANCA
    - Wegener's – specificity 85–95%
  - p-ANCA
    - PAN – specificity only 15%
- HLAB27, Lyme, ANA (SLE)
- Biopsy
  - If not resolving

Treatment

- Treat aggressively
  - Scleritis – sign of systemic disease progressing
- 1. Oral NSAIDs
  - +/– Topical steroids
  - Mild–moderate diffuse/nodular disease
  - No systemic disease
  - Small benefit in severe/necrotizing scleritis
- 2. Oral steroids
  - +/– Initial IV methylprednisolone pulse
  - Usually treat for 6–12/12
  - 1.5 mg/kg/d prednisolone
  - Indications
    - Severe disease, systemic association
    - Failed NSAIDs
  - Gastric & bone protection
- 3. Immunosuppression
  - Rheumatologist
  - Indications
    - Failed steroids
    - Too high steroid dose required
  - 1. Methotrexate
    - Best, 15–25mg po/wk
    - + Folic acid & monitor LFTs, FBC
  - 2. Azathioprine OR mycophenolate mofetil
  - 3. Cyclophosphamide
    - Underlying vasculitis – Wegener's, PAN
  - 4. TNF-alpha
    - Last resort, increase cancer risk
- Periocular corticosteroids
  - Controversial
    - Risk exacerbating scleral melt/perforation
    - Avoid in necrotizing disease
  - Subconjunctival/orbital floor
    - Methylprednisolone 0.5 mL, 40 mg/mL inferotemporal

Etiology Must Rule Out INFECTIOUS

- Investigate if unknown cause
  - Systemic disease in 40–57%
    - PAN, Wegener's, Relapsing polychondritis, RA, SLE
  - Inflammatory
    - PWRRS
    - IBD
  - Infectious
    - Toxoplasmosis, herpes zoster, Lyme disease
    - Prior ocular trauma, surgery
  - Other
    - Masquerade – neoplasia
    - Drugs – bisphosphonates

Types

- Anterior
  - D – diffuse
    - Common, mildest
  - N – nodular
    - Tender, elevated red
    - Immobile nodule in interpalpebral zone
  - N – Necrotizing
    - Inflammation
      - White avascular areas, surrounding scleral inflammation
      - Destructive
      - Sclera thin – underlying uvea brown
    - No inflammation
      - Scleromalacia perforans
      - Rare bilateral condition
      - Elderly women with longstanding RA
- Posterior
  - Inflammation posterior to ora serrata

Clinical

- Symptoms
  - Ocular history
    - Radiotherapy, mitomycin
  - Insidious onset 5–10 d
  - Moderate–severe pain
    - Radiating to forehead, jaw, temple, sinuses
    - +/– Prevent sleeping
    - Eye tender ++
  - Vision
    - Anterior – sometimes affected
    - Posterior – always affected
    - Keratitis, uveitis, glaucoma, cataract, fundus abnormality
- Signs
  - Decreased vision
  - Adjacent structures inflamed
  - Bluish-tinged sclera
  - Inflammation – does not blanch with 2.5%/10% phenylephrine
  - Posterior scleritis
    - Exudative retinal detachment
    - Choroidal folds or detachment
    - Disc, macular edema, subretinal mass
    - Restricted motility & proptosis

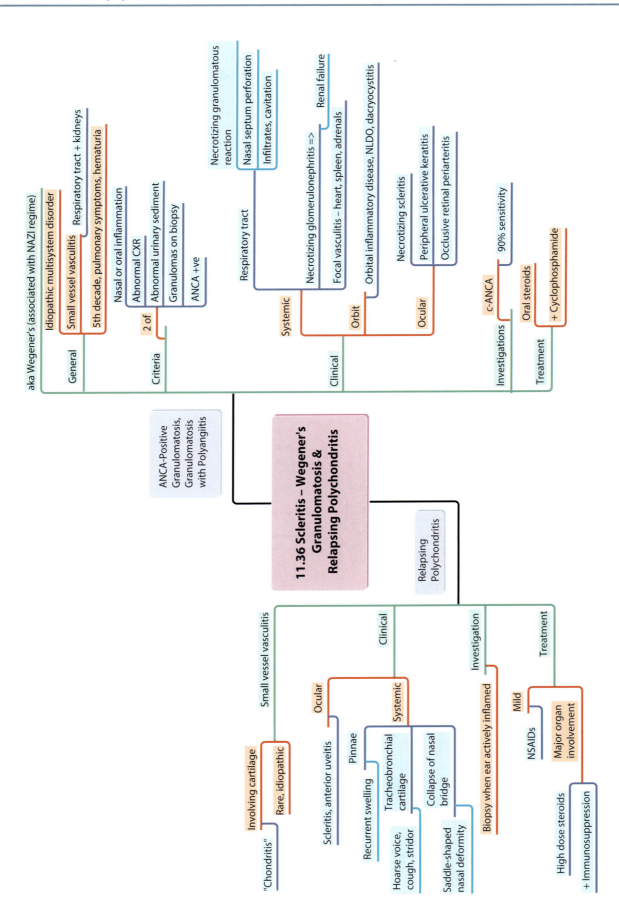

11.36 Scleritis – Wegener's Granulomatosis & Relapsing Polychondritis

ANCA-Positive Granulomatosis, Granulomatosis with Polyangiitis

General
- aka Wegener's (associated with NAZI regime)
- Idiopathic multisystem disorder
- Small vessel vasculitis — Respiratory tract + kidneys
- 5th decade, pulmonary symptoms, hematuria

Criteria — 2 of
- Nasal or oral inflammation
- Abnormal CXR
- Abnormal urinary sediment
- Granulomas on biopsy
- ANCA +ve

Clinical
- Systemic
  - Respiratory tract
    - Necrotizing granulomatous reaction
    - Nasal septum perforation
    - Infiltrates, cavitation
  - Necrotizing glomerulonephritis => Renal failure
  - Focal vasculitis – heart, spleen, adrenals
- Orbit
  - Orbital inflammatory disease, NLDO, dacryocystitis
- Ocular
  - Necrotizing scleritis
  - Peripheral ulcerative keratitis
  - Occlusive retinal periarteritis

Investigations
- c-ANCA — 90% sensitivity

Treatment
- Oral steroids
- + Cyclophosphamide

Relapsing Polychondritis

"Chondritis"
- Involving cartilage
- Rare, idiopathic

Small vessel vasculitis

Clinical
- Ocular
  - Scleritis, anterior uveitis
- Systemic
  - Pinnae — Recurrent swelling
  - Tracheobronchial cartilage — Hoarse voice, cough, stridor
  - Collapse of nasal bridge — Saddle-shaped nasal deformity

Investigation
- Biopsy when ear actively inflamed

Treatment
- Mild — NSAIDs
- Major organ involvement
  - High dose steroids
  - + Immunosuppression

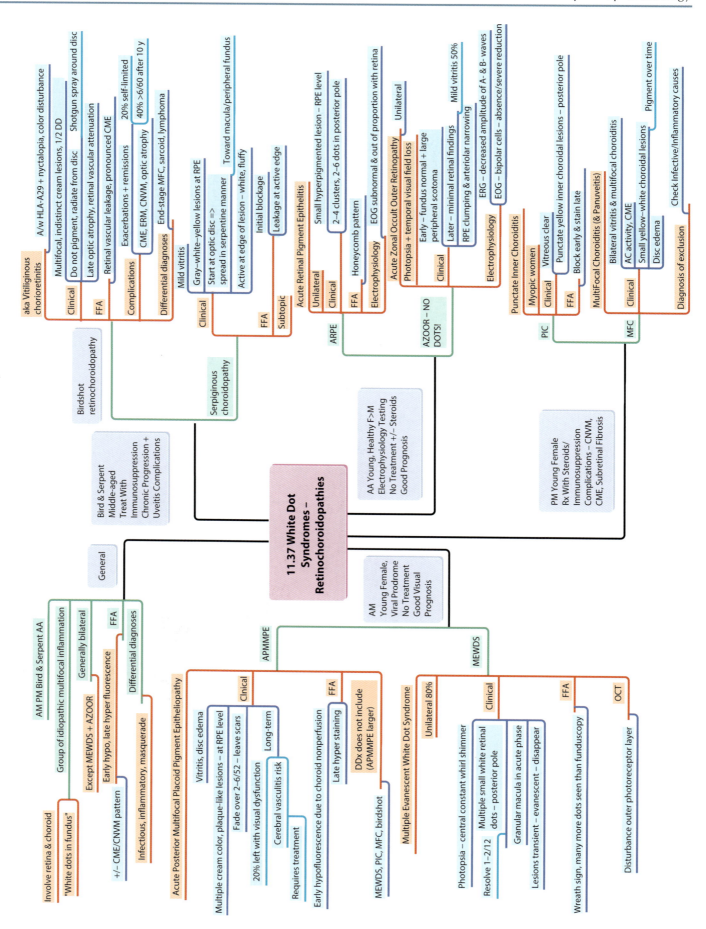

11.37 White Dot Syndromes – Retinochoroidopathies

Birdshot retinochoroidopathy (aka Vitiliginous chorioretinitis)

- Clinical
  - Multifocal, indistinct cream lesions, 1/2 DD
  - A/w HLA-A29 + nyctalopia, color disturbance
  - Do not pigment, radiate from disc
  - Shotgun spray around disc
- FFA
  - Late optic atrophy, retinal vascular attenuation
  - Retinal vascular leakage, pronounced CME
- Complications
  - Exacerbations + remissions
  - CME, ERM, CNVM, optic atrophy
  - 20% self-limited
  - 40% >6/60 after 10 y
- Differential diagnoses
  - End-stage MFC, sarcoid, lymphoma

Serpiginous choroidopathy
- Mild vitritis
- Clinical
  - Gray–white–yellow lesions at RPE
  - Start at optic disc => spread in serpentine manner
  - Toward macula/peripheral fundus
  - Active at edge of lesion – white, fluffy
- FFA
  - Initial blockage
  - Leakage at active edge
- Subtopic

Acute Retinal Pigment Epithelitis (ARPE)
- Unilateral
- Clinical
  - Small hyperpigmented lesion – RPE level
  - 2–4 clusters, 2–6 dots in posterior pole
- FFA
  - Honeycomb pattern
- Electrophysiology
  - EOG subnormal & out of proportion with retina

Acute Zonal Occult Outer Retinopathy (AZOOR – NO DOTS!)
- Unilateral
- Clinical
  - Photopsia + temporal visual field loss
  - Early – fundus normal + large peripheral scotoma
  - Later – minimal retinal findings
  - RPE clumping & arteriolar narrowing
  - Mild vitritis 50%
- Electrophysiology
  - ERG – decreased amplitude of A- & B- waves
  - EOG – bipolar cells – absence/severe reduction

Punctate Inner Choroiditis (PIC)
- Myopic women
- Clinical
  - Vitreous clear
  - Punctate yellow inner choroidal lesions – posterior pole
- FFA
  - Block early & stain late

MultiFocal Choroiditis (& Panuveitis) (MFC)
- Clinical
  - Bilateral vitritis & multifocal choroiditis
  - AC activity, CME
  - Small yellow–white choroidal lesions – posterior pole
  - Disc edema
  - Pigment over time
- Diagnosis of exclusion
  - Check Infective/Inflammatory causes

Birdshot retinochoroidopathy:
Bird & Serpent
Middle-aged
Treat With Immunosuppression +
Chronic Progression +
Uveitis Complications

ARPE:
AA Young, Healthy F>M
Electrophysiology Testing
No Treatment +/– Steroids
Good Prognosis

MFC:
PM Young Female
Rx With Steroids/
Immunosuppression
Complications – CNVM,
CME, Subretinal Fibrosis

MEWDS:
AM
Young Female, Viral Prodrome
No Treatment
Good Visual Prognosis

General
- Involve retina & choroid
- "White dots in fundus"
- +/– CME/CNVM pattern
- Group of idiopathic multifocal inflammation
- AM PM Bird & Serpent AA
- Generally bilateral
  - Except MEWDS + AZOOR
- FFA
  - Early hypo, late hyper fluorescence
- Differential diagnoses
  - Infectious, inflammatory, masquerade

Acute Posterior Multifocal Placoid Pigment Epitheliopathy (APMMPE)
- Clinical
  - Vitritis, disc edema
  - Multiple cream color, plaque-like lesions – at RPE level
  - Fade over 2–6/52 – leave scars
  - Long-term
    - 20% left with visual dysfunction
    - Cerebral vasculitis risk
    - Requires treatment
- FFA
  - Early hypofluorescence due to choroid nonperfusion
  - Late hyper staining
  - DDx does not include (APMMPE larger)
  - MEWDS, PIC, MFC, birdshot

Multiple Evanescent White Dot Syndrome (MEWDS)
- Unilateral 80%
- Clinical
  - Photopsia – central constant whirl shimmer
  - Multiple small white retinal dots – posterior pole
  - Resolve 1–2/12
  - Granular macula in acute phase
  - Lesions transient – evanescent – disappear
- FFA
  - Wreath sign, many more dots seen than funduscopy
- OCT
  - Disturbance outer photoreceptor layer

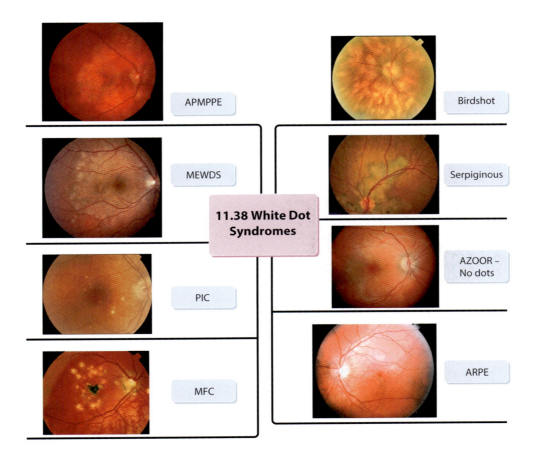

APMPPE

Birdshot

MEWDS

Serpiginous

11.38 White Dot Syndromes

PIC

AZOOR – No dots

MFC

ARPE

Index